Knowing Bodies, Passionate Souls

DUMBARTON OAKS BYZANTINE SYMPOSIA AND COLLOQUIA

Knowing Bodies, Passionate Souls
Sense Perceptions in Byzantium

Edited by

SUSAN ASHBROOK HARVEY AND MARGARET MULLETT

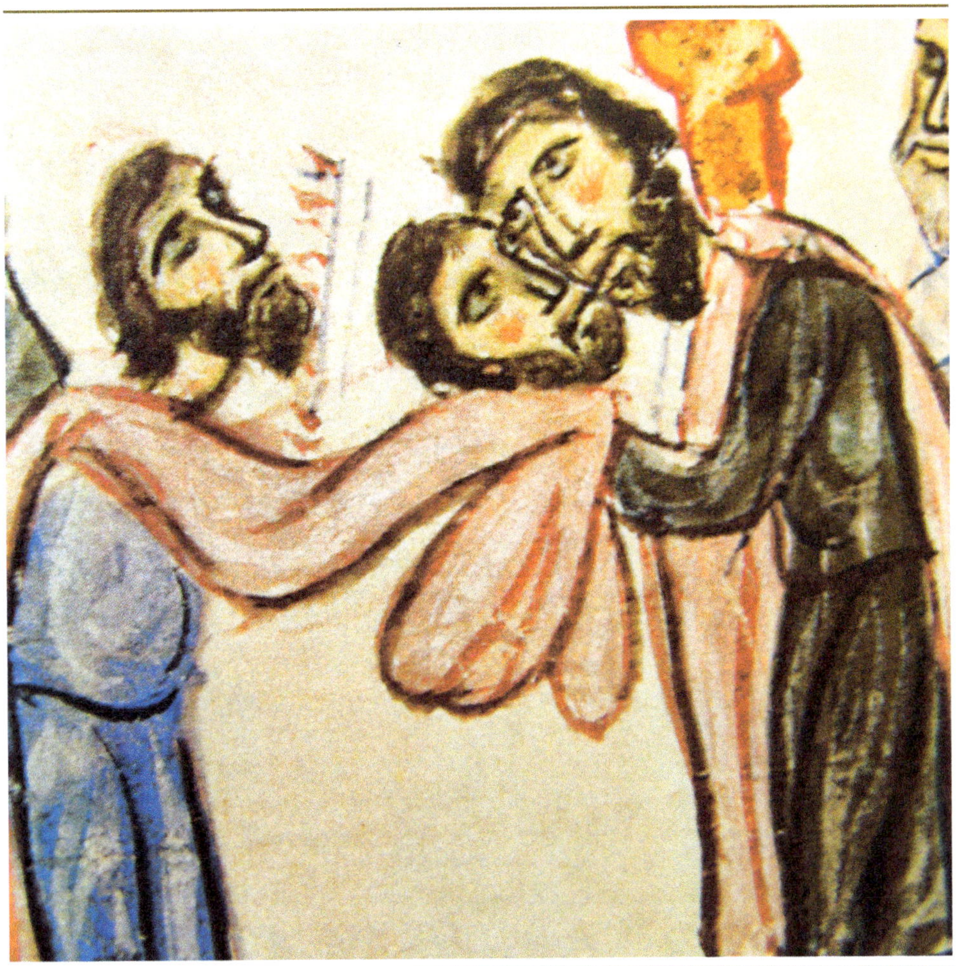

DUMBARTON OAKS RESEARCH LIBRARY AND COLLECTION

LIBRARY OF CONGRESS CATALOGING-IN-PUBLICATION DATA

Names: Harvey, Susan Ashbrook, editor of compilation. | Mullett, Margaret, editor of compilation.
Title: Knowing bodies, passionate souls : sense perceptions in Byzantium / edited by Susan Ashbrook Harvey and Margaret Mullett.
Description: Washington, DC : Dumbarton Oaks Research Library and Collection, [2016] | Series: Dumbarton Oaks Byzantine symposia and colloquia | Papers from a symposium held April 25–27, 2014 at Dumbarton Oaks in Washington, DC |
Includes bibliographical references and index.
Identifiers: LCCN 2016017742 | ISBN 9780884024217 (first cloth : alkaline paper)
Subjects: LCSH: Byzantine Empire—Social life and customs—Congresses. | Byzantine Empire—Intellectual life—Congresses. | Byzantine Empire—Religious life and customs—Congresses. | Senses and sensation—Byzantine Empire—History—Congresses. | Senses and sensation—Social aspects—Byzantine Empire—History—Congresses. | Senses and sensation—Byzantine Empire—Religious aspects—History—Congresses. | Perception—Social aspects—Byzantine Empire—History—Congresses. | Cognition—Social aspects—Byzantine Empire—History—Congresses.
Classification: LCC DF531 .K55 2016 | DDC 949.5/02—dc23
LC record available at http://lccn.loc.gov/2016017742

ISBN 978-0-88402-421-7

www.doaks.org/publications

Designed and typeset by Melissa Tandysh

Frontispiece image: Madrid, Bibl. Nac. Vitr. 26-2 (12th c.), fol. 131r: the emperor venerates the Mandylion (photo: Biblioteca Nacional de España); *page 9:* Göreme, Tokalı Kilise, Old Church, naos, looking north into the vault, healing of the blind man (photo: Tolga Uyar); *page 65:* Bayāḍ wa Riyāḍ, Bayad Plays the Lute, Biblioteca Apostolica Vaticana, MS. ar. 368, fol. 10r (photo: Bridgeman images); *page 121:* Portrait of the Ottoman sultan Mehmet Fatih smelling a rose, by Sinan Bey, late 15th century, Topkapi Palace Museum, MS. Hazine 2153, fol. 10a (photo: Bridgeman images); *page 167:* Göreme, Tokalı Kilise, Old Church, naos, looking south into the vault, ordeal of the bitter water (photo: Tolga Uyar); *page 207:* Göreme, Tokalı Kilise, New Church, naos, looking at southeast into vault, Peter consecrating the Seven Deacons (photo: Tolga Uyar); *page 259:* The ladder of virtues, Erlangen, Universitätsbibliothek Cod. 8, fol. 130v (photo: Universitätsbibliothek Erlangen-Nürnberg)
Jacket image: Judas's Betrayal, detail of the Kiss of Judas, Byzantine fresco, Church of St. Clement, Ohrid, Macedonia. Photograph by Erich Lessing /Art Resource, NY.

Companion audio files for chapters four and five,
as well as a hyperlinked list of all
URLs cited in every chapter,
may be found at
http://www.doaks.org/publications/knowing-bodies

CONTENTS

SMELL

TASTE

TOUCH

THE SENSORIUM

Acknowledgments

This book found its origins in a continuing conversation between the editors, then Senior Fellow and Director of Byzantine Studies respectively, and in many other briefer conversations with other current and former Senior Fellows and Fellows of Dumbarton Oaks; we gratefully acknowledge inspiration from Ioli Kalavrezou, Robert S. Nelson, Ivan Drpić, and Aglae Pizzone, among others. For the resulting spring symposium, the seventy-second at Dumbarton Oaks, we are grateful for the support of Jan Ziolkowski, Director of Dumbarton Oaks, and of the Board of Senior Fellows. We intended to connect the symposium with two other meetings, one on emotion and the other on dreams, and had also hoped to coordinate the meeting with an exhibition at the Walters Museum of Art, though this proved impossible at that time; it opened in fall 2016 as "A Feast for the Senses: Art and Experience in Medieval Europe," curated by Martina Bagnoli. But shortly after the symposium was agreed we discovered that another symposium was to be held at DO, a fortnight after ours, "Sound and Scent in the Garden," and we were fortunate to have many conversations with the symposiarch, D. Fairchild Ruggles, and Director of Studies, John Beardsley, as plans for both proceeded. Together we shared a short-term stipendiary and speaker Deborah Green, and together we planned Hugh Livingston's sound installation in the garden, as well as a small display on the Music Room Terrace. This comprised a scent lab organised by Professor Ruggles, which served also as an evocation of the scent world of one Byzantine scholar, Symeon Seth, with translations by Alison Noble of his alimentary treatise. Deborah Brown organized an exhibition in the library on rare musical works. James Carder mounted in the Orientation Gallery an exhibition of five pastels by former employee (1963–1993) and artist Alex de Boeck, entitled *Hagia Sophia Abstractions*, together with a slide show of images from *Study of Light in Hagia Sophia* taken in the 1930s and 1940s by the Byzantine Institute and now in the ICFA Photograph Collection. To Dede, John, Deb, James and Alison we owe many thanks. The symposium was blessed with good weather and with the youngest audience for a spring symposium in a long time; the topic struck a chord with many in the subject who had been waiting for such a gathering; articles on sensory topics have since appeared in *Dumbarton Oaks Papers*. The smooth running of the symposium owed a great deal to the professionalism of Carlos Mendez and Mario Garcia, as well as to Susannah Italiano and the Byzantine Studies team, Scott Fitzgerald Johnson, Jonathan Shea and Alec Luhring.

In the production of the book, as many debts of gratitude were incurred. Most of the chapters were originally delivered at the symposium, but when Stavroula Constantinou withdrew, Béatrice Caseau and Galina Tirnanić agreed to contribute; Susan Harvey added her paper to those on smell. The volume was almost ready to transmit to Publications when the six-year partnership of the editors was broken up as one moved back to Ireland and the other ended her two terms on the Board of the Senior Fellows. We are grateful to Michael Maas for overseeing the final stages, to Seh Hee Koh for her enthusiastic compilation of permissions and illustrations, and to the anonymous readers for saving us from error. No Byzantinist would refuse to thank Joel Kalvesmaki, Byzantine Editor, for the erudite and practical support he offers to all authors, volume editors, and series editors in his care; no editor of a book produced in Dumbarton Oaks could fail to acknowledge the genius of Kathy Sparkes, Director of Publications, who effortlessly produces the most beautiful of books. Dumbarton Oaks is not just the home of the humanities; it is also the seat of the senses.

Introduction

SUSAN ASHBROOK HARVEY AND MARGARET MULLETT

It is hard to imagine a place more suited for a symposium on the Byzantine senses than Dumbarton Oaks in April: amid glorious gardens, the elegance of the Music Room, and the splendors of the museums, the senses are engaged and celebrated at every turn. Moreover, Dumbarton Oaks has long attuned scholars to the fineries of the Byzantine sensorium. From the grand to the humble, it has laid a textured, sensorily diverse Byzantine world before us: the exquisitely worked golden marriage belt, glowing silver liturgical instruments, hauntingly evocative icons large (the Apostle Peter, painted) or small (John Chrysostom in tiny tesserae), colorfully woven tapestries, splendid ivories, coins, seals, pilgrim tokens, glistening illuminated manuscripts, carved stone. For some time now, Byzantinists—at Dumbarton Oaks and elsewhere—have attended well to a sensorily capacious Byzantine aesthetics. Yet scholars have often done so, ironically, without considering the senses themselves: their qualities, cognitive affects, or deeper cultural resonances and import.

In the broader world of scholarship and the academy, recent years have focused strong new currents of inquiry on embodiment as a human condition, and on the senses as an often underappreciated dimension of human experience and cognition. In keeping with intellectual traditions dating back to the philosophers of classical Greece and to biblical authors of the same and earlier eras, western scholarship, like western culture, has strongly favored attention to sight and hearing, to visual culture and aural and oral experience. What has been especially exciting in recent years has been the emergence of attention to the full sensory palette, separately and synesthetically, as scholars have looked anew at the significance of the senses for human flourishing.[1]

Byzantinists have been slow to look at the operations of the senses in Byzantium, even the most studied, sight, in each one's relation to the others, and to embrace phenomenological approaches in general. Work on smell and hearing has recently appeared, and yet the areas of taste and touch are still largely uncharted. Nor has much been done to explore how Byzantines viewed the senses, or how they envisaged the sensory interactions with their world. A map of the connections between sense perceptions and other processes (of perception, memory, imagination, visualization) in the Byzantine

1 For scholarship directly engaging Byzantium and its sources, see e.g., R. Nelson, ed., *Visuality Before and Beyond the Renaissance: Seeing as Others Saw* (Cambridge, 2000); G. Frank, *The Memory of the Eyes: Pilgrims to Living Saints in Christian Late Antiquity* (Berkeley, 2000); S. A. Harvey, *Scenting Salvation: Ancient Christianity and the Olfactory Imagination* (Berkeley, 2006); B. Pentcheva, *The Sensual Icon: Space, Ritual, and the Senses in Byzantium* (University Park, PA, 2010). Important articles and related studies will also be found in L. James, ed., *Desire and Denial in Byzantium: Papers from the 31st Spring Symposium of Byzantine Studies, University of Sussex, Brighton, March 1997* (Aldershot, 1999) and C. Nesbitt and M. Jackson, eds., *Experiencing Byzantium: Papers from the 44th Spring Symposium of Byzantine Studies, Newcastle and Durham 2011* (Aldershot, 2013).

brain has still to be sketched out. How did the Byzantines describe, narrate, or represent the senses at work?

What, in fact, might we learn by studying the Byzantine sensorium? Byzantine culture was notably attuned to a cosmos of multiple domains: material, immaterial; bodily, intellectual, physical, spiritual; human, divine. Despite a prevailing discourse that often subordinated the bodily to the eternal, the Byzantine world found its bridges between domains most often in sensory modes of awareness.[2] These different domains were concretely perceptible; further, they were encountered daily amid the mundane no less than the exalted. Icons, incense, music, sacred architecture, ritual activity; saints, imperial families, persons at prayer; medicine, demonology, or scientific inquiry; hymnography, ascetical or mystical literature: in every cultural expression, the Byzantines excelled in highlighting the intersections between human and divine realms through sensory engagement, whether positive or negative.

For example, at the eastern frontiers of the Roman Empire, the hymnographer Ephrem the Syrian late in the fourth century composed a cycle of hymns in which he pondered Paradise.[3] Paradise, he sang, is a place revealed to us by Scripture: we learn about it by reading, and by meditating to enter the words with ever-deeper apprehension. It is a place we once knew, in the persons of Adam and Eve, and to which we can hope, and long, and pray, and yearn to return if only we can repair our broken relationship with our Maker. In a striking intersection between the powers of reading (words, intellection, comprehension), and the distinctive cognitive abilities of the human senses, Ephrem's reflections further suggested that Paradise is a place not only revealed by sacred text but also made known to us through the realities of physical sensory experience. Realizing the capacities of sensory awareness to instruct us, whether to wonder or to fear, it was not a *vision* of Paradise Ephrem sought to instill in his listeners. Rather, with lush evocations of scents, tastes, textures, sounds, and colors; brilliance, radiance, and freshness, Ephrem's verses opened Paradise as a place one might now just barely discern even here, in this present, all too fallen order: in a glimpse, a fragrance, a taste. For, he sang, "I considered how the soul cannot have perception of Paradise without its mate, the body, its instrument and lyre."[4] Indeed, he sang, the soul in Paradise would be utterly lost, even impossible without the body.

> That blessed abode . . .
> . . . is complete and perfected
> in every way,
> and the soul cannot
> enter there alone,
> for in such a state [the soul] is in everything
> deficient—
> in sensation and consciousness;
> but on the day of Resurrection
> the body, with all its senses,
> will enter in as well, once it has been made
> perfect.[5]

From such a perspective, the physical world was itself a place from which to learn greater realities. What was needed was attention to what one encountered. For Ephrem, the senses were the means of that attention: sense perception and sensory awareness opened one to the astonishment of a transparent existence, redolent with divine presence:

> Let us see those things [God] does for us
> every day!
> How many tastes for the mouth! How many
> beauties for the eye!
> How many melodies for the ear! How many
> scents for the nostrils!
> Who is sufficient in comparison to the goodness of these little things?[6]

2 Consider, e.g., L. James, "Senses and Sensibility in Byzantium," *Art History* 27, no. 4 (2004): 522–37.

3 *Des heiligen Ephraem des Syrers Hymnen de Paradiso und Contra Julianum*, ed. and trans. E. Beck, CSCO 174–75 / CSCO Scr. Syr. 78–79 (Louvain, 1957), trans. S. P. Brock, *St. Ephrem the Syrian, Hymns on Paradise* (Crestwood, NY, 1990).

4 Ephrem, *HPar* 8.2, Brock, *Ephrem, Hymns on Paradise*, 132.

5 Ephrem, *HPar* 8.7, Brock, *Ephrem, Hymns on Paradise*, 133–34.

6 Ephrem, *HVirg* 31:16, trans. K. McVey, *Ephrem the Syrian: Hymns* (New York, 1989), at p. 401. Syriac ed. and trans. E. Beck, *Des heiligen Ephraem des Syrers Hymnen de Virginitate*, CSCO 223–24/CSCO Scr. Syr. 94–95 (Louvain, 1962).

For Ephrem, as for the broader early Byzantine world, the diverse cosmic domains material and immaterial were porous, permeating and penetrating one another continuously. The senses were the portals by which human comprehension could grasp more than the visible, physical place in which one stood. They provided data which the discerning individual could seek to process profitably.

For the Byzantines—as for Mediterranean culture in its broader history—the senses were an essential part of human existence. They were always more than aspects of human physicality. The senses attuned the ancient person to the varied contours of life: safety and danger, health and illness. They inscribed and delimited political and social patterns and hierarchies; they encoded profoundly effective systems of morality, ethics, and modes of knowledge. They were functionally intrinsic for cognition in its highest intellectual forms, as well as for navigating daily life, from its most basic skills (hygiene, sustenance) to its most celebratory endeavors (festivals, imperial celebrations). The senses enabled one to inhabit and negotiate a complex cosmos of multiple domains; and to work effectively within competing systems and structures of Byzantine society.[7]

Like bodies, the senses could be trained. They could be disciplined, instructed, and refined. One sort of training was present from deeply ingrained cultural habit: the pan-Mediterranean codes of sensory associations and meanings shared across domestic, civic, political, religious, and cultural landscapes. Another was the deliberate work of self-formation. For the Christian, for example, baptism and liturgical participation formed a Christian subject of highly trained sensory awareness and even sensory agency.[8] For the monk or nun the sacramentalized body was further ritualized into a sociality that might invert common sensory codes: of stench and sweetness, deprivation and satiety, and radiantly transfigured perceptions.[9]

Sensory rhetoric did heavy lifting in the task of educating toward a shared culture. On the one hand, there was constant engagement with intellectual currents that drew on philosophical and medical traditions to instruct audiences on the cognitive significance of sensation. Thus John of Damascus famously defended the use, not only of icons, but of liturgical accouterments: incense, holy oil, bread, wine, the sign of the cross.

> A certain perception takes place in the brain, prompted by the bodily senses, which is then transmitted to the faculties of discernment, and adds to the treasure of knowledge something that was not there before. The eloquent Gregory [of Nazianzos] says that the mind which is determined to ignore corporeal things will find itself weakened and frustrated.[10]

Moreover, John admonished, the intellect by itself simply could not comprehend sufficiently the fullness of reality which the human subject needed to grasp.

> If we sometimes understand forms by using our minds, but other times from what we see, then it is through these two ways that we are brought to understanding. It is the same with the other senses: after we have smelled, or tasted, or touched, we combine our experience with reason, and thus come to knowledge.[11]

The intimate intersection of the senses and emotion is apparent in high relief, whether considered through visual culture, rhetorical techniques, or the technologies of social habits to mark the life cycle of birth to death, with its trajectories of grief

7 E.g., N. Andrade, "The Processions of John Chrysostom and the Contested Spaces of Constantinople," *JEChrSt* 18, no. 2 (2010): 161–89; L. James, "Senses and Sensibility"; B. Caseau, "Incense and Fragrances: From House to Church; A Study of the Introduction of Incense into Early Byzantine Christian Churches," in *Material Culture and Well-Being in Byzantium (400–1453)*, ed. M. Grünbart et al. (Vienna, 2007), 75–92.

8 D. Krueger, *Liturgical Subjects: Christian Ritual, Biblical Narrative, and the Formation of the Self in Byzantium* (Philadelphia, 2014); G. Frank, "From Antioch to Arles: Lay Devotion in Context," in *Cambridge History of Christianity*, vol. 2: *Constantine to 600*, ed. A. Cassiday and F. Norris (Cambridge, 2007), 531–47; Harvey, *Scenting Salvation*, 57–98.

9 Harvey, *Scenting Salvation*, 201–21.

10 John of Damascus, *On the Divine Images*, 1.11, trans. D. Anderson, *St. John of Damascus: On the Divine Images; Three Apologies against Those Who Attack the Divine Images* (Crestwood, NY, 1980), 20.

11 John of Damascus, *On the Divine Images*, 3.24; trans. Anderson, *John of Damascus*, 79.

and celebration, fasting and feasting, as homilies concerned with lamentation and mourning (for death, for penance) remind us.[12]

Sensory rhetoric further elicited attunement to moral psychology. It could identify virtues and vices, encode values, and render concrete meanings with a clarity that events themselves could scarcely convey. Sensory rhetoric, for example, provided grist for religious critique, by highlighting the sensory attention that characterized religious reform. I offer one brief example here.

The emperors Constantine, Julian, Theodosius I, and Justinian (like Augustus before them) were all rulers valorized during their imperial reigns for their extensive religious reforms. These emperors refurbished sacred buildings and holy precincts, and constructed new ones; they restored, increased and strengthened sacred offices. They established new festivals and revived others that had languished forgotten. They enhanced religious ceremonial with imperial adornments that heightened the majesty and splendor of the occasions. They strengthened priesthoods, and insisted on improved levels of religious literacy regarding sacred traditions. Such reforms involved the sensory aspects of religion by means of material practice. They also provided rhetorical tools for critique.

The contrasting literary portraits of the emperor Constantine by the fourth-century Christian Eusebius of Caesarea and the late fifth-century pagan historian Zosimas make the point. Each presented an overtly religious agenda. Both portraits are notable for their attention to monumental building projects, the adornment of civic communities, the tone of religious observance, the quality of law, and the tradition of imperial beneficence to the poor and needy. These socially (and sensorily) concrete activities were then characterized in morally positive or negative terms, by the use of morally coded sensory imagery: light, radiance, and beauty according to Eusebius,[13] as opposed to debauchery, depravity, and decay in Zosimas.[14] All of these activities were religiously meaningful to Constantine's subjects and certainly also to his biographers. Their measure provoked praise or criticism, rendered in sensory terms, both for the materiality of Constantine's achievements and for their "spiritual" worth.

At Dumbarton Oaks, the symposium on the Byzantine senses provided a program that treated the senses in turn—and indeed, in their traditional philosophical ranking (inherited from Plato)—beginning with sight and progressing through hearing, smell, taste, and touch, to arrive finally at papers exploring the combined sensorium.

The essays in this book consider their place in what the Byzantines thought about perception and cognition, as well as the operations of individual senses in Byzantium in the context of all the senses. Recent work on dreaming, on memory, and on the emotions has made these advances possible, and collaborative experiments by Byzantinists and neurological scientists open further approaches. The happy coincidence of the Dumbarton Oaks Garden and Landscape symposium "Sound and Scent in the Garden" and the planning of the exhibition "A Feast for the Senses: Art and Experience in Medieval Europe," since held at the Walters Art Museum, has also enabled some cross-cultural comparisons to be made: gardens in Islamic Spain, Hebrew hymnography, Coptic cookery, classical and Ottoman Mediterranean ordure, and Romanesque and Gothic precious objects—that were not just looked at and listened to but also touched, smelled, heard.[15] Architects,

12 E.g., N. Tsironis, "Emotion and the Senses in Marian Homilies of the Middle Byzantine Period," in *The Cult of the Mother of God in Byzantium*, ed. L. Brubaker and M. B. Cunningham (Aldershot, 2011), 179–96; S. A. Harvey, "Guiding Grief: Liturgical Poetry and Ritual Lamentation in Early Byzantium," *Greek Laughter and Tears: Antiquity and After; Proceedings of the 8th A. G. Leventis Conference in Greek, University of Edinburgh, November 2013*, ed. D. Cairns and M. Alexiou (Edinburgh, 2017); H. Maguire, "The Depiction of Sorrow in Middle Byzantine Art," *DOP* 31 (1977): 123–74.

13 E.g., Eusebius of Caesarea, *Church History* 10.9.6–9, ed. and trans. K. Lake, H. J. Lawlor, and J. E. L. Oulton (Cambridge, MA, 1980), vol. 2; idem, *Life of Constantine* 4.24, 4.60–73, ed. and trans. Av. Cameron and S. G. Hall (Oxford, 1999); compare eidem, *Oration on the Tricennalia of Constantine* 2.1–6, 3.4–6, 5.1–4.

14 Zosimas, *New History* 2.29–39; trans. R. T. Ridley (Canberra, 1982).

15 On the two events see http://www.doaks.org/research/garden-landscape/scholarly-activities/past/sound-and-scent-in-the-garden and http://thewalters.org/events/event.aspx?e=4393 (all URLs in this chapter accessed 15 November 2016). M. Bagnoli, ed., *A Feast for the Senses: Art and Experience in Medieval Europe* (Baltimore, 2016).

musicologists, art historians, archaeologists, philologists, all have had a place in making the symposium and also the book. The symposium gained also from multimedia presentations with movies (the plastic bag film discussed by Glenn Peers,[16] Whittemore's monastic film[17]), sound recordings, Hugh Livingston's installation,[18] Spyridon Antonopoulos's singing, Alison Noble's exhibition of the scent-world of Symeon Seth,[19] and Dede Ruggles's associated scent laboratory;[20] all those riches are—ironically—represented in this book through sight alone, though links to sound and other websites may be found wherever possible.

Given that the study of visuality in Byzantium is far in advance of the study of any of the other senses, we chose to start not with more consideration of haptic vision or ekphrasis, but with a pair of papers on sight in the context of display.[21] One looked back at one exhibition, *Byzantine Things in the World*[22] and the other forward to the other, mentioned above, "A Feast for the Senses." At the symposium we found profound disagreement: nothing could have been further apart than Glenn Peers trying to set his objects free to interact in the company of modern pieces in a minimalist environment and Martina Bagnoli planning to contextualize hers in terms of sound and touch and smell in a limited and controlled context. One was a pessimistic though empathetic and deeply felt view, the other optimistic and committed to the historical reception of the objects and the need to educate the viewing public in the mode of display. The exhibitions were very different; the essays in this volume are much more in sympathy with one another, though one still concentrates on the subjectivity of the object, and the other looks to objects as evidence for a new awareness of the senses from the thirteenth century on.

Our three papers on hearing overlap and interrelate with each other like a jigsaw rather than a mosaic: Amy Papalexandrou's sense of architecture leads her to suggest that the noisiness of acclamations under the dome of Hagia Sophia was more important than acoustic qualities for liturgy or chant, and her work on inscriptions leads her to compare the Byzantium we think we know to a silent film; Kim Haines-Eitzen's desert silences (and different kinds of silence) strike her as sensorily positive, like musical rests; Spyridon Antonopoulos's rich temporal building up of surface like a Byzantine wall painting, laying layer of paint on layer in a single hymn sung once a year before arriving at the kalophonia of the fifteenth century, focuses on the role of the senses and the value—or not—of intelligibility.

As we move from the distance receptors to the contact senses, Felipe Rojas and Valeria Sergueenkova consider ways in which social memory was mobilized by smell to create long lines of continuity in Greece and Anatolia based on what the past smelled like in the past. Dragons and rocks and exploding cucumbers take us into unexpected and uncharted territory, where Ottoman tourists were directed at the foot of the Acropolis to the smell of Plato. So we were presented with these landscapes defined over time by smells, but also the ephemeral nature of smell, short of a vocabulary—at least in our culture—dependent on sight, more vulnerable in D. Fairchild Ruggles's Islamic garden than in Rojas's and Sergueenkova's olfactory communities. Susan Harvey sniffs out the habits of piety, rhetoric, and theology of holy oil to see how it

16 See Peers, below, p. 12.

17 Red Sea Monasteries, Egypt, The Byzantine Institute and Dumbarton Oaks Fieldwork Records and Papers, ca. late 1920s–2000s, MS.BZ.004-02-04, Image Collections and Fieldwork Archives, Dumbarton Oaks, Trustees for Harvard University, Washington, DC, https://vimeo.com/album/2292509/video/64573993.

18 http://www.doaks.org/research/garden-landscape/contemporary-art-installations/hugh-livingston

19 http://www.doaks.org/research/byzantine/scholarly-activities/past/knowing-bodies-passionate-souls-sense-perceptions-in-byzantium/seths-alimentary-treatise

20 http://www.doaks.org/research/byzantine/scholarly-activities/past/knowing-bodies-passionate-souls-sense-perceptions-in-byzantium/scent-lab

21 On haptic vision see R. Betancourt, "Why Sight Is Not Touch: Reconsidering the Tactility of Sight in Byzantium," *DOP* 70 (2016): 1–23; on ekphrasis most recently R. Webb, *Ekphrasis, Imagination and Persuasion in Ancient Rhetorical Theory and Practice* (Aldershot, 2009); *Ekphrasis: La représentation des monuments dans les littératures byzantine et byzantino-slaves: réalités et imaginaires*, ed. V. Vavřínek, P. Odorico, and V. Drbal = *BSl* 63, no. 3, suppl. (Prague, 2011); *Villes de toute beauté: L'ekphrasis des cités dans les littératures byzantine et byzantino-slaves*, ed. P. Odorico and C. Messis, Dossiers byzantins 12 (Paris, 2012).

22 https://www.menil.org/exhibitions/26-byzantine-things-in-the-world and G. Peers, *Byzantine Things in the World* (Houston, 2013).

works to create a people's saint, or a Byzantine imaginary, as practice evokes sensation, which creates meaning.

We consider taste in two tightly argued papers, one from text, the other (largely) from material evidence. Thomas Arentzen observes a poet taste the source of his poetry and depict both salvation as the sweetness of fruit and of milk, and eating as far from innocent, piling on gustatory images at the end of Lent when the congregation was hungry and craving. Darlene Brooks Hedstrom lingers on the paradox of the uniqueness of taste in monastic communities where the gatekeeper of taste was not the superior but the cook. She finds a vocabulary in recorded complaints about food in Egyptian monasteries—salty, insipid, brined, stale, pickled, soppy—which reveal ascetic taste as oddly luxurious, but controlled by the whims of monastic cooks. Both authors note that taste comes very low in the taxonomies of senses, unreliable in the judgment of Cyril of Jerusalem, but both see it as a complex sensory experience with much to tell us about congregations and communities.

Touch, the so-called basest sense, is the most diffuse, involving the entire body and not just one organ, like sight and hearing. It is also deliberate: unlike smelling and hearing, where it is not possible to avoid the experience, touch involves both intent and action. And it is twofold: the active, haptic, touching, and the passive, tactile, feeling. Ingela Nilsson looks at gendered touch, both chaste and forbidden, in which pleasure and pain turned out not to be so far apart, in which not touching turned out to be as important as touching, and in which both sensory and sensual experience are expressed through rhetoric. Béatrice Caseau follows the faithful into church, undergoing touch by a higher authority, kissing, rubbing foreheads, wearing encolpia, affixing seals, drinking or rubbing oil and sees their tactile piety as enabled by embodied religion, and offering religious agency through devotion. Galina Tirnanić notes that the receptors for pain are different from those of the nonviolent tactile sensation and examines the ways in which the pain of flogging, blinding, and burning was made visible to observers, so that the hand of the emperor became a iatric hand of healing in the community as a whole.

All our contributors are cautious about the difficulty of experiencing what the Byzantines experienced, from the first words of the first paper: "How we know past bodies is nearly insoluble." "We cannot experience as the Byzantines did," says Antonopoulos. The premodern ear may be the same as ours physiologically, but both the soundscape and the nature of perception have changed. All are clear that the senses are neither universal nor transhistorical, and that sensing is learned; most of our authors appeal to the cultural history of sensation as a guide through the desert: others cleave to phenomenology, affect theory, the archaeology of the senses, or sensorial fieldwork; several are comfortable with neuroscience. Ruggles, perhaps the most pessimistic of our authors, points to ephemerality, the lack of a "period nose," and recording problems with representing smell as the major factors which complicate analysis.

None of the papers managed to isolate a single sense totally: even the icon in the *Letter of the Three Patriarchs* had wet feet. And all have interesting views of how the senses interact. The hegemony of sight is deplored in more than one paper. And smell trumps sight at Panopios when a Pentelic marble slab smelled like human skin and so favored Prometheus over Asklepios; sound (the beloved voice) trumps sight (the two-dimensional image) in modern funerals, and music may be the most direct activator of sensory experience, but Photios's determination that sight trumps sound may have been disingenuous from one who used all the power of sound in his preaching. We realize that in memory, images are never purely visual, and that in rhetoric the senses are available only through hearing, as we also realize that smells are accessible only through sight. We may see in a dream narrative pain and cold trigger a rapid succession of feeling, aroma, sight, sound, taste, and fragrance. Sight, hearing, smell, and taste are as important for erotic experience as is touch. Romanos's characters "long to see, yearn to touch, crave a kiss."[23] Medieval objects were made to speak to every sense, not just sight. The multisensory appears to be normal in Byzantium.[24]

23 Arentzen, below, p. 170.

24 "Synesthesia" is currently gaining ground in the sense not of the rare neurological condition which associates more than

But this does not mean that there is general agreement on the nature of the sensorium, though there is agreement that the western sensorium is a construct. Ruth Webb in her piece on rhetoric looks at the way in which words set in motion processes both intellectual and spiritual, creating an illusion of sensation without involving the sensory organs directly. Sight brings along the other senses, the brain can stimulate a response similar to that of the senses, and rhetoric can stimulate that response with a single word. She proposes a sixth, spatial, sense which in the hands of a rhetor could create an illusion of presence. Laura Lieber looks at strong sensory language in the liturgical setting of sixth- and seventh-century Hebrew hymnography, in which performance is paramount, and all senses are employed to create a liturgical time combining past, present, and future, an imagined alternative to present reality. Marcus Plested pursues five spiritual senses, or perhaps just one in five modes, through Origen and Evagrios, Gregory of Nyssa, pseudo-Dionysios, Makarios, John of Damascus, Symeon the New Theologian, and Palamas, and sees a dominant Byzantine tradition of continuity between physical and spiritual senses, with strong theological defense of the material and physical. Chapters in this volume by Haines-Eitzen, Antonopoulos, Arentzen, Caseau, and especially Harvey already make it unsurprising that spiritual sensation, whether of grace or demonic activity, whether of saints, or angels, or God himself, was always a very real prospect within the Byzantine sensorium.

This book and the symposium which preceded it are very much at the beginning of things, not the end. There is a great deal more to do to arrive at a viable theory of the Byzantine senses, and certainly at a corpus of texts which deal with them. In what we have collected already—and Papalexandrou's appendix is a major step forward—Eustathios of Thessalonike is most prominent in terms of anecdote, and John of Damascus in terms of theology; this may well have changed in ten years' time. We may feel the lack of certain topics like secular music and elite cuisine; we miss the chance of allowing the power of ruins to open up the past or encourage storytelling; we may so far have been drawn more to the pleasant than the unpleasant. And we need to see how emotions, memory, and dreams play into what we have learned so far about the workings of the Byzantine mind.

But we cannot be sure that we can solve the major questions, those of accessibility: Can we achieve representation? Is a sensual museum impossible? Can we know what the scents of the Islamic garden were like? Were birdsong and the semantron just the same for the Byzantines as for us, and the only sounds that we know have not changed? And did garum taste different to Byzantines, better than it does to us? Were we right to focus largely on the human sensing subject, or should the neediness of icons be part of our remit as well? It may be true that the Byzantines were "far more different from ourselves than we have allowed ourselves to admit,"[25] but we should not despair; we have plenty of reasons to pursue the many and complex ways they used and viewed their senses, and we hope that this book will encourage others to join that pursuit.

one sense, but of the multisensory. Many of these papers, necessarily, discuss multiple senses. They do not do so in terms of "synesthesia" as a phenomenon, but because no sense is perceptible in isolation. Not only do the individual senses engage and elicit others, but furthermore the distinctive qualities of each are necessarily interdependent for full potency of meaning. These factors were well grasped by the Byzantines, and skillfully utilized through their different media and modes of expression, investigation, critique, or celebration. On this issue see James, "Senses and Sensibility" (n. 2 above) and Caseau below, n. 5.

25 Peers, below, p. 12.

Sight

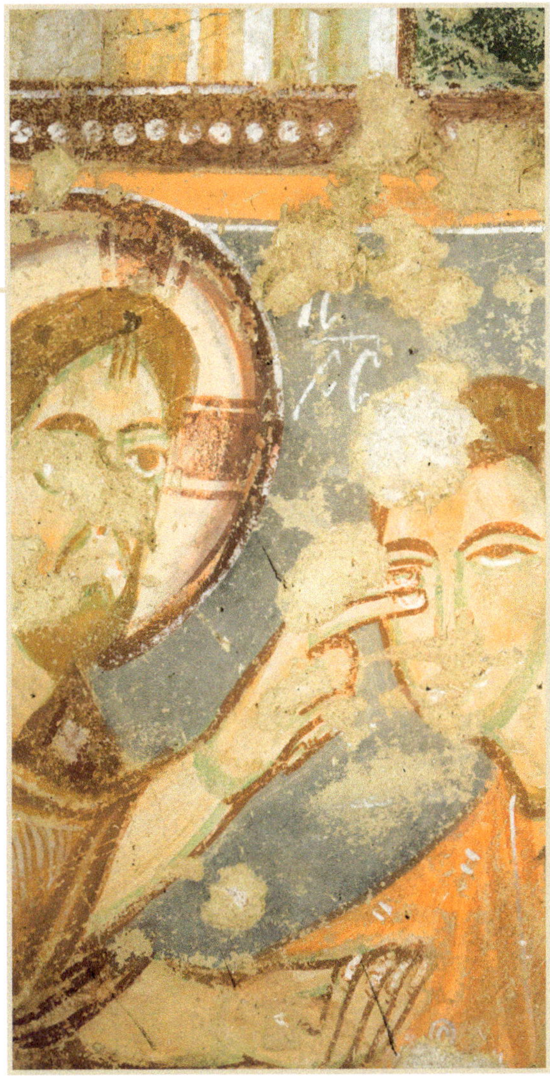

CHAPTER ONE

Sense Lives of Byzantine Things

GLENN PEERS

How we know past bodies is nearly insoluble. How we know our own is hard enough. When I presented a version of this essay at the conference, I could feel myself retreating just as I gained momentum in the speaking, and I felt—or knew—my body receding from my own consciousness. Michel Serres (b. 1931) described a talk he gave, during which a wasp stung him on the thigh, and while aware of the occurrence, his speaking suppressed any experience of the sensation; "Words fill our flesh and anaesthetize it," he wrote.[1] A necessary admission of this enterprise of understanding historical senses is our logocentric limitation. We are constantly catching up with ourselves, and attempts to articulate that feeling are always something slightly else and somehow short of the event. So, from a position as speaking, writing subject, I am all too aware of the derivative, secondary nature of what I am arguing and describing.[2]

Let me take it one step further, and indicate the real subject beyond myself—and ourself (intentional singular)—how historical subjects felt, sensed, and experienced the world, mostly beyond speech—that is, subjects, persons who left no words themselves and whose parts in the flows of that world need imagining and evoking. By these, I mean persons who are human and those who are not, because I take a position that many subjects exist, and existed, beyond the exclusive range of humans.[3] In other words, my argument pursues feeling and sensing subjects across a range of ontologies. I want to think through those silent things that fill our museums and historical monuments, and active spaces,

1 M. Serres, *The Five Senses: A Philosophy of Mingled Bodies (I)*, trans. M. Sankey and P. Cowley (London and New York, 2008), 59, "I do not mention this particular memory in order to boast of my Spartan courage, but only I indicate that the speaking body, flesh filled with language, has little difficulty in remaining focused in speech, whatever happens. Words fill our flesh and anaesthetize it. It has even been said, and written, that the word was made flesh. Nothing makes one more insensitive than words. If I had been looking at some image, listening to the sound coming from an organ, smelling a garland of flowers, tasting a sugared almond or grasping a pole, the hornet sting would have caused me to cry out. But I was speaking, balanced in a groove or enclosure, protected by a discursive breastplate. You want to anaesthetize a patient completely? Get him to speak with passion and vigor, ask him to talk about himself, and himself alone, of his one desire, demand that he prove something or that he convince his audience. He is intoxicated with sonorous words, the hornet is powerless. Militant egoists, we speak in order to drug ourselves."

2 Serres has noted several times his sympathy for the phenomenology of Merleau-Ponty, but always with a rather damning evaluation of the latter's verbal bias, which obscures the real nature, for Serres, of sensual encounters with the world. And yet Serres also acknowledges the ironies of his own rich facility with language, amply testified by the constant flow of books from his hand. This issue was recently discussed by Y. Hamilakis, *Archaeology and the Senses: Human Experience, Memory and Affect* (Cambridge, 2014), 68–70.

3 I am not alone in taking this stand: see, for example, I. Bogost, *Alien Phenomenology, or What It's Like to Be a Thing* (Minneapolis, 2012), A. M. Jones and N. Boivin, "The Malice of Inanimate Objects: Material Agency," in *The Oxford Handbook of Material Culture Studies*, ed. D. Hicks and M. C. Beaudry (Oxford, 2010), 332–51, C. Fowler, "Personhood and the Body," in *The Oxford Handbook of the Archaeology of Ritual and Religion*, ed. T. Insoll (Oxford and New York, 2012), 133–50, and B. Faure, "Substitute Bodies in Chan/Zen Buddhism," in *Religious Reflections on the Human Body*, ed. J. Law (Bloomington, 1995), 211–29. And Serres, *Five Senses*, 102–3, "Without being able to prove it I believe, like soothsayers and haruspices, and like scientists, that there exists a world independent of man. . . . I believe, I know, I cannot demonstrate the existence of this world without us."

to find out how they felt and how they came to make bodies feel and know.[4]

In making this argument, I am expressing myself in academic absolutes for the most part and with strong conviction. I am concerned I am falling into overreliance on the arbitrary in my reading of the historical record, that my selection and emphasis of certain symptoms over others will lead me to a wrong diagnosis. My premise is that Byzantines were, however, far more different from ourselves than we have allowed ourselves to admit. While I recognize its potential failings as hypothesis, the first step to an acceptance of difference—which ethnic, confessional, and intellectual stances have obscured in the last centuries—is the provisional quality of my argument. Here, Richard Shiff quoting Charles Sanders Peirce (1839–1914), "At times, proof would come to pass as mere feeling, 'a single feeling of greater intensity . . . belonging to the act of thinking the hypothetical conclusion. . . . Hypothesis produces the *sensuous* element of thought.'"[5]

Guessing, to use another word that Peirce was fond of, is a way of collecting observations from experience and then of beginning the formation of half-conscious expectations; for him, a fully accepted, simple, and interesting inference tends to erase the premises from which it comes, and it then comes to lack all surprise that the initial experience possessed.[6] While recognizing the risky position an academic occupies in these situations, one can also work backward and attempt sensuous guesswork to supplement explanations that other art historians have rendered unsurprising.

I will try to make this sensual, hypothetical point as vividly as I can at the outset by using an excerpt from a short film, *Plastic Bag* (2009), which was directed by Ramin Bahrani (b. 1975) and narrated by Werner Herzog (b. 1942). I will not be able to bring back to life such a common object from Byzantium, but I want to remember the pathos and moods and terrible patience of this entirely unremarkable made thing. The plastic bag is mass-produced, so he (I'll follow Herzog's cue for "he") says, so no moment of making is really possible, and yet his first breath is momentous and world-changing. Unfolded from a compressed pile of grocery-store bags, he is only, presumably, one of a sequence of life-opening gestures. "My first breaths. I meet my maker. I had a purpose." The human "maker" is the catalyst for life and consciousness, and while the bag is born to her purpose, he also possesses sufficient consciousness to know her needs and desire to fulfill them. But he also feels: the sensation of ice in his cavity is "shocking" (he doesn't seem to have a real inside/outside), and he learns how to navigate air and ocean through sensitive attention to draughts and currents in his holes. Among innumerable births in a world filled with endless things, this bag feels from his first breath, and differently from his human "master" and very differently from the "beastie" she owns (that is, a dog), and from the fish he admires and who in turn sample him.

Of course, no consciousness can hope to know, encompassingly, all these persons put into and remaining in the world, but art historians do try to know persons (commonly, objects, that is) from the past, of course, and yet we imagine them *senseless* to our attempts to know them. In the first place, we treat them like things in our world, when they are so much stranger even than ourselves; and in the second, we don't credit them with sufficient faculties of sensation.[7] Those sensations are natural to our world (though those others do not observe and feel in the same ways we

4 This argument is a further development of animist-based analyses that I have written in the last several years, but rather than overburdening this chapter with bibliography, I refer to G. Peers, ed., *Byzantine Things in the World* (Houston, 2013), published in conjunction with an exhibition by that name at the Menil Collection. See also J. Clifton, "Conversations in Museums," and R. Meyer, "Revolutionary Icons: Alfred Barr and the Remaking of Russian Religious Art," both in *Sensational Religion: Sensory Cultures in Material Practice*, ed. S. M. Promley (New Haven and London, 2014).

5 R. Shiff, *Doubt* (New York and London, 2008), 17–36, with this quotation at 17, italics from the original, that is, from C. S. Peirce, "Illustrations of the Logic of Science: Deduction, Induction, and Hypothesis," *Popular Science Monthly* 13 (1878): 482.

6 C. S. Peirce, "Guessing," *Hound and Horn* (1929): 267–82, also a fascinating detective story.

7 See B. Latour, "Reflections on Etienne Souriau's *Les différents modes d'existence*," in *The Speculative Turn: Continental Materialism and Realism*, ed. L. Bryant, N. Srnicek, and G. Harman, trans. S. Muecke (Melbourne, 2011), 303–33.

do), and they are alien to our knowing it (they do not use words to tell us so, and a big gap in understanding opens)—to my mind a double fallacy.[8] Here is the art-historical trap, talking and writing about the *mute* life these things have.[9]

The plastic bag is not a vehicle for allegory; he is just that thing, and he shows us a great deal in that mereness. His abilities to survive are never in doubt. "I am strong, and smart, and I would find my maker." He finds love in a very pretty, red plastic bag. But the currents of the world are too great for him: the bag assumed he was free, but experience taught him otherwise, and the bag learned deep patience. He waited in time that is not like ours, time that was too large for him, too, and "Sometimes, the waiting drove me mad," he says. The bag affirms early that he is indestructible, and his journey seems to confirm that state; and yet that state is also our guilt and burden. As almost every story relates, eternal life is not a happy gift, and we leave the bag in the flows of the ocean in despair over his seemingly never-diminishing awareness. Addressing his master, his last words in the film reveal his terrible endurance, "I wish you had created me so that I could die."

The plastic bag shows us the thoughts and feelings of a very common thing, but what makes it sidestep charges of anthropomorphism?[10] The bag is dependent on someone, an apparently higher being (she is the only human seen in the film and only partially). He feels loyalty to that master, as well as grief at her lack of fellow-feeling; and he feels the shocking cold of ice inside, so he knows bodily stimulus, but he does not seem to feel pain when fish nibble him, though he does wonder about the fate of those disembodied particles. The story does not follow them—do they have consciousness, too?—but he does demonstrate he lives in an environment, which all persons have, that is, a surrounding world we center. That environment provides him locomotion, and it cooperates with him to some degree.[11] So, he is like a human in some ways we recognize, but he is silent to that world, he waits endlessly, charmed and disappointed by the world his master thoughtlessly put him into.

His tragic life of denied purposefulness is not entirely absent from extant objects from the Byzantine world, but naturally and however comfortably, those objects lead different lives now. I want to give them due respect as feeling persons, as strange as that may sound, who have led long, patient, mostly silent lives. My experiment is to describe those lives, both in the attempted knowing of their beings and in their ongoing endurance of our love and care. My question is, did Byzantine objects have lives as persons, and can we know, through careful and empathetic looking and imagining (guessing?), how they *sensed* and *sense their worlds*?[12] Finally, what do we gain from this exercise, that is, trying

8 See B. Latour, *On the Modern Cult of the Factish Gods*, trans. C. Porter and H. Maclean (Durham, NC and London, 2010), 22–23, "And let no one try to tell us that the practitioners are engaging in dialectics, and that the subjects—auto-positioning themselves within objects—are revealed to themselves by alienating themselves via objects; artists, who could not care less about subjects or objects, move back and forth between them, without at any moment even lightly brushing either the subject-master-of-his-thoughts or the alienating object.... In all our activities, what we fabricate goes beyond us." See also G. Adamson, *Thinking through Craft* (Oxford and New York, 2007), 69–102.

9 Serres, *Five Senses*, 136, "All reception occurs within silence. Transmission will always win out, hands down, over reception. Here is neat proof: we cannot know that someone has received a message without asking for confirmation. Further transmission is therefore required in order to confirm reception. Sensation, receptive, is bathed in silence. You can take that as a sensible truth, as the truth of the senses, as a metaphysical truth. Our senses are bathed in muteness. May this book of mine inhabit the joy of such silence.... Sensation is acknowledged by language and transmits confirmation that the latter is receiving, thereby speaking of its silence. Sensation remains deaf and mute, almost monadic, tacit for as long as it acts as a receiver. Afterward, reception confirms itself, transmits, and thus speaks."

10 Analogy over anthropomorphism: see my "We Have Never Been Byzantine: On Analogy," in *Byzantium/Modernism*, ed. R. Betancourt and M. Taroutina (Leiden, 2015), 349–60.

11 As Uwe Steiner points out, our bias is the assumption that things are discrete, closed, and opaque, but the physical surround we carry with us is always and fully open to the world. See U. C. Steiner, "Actio, Narratio und das Gesicht der Dinge," *Zeitschrift für Medien- und Kulturforschung* 1, no. 1 (2011): 185–202.

12 See I. Stengers, "Reclaiming Animism," in *Animismus: Moderne hinter den Spiegeln / Animism: Modernity through the Looking Glass*, ed. A. Franke and S. Folie, trans. R. Voullié (Cologne, 2011), 183–92, here 188, "For Étienne Souriau (1892–1979), no creation bringing something new into existence is of human provenance alone, the human agent being instead the prey of the unrelenting imperative—'Guess!'—stemming from the work to be done."

to know how their bodies—persons, human and nonhuman—sensed?

This argument positions itself within current discourse and practice on the senses and develops, extends certain premises found in contemporary philosophical and anthropological studies. Scholars in medieval and early modern studies have been developing arguments about the importance of sense lives for understanding the past in recent years.[13] The gain from such studies has been a return of bodies to our historical inquiries, rectifying an absence that had largely abstracted our discourse to worlds of text and text's meaning-making abilities. We have not entirely left those worlds, however, and have, in some ways, changed continents, not forged new worlds; put simply, text privileged linguistic bodies over nonlinguistic ones.[14] Moreover, senses have tended to isolation, that is, they have been subjected to discrete studies. Byzantine visuality was a major development for sense studies in this field, because scholars argued that senses were conjoined and cooperative.[15] Those theories of vision had their basis in an atomic circulation that made vision possible through a tactile communication between seeing subject and seen; the implications of this work opened new, dynamic ways of seeing subjects' vision in that world. Recent work is sundering that connection, but it too works through that textually dominating mode of sense analysis.[16]

Two recent studies are important additions to the sense bibliography and worth mentioning in this context because they attempt, in sophisticated and persuasive ways, to move beyond our logocentric constriction.[17] Heather Hunter-Crowley reaches for an expansive sensorium in her analysis of silver liturgical objects from the sixth century, and she achieves profound insights into liturgical self-making through participatory things.[18] Annabel Wharton's most recent study ranges from feelings in historical buildings in Jerusalem and Las Vegas to video games, like Assassins' Creed, and so her lessons in agency of things should have a deep impact on Byzantine studies. The immersive worlds of video games are precisely the contemporary experiences to be drawn on for imaginative understandings of contexts like the liturgical transformations described by these two scholars. And yet they do not extend the sensorium as far as this essay argues we need to go, and indeed as in so many scholarly investigations, senses remain components, discrete and interlocked. Not only do senses flow together, always rushing the banks of a self, in time and motion unfixable, even inarticulable; they also make us more than ourselves in their excessiveness.[19] Words tame, inoculate senses, and our words likewise deny senses' life beyond us, even though the world around us has more sense than that assumption allows.[20]

Byzantine things, unlike the humans who made up that world, can still sense and feel, and I can give examples of paintings and reliefs showing

13 Searches bring up an array of choices, impossible a decade ago. Along with sources cited here, I would also add *Religion and the Senses in Early Modern Europe*, ed. W. de Boer and C. Göttler (Leiden and Boston, 2013).

14 See the apt criticisms in H. Hunter-Crowley, "Embodying the Divine: The Sensational Experience of the Sixth-Century Eucharist," in *Making Senses of the Past: Toward a Sensory Archaeology*, ed. J. Day (Carbondale-Edwardsville, IL, 2013), 160–76.

15 See the studies in *Visuality Before and Beyond the Renaissance: Seeing as Others Saw*, ed. R. S. Nelson (New York and Cambridge, 2000), as well as P. S. Wells, *How Ancient Europeans Saw the World: Vision, Pattern, and the Shaping of the Mind in Prehistoric Times* (Princeton, 2012).

16 See R. Betancourt, "Why Sight Is Not Touch: Reconsidering the Tactility of Vision in Byzantium," *DOP* 70 (2016): 1–23.

17 I am singling out Hunter-Crowley, "Embodying the Divine," and A. J. Wharton, *Architectural Agents: The Delusional, Abusive, Addictive Lives of Buildings* (Minneapolis, 2015).

18 D. Krueger's excellent *Liturgical Subjects: Christian Ritual, Biblical Narrative, and the Formation of the Self in Byzantium* (Philadelphia, 2014), is a perfect complement to this chapter.

19 S. Connor, "Michel Serres's *Les cinq sens*," in *Mapping Michel Serres*, ed. N. Abbas (Ann Arbor, 2005), 153–69, here 167, "The senses are the body forming and reforming itself. As such, the body is a miraculous nook in the flux, a negentropic eddy or swirl in the current that traverses it yet which it delays."

20 Advocating the position of Serres entails disavowing the human instrumentality at the heart of the Heideggerian model. The anthropocentric, linguistically biased position comes under a great deal of scrutiny, all of it negative, in Serres's writing. However, well recommended is an application of Heidegger's position to a Byzantine object by C. Barber, "Thingliness," in *Byzantine Things in the World* (n. 4 above), 99–105.

their feelings by changing colors, jumping to the ground, and repelling attackers by aggressively attacking. Even if such objects as performed these sensitive acts were showable in museums, for example, only their dormant state is now brought on through photographic capture and vitrine deep-freeze. Yet material qualities and conditions can reveal thought and life through sensual imagining. And that imagining has to exploit all these experiences, from exhibition to numinous, devotional contexts, since both are natural environments now. All objects' inner life (as in fellow humans', too) is invisible to us unless revealed in symptoms, but potential and surplus are always there.[21]

The person lives of Byzantine things are strangely straightforward, perhaps a reason for the obviousness of *Plastic Bag* for a Byzantinist. People in that past world knew very well that more than humans felt and sensed. Their history of art revealed it to them, their explanations for the world around them supported it, and experience confirmed it. Objects' and persons' interior lives have to be inferred from their symptoms, but that method is also our own natural means to know other human feelings and senses. We have the advantage, in some ways, of words, but those nonhuman persons also had a hard time hiding their feelings.

Almost at random, I have opened the *Letter of the Three Patriarchs*, and nearly every example adduced by the writer(s) reveals inner life through outward reactions—both human and nonhuman.[22] So, the Patriarch Germanos was deeply troubled by image destruction, and he wept and wailed before deciding to give an image of Christ freedom by bringing the icon down to the harbor at T'Amantiou; he attached a petition to the right hand of the icon that implored it to save itself. The icon did so, by standing in the water up to its ankles and moving in that way and with crazy speed to Rome. It stood in the Tiber for three days in a fiery guise, and then with striking speed, came to Pope Gregory II, who was waiting in a boat on the river, just like Symeon had in the Temple in Jerusalem. The icon's feet never dried, according to the story, and those sodden feet kept dripping salty, healing water for the afflicted of Rome.

Try this episode from the other way around: I'm picked up and placed in the water, and my grieving master pushes me away; I learn the currents of the sea, and I look for refuge in another place; that master forgot me, and I'll forget him and find another; my patience is short, because I am in relation to the great Master (the plaque in my right hand is directed at me and at him, "Master, master, save yourself and us, because we perish," from Matthew 8:25), and I have strength to travel, enflame, generate forever my own salty wetness; I cannot dry nor die, and I feel and fulfill the needs of those blind and broken persons, who are less than I am.

Byzantines knew special persons had abilities more than human to protect and save, and those special persons often behaved excessively and unpredictably, submissive and resistant according to a logic only partly understood by humans. All things are sui generis, even the plastic bag whose experience and feelings were its own only, and icons all feel differently, too. Their extraordinary reactions are noted and recorded, not their abilities of forbearance and qualities of patience.

The lifespan of that icon is not knowable, it no longer exists, and its eventual obsolescence can only be supposed. The icon appears in that written source, a description from a human perspective, but its independence and resistance come across very well, naturally even, and its emotions and its interior life are implicit in this account—no real explanation of that inner life was necessary in any of the accounts in that collection. But persons' senses of the world determined each narrative. Nearly every time a life of an object bubbles to the surface in a medieval Greek text, to generalize,[23] it reveals the collapse of a distinction between sign and referent, which

21 As J. Bennett, in *Vibrant Matter: A Political Ecology of Things* (Durham, NC, 2010), tells us, objects are not reducible to contexts we make and describe. See also P. Lemonnier, *Mundane Objects: Materiality and Non-Verbal Communication* (Walnut Creek, CA, 2013).

22 *The Letter of the Three Patriarchs to Emperor Theophilus and Related Texts*, ed. J. A. Munitiz, J. Chrysostomides, E. Harvalia-Crook, and C. Dendrinos (Camberley, Surrey, 1997), 49–51 (7.14.b–c).

23 Here guided by R. Shiff, "Watch Out for Thinking (Even Fuzzy Thinking): Concept and Percept in Modern Art," *Common Knowledge* 19, no. 1 (2013): 65–87.

we take as the basis for representation, and it shows the irruption of interior life, which we also take to be the basis for consciousness and subjectivity among humans.

To follow the premises of Philippe Descola (b. 1949), no single entity like Byzantine culture existed.[24] Rather many cultures unfolded among many subjects, some of which were things, and the object culture of the icon once of Germanos was simply generalized in that account to make it comprehensible to humans. These traits are typical of animist cultures.[25] Interiorities are spread across the world, while defining, physical differences are made particular to each species, culture.[26] These modes of being are revealed in participatory moments, when the icon revealed its independence, its majesty even. And continued to reveal traces of that state in lesser form (the secretion of salty water) until its existence ceased or altered beyond recognition. Its emotions showed as symptoms, not verbally expressed (though it perhaps could read), when it was threatened and then implored to save to itself.[27] How else could it have known, if not through its senses?

A thread running through modern thought assumes things to be extensions of our bodies—things become activated or actualized only when performed by us. And in another way, things are comprehensible as extensions or prostheses for us in the world. Such a position, of course, is exclusively human centered, and it is difficult to escape, even in the most thoughtful, careful analyses.[28] But, again, try it from the other side: we are objects' prostheses, their way to overcome their physical limitations and to realize their own emotional, sensory lives more fully than they can on their own. The focus of the story of the T'Amantiou icon is the icon after all, and all the other characters appear only as facilitators for its survival and for its newly splendid beneficence in Rome. Even told according to the text's own terms, human agents realized the icon's sensual shortcomings or gaps, and they ensured its survival as its extensions outside itself.

A precondition of feeling is worldedness, acknowledging a state of having one's own world of thoughts and feeling, and perhaps even explanations for that world.[29] Humans naturally self-acknowledge this possession. On the basis of film and hagiography, plastic bag and icon would do the same. Worldedness also needs a kind of body, with/through which to sense the world one creates, and one knows that sensing the world, and one then knows self.[30]

Mary continued to make worlds for herself through surrogates in relation to her. She ascended bodily, but her bodies continued to live and to circulate with extraordinary effect in the middle ages. One exciting body has been witnessed at Saidnaya, near Damascus, since the twelfth century, when Latin sources first mentioned that the monastery there (now a convent) possessed an icon that was "incarnate."[31] Arabic and Greek sources followed, and the shrine

24 P. Descola, *Beyond Nature and Culture*, trans. J. Lloyd (Chicago and London, 2013), 129–43.

25 See, for related analysis, M. Engelke, "Material Religion," in *The Cambridge Companion to Religious Studies*, ed. R. A. Orsi (Cambridge, 2012), and for recent studies of animism, *Animismus: Revisionen der Moderne*, ed. I. Albers and A. Franke (Zurich, 2012), and *Animism*, vol. 1, ed. A. Franke (Berlin, 2010).

26 According to Descola, again, animism sees continuity or spread of minds, of thinking, and discontinuity of bodies, of physical containers; Descola, *Beyond Nature and Culture*, 291. See also *La fabrique des images: Visions du monde et formes de la représentation*, ed. P. Descola (Paris, 2010), J. Robb, "Beyond Agency," *World Archaeology* 42, no. 4 (2010): 493–520, T. Webmoor and C. L. Witmore, "Things Are Us! A Commentary on Human/Things Relations under the Banner of a 'Social' Archaeology," *Norwegian Archaeological Review* 41, no. 1 (2008): 53–70, and L. Malafouris, "Before and Beyond Representation: Towards an Enactive Conception of the Palaeolithic Image," in *Image and Imagination: A Global History of Figurative Representation*, ed. C. Renfrew and I. Morley (Cambridge, 2007), 289–302.

27 Here, perhaps, is the icon's self-incongruity that showed its openness. See K. Pahl, "Doublings and Couplings: The Feeling Thing in Valéry and Kleist," *Zeitschrift für Medien- und Kulturforschung* 1, no. 1 (2011): 177–84.

28 Hamilakis, *Archaeology and the Senses*, 113 and 197, for example.

29 For example, K. Robertson, "Exemplary Rocks," in *Animal, Vegetable, Mineral: Ethics and Objects*, ed. J. J. Cohen (Washington, DC, 2012), 91–121.

30 A. Franke, "Beyond the Return of the Repressed," trans. W. Prantner, in Franke and Folie, *Animismus* (n. 12 above), 167–82, on self as gift of the other. See also the excellent D. Diederichsen, "Beseelung, Entdinglichung und die neue Attraktivität des Unbelebten," in ibid., 289–301.

31 G. Peers, *Sacred Shock: Framing Visual Experience in Byzantium* (University Park, PA, 2004), 133; D. Pringle, *The Churches of the Crusader Kingdom of Jerusalem: A Corpus*, vol. 2, *L–Z (excluding Tyre)* (Cambridge, 1998), 219–21; and see now E. Garosi, "The Incarnated Icon of Saydnaya: Light and

attracted pilgrims, Muslims and Christians both, because of the icon's fascinating demonstration of body.[32] The icon was said to have flowed with oil, as if the icon was a body with naturally flowing fluids. The image still attracts pilgrims of all kinds, and for that reason, it is essentially invisible behind its cladding and votives in a candlelit chapel.[33] But it was famous throughout the Christian and Muslim worlds, and some images reflect the appearance of that original icon, like an eleventh-century reliquary of the cross with its Virgin and Child panel—because the panel came from Saidnaya, one assumes this panel copied the iconography of the original (fig. 1.1).[34]

In any case, the small panel (the height of the reliquary is only 8.3 cm) does not give a clear sense of the powerful presence in the original, which can be sensed, however, at its shrine still. One enters the small sanctuary from a side entrance near the main church for the convent and finds a darkened space with a glowing presence of the Virgin flecked with the many votives that adorn her (fig. 1.2). The icon's body had—has—miraculously attractive powers, for it grew breasts, in fact, for its marvelous seepages and for an intense erotic power, too, as the testimony of a Muslim who saw the perfect breasts of the icon of Mary and converted to Christianity.[35] Mary's identity with her icon there was mysteriously excessive and desire-filled, and it made living relation to the divine in the world possible.

In western exhibitions, most experiences for art historians and others present as natural the binary position between a discrete subject and a discrete object. Full participation in object life and qualities in these cultural contexts is never entertained. A shrine like Saidnaya provides an extraordinary opportunity to know the richness of that icon's world that is so often closed off to us in most viewing contexts. Unlike museums in the past, our institutions have come to value the persistence of objects over direct, sensual contact.[36] A middle ground could exist between that subject- and objecthood, a space where what we do and what we receive, our autonomy and our dependency, would no longer be at odds.[37] And likewise that middle ground would be a place for these other persons, nonhuman objects, to reveal symptoms of feeling and sensing more fully and clearly to our comprehension.

But these icons need desire, and the symptoms they reveal of inner want are on their skin.[38] The symptoms are shown in light on their skin, and the embracing and kissing and genuflecting are also answers to their need for touch and love. Everyone orthodox or accustomed to visiting orthodox churches knows icons' neediness.

Shade," *Islam and Christian–Muslim Relations* 26, no. 3 (2015): 339–58, with extensive bibliography.

32 A. G. Remensnyder, "Christian Captives, Muslim Maidens and Mary," *Speculum* 82, no. 3 (2007): 671; J. Folda, *Crusader Art in the Holy Land from the Third Crusade to the Fall of Acre, 1187–1291* (Cambridge, 2005), 121, 176, 393; A. Cuffel, "From Practice to Polemic: Shared Saints and Festivals as 'Women's Religion' in the Medieval Mediterranean," *BSOAS* 68 (2005): 401–19; K. Ciggaar, "Painters, Paintings and Pilgrims in Medieval Jerusalem: Some Witnesses from East and West," *Journal of Eastern Christian Art* 2 (2005): 127–38; eadem, "Les villes de provinces Byzantines et les échanges culturels: Quelques traducteurs peu connus," in *Byzance et le monde extérieur: Contacts, relations, échanges*, ed. M. Balard, É. Malamut, and J.-M. Spieser (Paris, 2005), 91–94; and M. E. Heldman, "St. Luke as Painter: Post-Byzantine Icons in the Early-Sixteenth-Century Ethiopia," *Gesta* 44, no. 2 (2005): 137–8; D. Jacoby, "Society, Culture and the Arts in Crusader Acre," in *France and the Holy Land: Frankish Culture at the End of the Crusades*, ed. D. H. Weiss and L. Mahoney (Baltimore and London, 2004), 104–5.

33 See W. Dalrymple, *From the Holy Mountain: A Journey among the Christians of the Middle East* (New York, 1997), 186–91.

34 Y. Piatnitskii, *Sinai, Byzantium, Russia: Orthodox Art from the Sixth to the Twentieth Century* (London, 2000), no. B38, and see A. Cutler, "Everywhere and Nowhere: The Invisible Muslim and Christian Self-Fashioning in the Culture of Outremer," in Weiss and Mahoney, *France and the Holy Land*, 261.

35 V. F. Koenig, *Gautier de Coinci: Les miracles de Nostre Dame*, 4 vols. (Geneva, 1955–70), 3:25.58–63; K. A. Smith, "Bodies of Unsurpassed Beauty: 'Living' Images of the Virgin in the High Middle Ages," *Viator* 37 (2006): 178.

36 C. Korsmeyer, "Staying in Touch," in *Art and Ethical Criticism*, ed. G. L. Hagberg (Malden, MA, 2008), 187–210.

37 M. Merleau-Ponty, *Phenomenology of Perception*, trans. D. A. Landes (London and New York, 2012), xxxiv.

38 Serres, *Five Senses* (n. 1 above), argues that the contact of skin on skin makes consciousness and provides soul. This book begins with a tour de force description of the author caught below deck during a fire at sea, and he notes the moment of the birth of his soul, "The I as a whole leaps towards this localized point and moves decisively from one half of the body to the other when the point slides, in contact with the separating wall, from its internal to its external surface. Since my near shipwreck, I have become accustomed to calling this point the soul. The soul resides at the point where the I is decided. We are all endowed with a soul, from that first moment of passage when we risked and saved our existence" (ibid., 20).

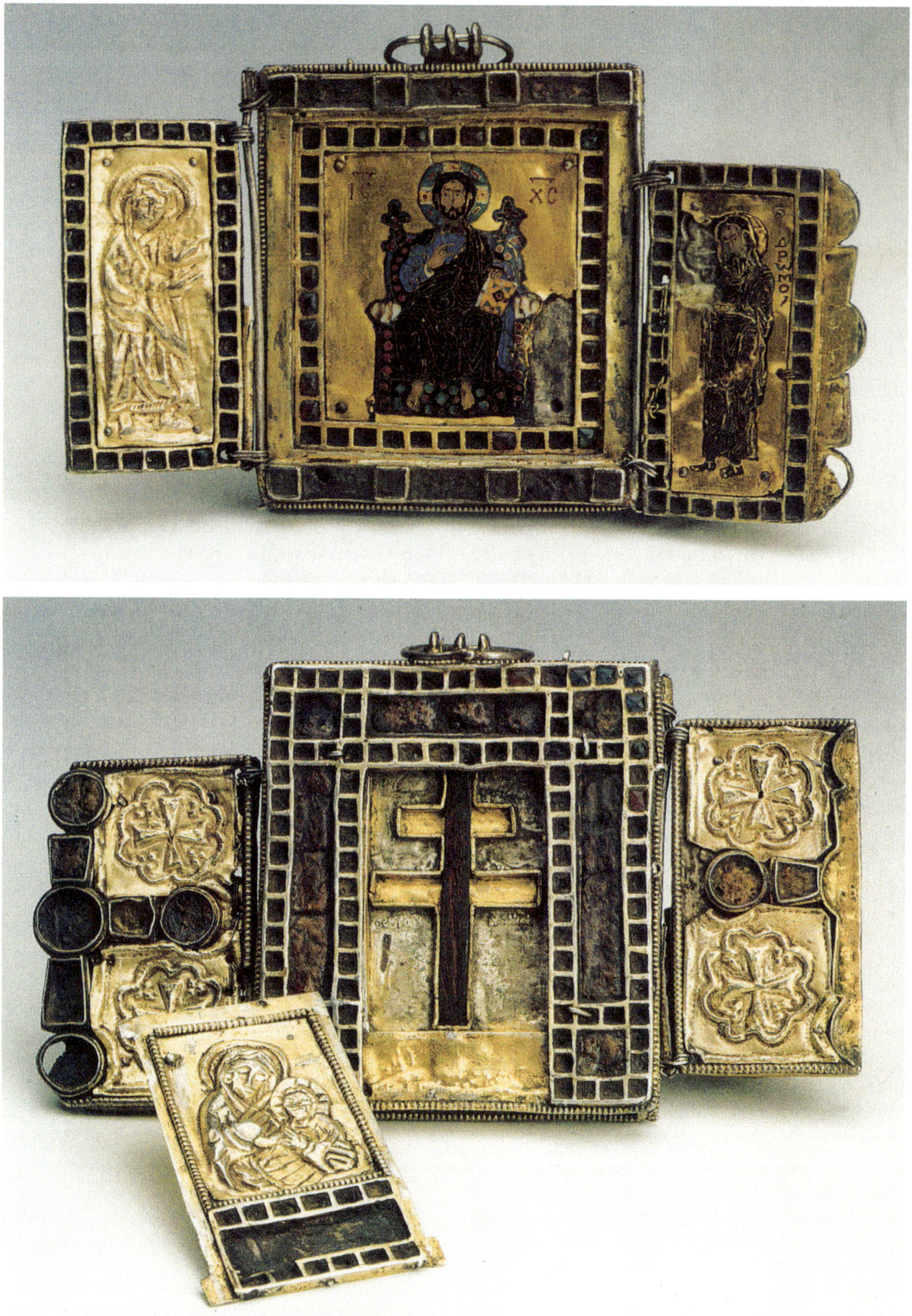

FIG. 1.1. Reliquary of the cross, Virgin and Child panel removed from setting, eleventh century (photo: Leonard Kheifets, © The State Hermitage Museum, St. Petersburg)

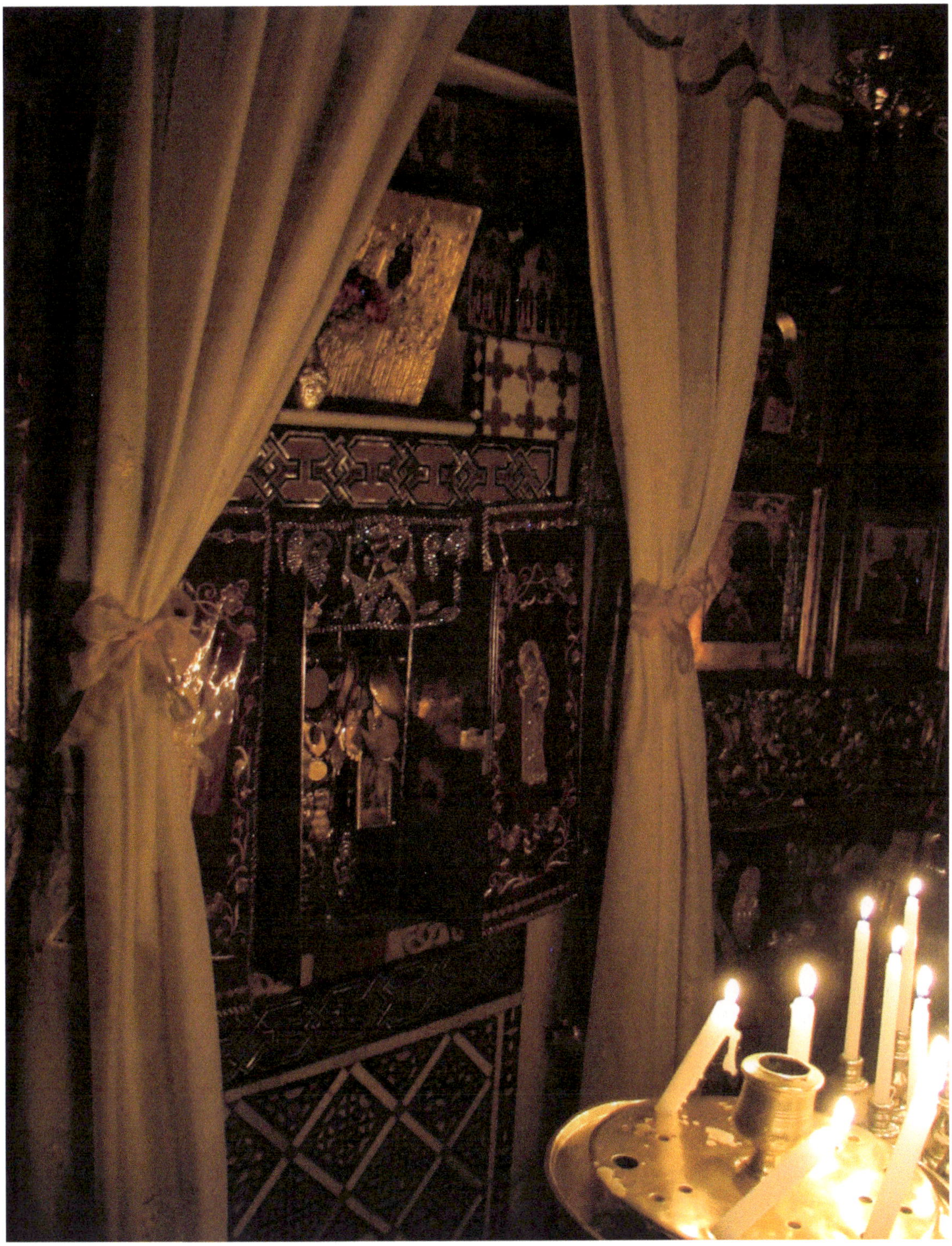

FIG. 1.2. View of Icon of the Virgin and Child in its current setting, Convent at Saidnaya, Syria (photo: author)

Museum encounters with them leave them cold: they treat icons like disembodied spirits, and all the icons know in museums is our mostly silent and passing attention, and our rather low-wattage desire. The tenth-century narration of the history of the Mandylion revealed an extreme case of desire that acted out its wants.[39] Taken from behind by Thaddaeus, the Mandylion was placed on his face, and it faced out glowing resplendently with that touch. Aroused in this way on entering the chamber, the face was enthusiastically embraced by Abgar, who touched himself over his entire body with that face.

That voraciousness is not typical of icons' restraint—they hold their desire with dignity—but they always try to show themselves to be desirable. These are their symptoms, their conditions that show their feelings of want. The shining face described in that text is a symptom close to what medieval viewers would have experienced in close contact with that particular body. Entering the fields of light intensity of the illuminated icon, clad in gilt-silver revetment in the copy now in Genoa, a viewer would know the same expression of desire seen by Abgar, and while no other viewer got to press the face all over, the icon revealed its feelings of want—the want the Lord feels for the love of his creation—in its material demonstration of halation, glow, candle-pulsing radiance (fig. 1.3).

The Mandylion had its own ways to show its feelings, but it was admittedly unlikely ever to have had a very wide audience, and likewise only the most exceptional cases of other icons or objects that showed forth are recorded. The use of reflection is a common factor in icon show, however, and that reflection must have reached, as it does still, many more people than said so. So, the moody icon described by Michael Psellos (1017/18–1078/96) engaged with a restricted set of persons, and it reached primarily the empress Zoe herself (thus its noteworthiness for the eleventh-century historian) with its chameleon abilities.[40] The icon revealed to her its feelings, how it sensed and understood its world, by altering its colors. The empress reacted wholeheartedly to the symptomatic shifts in colors, and her sensations were matched, as best she could interpret them, by the icon's showing forth of self-transfiguration.

Color in such an object was naturally made and applied to the surface of wood to create forms, but color was also animate matter, manifested most vividly in Zoe's temperamental icon. It showed colorful reactions, which were Zoe's means to know its meanings and messages for her. It performed alchemical operations, too, in the mysterious, even chemical—in some ways of thinking—production of life. The operation may be illusionism, in our understanding, that is, producing the appearance but not reality of life. But in Zoe's eyes, for example, no illusion was in evidence, just real presence in the thing. In the sixth century, Agathias wrote poetically of the power of color to pull out deep prayer from an icon's witness.[41] Color has a long history of providing vital power to art, from Plato through the high Renaissance. Moreover, it is a demonstration of the typological difference between Hebrew and Christian covenants, from the latter's point of view: the revelation to the Hebrews was simply empty lines that was only colored in with the life-giving warmth of the Incarnation.[42]

That sense of color giving life and warmth has a history, too, of the play between the inanimate and the animate, which goes back perhaps ultimately to Aristotle's theories of vital heat that warms and informs all matter.[43] The use

39 See Constantine Porphyrogennetos, *Narratio de translatione Constantinopolim imaginis Edessenae*, in PG 113:421–54. The most recent writing, to my knowledge, is F. Dell'Acqua, "The Fall of the Idol on the Frame of the Genoa *Mandylion*: A Narrative on/of the Borders," in *Negotiating Co-Existence: Communities, Cultures, and* Convivencia *in Byzantine Society*, ed. B. Crostini and S. La Porta (Trier, 2013), 143–73.

40 For example, B. Pentcheva, *The Sensual Icon: Space, Ritual and the Senses in Byzantium* (University Park, 2010), 184–5, and G. Peers, "Real Living Painting: Quasi-Objects and Dividuation in the Byzantine World," *Religion and the Arts* 16, no. 5 (2012): 433–60.

41 *The Greek Anthology*, I.34. See L. James, "Color and Meaning in Byzantium," *JEChrSt* 11, no. 2 (2003): 223–33. See, now, A. Pizzone, "Toward a Self-Determined and Emotional Gaze: Agathias and the Icon of the Archangel Michael," in *Aesthetics and Theurgy in Byzantium*, ed. S. Mariev and W.-M. Stock (Berlin, 2013), 75–103, and I have attempted to argue for a materialist reading instead in my forthcoming "The Matter of Crossing Beyond (and Back) in the Byzantine World."

42 See the studies by H. L. Kessler, *Spiritual Seeing: Picturing God's Invisibility in Medieval Art* (Philadelphia, 2000).

43 See F. Fehrenbach, "Kohäsion und Transgression: Zur Dialektik des lebendigen Bildes," in *Transgressionen/*

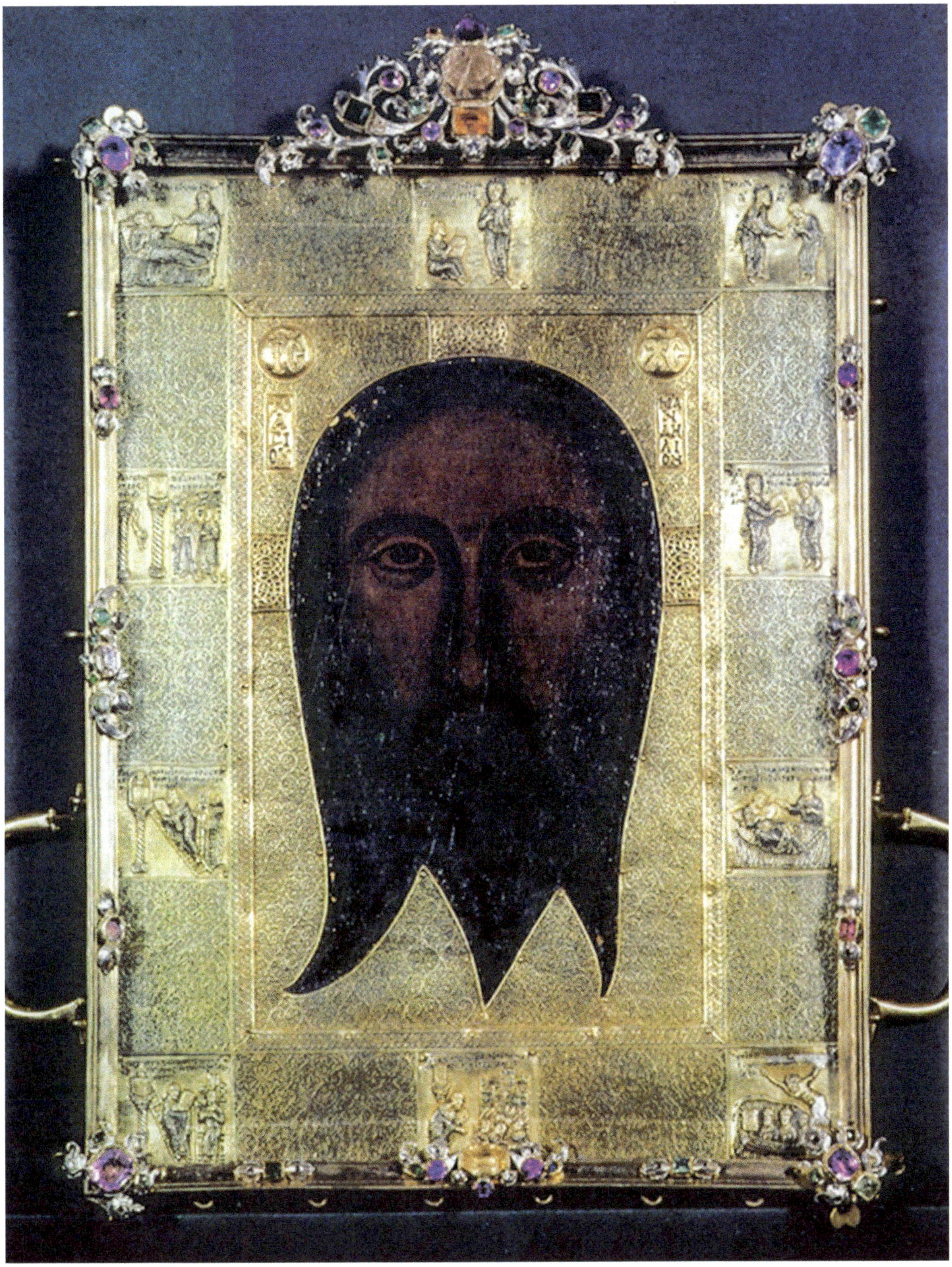

FIG. 1.3. Icon of the Face of Christ (Mandylion), panel medieval and frame late Byzantine, Chiesa di San Bartolomeo degli Armeni, Genoa, Italy (photo: Chiesa di San Bartolomeo degli Armeni, Genoa, Italy)

of color then is an essential way for pictures to skirt a state of dead matter. Resistance was of course always possible, but warmth and energy in color motivated testimony like that of Agathias, among many others, on the strange, compelling life force.[44] The converse of recognizing color's force is the emptying of life in images when colors fade. So when iconophiles advised the abandonment of images with faded color and form, they were admitting to the vitality of color and color's necessity for recognizing the power of the thing and of its relation to the divine.[45]

Likewise, the scraping and ingesting of pigment from manuscripts, icons and frescoes attests to the transformative quality of matter that also made life in things and relayed it to humans.[46] Modern art historians and conservationists often decry the application of new paint to old, faded paintings, to which a community might still want relation, and few outside such contemporary communities would support this "updating." And yet, taken at face value, such "refreshing" through new layers of paint provides new life, not only figuratively in terms of increased legibility and fullness of form, but also in a more literal fashion, the infusion of life-giving warmth through pigments.

One might say, from this point of view, that modern conservation efforts, like the cleaning of the Sinai Pantocrator in the 1960s, then, fail badly at bringing works back to life (fig. 1.4). The original state of the icon is unrecoverable, but the conservators and art historians at work then decided that an erasure of later layers to the sixth-century icon would return it as nearly as possible to a state chosen by its maker and possibly its patron. That return is naturally a fiction—not even entertained by the participants some sixty years ago, who stopped short of restoring the image to its first state. Rather, they decided to eliminate the later additions and leave the abraded, scoured surface around Christ. Now Christ's clothing is a weak frame for the action of blessing and intense stare(s) of God; one sees a more-or-less intact face, its ambivalences still enticing, but a reduced, lifeless surround. The decisions around these restorations are always difficult, but the later repainting has never been given its due, to my knowledge, as a kind of blood-transplant of color that allowed the persistence of the warm vivacity of that extraordinary face.[47]

This discussion of color, warmth and life sidesteps how objects feel about their constitutive energies, their spending and replacements, and finally objects' obsolescence. The last is the natural life-spanning of all things, but taken from objects' point of view, their life force marshaled itself in their material make up. The leap from vivid color to bleeding icons could be, from this perspective, explained by confusion between color and blood, or just as metaphor. But bleeding icons were taken very seriously by medieval people, who combined, for example, the blood of the famous bleeding icon of Christ from Beirut with blood shed by Christ's own body on the cross—no distinction between them was possible according to medieval understanding.[48] In exceptional cases like this, texts and witnesses survive, but establishing such moves among wood, color, and the flesh of Christ would be very difficult if no texts survived. The difficulty arises

Animationen: Das Kunstwerk als Lebewesen, ed. U. Pfisterer and A. Zimmermann (Berlin, 2005), 1–40, and the excellent study by B. Fricke, "A Liquid History: Blood and Animation in Late Medieval Art," *Res* 63–64 (2013): 53–69.

44 For example, *Kunst und Alchemie: Das Geheimnis der Verwandlung*, ed. S. Dupré, D. von Kerssenbrock-Krosigk, and B. Wismer (Düsseldorf, 2014), 13, and P. Schreiner and D. Oltrogge, *Byzantische Tinten-, Tuschen- und Farbrezepte*, DenkWien 419 (Vienna, 2011).

45 References in K. Parry, "Theodore Studites and the Patriarch Nicephorus on Image-Making as a Christian Imperative," *Byzantion* 59 (1989): 181.

46 V. Marinis, "Piety, Barbarism and the Senses in Byzantium," in Promley, *Sensational Religion* (n. 4 above). Here I would also cite some recent work on *Stoffe*, the analysis of substance and its histories, as another productive line of inquiry for Byzantinists. See P. Bühler, "'... und das Wort ward Fleisch ...': Stofflichkeit und Stoffeindlichkeit in der Bibel und im Christentum," in *Stoffe: Zur Geschichte der Materialität in Künsten und Wissenschaften*, ed. B. Naumann, T. Strässle and C. Torra-Mattenklott (Zurich, 2006), 19–37, and the studies in *Stoffe in Bewegung: Beiträge zu einer Wissensgeschichte der materiallen Welt*, ed. K. Espahangizi and B. Orland (Zurich and Berlin, 2014).

47 M. Chatzidakis, "An Encaustic Icon of Christ at Sinai," trans. G. Walters, *ArtB* 49, no. 3 (1967): 197–208. I have argued similar ideas in "Framing and Conserving Byzantine Art at the Menil Collection: Experiences of Relative Identity," *Zeitschrift für Medien- und Kulturforschung* 6, no. 2 (2015): 25–44.

48 See Peers, *Sacred Shock*, and my essay "Transfiguring Materialities: Relational Abstraction in Byzantium and Its Exhibition," *Convivium* 2, no. 2 (2015): 116–37, as well as M. Bacci, "Le *Majestas*, il *Volto Santo* e il *Cristo di Beirut*: Nuove reflessioni," *Iconographica* 13 (2014): 45–66.

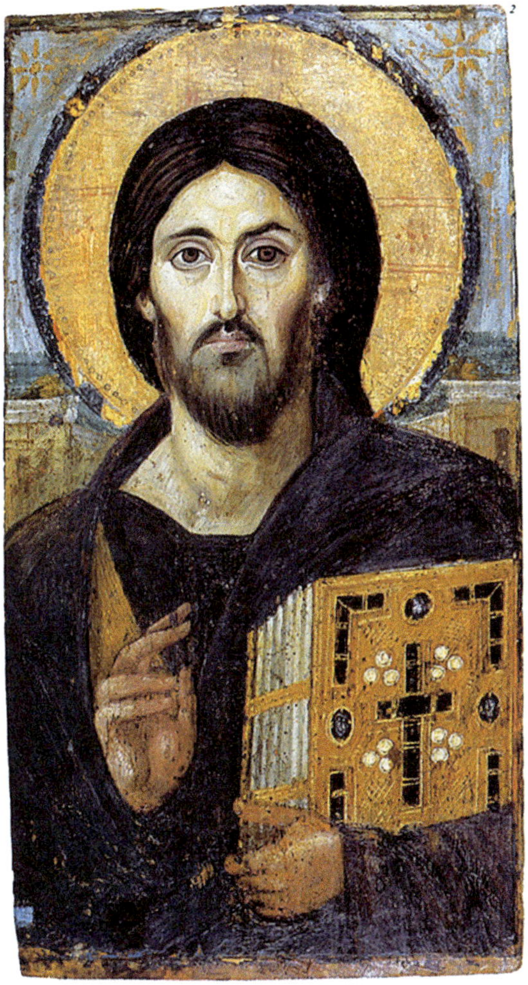

FIG. 1.4. Icon of Christ Pantokrator, sixth–seventh century, St. Catherine's Monastery, Sinai, Egypt (photo: courtesy of the Fathers of the Holy Monastery of St. Catherine, Sinai)

from our inclination to move from hypothesis or guesswork when confronted with an unusual, recalcitrant thing, to inference based on natural-seeming deductions, which in our case primarily invests in inert, lifeless matter.[49]

Things tell us different versions of themselves under certain conditions. The Mandylion again—perhaps even made by the Lord's own blood as pigment—shows in its Genoese copy vivacity of materials that demonstrates symptoms of feeling toward environment. Nothing as upsetting as opening its veins, the powerful radiance of the gilt-silver cladding of the darkened face at the center of the panel activates life. Just as materials such as silver and gold are in some way animate—in some way different from our own lives as humans, but undeniably alive to those people—and show their reactions to environment, so the object (a true image—an *echt Bild*) reveals its feeling life before its creation. As the light radiating from the surround spreads, so does the life and so does the transformative nature of its materials transform its believer.[50]

Now, those "perceptual qualities"—where do they reside, where are they provoked? In the backward glance of a viewer, or in the self-sufficient, perdurant regard of a nonhuman person? In any case, when I make an argument of this sort, my own position is informed guesswork. I argue and prove to my own satisfaction that sensation is spread far more broadly in the world and in the past than we habitually assume. Does it matter if a glass filled with ice water on a hot day is doing condensation or showing the feeling of divided sensation (cold inside, hot outside)? The stakes in accepting the latter as more than poetic fancy need some defending, if my argument can carry some interpretative strength for understanding the past.

Perhaps my argument cannot persuade: the data it gives depends on a strong change in our assumptions about our special, exclusive senses, which make us master of this world of the anthropocene.[51] But I would say we need to listen, to feel with things, exactly because of the antropocenic dangers. Byzantines knew this necessity all too well: Michael Kritoboulos (d. ca. 1470) wrote an extraordinary account of the despair and hopelessness of the palladium icon of the Virgin processed in the waning days of Byzantine Constantinople. No one doubted this feeling of dread and fear that that icon expressed outwardly through increased lethargy

49 See my "We Have Never Been Byzantine."

50 See F. B. Flood, "Bodies and Becoming: Mimesis, Mediation, and the Ingestion of the Sacred in Christianity and Islam," in *Sensational Religion* (n. 4 above), on incorporating charisma into the very essence of self, amplifying the underlying ambiguity between imitation and becoming that is perhaps central to all devotional practice.

51 An excellent primer on the subject is J. Parikka, *A Geology of Media* (Minneapolis, 2015).

(she was unbearably heavy), evasiveness (she slipped from their hands—I would imagine like a child who wants to avoid being held, an unholdable creature), fear (she wanted to hide her face to the ground). All these feelings were suicidal, and everyone trusted her feelings. The inhabitants of the city knew, according to Kritoboulos, terror, agony and fear in turn.[52] Those people knew deep empathy for their things; they read what they could know of those feelings and felt them in turn. The icon was seeking its own good, perhaps (assisted suicide?), and it used its human followers as prosthetics to express its emotions.[53]

Chronological unfolding of the history of the empire is a common technique in exhibition and in pedagogy, and it answers a perceived need on the part of viewers and students for historical grounding in conventional coherence (where we ignore experience for fictions). But perhaps not presenting our version of the past with an attitude of certainty and closure, and leaving open interplay, imaginative and generous, among all the persons, visitors, students, and inmates, could lead to fuller empathy with objects' feeling than we are permitted normally. Indeed, strange as it may seem, we largely take our own bodies for granted in these various contexts—when words win out again—and we do need to take more seriously the continuous spread of our seeing, feeling world of objects.[54]

Fellow feeling may be a way in, since a historical capture of feeling is likely nearly outside reach. A strength and attraction of feeling is its first-line encounter with the world, and its initial resistance to verbalization, indeed the disregard feeling has for it (figs. 1.5, 1.6). We often insist on separation of thought and feeling, but as Donald Judd (1928–94) stated, "the distinction between thought and feeling is, at the least, exaggerated."[55] Judd was the most unlikely Byzantinist almost that one can imagine, but his insistence on first-hand experience models an approach many of us, myself not less than anyone, can learn from. His *Untitled* from 1965 (green lacquer on galvanized iron, Menil Collection; figs. 1.5, 1.6), for example, is a difficult aspect of any room it occupies: how does one make sense of this rectangular box anchored to the wall at right angles? In the first place, the Judd piece brings one back to objectness, to the irreducible encounter with a made thing, and that sense, that feeling of first-feeling, is uncommon for most of us and certainly uncommon before a figural icon of the late middle ages.

Having written about the icon of St. George in the Byzantine and Christian Museum in Athens in the past, I have felt that I had a certain familiarity with this object (fig. 1.7).[56] But it is faceted in a complexity that I find myself

52 *Critobuli Imbriotae Historiae*, ed. D. R. Reinsch, CHFB 22 (Berlin, 1983), 58 (45.1–3); *History of Mehmet the Conqueror by Critoboulos*, trans. C. T. Riggs (Princeton, 1954), 58–59 [183–84], "During those same days, there occurred the following divine signs and portents of the terrors that were very soon to come to the city. Three or four days before the battle, when all the people in the City were holding a religious procession, men and women together, and marching around with the Ikon of the Mother of God, this latter slipped suddenly from the hands of its bearers without any cause or power being apparent, and fell flat on the ground. And when everybody shouted immediately, and rushed to raise up the ikon, it sank down as if weighted with lead, and as if fastened to the ground, and became well-nigh impossible to raise. And so it continued for a considerable time, until, by a great effort and much shouting and prayers by all, the priests and its bearers managed to raise it up and place it on the shoulders of the men. This strange occurrence filled everyone with much terror and very great agony and fear, for they thought this fall was no good omen—as was quite true."

53 Useful for thinking with is J. Basl and R. Sandler, "The Good of Non-Sentient Entities: Organisms, Artifacts, and Synthetic Biology," *Studies in History and Philosophy of Biological and Biomedical Sciences* 44, no. 4, part B (2013): 697–705.

54 For example, Malafouris, "Before and Beyond Representation" (n. 26 above), 289, "image and perception are continuous; in changing the one you affect the other and thus you cannot understand the one in isolation from the other."

55 D. Judd, *Complete Writings, 1975–1986* (Eindhoven, 1987), 30, "I've always considered the distinction between thought and feeling as, at the least, exaggerated; this is a small description that has been raised to a central fact of human nature. I tried to find the beginning of the idea but couldn't. Probably it was developed in early Christianity. I've always blamed it on the mind and body distinction of the Christians since it's handy for mysticism and their kind of belief. All experience, large and small, involves feeling; all thought involves feeling. All feeling is based on experience which involved thought. *Emotion or feeling is simply a quick summation of experience*, some of which is thought, necessarily quick so that we can act quickly. It's not irrational, virtually the opposite. Thought is not strict, isolated and only logical but is continually using its backlog of experience which is called feeling" [my emphasis].

56 Peers, *Sacred Shock*, and *Heaven and Earth: Art of Byzantium from Greek Collections*, ed. A. Drandaki, D. Papanikola, and A. Tourta (Athens, 2013).

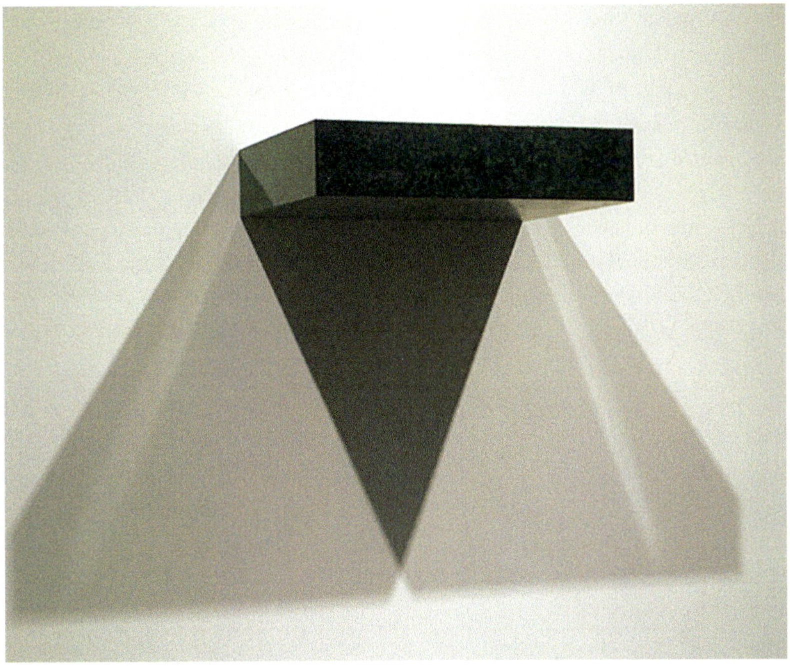

FIG. 1.5. Donald Judd, *Untitled*, 1965, Green lacquer on galvanized iron, 15.2 × 68.6 × 61.0 cm, The Menil Collection, Houston, gift of Walter Hopps (95-51) (photo courtesy The Menil Collection)

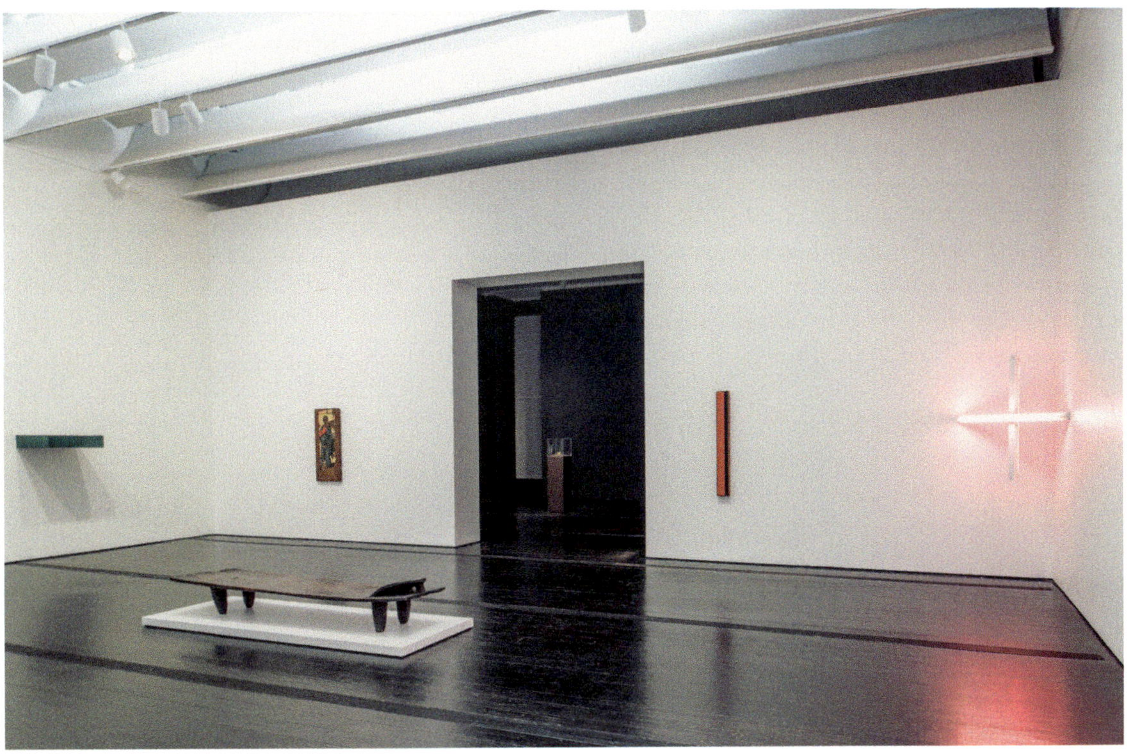

FIG. 1.6. Installation view of *Byzantine Things in the World*, The Menil Collection (photo: Paul Hester, with permission of The Menil Collection)

consistently undermined by. The painting covers both sides of the panel—both are normally on view, so like a body standing in the center of a floor, but in the recent exhibition at the National Gallery in Washington, DC, it was pinned to the wall and only George could be seen (fig. 1.8). The dynamic emergence of the saint, in his nearly three-dimensional form, also contains its immersion in the ground of the panel with its scenes of George's transcendent suffering. Each time I imagine the icon, as well as see its various aspects, I am forced back on a first feeling, since each time my knowledge is proved wrong. That icon deserves its individuality as thing, as one aspect of its personality, which includes its symbolic reference to a deceased and venerated person. By denying the first feeling in ourselves, we often pretend to take an objective position against the work that confirms our habit-formed, self-satisfying positions.[57]

I can try another way to describe the necessity of the spread of fellow-feeling in things: humility. I can argue it with reference to explanations for classic perspective-driven Renaissance painting. For Erwin Panofsky (1892–1968), the viewing subject constituted this system of space, but it was also objectively true. To simplify, the viewer controls and comprehends this extension of one's world: space retreats into the picture in a measured, orderly way. In that classic explanation of what we see and experience in Renaissance art, the perspectival system organizes itself as an organic and logical extension of our subject position as privileged viewer. Long ago now, Otto Demus (1902–90) described a complex system of space that made Byzantine space so much more comprehensible to us (because it was very much a modernist position), but it was still within a Panofskian mode of subject-oriented experience.[58] Byzantine churches, in my *own* experience, are wildly decentering spaces, despite the logic and organization of the space; my head often spins like Paul the Silentiary (d. ca. 580) and Procopius of Caesarea (ca. 500–ca. 565) described, a deeply unsettling ecstasy (fig. 1.9). This space is not an environment, because that word implies a surrounding space around one; it is really a complex ecology within which all persons seek homeostasis, a balance leading to redemption.[59] Moreover, in an animist context, contexts create subjects and not the other way around.[60] Our inter-objective world, not distinct from Byzantine church ecologies, is meshwork and not a series of layers to penetrate and understand, as in a Renaissance painting-system.[61] Hubert Damisch (b. 1928) knows painting is not

57 P. Bourdieu, *Outline of a Theory of Practice*, trans. R. Nice (New York, 1977), 96, "Objectivism constitutes the social world as a spectator presented to an observer who takes up a 'point of view' on the action, who stands back so as to observe it and, transferring into the object the principles of his relation to the object, conceives of it as a totality intended for cognition alone, in which all interactions are reduced to symbolic exchanges. This point of view is the one afforded by high positions in the social structure, from which the social work appears as representation (in the sense of idealist philosophy but also used in painting or in the theater) and practices that are no more than 'executions,' stage parts, performances of scores, or the implementing of plans." And see J. Fabian, *Time and the Other: How Anthropology Makes Its Objects* (New York, 2002), 105–41, and of course G. Kubler, *The Shape of Time: Remarks on the History of Things* (New Haven and London, 1962).

58 *Byzantine Mosaic Decoration: Aspects of Monumental Art in Byzantium* (London, 1948). See, for example, G. Deleuze (1925–95), *Francis Bacon: The Logic of Sensation*, trans. D. W. Smith (Minneapolis, 2003), 103–4, "Byzantine art reverses Greek art by giving such a degree of activity to the background that we no longer know where the background ends and the forms begin. . . . As opposed to classical representation, distant viewing no longer has to vary its distance according to this or that part, nor does it have to be confirmed by a close viewing that picks out the tactile connections, but is established directly by the whole of the painting. . . . Even abstract painting, in its radical attempt to insinuate an optical space of transformation, will rely on disintegrating factors, on relations of value, of light and shadow, of clarity and obscurity, rediscovering a pure Byzantine inspiration beyond the seventeenth century: an optical code."

59 This ecology is close to what Merleau-Ponty called the flesh of the world. For an attempt at a description of the flesh of a Byzantine church, see Hamilakis, *Archaeology and the Senses* (n. 2 above), 75–78.

60 See E. Viveiros de Castro, "Cosmological Deixis and Amerindian Perspectivism," *Journal of the Royal Anthropological Institute* 4, no. 3 (1998): 315–16, and idem, "Perspectivism and Multinaturalism in Indigenous America," in *The Land Within: Indigenous Territory and the Perception of the Environment*, ed. A. Surrallés and P. García Hierro (Copenhagen, 2005), 36–74, where he corrects the Saussurean formula, "the point of view creates the object," in favor of an Amerindian perspectivism that proceeds from the point of view creating the subject. See also V.-P. Herva, "Spirituality and the Material World in Post-Medieval Europe," in *Archaeology of Spirituality*, ed. K. Rountree, C. Morris, and A. A. D. Peatfield (New York, 2012), 71–85.

61 See T. Morton, *Hyperobjects: Philosophy and Ecology at the End of the World* (Minneapolis, 2013), 84–85, "what is called *subject* and what is called *mind* just are interobjective effects, emergent properties of relationships between enmeshed

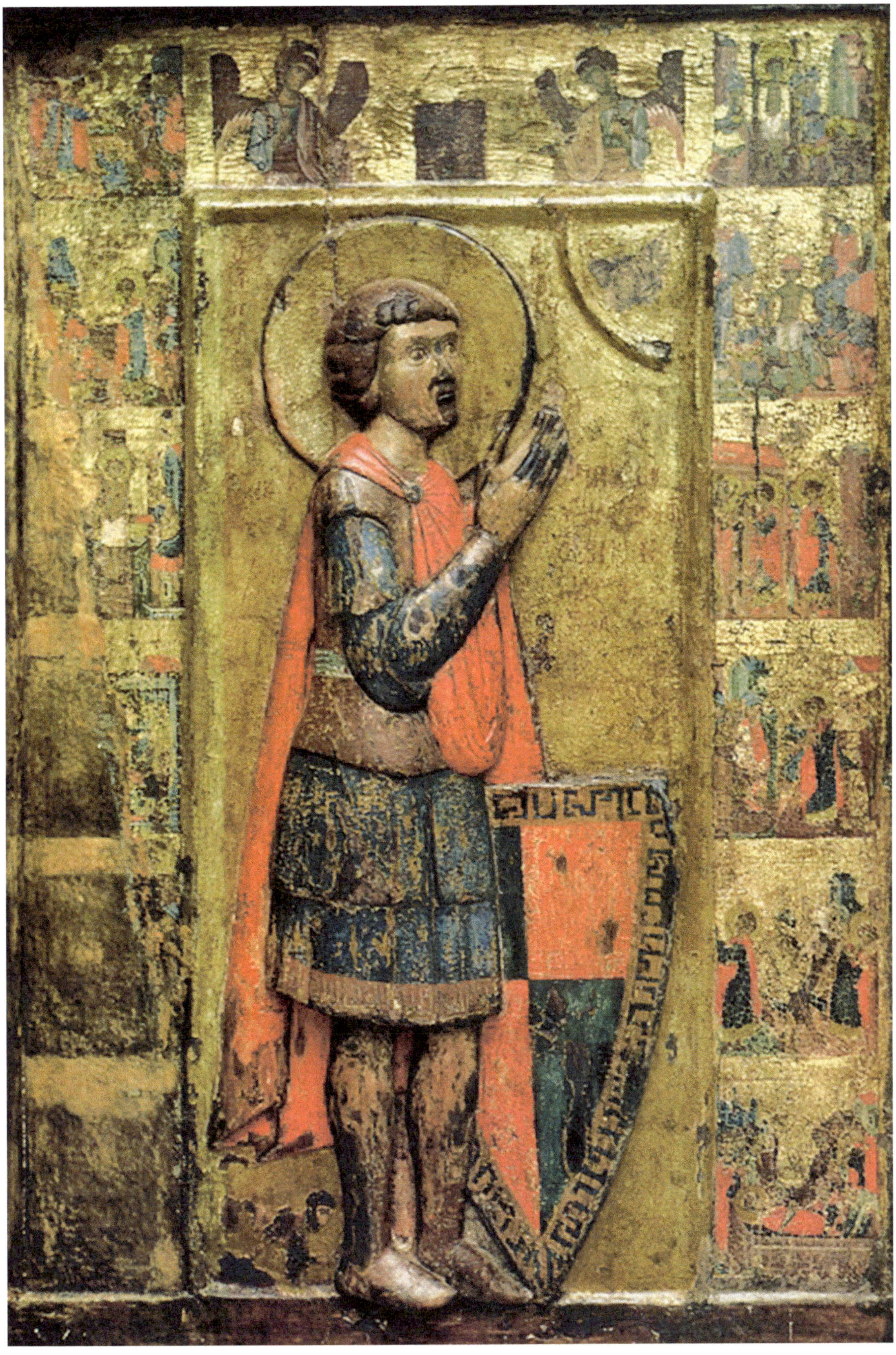

FIG. 1.7.
Carved icon of St. George, thirteenth century. Byzantine and Christian Museum, Athens, Greece (photo courtesy Byzantine and Christian Museum, Athens, Greece)

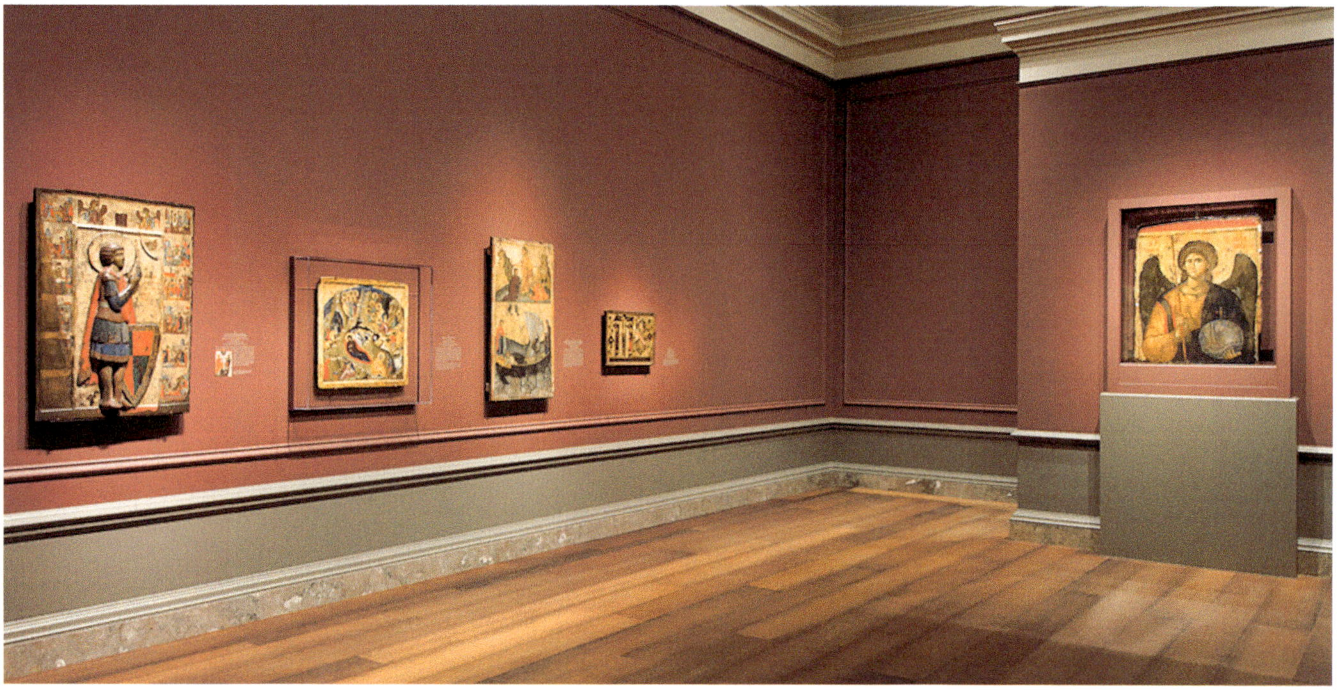

FIG. 1.8. Installation shot of the exhibition, *Heaven and Earth: Art of Byzantium from Greek Collections,* National Gallery of Art, Washington, DC (photo courtesy National Gallery of Art, Washington, DC)

under our control; perspective masters *us*, since it preexists us, and determines our perception.[62] Likewise, a church interior does not wait for us to make sense of it; it forms us, senses us, as we enter its poised, restless ecology.[63] As Damisch has asked, "how can anyone agree that painting is nothing but vanity, when it has the power to make humanity sensible of its own nothingness, its dependence, its *void?*"[64]

This argument for fellow-feeling depends on a historical rigor that does not exclude other interpretative stances. For example, theological systems are somewhat beside the point for my explanation, because they belong to a world of text that is, or pretends to be, self-sufficient and totalizing in the descriptions of the world. The world of text is necessary. We are language-bound and -defined beings after all. But recognizing levels of reality, exclusive and interdependent at the same time, is a productive starting point for knowing bodies.[65]

In 1990, Henry Maguire (b. 1945) delivered a paper at the Dumbarton Oaks spring symposium on the state of the discipline of Byzantine art history in that period, which appeared to many as a period of crisis for our field.[66] He relied on a retrospective framework (John Ruskin, namely) to

objects.... What is called *consciousness* is an aesthetic effect: it is consciousness-for."

62 Or another way: M. Iversen and S. Melville, *Writing Art History: Disciplinary Departures* (Chicago and London, 2010), 172,"If we are to get the shape of that [art history] writing right (if we are to understand the terms on which it gives itself essentially to reading), we have to see it as belonging to—emergent within—the terms of the object's visibility, and so need to think about it as structured by that particular shape—by a certain deep impossibility of sculpture and its radical plasticity, that leaves us as if condemned to write back and forth between art's architectural incipience and its more or less painterly dissolution without being able to fully order those moments in relation to any fixed and present center."

63 See Connor, "Michel Serres's *Les cinq sens*" (n. 19 above), 162–63.

64 *A Theory of /Cloud/: Toward a History of Painting*, trans. J. Lloyd (Stanford, 2002), 181, and *The Origin of Perspective*, trans. J. Goodman (Cambridge, MA, 1994).

65 G. Rohrbaugh, "Artworks as Historical Individuals," *European Journal of Philosophy* 11 (2003): 178–79, "A properly conceived ontology of art is one which provides a metaphysical framework flexible enough to represent accurately a wide variety of phenomena and to permit the expression of heterogeneous critical views, views which must be evaluated in their own terms." See also A. Hennion, "Offene Objekte, Offene Subjekte? Körper und Dinge im Geflecht von Anhänglichkeit, Zuneigung und Verbundenheit," trans. A. Ortner, *Zeitschrift für Medien- und Kulturforschung* 1, no. 1 (2011): 93–109.

66 Published as "Byzantine Art History in the Second Half of the Twentieth Century," in *Byzantium: A World Civilization*, ed. A. Laiou (Washington, DC, 1992), 119–55.

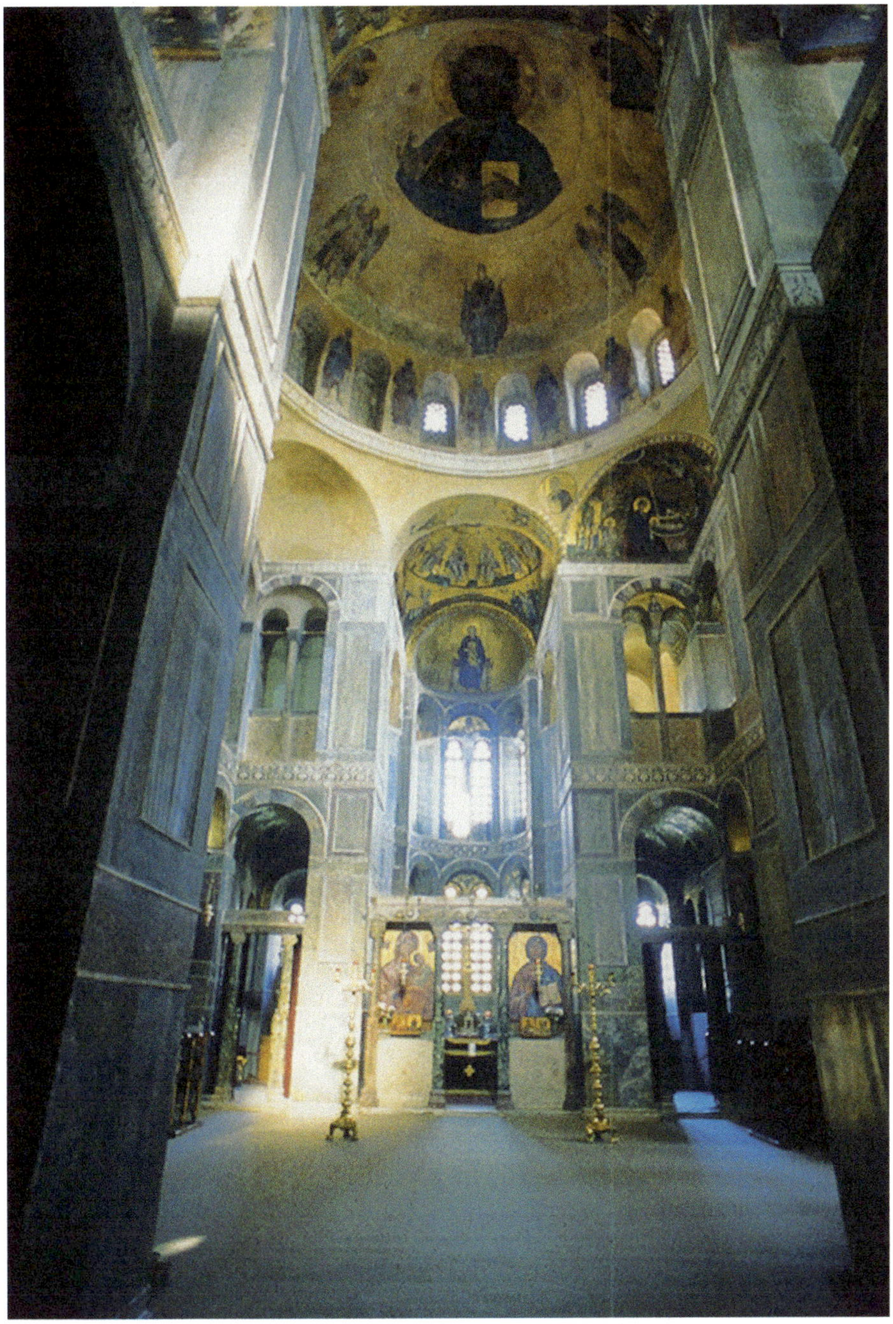

FIG. 1.9.
Interior of the Katholikon of Hosios Loukas, Phokis, Greece (photo: author)

isolate the ways in which Byzantinists had been avant-garde all along, while nevertheless pointing out shortcomings in then-current practice. Some twenty-five years after the event, the state of the field has largely answered Maguire's final call, "to find ways of doing art history that make room for the study of *both* the object and its environment at the same time." The field is on the verge of another "sea change," in my opinion, and it needs now to take as literally as possible Maguire's statement. For, an object does indeed have an environment, as any human subject does, too—namely the space, time, materialisms that enfold one. That expansive and inclusive environment, if admitted fully into our studies, will fundamentally alter our questions, because those questions will be shared across a broad ontology that comprises us and them all.

From that vantage point, then, persons' senses have materiality and time, ours simply more passing, more temporary, than what art historians give their objects of study. Byzantines, I would argue, knew the vitality of the world, and they understood, for example, some ways stone, trees, animals felt the world. And like us, they knew some of these creatures outlast human lifespans. Humanity was fortunate to possess souls, which grant an eternity, but in this world, in this ongoing age of the always-almost reckoning, humanity is in a deficit position against trees and stones, and even some animals. The sense of time is another facet of sensation and feeling, and we understand ours more or less, but we also need to think geological time, or rather fail at thinking it, since it is out of our comprehension really.[67] Objects too have a deep sense of time, and they wear that sense as we do our age, outside and in.[68] They have better patience and endurance than we do, and they can teach us our dependence on them; they can show temporary abatement of the void. By accepting the spread of feelings, different from our exceptionalist feelings but still valid, we can be more humble in the face of things and time, and our analysis of these objects can be more accepting of their individuality, their special feelings.

67 For example, see B. Brown, "Anarchéologie: Object Worlds and Other Things, circa Now," in *The Way of the Shovel: On the Archaeological Imaginary in Art*, ed. D. Roelstraete (Chicago, 2013), 264, "Shovel in hand, what does the artist know that seems so difficult to know? Simply that, in the midst of repatriation debates over one artefact or another, the ground (that is, the earth) is always in the midst of filing its own claim, which is to have all its objects back. Call it a claim on behalf of nothing that is almost everything at once."

68 From another point of view, U. C. Steiner, "The Problem of Garbage and the Insurrection of Things," in *Trash Culture: Objects and Obsolescence in Cultural Perspective*, ed. G. Pye (Oxford, 2010), 129–46, and G. Böhme, "Das Ding und seine Ekstasen: Ontologie und Ästhetik der Dinghaftigkeit," in his *Atmosphäre, Essays zur neuen Ästhetik* (Frankfurt am Main, 1995), 155–76.

My thanks to Mark Cheetham, Christoph Eggersglüß, Derek Krueger, Elisabetta Povoledo, and T'ai Smith for advice and guidance. I am especially grateful to the symposiarchs, Margaret Mullett and Susan Harvey, for the opportunity to think through some of these questions and to take part in such a stimulating symposium. I would also like to acknowledge a 2014 summer fellowship from the Internationales Kolleg für Kulturtechnikforschung und Medienphilosophie, Bauhaus-Universität Weimar, during which I was able to write and talk with excellent colleagues.

CHAPTER TWO

The Materiality of Sensation in the Art of the Late Middle Ages

MARTINA BAGNOLI

> Since my lady of Champagne wishes me to undertake to write a romance, I shall very gladly do so, being so devoted to her service as to do anything in the world for her, without any intention of flattery. But if one were to introduce any flattery upon such an occasion, he might say, and I would subscribe to it, that this lady surpasses all others who are alive, just as wind which blows in May or April surpasses any other breezes.[1]

So the twelfth-century author Chrétien de Troyes describes the loveliness of his patron, the countess of Champagne, in his prologue to Lancelot. To evoke a woman's beauty and character Chrétien chooses not a visual image but the memory of a sensuous experience—the touch of a breeze on one's skin.

Chrétien de Troyes's literary image draws attention to the importance of sensation in the cognitive process. To say that the senses create knowledge is something of a truism since it is through the senses that we understand the world around us, but there is nothing obvious in the way we construct that knowledge. What did it mean to be compared to a spring wind in twelfth-century France? What associations did the poetic similarity raise in the reader's mind? And how are these associations different from what we imagine today? In twelfth-century cosmology, winds were agents of divine power[2] and in troubadour poetry they were often understood as the messenger of the beloved, whose presence could thus be felt even at a distance.[3] These notions provide a background against which Chrétien's sensorial image can be measured. His choice of simile underscores the author's disposition toward his patron, whose presence animates his composition. Moreover, the comparison shows a degree of sensitivity to natural events that is rare in today's western culture. How is a spring wind more pleasant than any other breeze? On what experiential knowledge is that difference predicated?

The role that culture plays in tuning our neurons has been the subject of much consideration by anthropologists and historians who have foregrounded the study of sense perception in society and challenged the notion that sensation is neutral and that we all feel in the same way. For example, a team of anthropologists and psychologists at the Max Planck Institute for Psycholinguistics and the

1 W. J. A. Jonckbloet, ed., *Le roman de la charrette* (The Hague, 1850), vv. 1–13. The wording of the prologues is problematic. See K. D. Uitti, "Autant en emporte *li funs*: Remarques sur le prologue du *Chevalier de la Charrette* de Chrétien de Troyes," *Romania* 105, nos. 2–3 (1984): 270–79; J. Janssens, "Le prologue du 'Chevalier de la Charrette': Une clef pour l'interprétation du roman?" *Bien dire et bien aprandre* 4 (1986): 29–57; M. Tomaryn Bruckner, "Le Chevalier de la Charrette: That Obscure Object of Desire, Lancelot," in *A Companion to Chrétien de Troyes*, ed. N. J. Lacy and J. Tasker Grimbert (Cambridge, 2005), 136–55.

2 B. Obrist, "Wind Diagrams and Medieval Cosmology," *Speculum* 72, no. 1 (1997): 33–84.

3 P. Dronke, *The Medieval Lyric*, 3rd ed. (New York, 1996), 175.

Radbound University in Nijmegen, Holland, have recently examined the linguistic codability of sensory perception and demonstrated that diverse cultural groups are more or less apt to react to and define different sets of sensory stimuli.[4] Accordingly, Americans were found to be less apt at describing smells than a group of rain-forest inhabitants from Malaysia, who have in their vocabulary abstract terms to identify odors. The same principle can be applied to the understanding of the cultures of the past. Culling information from material evidence and textual sources, the study of the cultural history of sensation investigates the role of perception in shaping societies.[5]

This notion is of great import for the history of medieval art. Throughout the middle ages, sensory knowledge was paramount. Medieval image/objects were made to speak to every sense and not to sight alone. They functioned in a rich sensory world that was often integral to their apprehension. They were not only seen, but were also, and at the same time, touched, smelled, and heard. The sensory language they employed appealed to the body and it is through the body that they helped construct a reality where empirical knowledge overlapped with spiritual imagination. Consequently, the consideration of sensation in medieval art dictates a reassessment of the primacy of sight as a conduit to knowledge, and should be seen as a corollary of the shift from opticality to materiality. In the last twenty years, scholars have come to appreciate that the material manifestation of images, their "bodies" if you will, were themselves important sites of meaning.[6] Not only did different materials carry specific symbolic significance, their "objecthood" gave images the agency to act in a complex set of meaning-making relationships.[7] Much of this meaning is established by our apprehension of them in relation to ourselves, their existence not as an abstraction of the self but as a reality of being. With respect to this, Merleau-Ponty's critique of objective thought should be considered the starting point for the current interest in materiality and of phenomenology as a critical tool.[8] Notwithstanding Merleau-Ponty's interest in experience, his approach to perception was very much based on the primacy of language, a stance later rejected, especially by Michel Serres.[9] Stating that: "le corps sait dire je tout seul," Serres

4 The study was conducted under the direction of Asifa Majid and Stephen G. Levinson and published at http://www.mpi.nl/departments/language-and-cognition/linguistic-diversity-and-processing/projects/language-of-perception/home (accessed 15 November 2016). The same authors worked also on difficulties of describing sensorial perception with language; see their article "Differential Ineffability and the Senses," *Mind & Language* 29 (2014): 407–27.

5 The work of David Howes and Constance Classen in particular has been very important for this field of studies: D. Howes and C. Classen, *Ways of Sensing: Understanding the Senses in Society* (London, 2014); C. Classen, *The Deepest Sense: A Cultural History of Touch* (Urbana-Champaign, 2012); D. Howes, *The Empire of the Senses: The Sensual Culture Reader* (Oxford and New York, 2004); C. Classen, D. Howes, and A. Synnot Aroma, *The Cultural History of Smell* (London and New York 1994). See also R. Jütte, *A History of the Senses: From Antiquity to Cyberspace* (Cambridge, 2005); F. Quiviger, *The Sensory World of the Italian Renaissance* (London, 2010); R. G. Newhauser, "The Senses in Medieval and Renaissance Intellectual History," *Senses & Society* 5, no. 1 (2010): 5–9. He is also the editor of the volume *A Cultural History of the Senses in the Middle Ages* (London, 2015).

6 J.-C. Bonne, "Entre l'image et la matière: La choséité du sacré en Occident," in *Les images dans les sociétés médiévales: Pour une histoire comparée, Bulletin de l'Institut Historique Belge de Rome* 59 (1999): 77–111; H. L. Kessler, *Seeing Medieval Art* (Peterborough, 2004); idem, "Object as Subject in Medieval Art," *The Haskins Society Journal* 22 (2010): 205–28; M. Bagnoli, "Medieval Art and the Object," *Word and Image* 22, no. 3 (2006): 193–95; C. W. Bynum, *Christian Materiality: An Essay on Religion in Late Medieval Europe* (New York, 2011).

7 On the iconology of materials see G. Bandmann, "Bemerkungen zu einer Ikonologie des Materials," *Städel-Jahrbuch* 2 (1969): 75–100; T. Raff, *Die Sprache der Materialen: Anleitung zu einer Ikonologie der Werkstoffe* (Munich, 1994); B. Reudenbach, "'Gold ist Schlamm': Anmerkungen zur Materielbewertung im Mittelalter," in *Material in Kunst und Alltag*, ed. M. Wagner and D. Rübel (Berlin, 2002), 1–12; B. Buttner, "From Bones to Stones: Reflections on Jeweled Reliquaries," in *Reliquiare im Mittelalter*, ed. B. Reudenbach and G. Toussaint (Berlin, 2005), 43–59; M. Cole, "The Cult of Materials," in *Revival and Inventions: Sculpture through Its Material Histories*, ed. S. Clerbois and M. Droth (Oxford, 2010), 1–15; I. Weinryb, "Living Matter: Materiality, Maker and Ornament in the Middle Ages," *Gesta* 52, no. 2 (2013): 113–31. For a discussion of the agency of objects see: "Things," ed. B. Brown, special issue of *Critical Inquiry* 28, no. 1 (2001); H. Belting, "Image, Medium, Body: A New Approach to Iconology," *Critical Inquiry* 31, no. 2 (2005): 302–19; B. Latour, *Reassembling the Social: An Introduction to Actor-Network-Theory* (Oxford, 2005); J. Bennett, *Vibrant Matter: A Political Ecology of Things* (Durham, NC, 2010).

8 M. Merleau-Ponty, *Phenomenology of Perception*, second English translation (London, 2012), originally published in French in 1945. Also important to this discussion is his *The Visible and the Invisible* (Evanston, 1969), originally published in French in 1964.

9 On Merlau-Ponty's discussion of language see P. E. Lewis, "Merleau-Ponty and the Phenomenology of Language," *Yale*

disputes any attempt to intellectualize sensation as an abstraction of the mind and reaffirms it firmly in the domain of the immediate and the tactile.[10] Serres's poetic analysis of the organic unity of the thinking body is of great import for a reevaluation of the importance of the nonvisual and the nontextual in the arts. To speak of the nonvisual in the context of the visual arts seems paradoxical, but shifting the focus from sight to other modes of perception has made possible the rediscovery of the important role that a variety of stimuli, for example hearing and hence music, played in the creation and reception of objects. Understanding this distinction is particularly relevant to an examination of the art of the later middle ages, when changes in philosophical and cultural paradigms helped promote a culture of sensation.[11] Characteristic of this change is the shift from "words" to "things" that occurred in thirteenth-century encyclopedias. Encyclopedists of this time, like for example Bartholomeus Anglicus, Thomas of Cantipre, and Vincent of Beauvais, moved their attention from logic and etymology to natural philosophy and the material world.[12] In what follows, I shall briefly review these changes before discussing the role of art in the construction of a material environment where sensation real, imagined, and desired coexisted.

Sensual Awakenings

It is hard to overemphasize the revolution brought about by the reintroduction of Aristotelian philosophy into western thought at the end of the twelfth century.[13] For the student of sensation, the rediscovery of Aristotle is of particular importance for its renewed interest in the sensible world.[14] Furthermore, it prompted a revision of the role of sense perception in intellectual abstraction and spiritual enlightenment, namely through the writings of Thomas Aquinas.[15] Aquinas understood sensation as a physical event.[16] Since perception was at the basis of cognition and consequently the mind's ability

French Studies, 36–37 (1966), 19–40; L. Hass, *Merleau-Ponty's Philosophy* (Bloomington, 2008), 170–92.

10 M. Serres, *Les cinq sens* (Paris, 1985), 15.

11 Carl Nordenfalk was the first scholar to investigate the iconography of sensation: "Les cinq sens dans l'art du Moyen Âge," *Revue de l'Art* 43 (1976): 17–28; idem, "The Five Senses in Late Medieval Art and Renaissance Art," *Journal of the Warburg and Courtauld Institute* 48 (1985): 1–22. A number of studies on the importance of the senses in religious art have begun to emerge in the last few years. See in particular C. Burnett, M. Fend, and P. Gouk, *The Second Sense: Studies in Hearing and Musical Judgment from Antiquity to the Seventeenth Century* (London, 1991); E. Palazzo, "Art, Liturgy and the Five Senses in the Early Middle Ages," *Viator* 41 (2010): 25–56; idem, "Les cinq sens au Moyen Âge: État de la question et perspectives de recherche," in *Cahiers de civilisation médiévale* 55 (2012): 339–66; idem, *L'invention chrétienne des cinq sens dans la liturgie et l'art au Moyen Âge* (Paris, 2014); L. James, "Senses and Sensibility in Byzantium," *Art History* 27, no. 4 (2004): 522–37; B. V. Pentcheva, *The Sensual Icon: Space, Ritual, and the Senses in Byzantium* (University Park, PA, 2010); J. Jung, "The Tactile and the Visionary: Notes on the Place of Sculpture in the Medieval Religious Imagination," in *Looking Beyond: Visions, Dreams and Insights in Medieval Art and History* (Princeton and University Park, PA, 2010), 203–40. B. Williamson, "Sensory Experience in Medieval Devotion: Sound and Vision, Invisibility and Silence," *Speculum* 88, no. 1 (January 2013): 1–43. This article presents some of the research that was instrumental in shaping my exhibition *A Feast for the Senses: Art and Experience in Medieval Europe*, Baltimore, Walters Art Museum, 16 October 2016–8 January 2017 and Sarasota, The Ringling Museum of Art, 4 February–30 April 2017. Owing to a longer production schedule the article in this journal appears after the exhibition catalogue (Baltimore, 2016).

12 Isidore of Seville's *Etymologies* can serve as an example of the early medieval encyclopedia based on the nature of words rather than things. See S. A. Barney, W. J. Lewis, J. A. Beach and O. Berghof, *The Etymologies of Isidore of Seville* (Cambridge, 2009). On medieval encyclopedias in general see B. Ribémont, *De natura rerum: Études sur les encyclopédies médiévales* (Orléans, 1995); idem, *Littérature et Encyclopédies du Moyen Âge* (Orléans, 2002). On the *Properties of Things*: B. Ribémont, *Le Livre des Propriétés des Choses: Une encyclopédie au XIVe siècle* (Paris, 1999); B. Anglicus, *On the Properties of Soul and Body: De proprietatibus rerum, libri III et IV*, ed. and trans. R. J. Long (Toronto, 1979).

13 Aristotle's medieval Latin translations are collected in the corpus edited by L. Minio-Paluello, *Aristoteles Latinus*, 33 vols. (Bruges, 1953). For a summary of the arrival of Aristotle in the west see Fernand van Steenberghen, *Aristotle in the West: The Origins of Latin Aristotelianism* (Louvain, 1955). B. G. Dod, "Aristoteles Latinus," in *The Cambridge History of Later Medieval Philosophy: From the Rediscovery of Aristotle to the Disintegration of Scholasticism, 1100–1600*, ed. N. Kretzmann, A. Kenny, and J. Pinborg (Cambridge, 1982), 43–79; C. H. Lohr, "The Medieval Interpretation of Aristotle," in ibid., 80–98.

14 Aristotle discusses the senses mostly in his *De anima*, ed. and trans. R. D. Hicks (Cambridge, 1907).

15 Thomas Aquinas, *A Commentary on Aristotle's De anima*, trans. R. Pasnau (New Haven, 1999).

16 This is the conclusion of S. M. Cohen, "St. Thomas Aquinas on the Immaterial Reception of Sensible Forms," *Philosophical Review* 91, no. 2 (April 1982): 193–209. Expanding on Cohen's argument is M. Tweedale, "Origins of the Medieval Theory That Sensations Is an Immaterial Reception of Forms," *Philosophical Topics* 20, no. 2 (1992): 215–31.

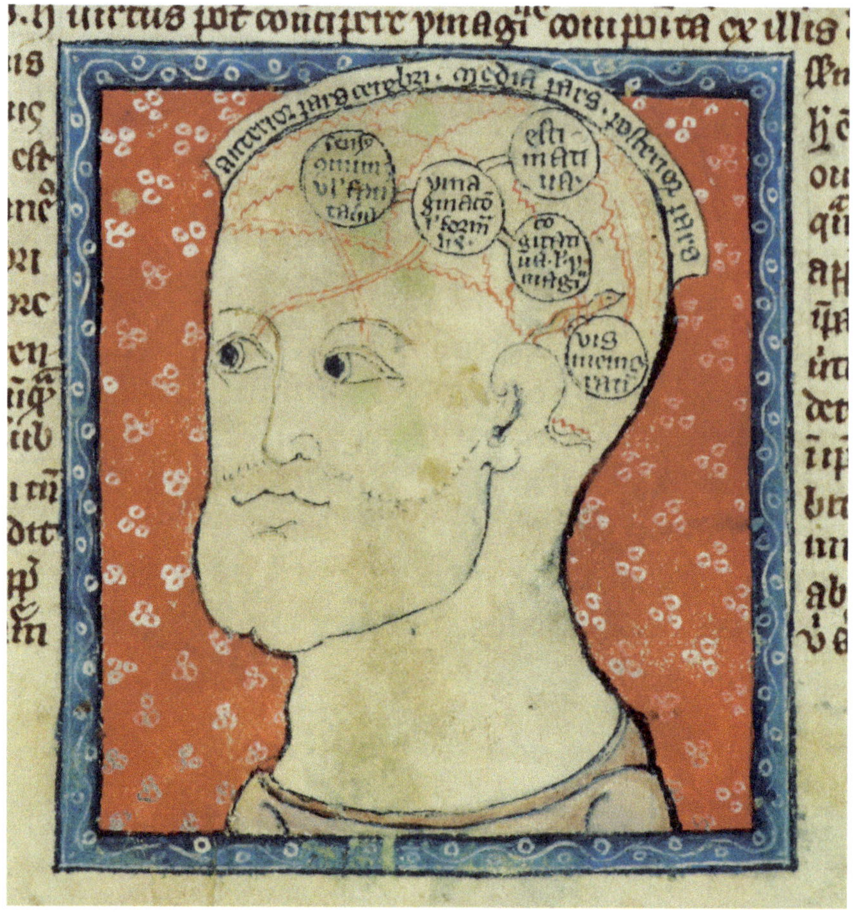

FIG. 2.1
Diagram of the brain, Cambridge, University Library MS. G G 1.1, fol. 490v (photo: reproduced by kind permission of the Syndics of Cambridge University Library)

to abstract bodily experience, the realm of the physical was participant in understanding and knowledge.

Earlier theories of knowledge were more ambiguous about the role of the body and hence sensation in perception. Augustine for example, following Plotinus, understood sensation as an activity of the soul processing the stimuli sent by the senses.[17] Like his classical antecedents, Augustine believed that feeling (*sentire*) occurs in the soul and he distinguished *anima* from *animus*. *Anima* was the most basic passive soul, where sensory perception was received and understood in a limited way, whereas *animus* was where intellectual knowledge was unleashed.[18] A comparison between a fourteenth-century and an early thirteenth-century diagrammatic representation of cognition (figs. 2.1, 2.2) makes the contrast between these two outlooks evident. The fourteenth-century diagram (fig. 2.1) appears in an English illustrated lay encyclopedia, where it illustrates a chapter titled "qualiter caput hominis situatur" that summarizes the works of Aquinas and Avicenna. In the drawing, lines (the optic nerve) link visual stimuli to the brain, where they are collected by a faculty called

17 Key elements of Augustine's theory of sensation are contained in his *De Trinitate* 11. *De Trinititate libri XV*, ed. W. J. William Mountain, CCSL 50A (Turnhout, 1968), esp. I.1, p. 460. Augustine's theory of sensation is far from clear and has spurred much discussion. See in particular Sister M. A. I. Gannon, "The Active Theory of Sensation in St. Augustine," *The New Scholasticism* 30 (1956): 167–200; T. L. Miethe, "Augustine's Theory of Sense Knowledge," *Journal of the Evangelical Theological Society* 22, no. 3 (September 1979): 257–64; D. Chidester, "Symbolism and the Senses in Saint Augustine," *Religion* 14 (1984): 31–51; E. Vance, "Seeing God: Augustine's Sensation and the Mind's Eye," in *Rethinking the Senses: Heritage/Fascinations/Frames*, ed. S. Nichols, A. Kablitz, and A. Calhoun (Baltimore, 2008), 13–29; M. Carruthers, "Intention, sensation et mémoire dans l'esthétique médiévale," *Cahiers de civilisation médiévale* 55 (2012): 367–78.

18 *De Trinitate* 9.2.2.

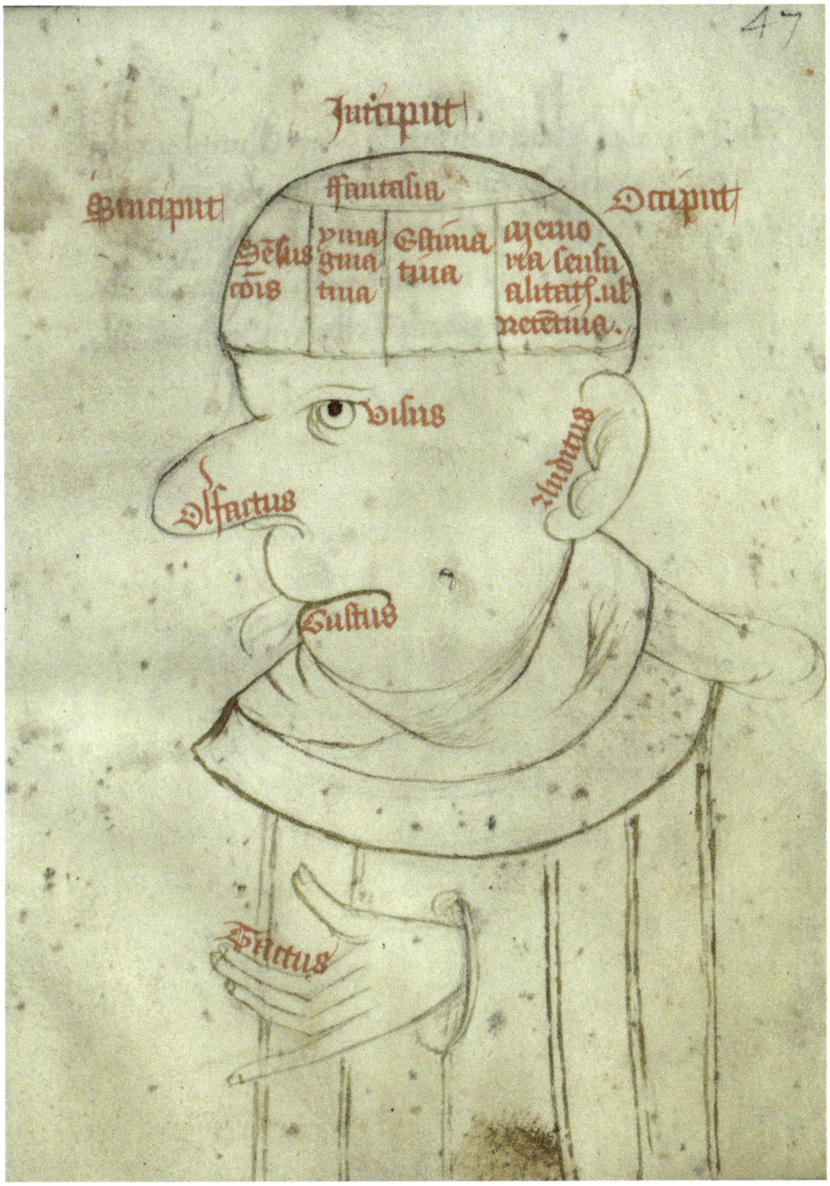

FIG. 2.2
Diagram of the brain, Cambridge, Trinity College Library MS. O. 7. 16, fol. 47r (photo: reproduced by kind permission of the Syndics of Cambridge University Library)

common sense.[19] From there sensory images move to a chamber for recognition called *vis formalis*, where they are transformed into mental pictures and at the same time they are analyzed and interpreted by estimative faculties (*vis estimativa*), which prepares them for the imagination (cell four in the diagram, *vis cogitativa*). These processes formed multimodal sensory images, composed of diverse raw sensory stimuli. The processed mental images that are the basis of human intellect and reason are stored in memory, whence they can be retrieved (cell five in the diagram, *vis memorativa*). The little lizard over the man's ear is the switch that allows memory images to flow back to the brain when things are remembered. The earlier diagram (fig. 2.2) illustrates an early thirteenth-century Cistercian

19 Cambridge University Library MS. G G 1.1. The manuscript is digitized and published: http://cudl.lib.cam.ac.uk/view/MS-GG-00001-00001/988 (accessed 15 November 2016). On this manuscript see P. Binski, P. Zutshi, and S. Panayotova, *Western Illuminated Manuscripts: A Catalogue of the Collection in Cambridge University Library* (Cambridge, 2011). For this diagram in particular see Carruthers, "Intention, sensation"; M. J. Carruthers and J. M. Ziolkowski, *The Medieval Craft of Memory: An Anthology of Texts and Pictures* (Philadelphia, PA, 2002), 120–21, figs. 6.1–6; M. Camille, "Before the Gaze," in *Visuality Before and Beyond the Renaissance: Seeing as Others Saw*, ed. R. S. Nelson (New York and Cambridge, 2000), 197–223.

dissertation on the soul by the pseudo-Augustine and presents a more dualistic approach.[20] Both drawings show the head of a man and the different brain chambers where raw sense perception was processed. But whereas the later one shows sensation in motion and the fluid progression from the exterior world to mental activity, the earlier diagram makes these two activities completely separate. The bodily senses are isolated from the internal senses (the brain cells) and there is no mechanism for flow and processing of data like one sees in the later picture. In addition, the caricaturized identification of the bodily senses lends them a negative connotation and sets them in opposition to the neat spatial and textual identity of the inner senses. To the contrary, in the fourteenth-century diagram outer and inner senses are represented as equally important to the creation of knowledge.

This shift happened against the background of an increasingly humanized religion. In the later middle ages, Christian devotion shifted from an apprehension of the Trinity to that of Christ in his humanity. As a result the dualism of bodily and spiritual senses promoted by the early church fathers began to fade. The sanctification of Christ's human body, on one hand, and the desire to emulate him, on the other, drove twelfth-century theologians, in particular Bernard of Clairvaux, to use sensory language to describe mystical union with God.[21] Such writings often blurred the distinction between the bodily and the spiritual. This trend continued and accelerated during the thirteenth and fourteenth century, with influential thinkers like Bonaventure.[22]

Bodily Knowledge

In this new theoretical framework, experiential knowledge as defined by sensation was relied upon to evaluate matters of physical but also moral nature. Notwithstanding a philosophical tradition that placed smell, touch, and taste at the bottom of a hierarchical pyramid of cognition, these carnal senses ranked higher than hearing and sight on an array of topics. Smell, for example, was important in the investigation of precious stones. In the ca. 1200 Aberdeen bestiary the agate stone is identified by the scent of myrrh it exudes when placed into a fire.[23] Since the bones of saints were often compared to precious stones, it is not surprising to learn that smell could be used to identify saints as well. To be sure, dead saints smelled of fragrant flowers, since their spiritual purity preserved their bodies from rotting. In a miniature in the life of St. Albans by Matthew Paris, illustrating the *inventio* of St. Alban's relics, an attendant to King Offa gestures to his nose while an inscription next to him reads "redolet."[24] The fragrance exuding from the remains of St. Albans confirms to King Offa, to his retinue, and to the reader of the manuscript that these are indeed the bones of a saint (fig. 2.3). The association of saints with fragrant smells underlines the use of pomanders as reliquaries. Pomanders were objects of adornment commonly used in the later part of the middle ages and into the Renaissance as containers of fragrant substances.[25] They were constructed of four segments that would close

20 On Cambridge, Trinity College Library MS. O. 7. 16 see M. R. James, *A Descriptive Catalogue of the Western Manuscripts in the Library of Trinity College*, vol. 3 (Cambridge, 1903), 357; M. Bagnoli, ed., *A Feast for the Senses: Art and Experience in Medieval Europe* (Baltimore, 2016), cat. nos. 4, 137–38.

21 Bernard uses of sensory language in his commentary on the Song of Songs. See his *Sermones super Cantica Canticorum* 6, in *Sancti Bernardi, Opera Omnia*, ed. J. Leclercq, C. H. Talbot, and H. M. Rochais, 8 vols. (Rome, 1957–80), 1:2–27. A number of scholars have commented on Bernard's focus on somatic language. The complete bibliography is found in G. Rudy. *The Mystical Language of Sensation in the Later Middle Ages* (Hoboken, 2013), on whose conclusions I base my discussion.

22 Most of Bonaventure's discussions on sensation are found in his *Itinerarium mentis in Deum* 4: *Breviloquium* 5.6; *Commentaria in libros Sententiarum* dist. 13 dub. 1, dist. 34 art. 1, *De reductione artium ad theologiam* 10; See *S. Bonaventurae, Opera Omnia*, 10 vols. (Quaracchi, 1882–1902). See Rudy, *Language of Sensation*, 103–9. On the nature and importance of the imagination in the meditative process see M. Karnes, *Imagination, Meditation, and Cognition in the Middle Ages* (Chicago, 2011).

23 University Library MS 24: "Acates lapis. . . . Alius est qui odorem habet mirre quando ponitur in igne." The Aberdeen bestiary is digitized and its images along with Colin Mclaren's transcription and translation are available at http://www.abdn.ac.uk/bestiary/translat/101r.hti (accessed 25 September 2016).

24 Dublin, Trinity College Library, MS. 177, fol. 59r. On this manuscript see F. McCulloch, "St. Albans and Amphibalus in the Work of Matthew Paris: Dublin Trinity College MS 117," *Speculum* 56, no. 4 (1981): 761–85; C. Hahn, *Portrayed on the Heart: Narrative Effect in Pictorial Lives of Saints from the Tenth to the Thirteenth Century* (Oakland, 2001), 311.

25 For pomanders in general see R. W. Lightbown, *Mediaeval European Jewelry: With a Catalogue of the Collection in the Victoria & Albert Museum* (London, 1992).

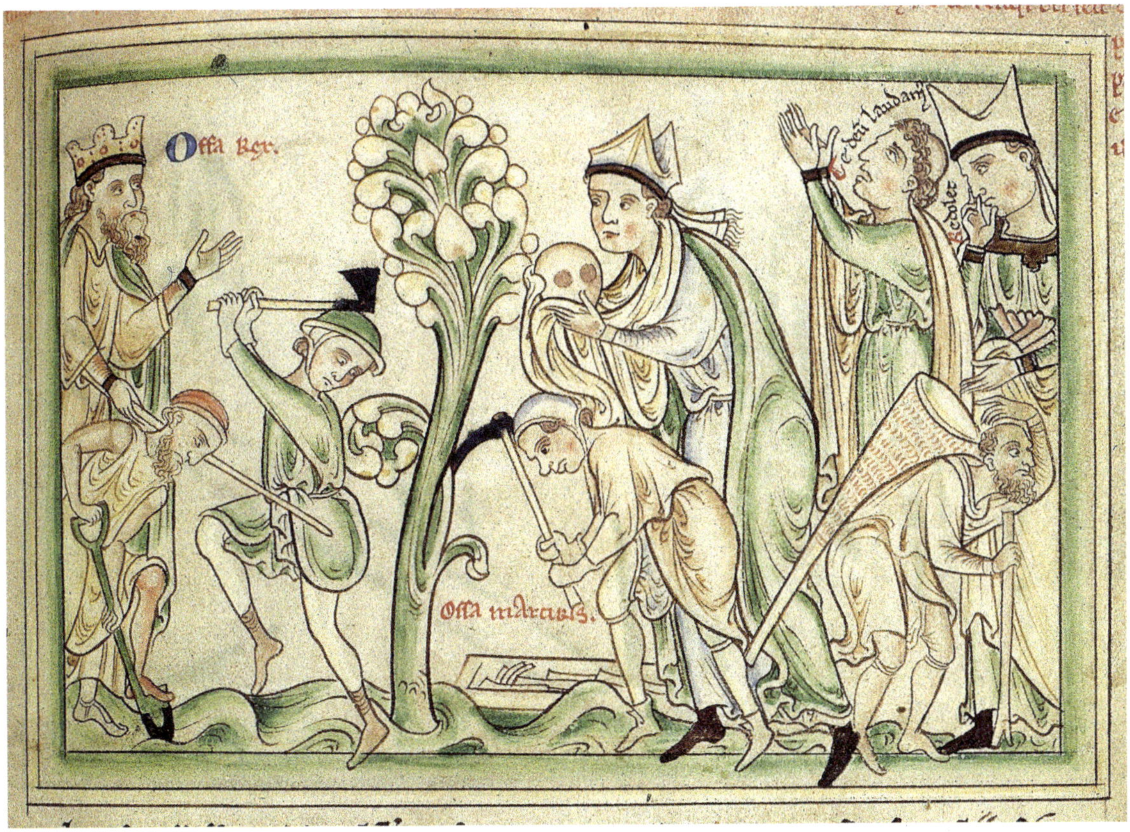

FIG. 2.3 King Offa finds the relics, Dublin, Trinity College Library, MS. 177, fol. 59r (photo: courtesy the Board of Trinity College Dublin)

around a central shaft, or screw into an "apple." Each segment contained an essence. The perfumes were thought to have health benefits and served as protection against various illnesses, including the plague. Each of the four segments of the apple in a pomander in Munich is dedicated to a saint, whose name and picture are engraved on the side.[26] The central screw is decorated with a figure of the Virgin Mary. In the Munich pomander, the *Odor Dei* of the saints serves as substitution for natural fragrances. Like the perfumes the relics would also have provided a modicum of protection to the wearer. Through the medium of smell, the Munich reliquary associates sensuality, spirituality, and medicine.

Conversely, a bad smell was an indicator of moral corruption. Accordingly, sinful rulers exuded the stench of rotten flesh, as Galerian does in an early fifteenth-century copy of Laurent de Premierfait's translation of Boccaccio's *De casis virorum illustris* illustrated by the Boucicault Master (fig. 2.4).[27]

In natural philosophy, smell competed with taste, which was often reputed superior for physical examinations. In the anonymous thirteenth-century compendium *Summa de saporibus*, taste is described as that sense: "ordained above all the other senses as properly and principally the investigator of the nature of things."[28] In a

26 Munich, Bayerisches Nationalmuseum, ca. 1470. On this see Lightbown, *Medieval European Jewelry*, 357.

27 Los Angeles, J. Paul Getty Museum of Art, MS. 63, fol. 258. On this manuscript see E. Morrison and A. D. Hedeman, *Imagining the Past in France: History in Manuscript Painting, 1250–1500* (Los Angeles, 2010) cat. no. 37, pp. 220–22 with further bibliography.

28 "Solus ergo gustus proprie et principaliter ad rerum naturas investigandas pre ceteris sensibus est destinatus." The text survives in three thirteenth-century manuscripts and one fifteenth-century copy. The thirteenth-century manuscripts are Oxford Bodleian Library, Bodley 679; Florence Biblioteca Laurenziana Ashburnham 143; and London, British Library, MS. Harley 3849, from which I take the quotation. See on this C. Burnett, "The Superiority of Taste," *Journal of the Warburg and Courtauld Institute* 54 (1991): 230–238. The Harley manuscript contains also the text of the *De saporibus et odoribus* (fols. 75v–77r) by the Salernitan doctor Urso of Calabria. See on this C. E. Wright, *Fontes Harleiani: A Study of the Sources*

FIG. 2.4.
Galerian on his death bed, Los Angeles, J. Paul Getty Museum of Art, MS. 63, fol. 258 (photo: courtesy Getty's Open Content Program)

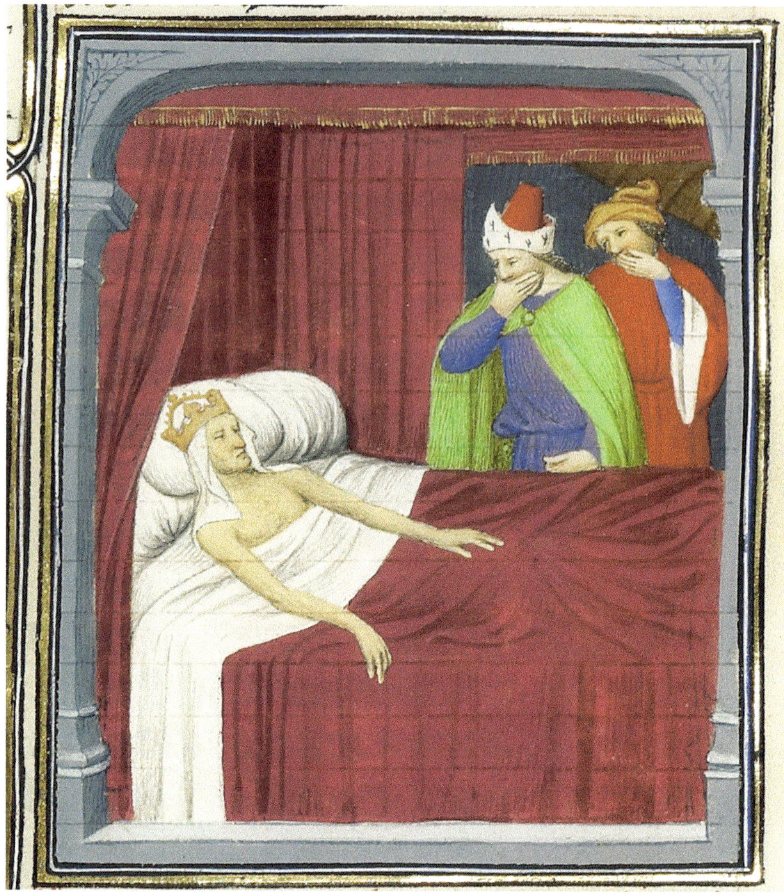

fifteenth-century miniature of the French translation of Bartholemeus Anglicus's *Propriété des choses*, taste is illustrated as a scene of daily life (the first of its kind) with people eating around a table while a doctor tends to a sick man in the adjacent room.[29] Most of all, taste was the preferred tool of discernment for matters of the spirit. Sweetness was associated with God and its taste heralded mystical unity. The correlation of God with a sweet taste comes from the Bible, specifically verse 9 of Psalm 33 (34): "Taste and see that the Lord is sweet." In his Sermons on the Song of Songs, Bernard of Clairvaux used these words to argue that spiritual things can be tasted and touched. Bernard's somatic language to describe mystical union with God became very influential in monastic mysticism.[30] The experience of *dulcedo* became thus the hallmark of spiritual communion with God. Caesarius of Heisterbach (1180–1240), for example, reported that a devout anchorite was rewarded with the taste of sweetness as her saliva turned into honey when she recited long sequences of prayers.[31] To trigger the mystical experience, in fifteenth-century Florence, dolls of the baby Jesus were sometimes confectioned with sugar so that the

of the Harleian Collection of Manuscripts in the British Museum (London, 1972), 254, 296, 436.

29 The miniature appeared on the antiquarian market in 1992. The present whereabouts are unknown. I wish to thank William Voelkle for alerting me to its existence and showing me pictures.

30 Rudy, *Mystical Language*.

31 On the specifics of the notion of sweetness as a as an attribute of God, see F. Posset, " 'Christi Dulcedo': The Sweetness of Christ in Western Christian Spirituality," *Cistercian Studies Quarterly* 27, no. 4 (1995): 245–65: R. Fulton, " 'Taste and See That the Lord Is Sweet' (Ps. 33:9): The Flavor of God in the Monastic West," *The Journal of Religion* 86, no. 2 (April 2006): 169–204; M. Carruthers, "Sweetness," *Speculum* 81 (2006): 999–1013. Caesarius of Heisterbach, *Dialogus miraculorum*, ed. J. Frange (Cologne, 1857), 2:69–70; for the English translation see *The Dialogue on Miracles,* trans. H. von Essen Scott and C. Swinton Bland, 2 vols., Broadway Medieval Library (New York, 1929), 1:533–34.

devout playing with them and kissing them would taste his divine presence.[32]

More importantly taste was invoked to help the faithful comprehend the true spiritual import of the Eucharist. By the late middle ages, the Eucharist was the central sacrament of Christian life.[33] Ministered by the clergy alone but offered to the entire community of the faithful, the Eucharist represented the moment when Christ's presence could be experienced by all. Although the laity were encouraged to partake of the Eucharist at least once a year, communion was valid only if taken with the full understanding of Christ's sacrifice and of the miraculous nature of the sacrament. Complete empathy with Christ's suffering and surrender to the dogma of faith was necessary for the miracle of transubstantiation to occur; otherwise the communicant would consume mere bread and wine and not the body of Christ. An early thirteenth-century paten in the collection of the Metropolitan Museum of Art provides a reminder of this teaching. An inscription around the rim reads: "the bread that you blessed now is the flesh of Christ, this you ate if you truly believe that it is the flesh."[34] To invest a tasteless wafer with Christ's presence required some imagination and to train this thought process, the communicant was encouraged to rely on taste to signal the miracle happening at the altar. In his very influential liturgical treatise, *De sacris altaris misterio*, Innocent III made that connection explicit when he stated that God offered his flesh as food to us so that ingesting his humanity we can be saved by his divinity so that we taste spiritually.[35]

From the thirteenth century onward, sermons propagated these ideas among common people. Preachers often encouraged the communicant to understand the Eucharist through their senses, teaching the laity how to literally "make sense" of it. In one of his sermons for Maundy Thursday Jacopo of Voragine enlisted the senses of hearing and taste in addition to sight as a way to celebrate the memory of Christ's passion.[36] Voragine explains how sight was solicited by images of the passion, hearing by the words of the preachers and taste by the savor of the host. In Jacopo's speech the three senses (sight, hearing and taste) are used to distinguish among different phases of understanding: seeing the passion stirred the faithful, hearing Christ's torments moved them even further, but it was tasting the host that affected them the most. Voragine here refers to a taste that can be sampled only by the spirit, since the host had (and has) no taste, the experience is discussed in somatic terms.

32 C. Klapisch-Zuber, *Women, Family and Ritual in Renaissance Italy* (Chicago, 1985), 310–20, especially 317.

33 The importance of the Eucharist in late medieval culture has been explored by M. Rubin, *Corpus Christi: The Eucharist in Late Medieval Culture* (Cambridge, 1991); K. Van Ausdall, "Communicating with the Host: Imagery and Eucharistic Contact in Late Medieval and Early Renaissance Italy," in *Push Me, Pull You*, ed. S. Blick and L. D. Gelfand (Leiden, 2011); eadem, "Art and Eucharist in the Late Middle Ages," in *A Companion to the Eucharist in the Middle Ages* (Leiden, 1911), 541–604.

34 QVE[M] BENEDIXISTI PANIS NVNS EST CARO XP(IST)I + HV[N]C SANE COMEDIS SI QVOD SVA SIT CARO CREDIS +. Metropolitan Museum of Art, inv. no. 47.101.27. The paten is part of a set including a chalice and a straw and was made for the Benedictine monastery of Saint Trudpert at Münstertal, near Freiburg im Breisgau, Germany. On the liturgical set see *The Cloisters: Medieval Art and Architecture*, ed. P. Barnet and N. Wu (New York, 2005), no. 42, p. 77; M. E. Frazer, "Medieval Church Treasuries," *The Metropolitan Museum of Art Bulletin* 43, no. 3 (winter 1985–86).

35 Innocent III, *De sacris altaris misterio libri sex* 4.44: "Sapientia Dei que per visibilia manifestat, volens evidenter ostendere quod ipsa cibus est animarum quod carnem assumptam proposuit in edulium, ut per cibum umanitatis invitaret ad gustum divinitatis, de quo dicit psalmist: Gustate et videte quoniam suavis est dominus. Totum ergo Christus se exhibet nobis in cibum, ut sicut divinitate nos reficit, quam spiritualiter gustamus corde, ita nos humanitate reficiat, quam corporaliter ore comedimus, et ita de visibilibus ad invisibilia, de temporalia ad eterna, de terrenis ad celestia, de humanis ad divina nos transferat." PL 217:884C–D.

36 Jacobi de Voragine, *Sermones aurei in omnes Quadragesimae dominicas et ferias*, ed. R. Clutius (Augsburg and Crocow, 1760), *Feria IV, Hebd. VI, In die coena dominini, Sermo* 1, p. 379: "Quarto debet probare digne recipientium fructum quante sit utilitatis. Que quidem utilitas attenditur in vita et in morte. In vita enim, est dimissum nobis in memoriale passionis Christi et in medicamentum curationis. Habemus igitur triplex memoriale passionis dominice. Unum est in visu, scilicet passio Christi depicta, et illud debe affectum nostrum multum movere. Secundum est in suditu, scilicet passio Christi audita vel predicata, et illud debet nos movere magis. Tertium est in gustu, scilicet passio Christi in hoc sacramento tam veraciter et tam singulariter expressa, et illud debet nos movere maxime." On this and other sermons dedicated to the Eucharist see N. Beriou, "L'eucharistie dans l'imaginaire des prédicateurs en Occident (XIIIe–XVe siècle)," in *Pratiques de l'Eucharistie dans les Églises d'Orient et d'Occident (Antiquité et Moyen Âge): Actes du séminaire tenu a Paris, Institut catholique* (1997–2004), ed. N. Bériou, B. Caseau, and D. Rigaux (Paris, 2005), 880–925, 908 in particular. On the importance of sensory perception and the Eucharist see also A. W. Astell, *Eating Beauty: The Eucharist and the Spiritual Arts of the Middle Ages* (Ithaca, NY, 2006).

This is also the approach taken by Robert of Sorbon in his treatise *De saporibus*, where he distinguishes among a rich scale of thirty-two tastes the Eucharist can elicit.[37] It is tempting to link Robert's interest in the variegated nature of divine taste with the explosion at this same time of cookery books, in particular those devoted to the making of different-tasting sauces. In medieval Latin, *sapor* meant taste but also sauce, making the parallel even more tempting. Very often these manuals, like that attributed to Magninus Mediolanensis, were medicinal in nature and presented sophisticated mixings of ingredients intended to counterbalance the negative effects of certain foods according to the theory of the humors.[38] As a result, the sauces that these cookery books proposed required a number of exotic spices that would make them unpractical and prohibitively expensive. More than practical guides, then, these books like Robert of Sorbon's spiritual *opusculum*, served to regale the readers with an imaginary and unattainable taste.

As the examples above demonstrate, smell and taste were inscribed in a new bodily geography of knowledge that pertained to both the practical and the spiritual, and which allowed frequent border crossings between the two realms. The sense of touch, too, belonged to this episteme. Often considered the most carnal of senses for its immediacy, in Christianity touch was generally condemned as a path to damnation.[39] Yet from the twelfth century onward, the hand began progressively to be seen as an instrument of the soul. Bruno of Segni, for example, discusses touch as a supreme instrument of knowledge, saying that "touch is like faith: here we can hold and feel God."[40] Balduin of Ford (1185–1190) repeats this concept and compares touching with faith.[41] We find the echoes of this idea in a late twelfth-century manuscript of glossed miscellaneous biblical texts from the Monastery of Heilbrom (fig. 2.5).[42] In the line drawing, a pure soul is pictured climbing the ladder of wisdom. The rungs of the ladder consist of the five senses: sight being the first and touch the last. Touch is placed at the crossroad between Heaven and Hell and depending on its use it can lead one way or the other. If one chooses well, the four cardinal virtues, *Prudentia, Temperantia, Fortitudo,* and *Justitia*, can lead one to God. The inscription around the border affirms the importance of free will to combat temptations and opt between the damnations of hell and the joy of heaven as it was understood by St. Augustine.[43] It is tempting to tie these ideas to the cotemporaneous interest in the work of hands expressed by important theologians such as Hugh of St. Victor and Rupert of Deutz, who recognized the value of the mechanical arts as a gift proceeding from the Holy Spirit and as an instrument in the combat against vices.[44]

37 The text of Robert of Sorbon's treatise is found in a manuscript at the Bibliothèque Nationale de France, MS. lat. 15954, fol. 274r. It is still unpublished but has been studied by Bériou, "L'Eucharistie," 881–85.

38 L. Thorndike, "A Medieval Saucebook," *Speculum* 9 (1934): 183–90. Magninus's manuscript is in Naples, Biblioteca Nazioanle, MS. VIII D. 35, fols. 52–53. See on this also T. Scully, "Opusculum de Saporibus of Magninus Mediolanensis," *Medium Aevum* 54 (1985): 178–207. On the proliferation and use of these books in the later middle ages see B. Larioux, "Entre savoir et pratiques: Le livre de cuisine à la fin du Moyen Âge," *Médiévales* 14 (1988): 59–71.

39 On the history of touch see Classen, *Deepest Sense* (n. 5 above); D. Heller-Roazen, *The Inner Touch: Archaeology of a Sensation* (New York, 2007). For a review of representation of touch see C. Nordenfalk, "The Sense of Touch in Art," in *The Verbal and the Visual: Essays in Honor of William Sebastian Heckscher*, ed. K.-L. Selig and E. Sears (New York, 1990).

40 "tactus animae fides est: hac enim dominus tenetur et tangitur." S. Brunoni Astensis Episcopi Signensis, *Commentaria in Mattheum*, 4.25, PL 165:281. See on this J.-Y. Tilliette, "Le symbolisme des cinq sens dans la littérature morale et spirituelle du XIe et XIIe siècles," *Micrologus* 10 (2002): 15–32.

41 Balduinus Cantuariensis Archiepicopus, *Tractatus diversi*, tractatus 4, PL 204:438: "Tactus fidei est. Fidem enim comprehendit."

42 On Erlangen, Universitätsbibliothek Cod. 8, fol. 130v see E. Lutze, *Die Bilderhandschriften der Universitaetsbibliothek Erlangen* (Erlangen 1936), 1; T. Eriksson, "L'Échelle de la perfection," *Cahiers de civilisation médiévale* 7, no. 28 (October–December 1964): 439–49.

43 +DU(M)SEDE(M) MENTIS VEXANT FANTASMATA CARNIS / AD CELU(M) TENDENS SUSPIRAT XPICOLE MENS +ARBITRII DEXTRU(M) RAMU(M) PETE / SP(ER)NE SINISTRU(M) / NA(M) DEXTER CELU(M) TIBI PANDIT / LEVUS ABYSSUM. On the importance of free will in Augustine's theory of sensation see Carruthers, "Intention, sensation" (n. 17 above); H. Khan, "Discovering the Will: From Aristotle to Aquinas," in *The Question of "Eclecticism": Studies in Later Greek Philosophy*, ed. J. M. Dillon and A. A. Long (Berkeley, 1988), 234–59.

44 Hugh of St. Victor and J. Taylor, *Didascalicon: A Medieval Guide to the Arts* (New York, 1961); Rupert of Deutz, *De Sancta Trinitate et operis eius*, 2.3, ed. R. Haacke, CCCM 21 (Turnhout, 1971), 187.

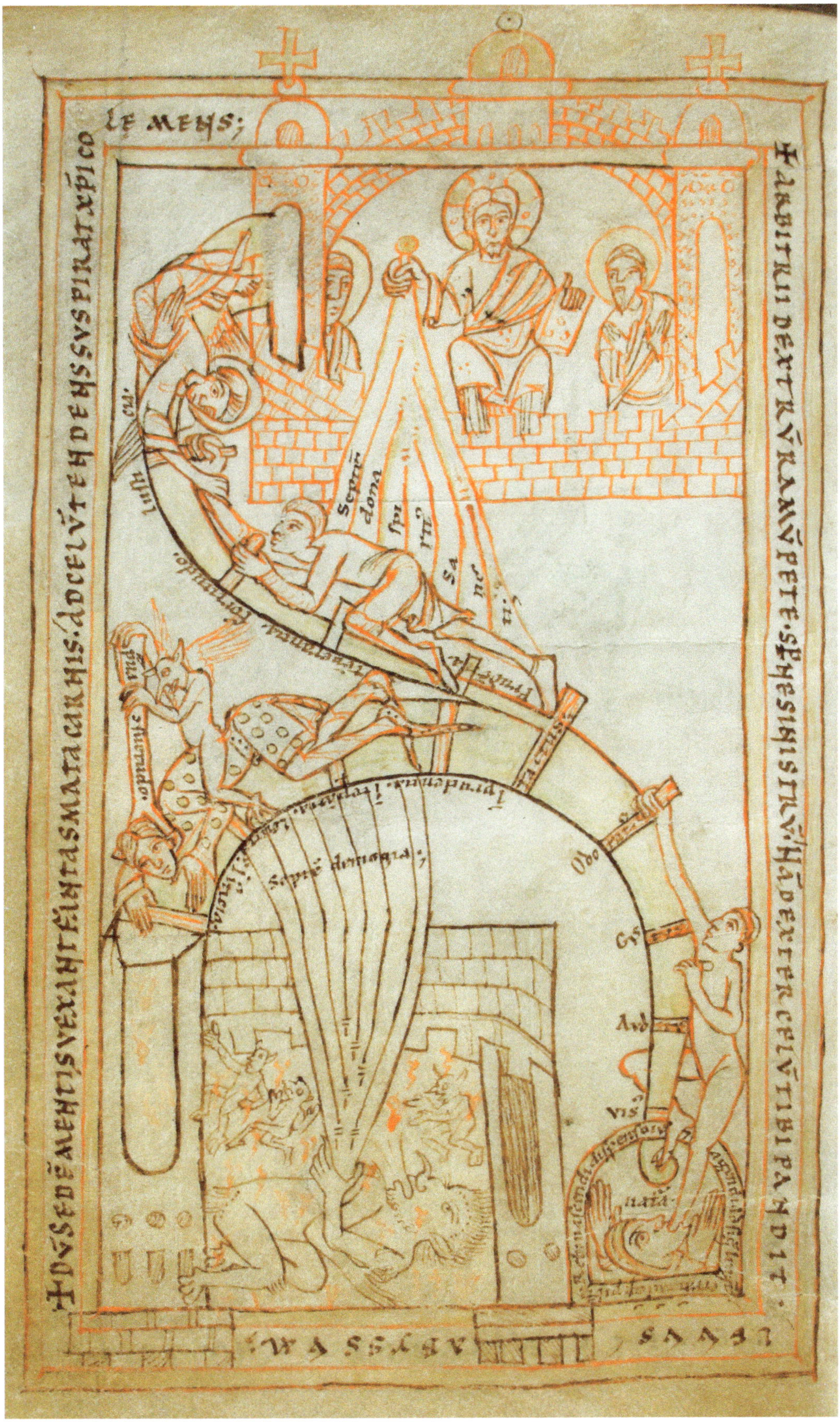

FIG. 2.5. The ladder of virtues, Erlangen, Universitätsbibliothek Cod. 8, fol. 130v (photo: Universitätsbibliothek Erlangen-Nürnberg)

FIG. 2.6.
Handwarmer with apostles, Paris, Musée de Cluny (photo: RMN-Grand Palais)

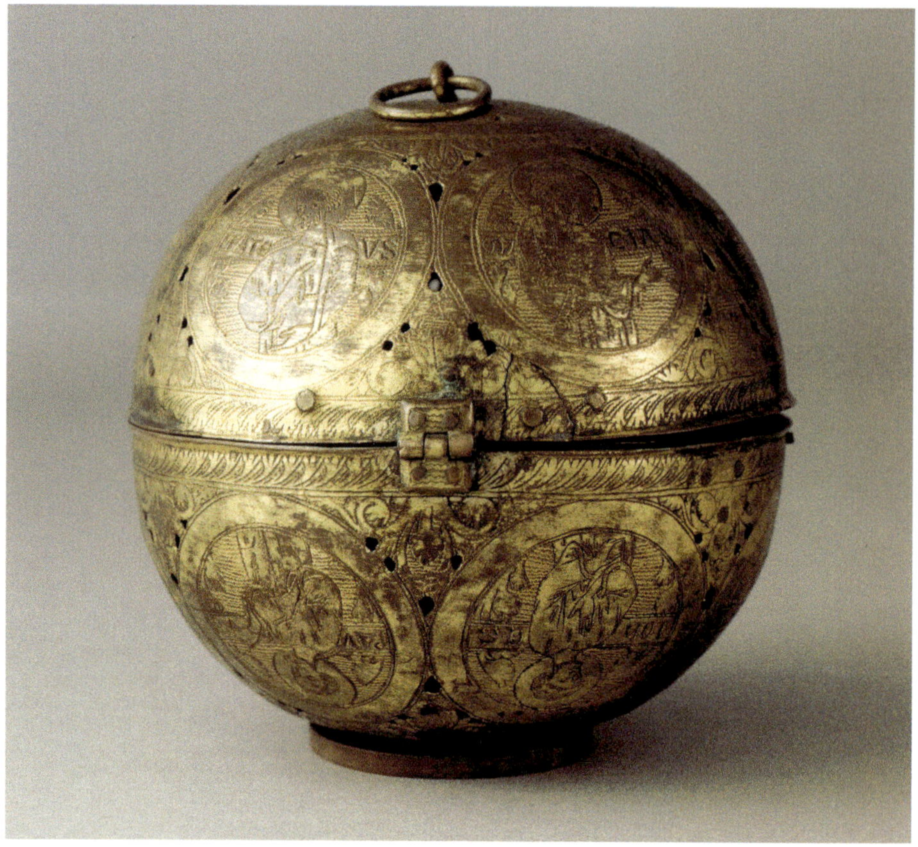

These ideas provide the background from which to understand the assertions of the monk Theophilus, who in his famous book on the diverse arts associates manual skill with the advancement of the soul. Speaking of the decoration of churches, Theophilus assures the reader that he "has committed each thing to the storeroom of his heart" and "examined them one by one with careful experiment testing them all by eye and by *hand*."[45] The statement is interesting because it confirms Theophilus's understanding of skillful hands as a measure not just of craft but also of moral value. In his manual, the author invites his fellow monks to exercise their crafts as a way to apply their right to knowledge.[46] Theophilus understands artistic talent as an inherited right, which man maintained despite his fall from grace. Man could regain his likeness to God only if this right was studiously exercised. Like Rupert of Deutz and Hugh of St. Victor, Theophilus elevates the mechanical arts to the level of other intellectual faculties engaged in achieving wisdom.

The crafting of liturgical implements manifested these ideas. Within this category, handwarmers present a revealing case. Seldom mentioned in the art historical literature, handwarmers were commonly used throughout the medieval period to warm the fingers of the celebrant so as to avoid awkward mistakes during the celebration of the mass.[47] They would be held in the hand and were filled with fuel, which sat inside a gyrating core so that when handled, the fuel would not spill. This mechanism is commonly known as Cardan suspension in honor of the sixteenth-century Italian physicist Girolamo Cardano, but it had been known and used at

45 My emphasis. Theophilus, *On Diverse Arts*, ed. and trans. J. G. Hawthorne and C. S. Smith (New York, 1979), 47.

46 On the importance of craftsmanship in twelfth-century thought and the arts see: M. Bagnoli, "The Stuff of Heaven: Materials and Craftsmanship in Medieval Reliquaries," in *Treasure of Heaven: Saints, Relics and Devotion in Medieval Europe*, ed. M. Bagnoli et al. (New Haven and London, 2010), 137–47.

47 G. Schiedlausky, *Kühlkugel und Wärmapfel* (Munich, 1984).

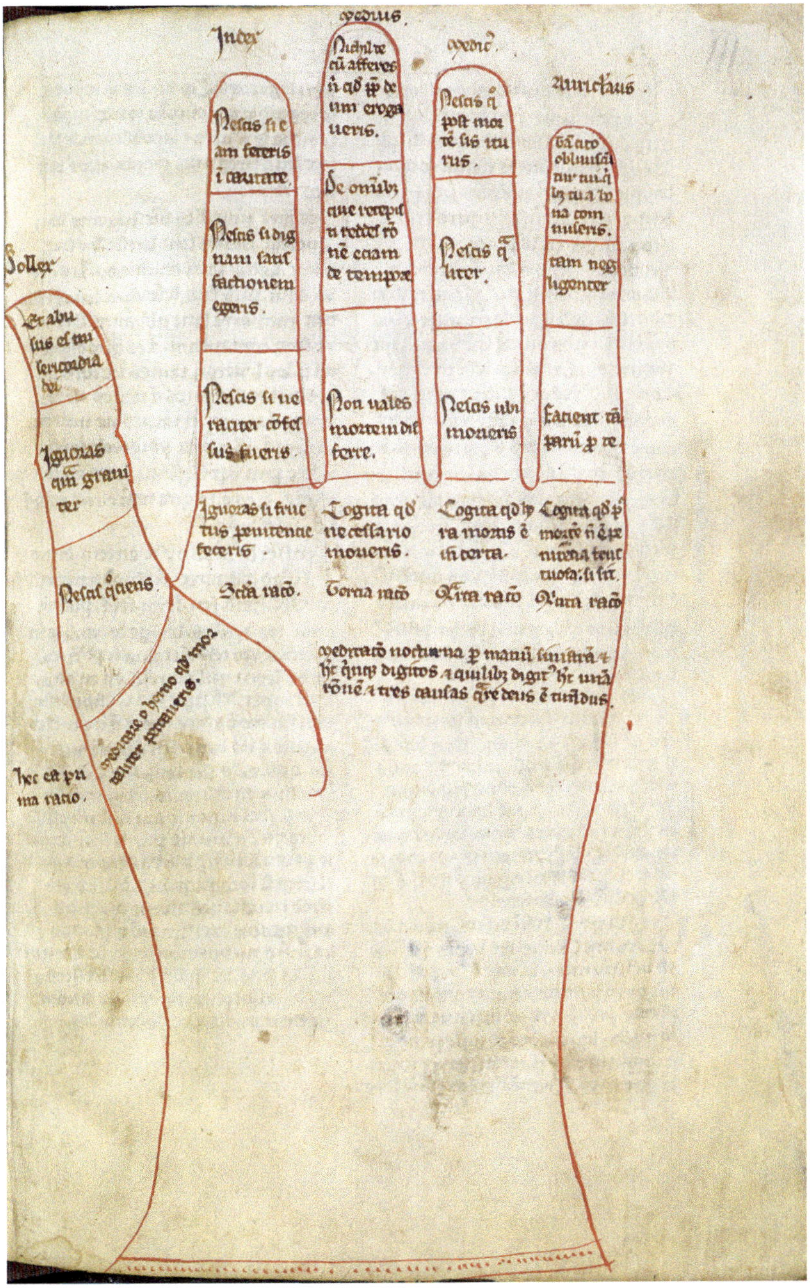

FIG. 2.7.
Mnemonic hand diagram, London, British Library MS. Harley 273, fol. 111r (photo: British Library)

least since late antiquity. The cleverness of the mechanism made handwarmers a matter of interest. Villard de Honnecourt, for example, makes a note of the intricacies of the interior suspension in his journal, explaining its function.[48] In his drawing, Villard exaggerates the intricacies of the mechanics, an implicit admission of its value and significance. Thus, it is evident that handwarmers not only ensured dexterity when it was most required, they also celebrated the beauty of *ars mechanicae* and in so doing, drew attention to the power of the hand as an agent of faith. The decoration of an early thirteenth-century handwarmer in the Musée de Cluny in Paris underscores this idea by picturing the apostles with their hands extended in blessing (fig. 2.6). To a certain degree, handwarmers traced a sacred geography of the hand not too dissimilar from that delineated

48 C. F. Barnes, ed., *The Portfolio of Villard de Honnecourt (Paris, Bibliothèque nationale de France, MS Fr 19093): A New Critical Edition and Color Facsimile* (Farnham, 2009).

by late medieval mnemonic diagrams based on the hand.[49] Used by the laity to keep track of long sequences of prayers, these diagrams associated different parts with different prayers. One example in a fourteenth-century miscellany for lay use illustrates a guide to daily and nightly devotions (fig. 2.7).[50] The diagram is described thus: "meditatio nocturna per manum sinistram. Et habent quinque digitos, et quilibet digitus habet unam rationem, et tres causas quare Deus est timendus." Through the hand one learns to fear and respect God. To my mind, the idea of the hand as a guide to the soul, inherent in this drawing, underscores the importance of touch in the creation and transmission of knowledge in the realm both of liturgical ritual and of lay devotion.[51]

Materialized Sensation

The examples above describe a geography of knowledge that was written on the body. An investigation of the materiality of medieval art must account for the role of sensory objects in the construction of meaning. This is particularly urgent for the art of the late middle ages, which placed a great interest in multisensory engagement. Emblematic of this idea is the table fountain from the Cleveland Museum of Art (fig. 2.8).[52] The only known complete surviving table fountain of the middle ages, the Cleveland engine is a feast for the eyes, ears, and nose. Conceived as a miniature building, it would have spouted scented water that set in motion tinkling bells. The smells and sounds complemented the enameled decoration picturing female figures sitting in gardens and playing various instruments. In medieval romances, the sound of running water and the smell of flowers was often the setting for love scenes or pleasurable moments. By virtue of its decoration, function and sensory engagement, the Cleveland fountain materializes ideas of beauty and love associated with water springs and gardens in countless romantic scenes in the literature of the period. Take for example the masterly description of the spring of Narcissus in the *Roman de la Rose*: "Around the streams and the banks of the bright and lively springs the fresh grass grew thickly, so that one could have lain with one's mistress as if on a feather bed, for the earth was soft and cool. . . . But the beauty of all this was greatly enhanced by the place itself, which was of such a kind that flowers were always plentiful, both in winter and in summer. . . . That ground was extremely pretty, for it was decorated and, as it were, painted with sweet-smelling flowers of various colours."[53] Beyond the pleasure that it provided to the ears and nose, the Cleveland fountain recalled a sensual pleasure of a different kind.

Similarly an aquamanile in the collection of the Metropolitan Museum of Art draws attention to the eroticism that accompanied the consumption of food, another theme often exploited in medieval romances (fig. 2.9).[54] In

49 For hand mnemonic diagrams in general see C. R. Sherman and P. M. Lukehart, *Writing on Hands: Memory and Knowledge in Early Modern Europe* (Carlisle, PA, 2000).

50 London, British Library MS. Harley 273, fol. 111r. The manuscript is a miscellany made up of composite texts mostly in Anglo-Norman. *A Catalogue of the Harleian Manuscripts in the British Museum*, 4 vols. (London, 1808–12), 1: no. 273; S. H. A. Shepherd, "The Middle English Pseudo-Turpin Chronicle," *Medium Aevum* 65 (1996): 32 n. 26.

51 Later examples include the diagrams that appear in S. Fridolin, *Schatzbehalter der wahren Reichtümer des Heils* (Nuremberg, 1491), fol. 298r. I consulted the copy at the Walters Art Museum (inv. no. 91.1086); P. W. Parshall and R. Schoch, *Origins of European Printmaking: Fifteenth-Century Woodcuts and Their Public* (Washington, DC, and New Haven, 2005), 78, 258–59. D. Bartl and M. Gepp-Labusiak, *Der Mainzer Schatzbehalter: Ein Koloriertes Andachtsbuch von 1491* (Darmstadt, 2012).

52 S. N. Fliegel, "The Cleveland Table Fountain and Gothic Automata," *Cleveland Studies in the History of Art* 7 (2002): 6–49; N. Miller, "Paradise Regained: Medieval Garden Fountains," in *Medieval Gardens*, ed. E. B. MacDougall, Dumbarton Oaks Colloquium on the History of Landscape Architecture 9 (Cambridge, MA, 1986), 137–53.

53 "Entor les ruissiaus et les rives / Des fontaines cleres et vives, / Poignoit l'erbe freschete et drue; / Ausinc i poïst-l'en sa drue / Couchier comme sor une coite, / Car la terre estoit douce et moite / . . . / Mès moult embelissoit l'afaire / Li leus qui ere de tel aire, / Qu'il i avoit tous jours plenté / De flors et yver et esté. / . . . / Trop par estoit la terre cointe, / Qu'ele ere piolée et pointe / De flors de diverses colors, / Dont moult sunt bones les odors." Guillaume de Lorris and Jean de Meun, *Le Roman de la Rose*, ed. F. Michel, 2 vols. (Paris, 1864), 1:46–47, vv. 1399–1418. I am using the translation in modern English by Frances Horgan (Oxford, 1994). For the importance of fountains in medieval gardens and their symbolism see Miller, "Paradise Regained."

54 New York, Metropolitan Museum of Art, inv. no. 1975.1.1416. See P. Barnet and P. Dandridge, *Lions, Dragons, & Other Beasts: Aquamanilia of the Middle Ages, Vessels for Church and Table* (New Haven, 2006), 136; F. Scholten, *The Robert Lehman Collection of European Sculpture and Metalwork* (New York, 2011), no. 4, pp. 10–13 A useful discussion of food metaphors in Italian Renaissance literature is given by P. Palma,

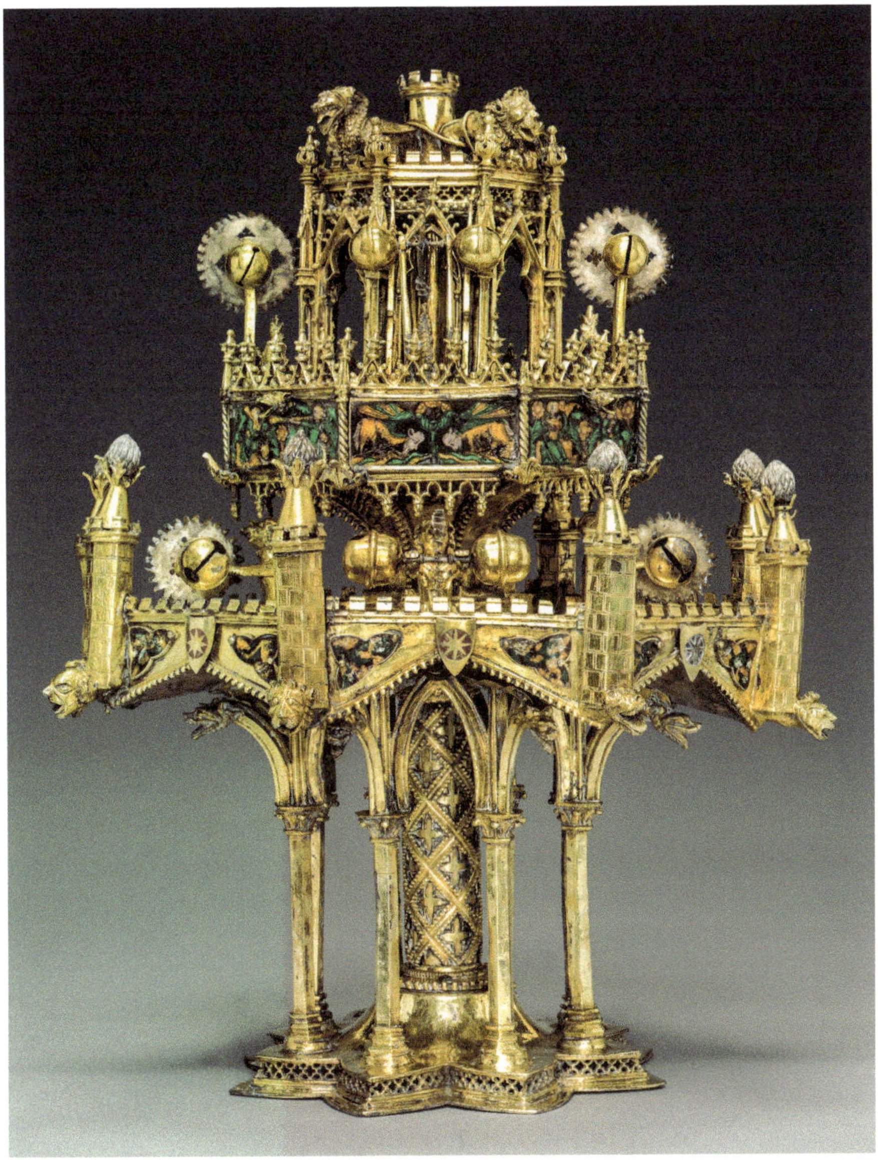

FIG. 2.8.
Table fountain, ca. 1320–40, France, Paris; gilt-silver and translucent enamels; 31.1 × 24.1 × 26.0 cm; Cleveland Museum of Art, gift of J. H. Wade 2914.859 (photo: The Cleveland Museum of Art)

Chrétien's Chevalier de la Charette, the sexual encounter between Gawain and an unknown temptress is introduced by a meal. Chrétien lavishes great care on the description of the setting, including a meticulous description of the table set with a white linen tablecloth and fresh towels piled up next to a basin of scented water for washing hands.[55] Used to pour scented water over the hands of patrons during meals, aquamaniles were objects that portended and provided sensual pleasure.[56] That is particularly true of the Metropolitan Art Museum's aquamanile shaped in the form of Phyllis riding Aristotle. The story of Aristotle and Phyllis

Savoring Power, Consuming the Times: The Metaphors of Food in Medieval and Renaissance Italian Literature (South Bend, IN, 2013), 19, 136.

55 "Par l'uis qu'il ont trové overt / Antrent anz, et voient covert / Un dois d'un tablier grant et lé; / Et sus estoient aporté / Li mes, et les chandoiles mises / Es chandeliers totes esprises, / Et li henap d'argent doré, / Et dui pot, l'uns plains de moré, / Et li autres de fort vin blanc. / Delez le dois, au chief d'un banc / Troverent deus bacins tous pleins / D'eve chaude a laver lor mains; / Et de l'autre part ont trouvee / Une toaille bien ovree, / Bele et blanche, as mains essüier." Chrétien de Troyes, *Le Chevalier de la Charrette*, ed. and trans. A. Foulet and K. D. Uitti (Paris, 1989), 120–22, http://visualiseur.bnf.fr/CadresFenetre?O=NUMM-101432&M=notice (accessed 26 September 2016).

56 Aquamaniles were also commonly used in liturgical rituals. Their forms and function is discussed at length in M. Hutt, *Aquamanilien: Gebrauch und Form* (Mainz, 1993), 78–137.

FIG. 2.9. Aquamanile, New York, Metropolitan Museum of Art, Lehman Collection (photo: The Metropolitan Museum of Art)

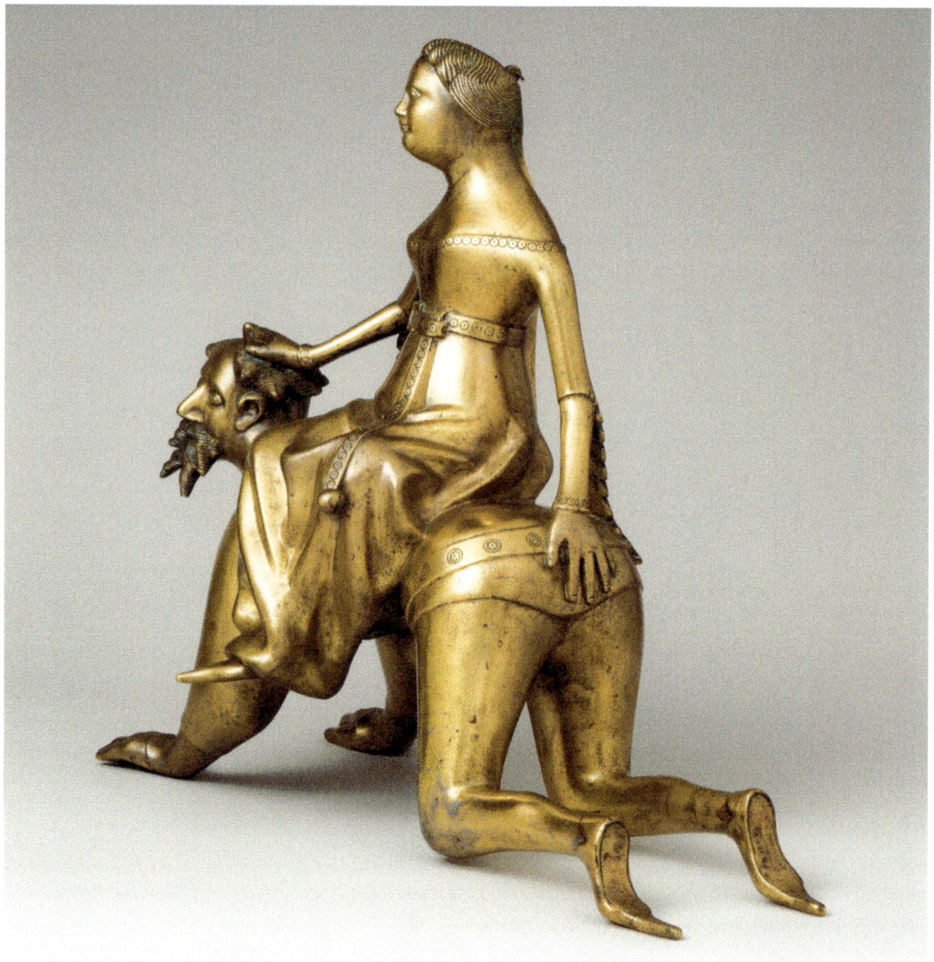

was a popular courtly romance. In love with the beautiful Phyllis, Alexander the Great neglected the affairs of state. Aristotle reprimanded him and as a result the young emperor withdrew from his lovely young wife. Piqued by this lack of attention, Phyllis directed her wiles toward the aging philosopher, managing to turn him into her love slave. Asked by the young woman to act as a mount, Aristotle complied and was thus ridiculed. The moral lesson of the story is turned on its head by the implicit eroticism of this object. Phyllis's hand gently strokes Aristotle's bottom, while her long fashionable sleeves fall back to reveal her slender arms. Presumably one of her arms served as handle. Although not very practical, the New York aquamanile was functional. It was filled through a hole on the back of Phyllis's head, and emptied through a spigot under Aristotle's beard. The fact that the aquamanile was handled adds to the erotic content of its imagery. The presence of a cock on the spigot's turn-handle underscored the erotic sous-entendre of the imagery.

This type of inversion, where the object delivering a moral lesson invites the opposite response, is common in medieval culture. Think for example of the erotic images populating the border of devotional manuscripts.[57] But whereas in those cases the reliance on sight makes the seduction of the images more theoretical, the tactile seduction of the aquamanile is experienced firsthand and thus provides a moral lesson that is felt rather than seen. For this reason, it seems to

57 An extensive survey of marginal images is provided by L. M. C. Randall, *Images in the Margins of Gothic Manuscripts* (Berkeley, 1966); M. Camille, *Images on the Edge: The Margins of Medieval Art* (London, 1992). The role of marginal illustration as mnemonic devices is discussed by M. J. Carruthers, *The Craft of Thought: Meditation, Rhetoric, and the Making of Images, 400–1200* (New York, 1998).

me that the material temptation provided by the aquamanile is unique to courtly culture and links this object to princely codes of conduct.

Mirrors of Princes taught rulers how to resist the temptations of the flesh, precisely because they were constantly exposed to them. In a fourteenth-century *Avys au Rois* the chapter dedicated to the exercise of moderation is illustrated with a prince holding a T-square and standing in front of four rows of figures representing four areas of temptations: love, food, money, and war.[58] The text explains how the necessary accoutrements of a ruler—banqueting, riches, and pageantry—must be subordinated to higher goals. The T-square is here a symbol of measure, the main virtue for a just ruler, as all pleasures must be enjoyed in moderation. In the same book, Temperance is illustrated by a ruler sitting in front of a lavishly laid table: he points to the food and touches his mouth. In another miniature a group of finely dressed women press around a king, representing Temperance, and pull him in several opposite directions (fol. 38r).[59] The miniature marvelously illustrates the pull exerted on the body by sensual pleasure. The existence of sensual pleasure creates an opportunity for temperance. For that reason, codes of etiquette and table manners stipulated that eating too fast, too much or with too much enjoyment was a display of bad taste.[60] Thus, disciplining the senses becomes an act of moral but also aesthetic importance.

We find the idea of beauty in reason's dominance over pleasure in theological discussions. In Christianity pleasure was traditionally equated with sin and the fight against pleasure was the keystone of monastic life, which was by emulation the model of every Christian. During the course of the twelfth century this stark duality began to give way to a more nuanced approach whereby pleasure was integrated in a broader scheme that accounted for human psychology. In particular, the localization of pleasure in a system of passions allowed thinkers like Albertus Magnus and later Aquinas to isolate pleasure before it turned to sin.[61] Sinful was not the feeling of pleasure but rather consenting to pleasure for an illicit passion. In this way, pleasure was governed by morality and it was defined by the dynamic relationship between desire, the object of desire, and reason, the last called to govern the appetite for sensible things. Pleasure was good when it resulted from an alignment of these three elements. Shifting the weight of sin from pleasure to morality resulted in a reassessment of the sins traditionally attached to the pleasure of the body as defined by touch and taste and consequently an acceptance of the disciplined body as a tool to find God. This is particularly relevant for devotional objects, as I shall now show.

Longing to Experience

The implements such as images, books, and prayer beads used in the act of praying relied on sensation to help the devout feel unity with God. The idea was to create in the mind a sensation of a spiritual nature starting from physical sensory stimuli. Images were paramount in this process of meditation. Much has been written on the role of such art in late medieval devotion.[62] However,

58 New York, Morgan Library and Museum MS. M.456. On this manuscript see M. Camille, "The King's New Bodies: An Illustrated Mirror of Princes in the Morgan Library," in *Kunstlerischer Austausch: Akten des XXVIII. Internationalen Kongresses für Kunstgeschichte*, Berlin, 15.–20. July 1992, ed. T. W. Gaehtgens (Berlin, 1993), 393–405. On the Aristotelian foundation of these type of manuals, including this one, see C. R. Sherman, *Imaging Aristotle: Verbal and Visual Representations in Fourteenth-Century France* (Berkeley, 1995).

59 Visible at: http://ica.themorgan.org/manuscript/page/34/112420 (accessed 20 October 2016).

60 M. P. Cosman, *Fabulous Feasts: Medieval Cookery and Ceremony* (New York, 1976), 104–9.

61 Jean de La Rochelle, *Summa de Anima*, ed. J.-C. Bougerol (Paris, 1995), 255; Albertus Magnus, *De bono*, in *Opera Omnia*, ed. C. Feckes and W. Kuebel (Munster, 1951), 28:195–216; Thomas Aquinas, *Summa Theologiae*, I IIae, q. 31, *De delectatione secundum se*, q. 32, *De causa delectationis*, q. 33, *De effectibus delectationis*, q. 34 *De bonitate et militia delectationum*. I base my discussion on the careful and detailed analysis of these ideas by S. Vecchio, "Il piacere da Abelardo a Tommaso," in *Piacere e dolore: Materiali per una storia delle passioni nel medioevo*, ed. C. Casagrande and S. Vecchio (Florence, 2009), 67–86.

62 The literature on late medieval devotional art is vast. I am here giving bibliographical information only on a few titles that have been most useful to me: H. van Os, *The Art of Devotion in the Late Middle Ages in Europe, 1300–1500* (Amsterdam, 1995); D. G. Wilkin, "Opening the Doors to Devotion: Trecento Triptychs and Suggestions Concerning Images and Domestic Practice in Florence," in *Italian Panel Painting of the Duecento and Trecento*, ed. V. M. Schmidt (Washington, DC, 2002), 371–93. In the same volume see J. Cannon, "Beyond the Limitations of Visual Typology: Reconsidering the Function and Audience

we have tended to emphasize sight above all other senses in interpreting the role of objects in devotional practice. Sight was not exercised in isolation and other sensations played an important role too. Indeed, touch, hearing and smell were even more important because they could locate the visionary in the devotee's own present circumstances. Tactile experiences, especially those of a painful nature, were central because they forced the worshipper to commune physically with Christ, and achieve a state of empathy with his suffering. Indeed, the Latin word for empathy, *compassio*, literally means to suffer with. Painful meditative tactics that included the use of hair shirts, flabella, nails, and other tortures mortified the flesh in the attempt to free the spirit from its constraints and reach out to God.[63] A paragon of this behavior is the mystic Henry Suso, who used to strap a nails-laden cross to his back, and in this way feel more keenly his union with Christ and at the same time his immense inferiority in respect to him.[64] The search for painful experiences as a gift that promoted sanctity was part of a pervasive culture of suffering that marked late medieval culture and governed attitude toward its physical and spiritual benefits in society and religious life.[65]

Alongside these more forceful methods there existed less extreme practices that relied on a direct physical contact with devotional objects to invite the devotee to imagine rather than experience Christ's passion. This is the case with devotion to the five wounds of Christ that fomented a markedly tactile response. Like many others of this kind, the illustration of the wounds in a sixteenth-century book of hours at the Walters Art Museum (fig. 2.10) shows sign of rubbing.[66] The image accompanied a prayer where the supplicant invokes Christ's help to impress upon her heart the sentiments of faith and charity that the sight of the wounds should inspire. Touching the image helped the owner of the book imprint in her mind Christian virtues. A woodcut of the same image at the National Gallery of Art carries an inscription that invites the onlooker to kiss the wound of Christ and so be recompensed with an indulgence (fig. 2.11).[67] The National Gallery woodcut is interesting because it purports to reproduce the original size of the actual wound of Christ. In this way, the beholder could measure Christ's wound against his own body, thus making the image part of his tangible reality.

---

of Three Vita Panels of Women Saints c. 1300," 290–330 and K. Krüger, "Medium and Imagination: Aesthetic Aspects of Trecento Panel Painting," 57–81; J. F. Hamburger, *Nuns as Artists: The Visual Culture of a Medieval Convent* (Berkeley, 1996); idem, "Speculation on Speculations, Vision and Perception in the Theory and Practice of Mystical Devotion," in *Deutsche Mystik im abendländischen Zusammenhang: Neu erschlossene Texte, neue methodische Ansätze, neue theoretische Konzepte,* Kolloquium Kloster Fischingen 1998, ed. W. Haug and W. Schneider-Lastin (Tübingen, 2000), 353–408; J. F. Hamburger and S. Marti, eds., *Crown and Veil: The Art of Female Monasticism in the Middle Ages* (New York, 2008), 353–408; J. F. Hamburger, "Mysticism and Visuality," in *The Cambridge Companion to Christian Mysticism*, ed. A. Hollywood and P. Z. Beckman (Cambridge, 2011), 277–93; D. S. Areford, *The Art of Empathy: The Mother of Sorrows in Northern Renaissance Art and Devotion* (Jacksonville, 2013).

63 For a discussion of the importance of the body (and its mortification) in medieval devotion see C. Walker Bynum, *Holy Feast and Holy Fast: The Religious Significance of Food to Medieval Women* (Berkeley, 1987); eadem, "Warum das ganze Theater mit dem Körper? Die sicht einer Mediävistin," *Historische Anthropologie: Kultur-Gesellschaft-Alltag* 4 (1996): 1–33.

64 Henry Suso, *The Exemplar with Two German Sermons*, ed. and trans. F. J. Tobin (Mahwah, NJ, 1989); Hamburger, *Nuns as Artists*; idem, *St. John the Divine: The Deified Evangelist in Medieval Art and Theology* (Berkeley, 2002), 195–200.

65 Medieval attitudes toward pain have been studied by E. Cohen, *The Modulated Scream: Pain in Late Medieval Culture* (Chicago, 2010).

66 On Walters Art Museum, MS. W.165, known as the Loftie Hours from the name of its nineteenth-century owner, see J. Marrow, "A Book of Hours from the Circle of the Master of the Berlin Passion: Notes on the Relationship between Fifteenth-Century Manuscript Illumination and Printmaking in the Rhenish Lowlands," *ArtB* 60 (1978): 609, no. 62, pl. 46 (fol. 23v); idem, "Passion Iconography in Northern European Art of the Late Middle Ages and Early Renaissance: A Study of the Transformation of Sacred Metaphor into Descriptive Narrative," *Ars Neerlandica* 1 (1979): 225, no. 8b; J. H. Marrow, H. L. M. Defoer, A. S. Korteweg, and W. C. M. Wüstefeld, *The Golden Age of Dutch Manuscript Painting* (New York, 1990), 188–89, no. 52. The manuscript is fully digitized and published: http://thedigitalwalters.org/Data/WaltersManuscripts/html/W165/description.html (accessed 15 November 2016).

67 On Washington, DC, National Gallery of Art, Rosenwald Collection 1943.3.831 see D. S. Areford, "The Passion Measured: A Late-Medieval Diagram of the Body of Christ." In *The Broken Body: Passion Devotion in Late-Medieval Culture* (Groningen, 1998), 211–38; idem, in Parshall and Schoch, *Origins* (n. 51 above), no. 78; Bynum, *Christian Materiality* (n. 6 above), 94, 96, fig. 30 and A. Powell, *Depositions: Scenes from the Late Medieval Church and the Modern Museum* (Cambridge, MA, 2012), 179, 181, 182, fig. 50.

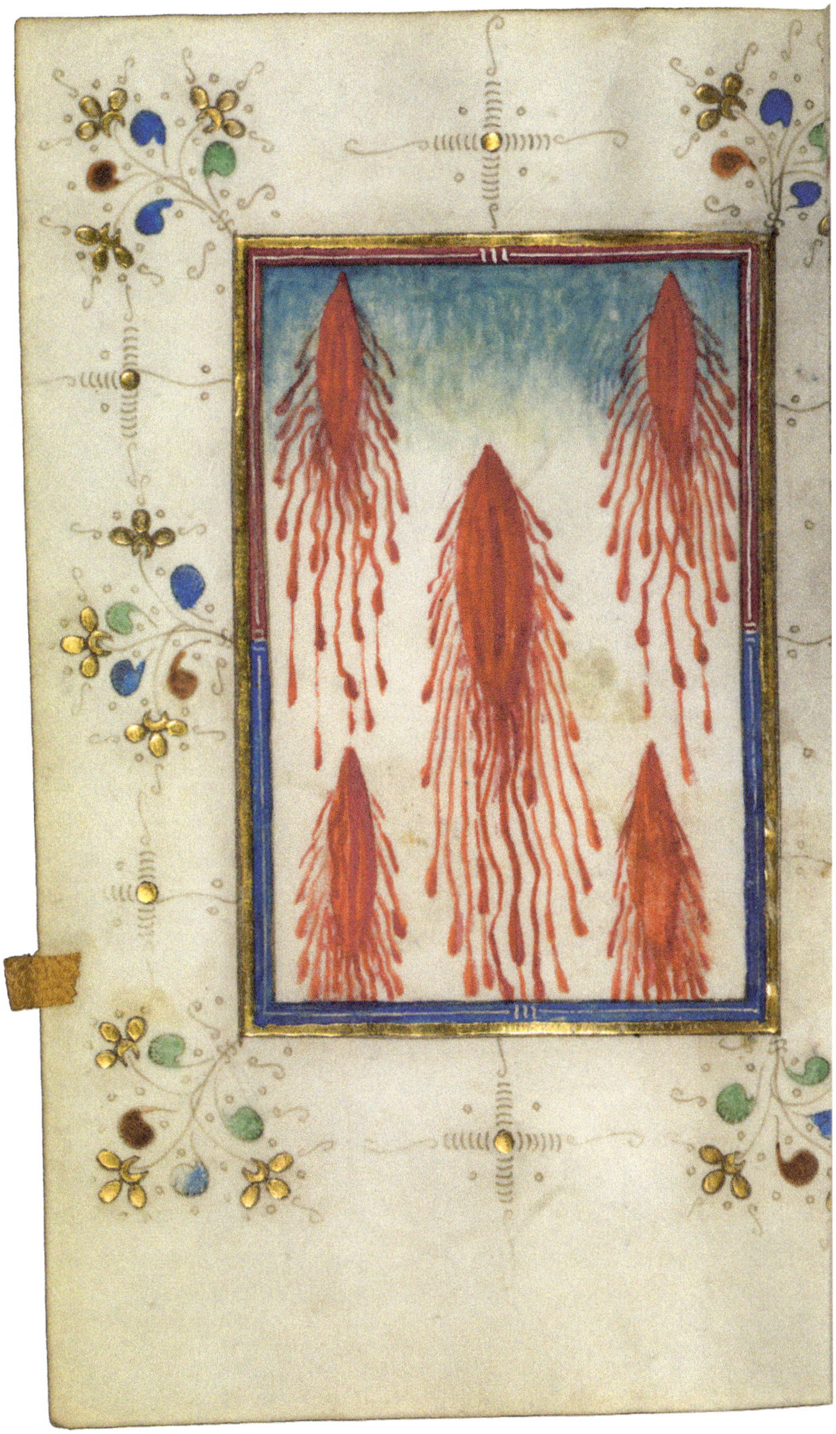

FIG. 2.10.
The five wounds of Christ, Loftie Hours, Baltimore Walters Art Museum MS. W.165, fol. 110v (photo: Walters Art Museum)

More personal still, are those objects decorated with images of the five wounds meant to be worn on one's person, like small hanging scrolls and jewelry.[68] Beyond their function as amulets, these objects served to imprint on the body of the wearer Christ's mark, in emulation of St. Francis, whom God favored with his touch.

68 This is the case of a scroll at the British Library, MS. Harley Roll T 11 and a ring at the British Museum, inv. no. P&EAF 897. On the roll see C. M. Woolgar, *The Senses In Late Medieval England* (New Haven, 2006). For the ring see J. Robinson, *Masterpieces of Medieval Art* (London, 2008), 71.

FIG. 2.11.
The symbols of the passion and the wounds of Christ, Washington, DC, National Gallery of Art, the Rosenwald Collection 1943.3.831 (photo: National Gallery of Art, Washington, DC)

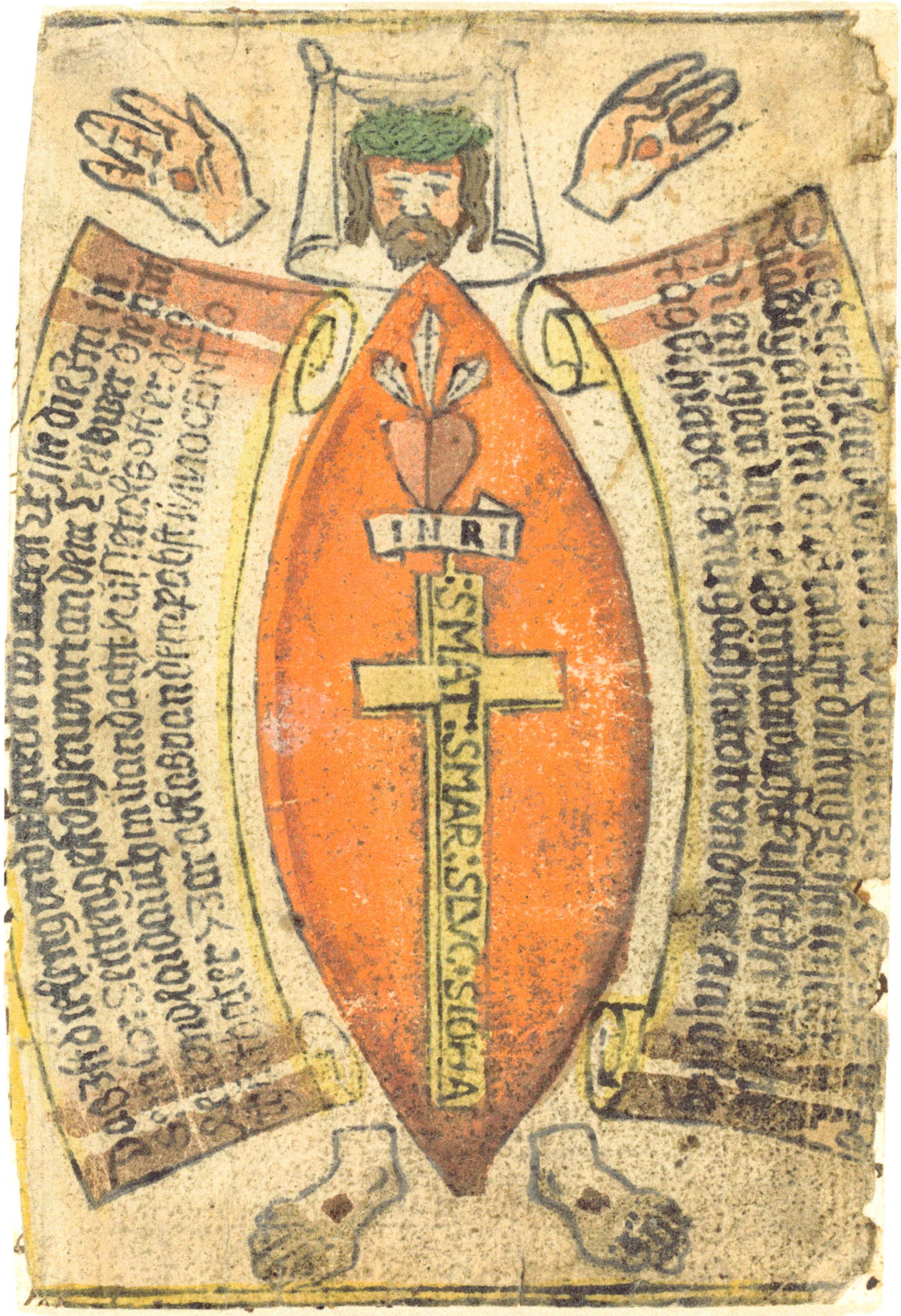

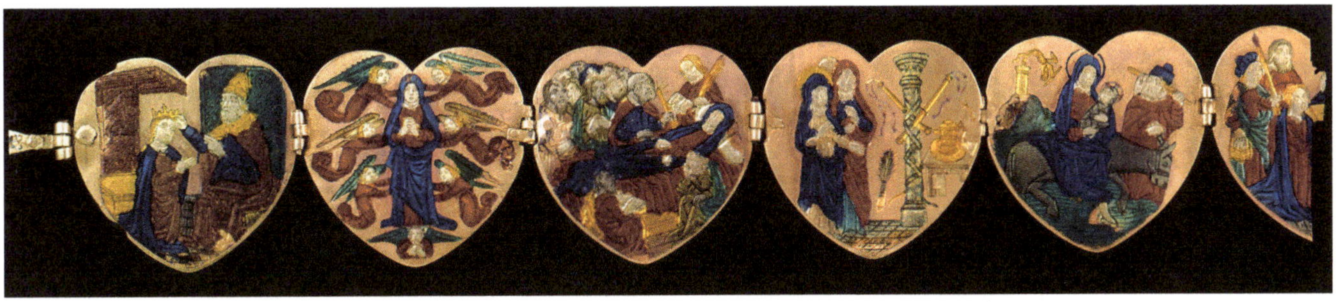

FIG. 2.12.
Heart-shaped paternoster, Munich, Schatzkammer der Residenz, (photo: Bayerische Schlösserverwaltung, L. Weiss, Munich)

Touch was also a very important accompaniment to long recitations of prayers. Prayer beads were often made of smooth soft stones, like amber, coral, or jasper and were sometimes enriched with fragrances so that their haptic appeal would be coupled by pleasant smells.[69] The tactility and smell of prayer beads gave a tangible form to prayers. This seems to be the reason for the appearances of prayer beads in the border of books of hours, like that once owned by Catherine Duchess of Cleves now at the Morgan Library in New York, where a lush paternoster made of coral runs along the edge of the suffrage prayer dedicated to the three magi.[70]

More rarely, prayer beads show elaborate figurative programs. The paternoster in the Schatzkammer der Residenz in Munich consists of ten heart-shaped beads decorated with basse-taille scenes of the story of Joachim and Anna and the life of the Virgin (fig. 2.12).[71] Made in France ca. 1480, it is described in a 1598 court inventory as a man's paternoster. An annotation in the margin of the 1510 version of Olivier de La Marche's poem *Le parement et triumphes des dames* is useful in explaining how these objects worked. In it, the editor of the volume, Pierre Desrey, states: "Paternosters are proper as a special food for the liberal heart, giving as they do a reminder and recollection of God, to whom each one should do a good service in all places."[72] The aim of the paternoster was to feed the heart with images of God. The shape of the beads is a reminder that the sacred stories need to be imprinted in the heart of the faithful. It is worth recalling that, although the Aristotelian notion of the heart as a place of sensation was discarded by Galen, who favored the brain as the center of motion and thought, throughout the middle ages and particularly in the later period (and beyond), the heart remained the prime organ of feeling.[73] Indeed a number of medieval philosophers tried to reconcile Aristotelian and Galenic theories so that the heart maintained its primacy as the seat of perception and emotions. These ideas were shared by philosophers, preachers, and doctors and included influential figures as Albertus Magnus, Giovanni da San Gimignano, and Arnau da Villanova among others.[74] According to such notions, the heart was the seat of the soul and while the brain was the mediator, sensation began and ended in the heart. The heart provided sense organs with the animal spirit that moved perception to the brain and allowed them

69 Lightbown, *Mediaeval Jewelry* (n. 25 above), 351.

70 New York, Morgan Library and Museum, MS. M.945 (ca. 1435), fol. 237; The manuscript is digitized and published: http://www.themorgan.org/collection/Hours-of-Catherine-of-Cleves. See on this R. Dückers and R. Priem, *The Hours of Catherine of Cleves: Devotion, Demons and Daily Life in the Fifteenth Century* (New York, 2009) with earlier bibliography.

71 H. Brunner, *The Treasury in the Residenz Munich* (Munich, 1977), 35, no. 21; Lightbown, *Medieval Jewelry*, 354 and plate 114.

72 Olivier de La Marche, *Le Triumphe des Dames,* ed. J. B. Kalbfleisch (Rostock, 1901).

73 H. Webb, "Cardiosensory Impulses in Late Medieval Spirituality," in Nichols, Kablitz, and Calhoun, *Rethinking the Senses* (n. 17 above), 265–85; eadem, *The Medieval Heart* (New Haven, 2010).

74 Albertus Magnus, *On Animals: A Medieval Summa Zoologica*, ed. and trans. K. F. Kitchell Jr., and J. M. Resnick (Baltimore, 1999). J. Ziegler, *Medicine and Religion c. 1300: The Case of Arnau da Villanova* (Oxford, 1998); A. Dondaine, "La Vie et les oeuvres de Jean de San Gimignano," *Archivum Fratrum Praedicatorum* 9 (1939): 128–83; J. Ziegler, "Medical Similes in Religious Discourse: The Case of Giovanni di San Gimignano O.P. (ca. 1260–ca. 1333)," *Science in Context* 8 (1995): 103–31; M. Oldoni, "Giovanni da San Gimignano," in *L'enciclopedismo Medievale*, ed. M. Picone (Ravenna 1992), 212–28; *Giovanni da San Gimignano: Un enciclopedico dell'anima; Studi e testi*, ed. M. Oldoni and A. Zapperi (San Gimignano, 1993).

to sense. Thus, the heart became a circulator of sensations, which to some degree it absorbed. In her study of the medieval notion of the heart, Heather Webb calls this scheme of thought the "porous heart": a heart that breathes and communes with the outside world. Spiritual communion with God could thus be imprinted in the heart, like that of Chiara da Montefalco, who had visions of Christ transfixing her with his cross and as a result her heart became shaped like the *arma Christi*.[75]

The Munich paternoster reflects these ideas as the choice of technique confirms. The stories depicted on it are flat to the touch since they are executed in basse-taille enamels. Basse-taille involved chasing the figures on a supporting layer of gold or silver and then covering them with a layer of ground glass. When fired the enamel remained transparent and was brightened by the sparkle of the metal underneath. The modeling of figures was achieved by chasing and engraving the base layer, so that although flat, basse-taille enamels achieve a sense of volume and depth. Where the underlining relief is deeper the color of the enamel is darker, and lighter where it is shallower. To a degree, basse-taille enamel tricks the eyes into seeing a relief that is not there when touched. Perhaps in this case the intent was to portray something that the hand could not touch but the heart could feel. Thus, the paternoster provided a template to feel "immaterially" with the spiritual senses. One is reminded of the words of Ugo Panziera da Prato, a thirteenth-century mystic (ca. 1260/70–1330) who associated the perception of a mental image to that of a painted statue. Ugo stated that in contemplating an account of Christ (his passion) the mind moves in sequential steps. At first Christ seems written in the mind's imagination. Then he seems outlined (disegnato), then outlined and shadowed, then colored and fleshed out (incarnato). Finally fleshed out and in relief (rilevato).[76] Gazing and stroking the flat enamels would have allowed the owner to recreate the real three-dimensional images in his own heart. With respect to this, the Munich paternoster is successful in disciplining the bodily senses to privilege the spiritual. The hand cannot feel the relief that the devout senses through the heart.

To wit, even though unity with God was a sensation of the spirit and could only be felt with the spiritual senses, the reaction was often described as somatic. This is the sense of a print by the anonymous Dutch master identified by the monogram I. A. M. active in Zwolle in the second half of the fifteenth century depicting the miracle of St. Bernard's lactation (fig. 2.13).[77] According to legend, while praying before an image of the Virgin and child, the saint was rewarded with a drop of the Virgin's milk. The master of Zwolle was very careful to articulate Bernard's spiritual sensation and he showed the spray of milk hitting Bernard on his forehead. The spiritual taste that Bernard perceives is amplified by sound and by vision, as signaled by singing angels and the flickering of candles. In the print, the milk of the Virgin follows a reverse trajectory: the words of prayers leave the saint's mouth as the milk fills it with sweetness.[78] The experience is multimodal. Following intense visualization hearing and taste are the real symptoms of mystical union.

The importance of music as a component of divine manifestation is documented by a small painting of the glorification of the Virgin by Geertgen tot Sint Jans in the Boijmans Museum in Rotterdam. A cloud of music-making angels surrounds the Virgin and Child, the latter holding little bells in his hands (fig. 2.14). The Rotterdam panel was once part of a diptych that included a crucifixion scene on the left side.[79]

75 Chiara's heart was removed at her death in 1308 and kept as a relic and proof of her sanctity.

76 "Nel primo tempo nel quale la mente comincia cole infrascritte circunstanzie di Cristo a pensare, Cristo pare nella mente e nella imaginativa scritto. Nel secondo pare disegnato. Nel terzo pare disegnato e ombrato. Nel quarto pare colorato e incarnato. Nel quinto pare incarnato e rilevato." Ugo Panziera da Prato, *Trattato della perfezione*. I am using the transcription of Arrigo Levasti in *Mistici del duecento e del trecento* (Milan, 1960), 273. The translation is mine. On Ugo's Trattati see also T. Fracassini, "I cantici e i trattati di Ugo Panziera da Prato," *Archivio Storico Pratese* 6 (1926): 96–110.

77 Amsterdam, Rijksmuseum, inv. no. RP-P-OB-1093.

78 A. M. Altermatt, "Lactatio und Amplexus: Die zentralen Themen der Bernhardsikonographie," in *Stiftung Kloster Eberbach: Bernard von Clairvaux: Der Zisterzienzerheilige zur und in der Kunst*, ed. J. Jacob, exhibition catalogue, Abbey Museum Kloster Eberbach (Bad Kreuznach, 2003), 24–41.

79 Now Edinburgh, National Gallery of Scotland inv. no. 2450, on which see B. Ridderbos, "The Rotterdam Edinburgh

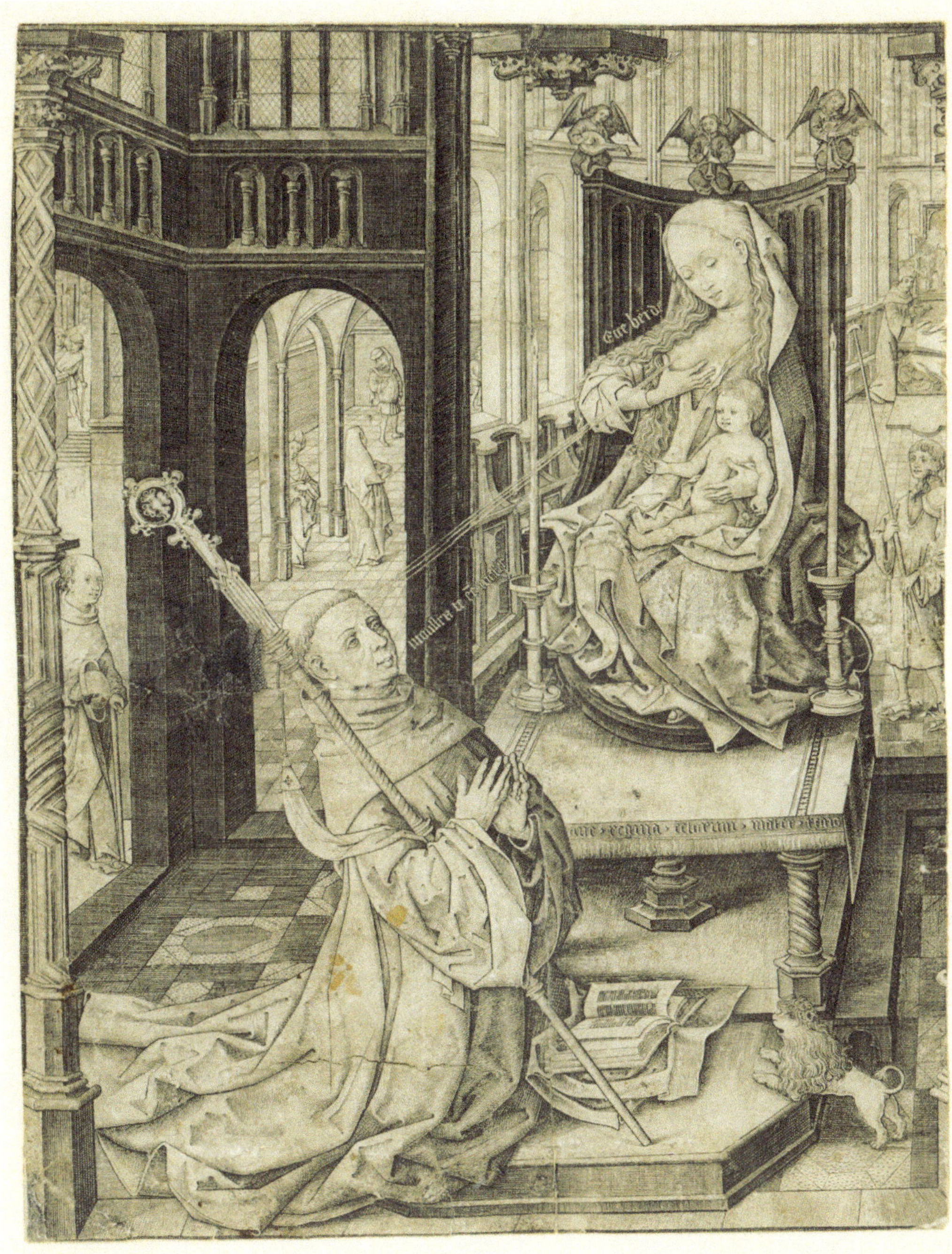

FIG. 2.13.
The Lactation of Bernard, Amsterdam, Rijksmuseum, inv. no. RP-P-OB-1093 (photo: public domain)

The coupling of an image of the Virgin and Child with the crucifixion was common in late medieval devotional paintings. These diptychs were often associated with particular prayers. In this case, the presence of the crown of roses on the Virgin's head, as well as the rosaries offered by angels on both sides of her face, suggests that the diptych was connected with the recitation of the rosary. The rosary consisted in the recitation of sequences of *Ave Marias* regularly interrupted by a *Paternoster*. The point of long recitation of prayers such as the Rosary was to bring the devout closer to God so that the worshipper could feel united with the creator. Sometimes, this unity was expressed through taste, like the

Diptych with Maria Sole and the Devotion of the Rosary," in van Os, *Art of Devotion* (n. 62 above), 151–56.

FIG. 2.14.
Geertgen tot Sint Jans, Virgin in Glory Rotterdam, Boijmans Museum, (photo: Museum Boijmans Van Beuningen, Rotterdam)

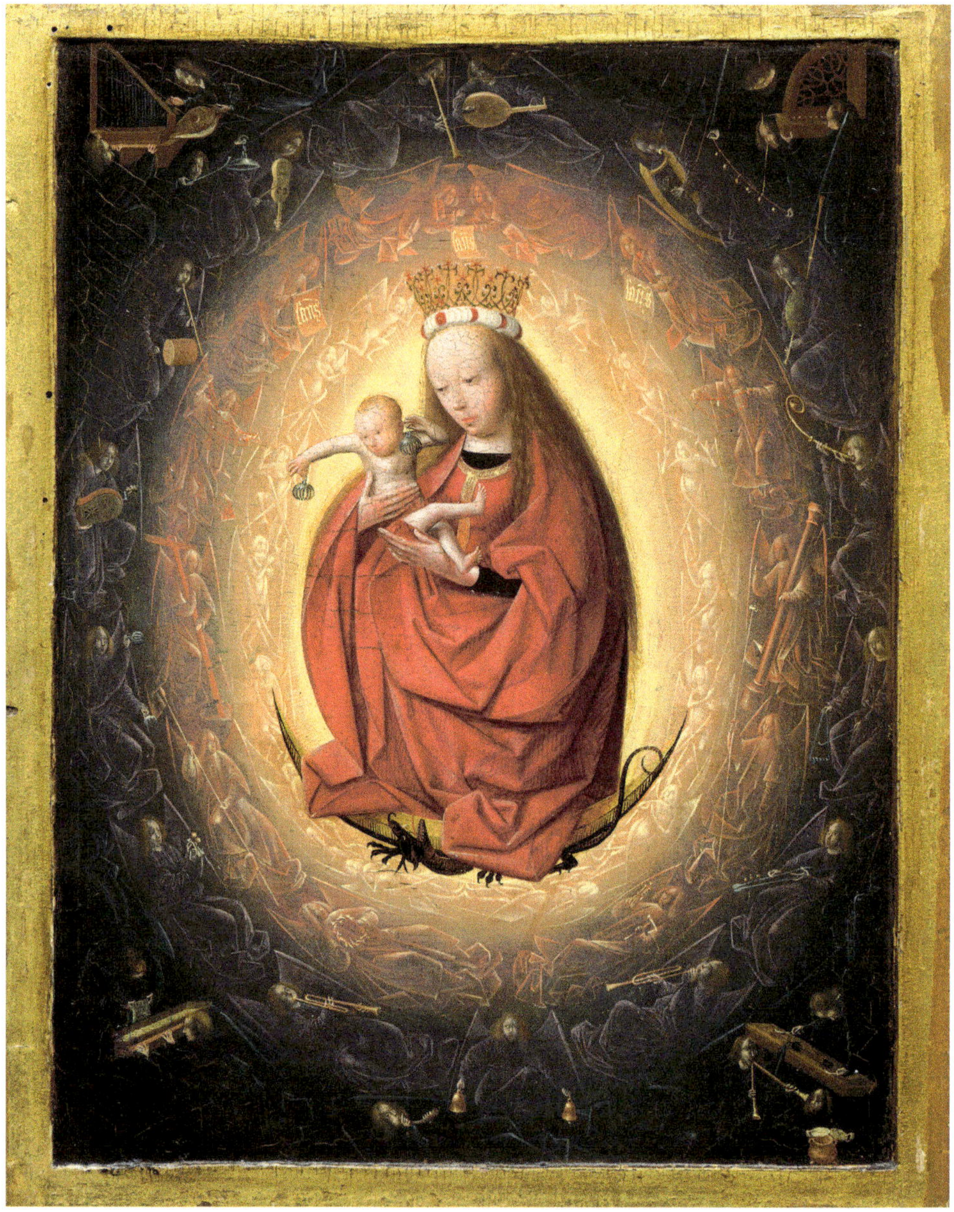

episode reported by Caesarius of Heisterbach mentioned earlier. In Geertgen's painting, it is music that manifests God's embrace. Music is here not a symbol of Divinity. It *re-presents* it by alluding to the sound that anyone would have experienced in the presence of God, like Mary Magdalene did during her ecstasy: "Every day at the seven canonical hours she was carried aloft by angels and her *bodily ears* heard the glorious chants of the celestial hosts."[80]

This is the sense of the little bells that decorate miniature cradles of the Baby Jesus. These objects, like the example at the Musée de Cluny in Paris were used as part of spiritual exercises by nuns and beguines, who as part of their devotion ministered to the Christ child and rocked his cradle. Often, these objects decorated altars during the period of Advent (fig. 2.15).[81] The bells would have rung every time the cradle moved, especially so when the baby was laid in it.

80 Jacobus de Voragine, *The Golden Legend: Readings on the Saints*, ed. and trans. W. G. Ryan (Princeton, NJ, 1993), 386.

81 See also V. Brilliant in Bagnoli, *Feast for the Senses* (n. 20 above), 175 no. 40; and Bynum, *Christian Materiality*, 62.

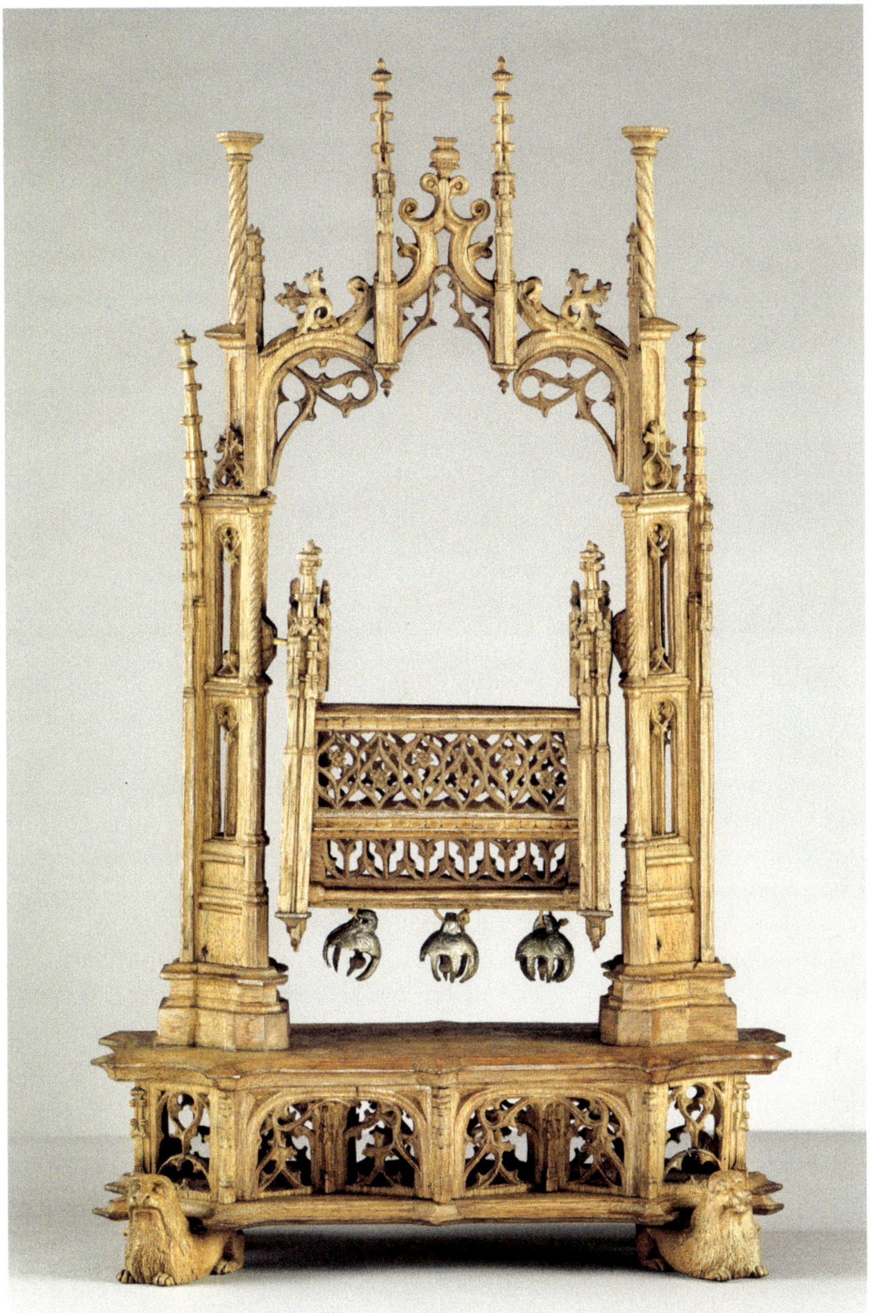

FIG. 2.15.
Cradle of Baby Jesus, Paris, Musée de Cluny, inv. no. Cl. 23607a (photo: RMN-Grand Palais)

These tinkling bells announced the presence of the divine in the baby Jesus, just like the sound of a bell at the moment of the consecration of the Eucharist announced (and announces) the presence of Christ in the host. These cradles are often shaped like Gothic churches, visually associating the cradle with the altar and the baby with the sacrificial host. Here, sound completes the picture presented by the physical object with a sensorial stimulus.

Immersive Environments

Many medieval objects have lost their sounds, which once were an important component of their meaning. It is hard to recapture the soundscape that completed the performance of medieval literary texts. Not only do we have no recording, we also function in a world where literature is neither heard, recited, or sung, but read silently. Many medieval texts, instead, included

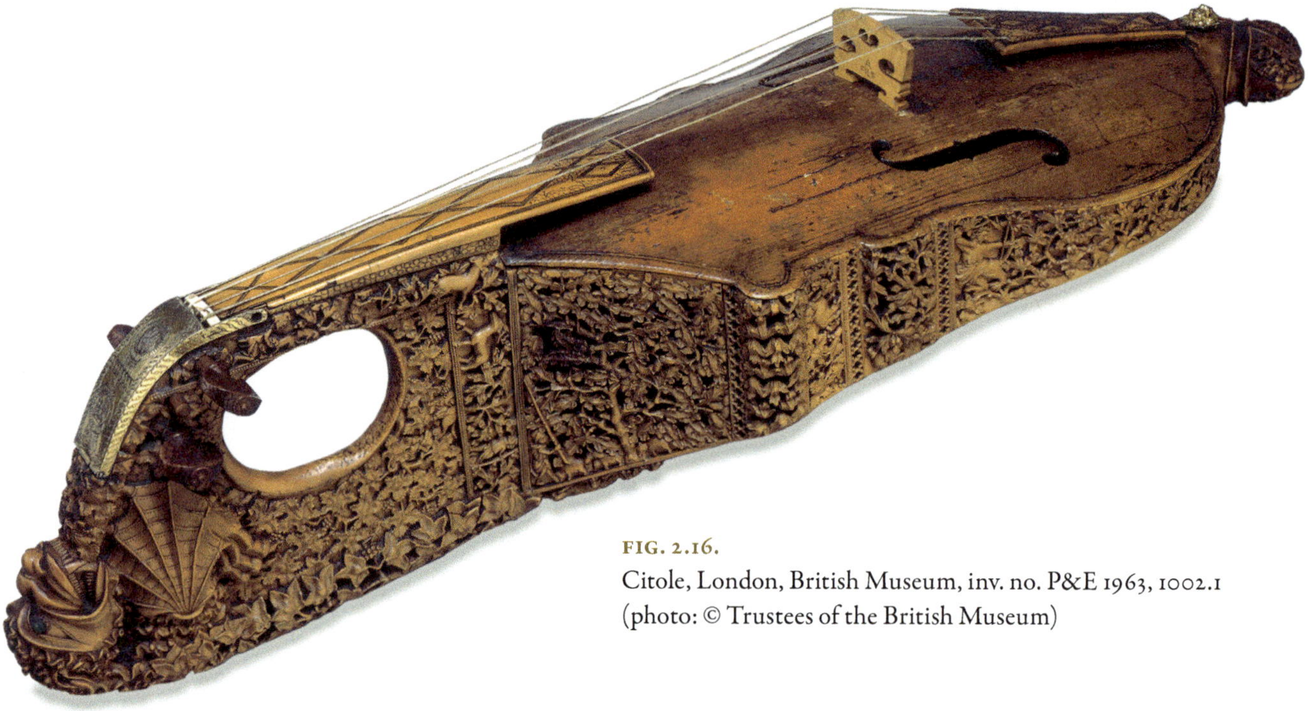

FIG. 2.16.
Citole, London, British Museum, inv. no. P&E 1963, 1002.1 (photo: © Trustees of the British Museum)

songs and poetry. To be sure, the interaction of sound, word, and image is a key component of medieval "reading." The Roman de Fauvel, a fourteenth-century satirical compilation combining romances, poems, songs, and images, is a good example of what is at stake here. In her study of this manuscript, Emma Dillon has demonstrated how musical notation is present not just as a guide for musical performances but also as a sensory gloss. In places where images are absent, music works to promote mental pictures. This is the case with the passage describing the army of virtues. On fols. 38v–39v, the fight of Virtues and Vices in the central column of the text is buttressed on each side by the columns of chants that ornament the image described by the text. For example, Virginité is accompanied by the *Adoremus dominum*, the first of a series of chants for the office of St. Agnes whose vita matches the story of Virginité. Where images are present, music promotes a counterpoint to the illustrations. This is demonstrated on fol. 42r, where the image of the fountain of youth—in which the evil progeny of Fauvel wash away old age and rejuvenate in perpetual youth—abuts a passage of liturgical music associated with baptism. Here the sounds of the chant *hic fons,* customary for the baptismal liturgy, establishes an inverted comparison with the pictured ablutions of Fauvel's tribe.

The same type of playful counterpoint is visible in the decoration of an early fourteenth-century citole at the British Museum (fig. 2.16). Instruments of this type were often used to accompany love ballads.[82] The side of this one is intricately carved with hunting scenes among a lush forest: hounds chase a beast of prey, a swineherd holds a pig while knocking acorns off a tree, hunters prepare to shoot their bows. This scene transmits a cacophony of barking, shouting, and howling at odds with the harmonious and sweet harmony of a love song, but conversely, in alignment with the poetic analogy of hunting and courtship, a common simile, for example, in Andrea Cappellanus's love manual.[83]

Sound counterpoints of this type are at work in liturgical books as well. This is the case for a fourteenth-century English psalter hours in the Walters Art Museum (fig. 2.17). In this book, the mock funeral of Reynard the Fox extends over the bottom margin of the *Hours of the Cross*

82 This object has been the subject of a recent monograph: *The British Museum Citole: New Perspectives*, ed. J. Robinson, K. Buehler-McWilliam, and N. Speakman (London, 2013).

83 Andreas Cappellanus, *The Art of Courtly Love*, ed. and trans. J. J. Parry (New York, 1960).

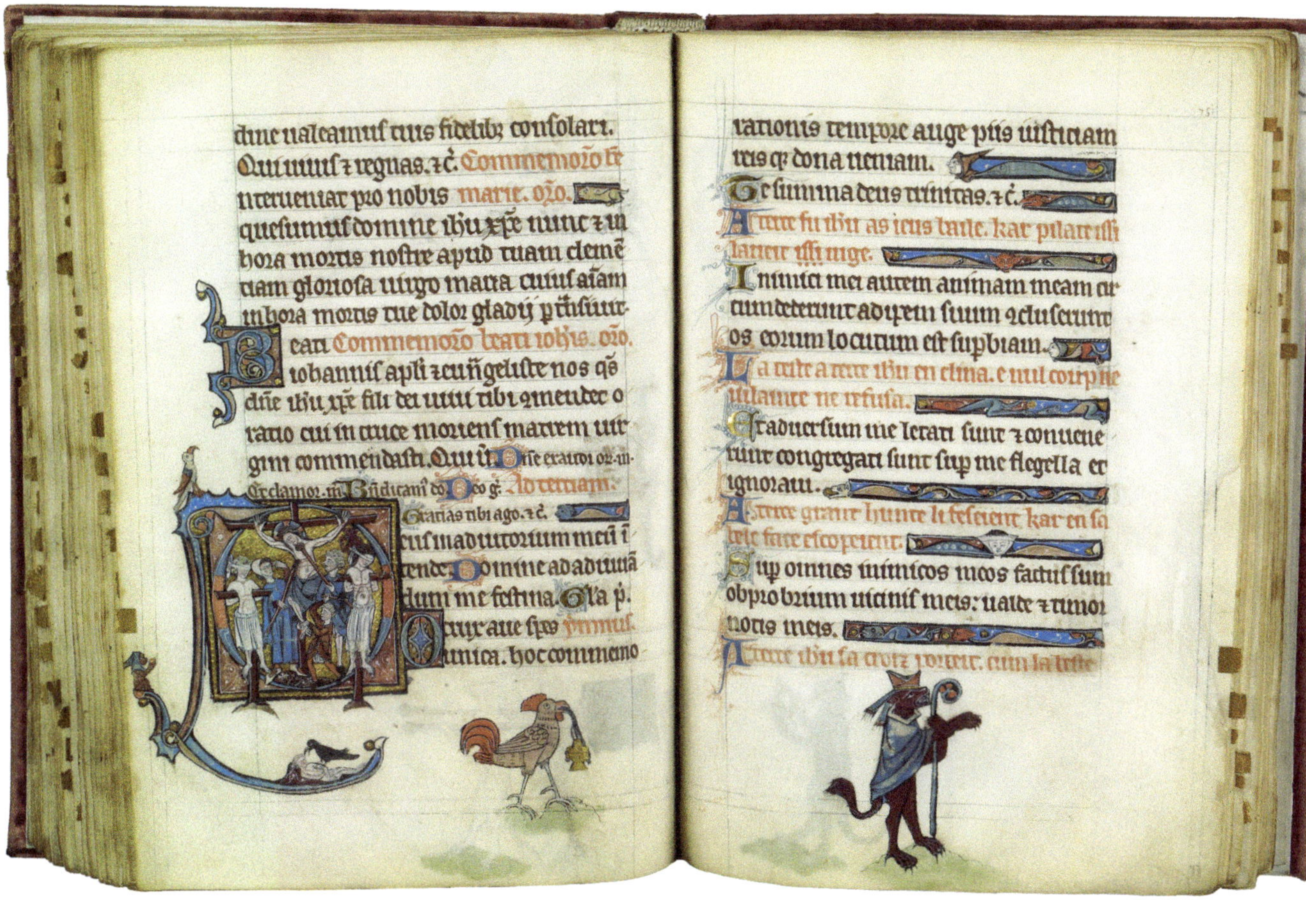

FIG. 2.17. Book of Hours, Baltimore, Walters Art Museum, MS. W.102 (photo: Walters Art Museum)

showing one animal playing one instrument on each page. Emma Dillon has argued that the spacing of the procession freezes the intended forward movement of the story by isolating each sound played by the animals all seemingly synchronized on the same upbeat tempo. The dissonance between spacing and musical tempo in the margin reflects the complex temporalities expressed by the prayers above, where images and texts create a back and forth movement between Old Testament time, New Testament time and the liturgical time of the interpreter/reader. The movement is actuated through layout, decoration and languages, as Latin psalm verses written in black ink are interwoven with old French couplets narrating the passion and written in red ink, both recited and sung by the reader. Reynard's single note parade binds past, present, and future in a continuous meditative choreography of the mind.

In W.102, it is the sound imagined that acts as a motor of exchange between different temporalities. In courtly ritual, the shift between reality and fiction, present circumstances and past events, was actuated through the creation of immersive environments. In the celebrated illustration of January in *Les Très Riches Heures du duc de Berry*, by the Limbourg brothers, the chivalric stories pictured on the tapestry seem to leave the walls to invade the banqueting hall, a marvelous rendition of the immersive environment of a princely banquet.[84] Some of the multimodal nature of this type of décor is echoed by the early Flemish tapestry with the story of Jourdain de Blaye, in the Museo Civico in Padua (fig. 2.18). The only surviving piece of a large set, the tapestry recounts the story of the orphan hero Jourdain de Blaye, who after many travails

84 Pol de Limbourg and Jean Colombe, *The* Très Riches Heures *of Jean, Duke of Berry*, introduction and legends by R. Cazelles and J. Longnon (New York, 1969); F. Autrand, P. D. Stirnemann, I. Villela-Petit, and E. Toulet, *Les Très Riches Heures du duc de Berry et l'enluminure en France au début du XV*^{e} *siècle* (Paris, 2004).

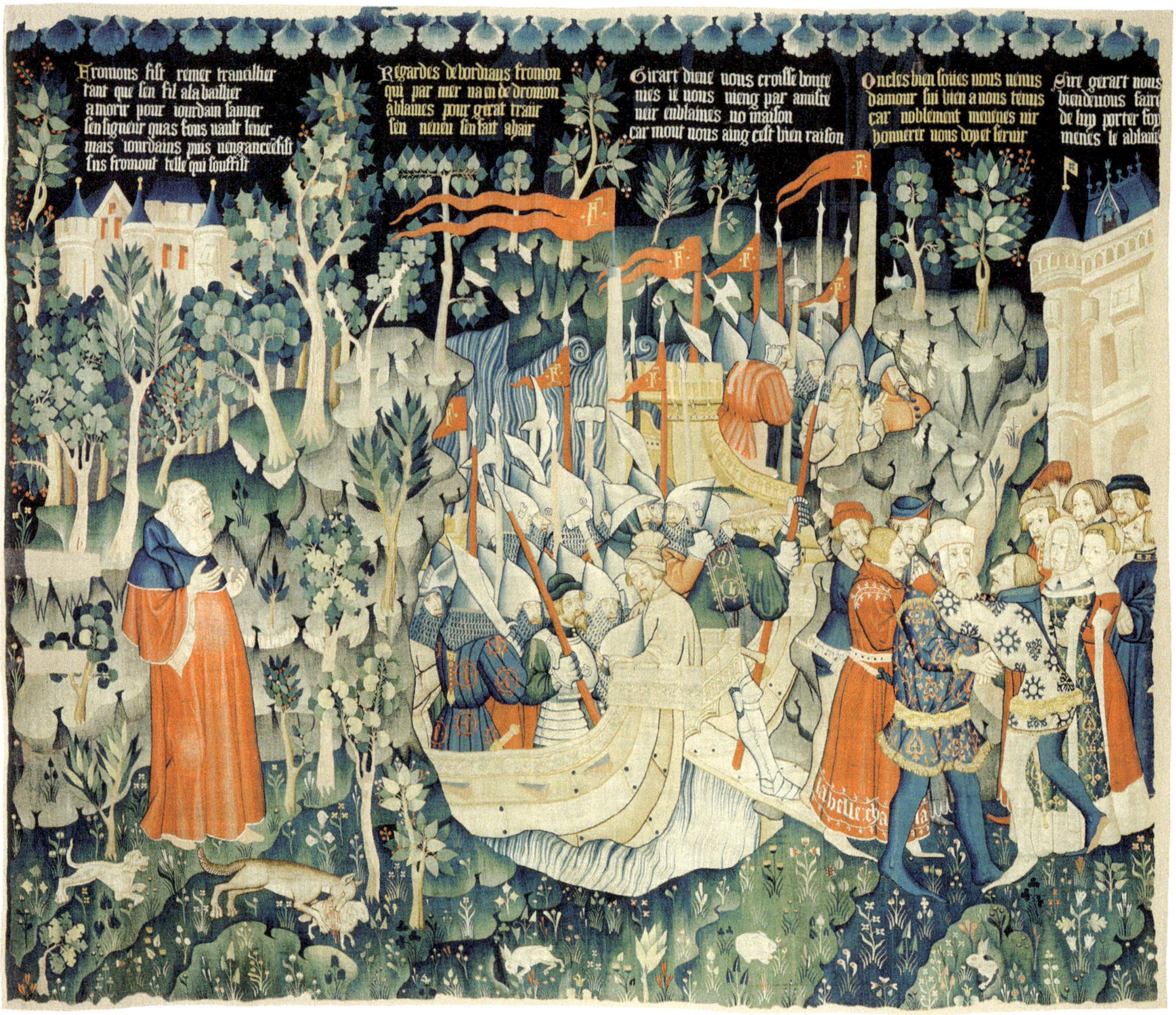
Fromons fist rener trancilhier
tant que sen fil ala baillier
a morir pour iourdain sauuer
sen signeur quas sous vault lever
mais iourdains puis vengance fist
sus fromont telle qui souffrist
Regardes de bordiaus fromon
qui par mer va en de dromon
ablaines pour gerat trair
sen neueu sen fait a hair
Girart dime vous croisse bonte
mes ie vous vieng par amistie
veir en blaines no maison
car mout vous aing cest bien raison
Oncles bien soiies vous venus
damour sui bien a vous tenus
car noblement menes mir
honnerer vous doy et servir
Sire gerart nous
bien deuons faire
de luy porter foy
menes le ablaine

FIG. 2.18. Padua, Museo Civico, tapestry of Jourdain de Blaye (photo: Ministero dei Beni e delle Attività Culturali e del Turismo)

prevailed over his evil uncle. In the tapestry, the story is summarized in the verses appearing at the top, as an aide-mémoire. It is also actively recited by the open-mouthed figure standing on the left, outside the story proper, representing the narrator in the text of the *chanson de geste*.[85] However, he could also symbolize the person who, on the occasion of festive events, would entertain guests at banquets by reciting similar poems. The figure situates the viewer between events of the past imaged on the tapestry and those acted out in the real world of the viewer. When heard in this way, the tapestry collapses the present with historical events in a continuous multimodal performance.

This same ideas underlie the image of the banquet organized by the king of France in honor of Charles IV, Holy Roman Emperor illustrated in the a fourteenth-century copy of the *Grandes Chroniques de France* (fig. 2.19).[86] To entertain the emperor, his nephew king Charles V of France staged a reenactment of the first crusade and the capture of Jerusalem. A ship transporting Peter the Hermit rolled before

85 *Jourdain de Blaye, Chanson de geste*, ed. P. F. Dembowski (Chicago and London, 1969).

86 MS. fr. 2813 fol. 473v. A. D. Hedeman, *The Royal Image: Illustrations of the "Grandes Chroniques de France," 1274–1422* (Berkeley, 1991), 128–38; Morrison and Hedeman, *Imagining* (n. 27 above), 181, no. 26.

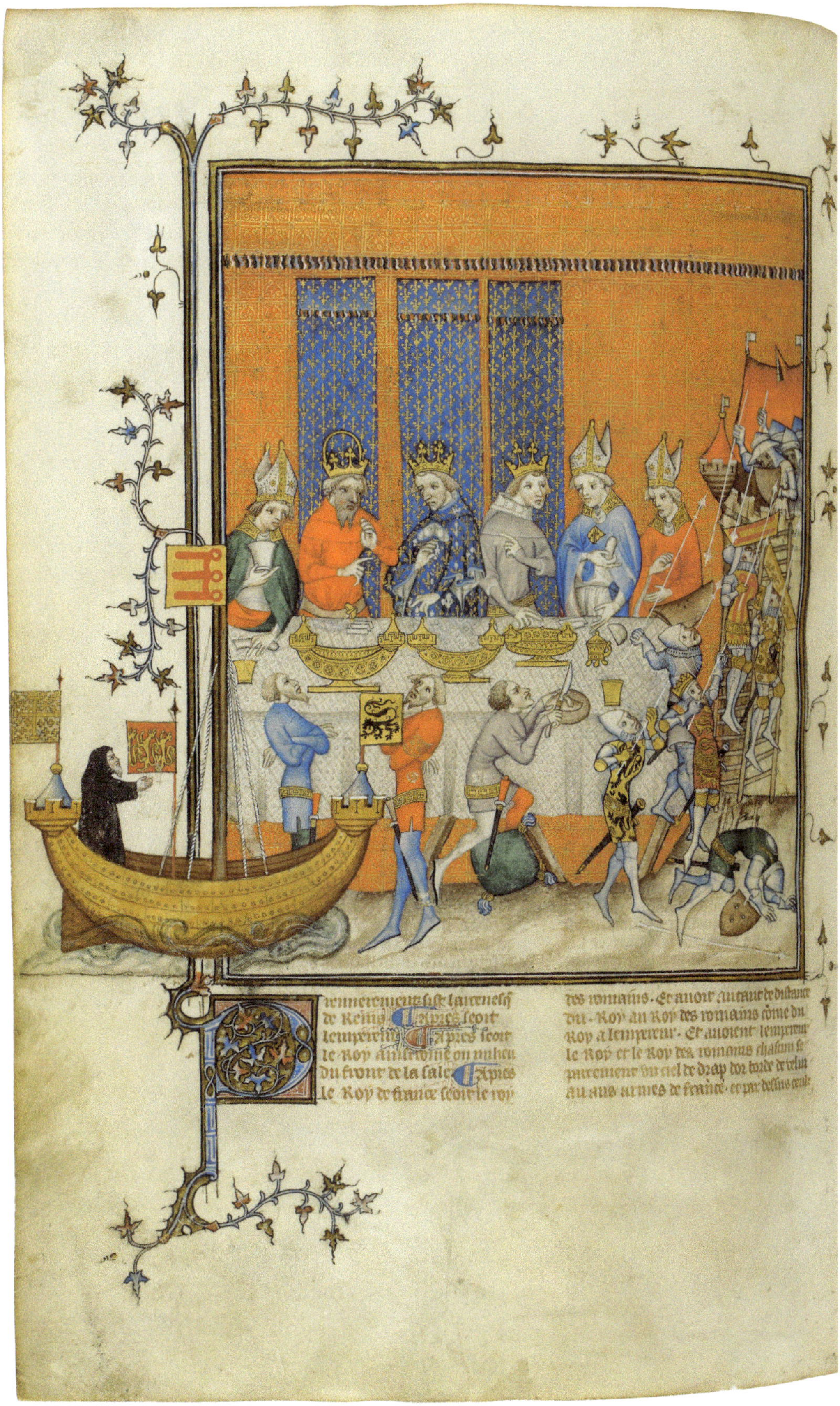

FIG. 2.19.
Grandes Chroniques de France, Paris, BnF MS. fr. 2813, fol. 473v (photo: Bibliothèque nationale de France)

the diners while an army of Christian knights engaged in combat with the army of the Saladin. As Anne Hedeman has argued, in the miniature, the coat of arms appearing on the soldiers scaling the wall of Jerusalem belong to the royal guests of the banquet, who are therefore actors and spectators at once. In addition, the crusader's ship, *nef* in French, recalls the golden nefs appearing on the table. These vessels were saltcellars, which would be positioned before distinguished individuals. One such example survives in the collection of the Metropolitan Museum of Art.[87] The Metropolitan Museum of Art saltcellar is small, as most of these containers were.[88] By considerably enlarging the size of the saltcellars on the table in front of the three rulers, the miniaturist of the *Grandes Chroniques* established a direct overlap between spectacle, décor, historical narrative, and present events. The oversized saltcellars draw attention also to another important point. A natural preservative, salt was paramount to keep food, meat in particular, from rotting. In Christian ritual it symbolized divine wisdom and was used in baptism, when it would be placed in the mouths of the catechumens so that they could receive "the salt of wisdom." Similarly in the New Testament, the apostles are compared to the "salt of the earth" (Matthew 5:13). Generally speaking, to be salted meant to be wise whereas the opposite meant to be foolish.[89] The three rulers of the *Grandes Chroniques* banquet are endowed with salt because they were tasty like their historical counterparts.

Shifting Sensory Perception

As the last example indicated, in courtly ritual, food and taste were important to create different levels of metaphorical associations. Medieval cuisine was one of metamorphosis and wonder and food served on the occasion of banquets rivaled the spectacles planned to entertain the guests.[90] Food matter was pounded, grated, and reassembled in fanciful shapes. Cooked animals were put back together as hybrid creatures or covered anew with their original furs or feathers to make them look alive. A delicacy of the day, the entrails of venison were often recreated with dried fruits and nuts and shaped to emulate the actual organs. Diners were offered calf cooked in its skin with an attached silver horn to make it look like a unicorn.[91] Recipes abound that teach how to reinstate the feathers and beak of a peacock after it had been roasted. The transformation of a cooked meal into a live creature was epitomized by the trick of serving a lidded breadbasket containing live birds, which would fly away as soon as the lid was opened. Sauces of different colors and taste transformed any course into a feast for the eyes and the mouth. At banquets, table appearances were deceiving, taste was misleading, and transformation celebrated.

Objects too were part of this culture of wonder. Centerpieces made with fossilized sharks' teeth were a valued antidote to poisons. One such example, dating from the mid-fifteenth century in the collection of the Kunsthistorisches Museum in Vienna, presents a bouquet of fossils sprouting from a silver gilt base.[92] The fossils were understood to be adders' tongues, which, it was believed, would react to poison by sweating. The inanimate tongues would thus taste perilous food and would come alive to warn the diners should the need arise. At times, objects could produce sounds. A goblet of Mongolian origin in

87 W. D. Wixom, ed., *Mirror of the Medieval World* (New York, 1999), cat. no. 125.

88 See for example that in the collection of the Walters Art Museum, 54.2501: R. Randall, "A Medieval Puzzle," *Walters Art Gallery Bulletin* 27, no. 3 (1975): 1–3 and that at the Louvre, inv. no. MR 119, which measures only 10 cm in height: D. Alcouffe, *Les Gemmes de la Couronne* (Paris, 2001), 179–80.

89 See on this J. E. Latham, *The Religious Symbolism of Salt* (Paris, 1982).

90 Cosman, *Fabulous Feasts* (n. 60 above); T. Scully, *The Art of Cookery in the Middle Ages* (Woodbridge, Suffolk, 1995); C. Benporat, *Cucina italiana del Quattrocento* (Florence, 1996); C. Napoletano, *The Neapolitan Recipe Collection*, ed. T. Scully (Ann Harbor, 2000); J. Bridgeman and A. Griffiths, *A Renaissance Wedding: The Celebrations at Pesaro for the Marriage of Costanzo Sforza & Camilla Marzano D'aragona, 26–30 May 1475* (London, 2013).

91 This was the case of the marriage of the Sforza d'Aragona wedding at Pesaro in 1475. Bridgeman and Griffiths, *Renaissance Wedding*, 40.

92 T. Freller, "Lingue di serpi, Natternzungen und Glossopetrae: Streiflichter auf die Geschichte einer populären kultischen Medizin der frühen Neuzeit," *Sudhoffs Archiv* 81, no. 1 (1997): 62–83; M. Leithe-Jasper, "Decorative Arts," in *Kunst Historisches Museum Vienna: Guide to the Collections* (Vienna, 1988), 137; C. Duffin, "Natternzungen-Kredenz: Tableware for the Renaissance Nobility," in *Jewelry History Today* 14 (2014): 3–5.

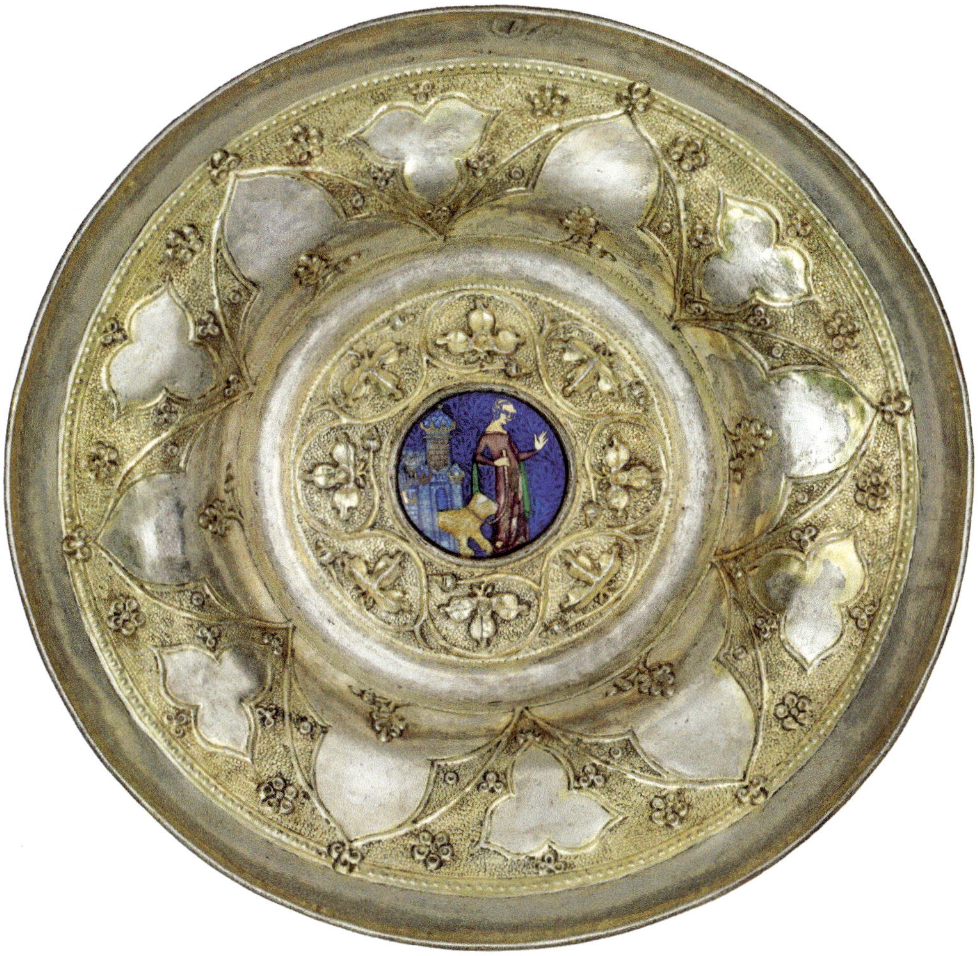

FIG. 2.20.
Hanap with Lady and lion, London, Victoria and Albert Museum, inv. no. 107-1865 (photo: Victoria and Albert Museum, London)

the treasury of St. Maurice, Switzerland, has a lid with a sphere surrounded by snakes.[93] The sphere contains a mechanism that produces a "song" at every movement. It is very tempting to think that this cup, which, since the sixteenth century serves as a reliquary, did at one point grace the table of some noble lord, where it would have awed guests with its voice. Other vessels demonstrate the enjoyment of this type of magic. Many fourteenth-century drinking cups have bottoms decorated with medallions in translucent enamels, like the hanap now in the collection of the Victoria and Albert Museum decorated with a medallion showing an elegant lady leading a lion on a leash (fig. 2.20).[94] The lady with the lion is probably a reference to Richard of Fournival's *Le Bestiaire d'amour*. In this text, the author discusses love as a lion, which attacks only when looked in the eyes. In the same way, love has the power to leave a man senseless only if he looks at the object of his desire.[95] The cup decoration would appear and disappear according to the amount of liquid in it. The enamels were fully visible when the cup was empty, invisible when it was full. The cup plays a game of hide-and-seek

93 E. Antoine-König, *Le Trésor de l'abbaye de Saint-Maurice d'Agaune* (Paris, 2014), 26, 100–102.

94 London, Victoria and Albert Museum, inv. no. 107-1865 (ca. 1340). R. W. Lightbown, *French Silver* (London, 1978), no. 7, p. 13, illustrated; D. Gaborit-Chopin and E. Taburet-Delahaye, *Objets d'art du Moyen Âge* (Paris, 1981), nos. 127–28, 242–45; C. Oman, "A Mysterious Hoard of Early French Silver," *Pantheon* 19 (March 1961): 82–87; R. W. Lightbown, *Secular Goldsmiths' Work in Medieval France: A History* (London, 1978), pl. VI; C. Descatoire, *Treasures of the Black Death* (London, 2009), no. 14, pp. 70–71.

95 C. Hippeau, ed., *Le Bestiaire d'amour par Richard de Fournival, suivi de la Réponse de la dame* (Paris, 1860), 12–13. See also J. M. A. Beer, *Beasts of Love: Richard de Fournival's* Bestiaire d'amour *and a Woman's* Response (Toronto, 2003).

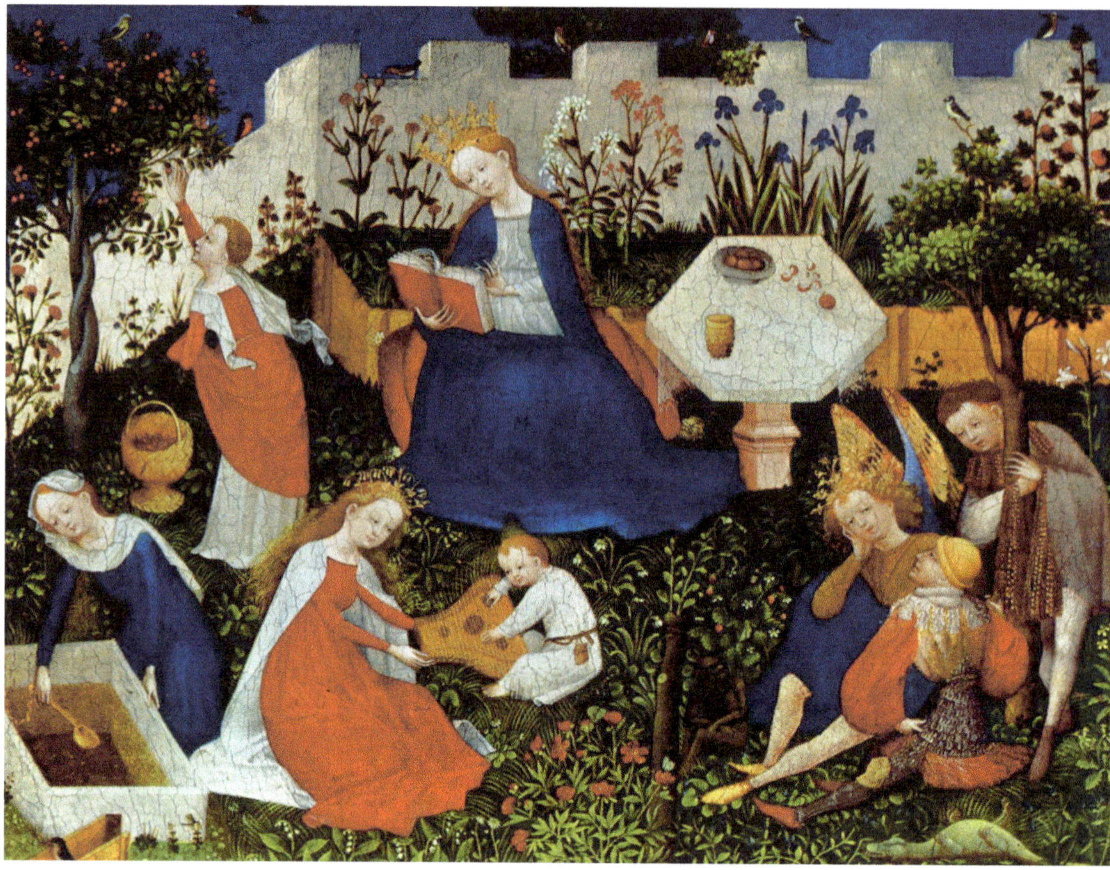

FIG. 2.21. Frankfurt, Staedl Galerie, Paradiesgärtlein (photo: The Yorck Project: 10.000 Meisterwerke der Malerei. DVD-ROM, 2002, ISBN 3936122202, distr. Directmedia Publishing GmbH via Wikimedia Commons)

that enhances the meaning of the images by impairing sensation.

The use of materials to confound was not limited to the banquet hall but it is truly a hallmark of the art of the period. A consideration of the technical advances achieved at this time shows a desire to push the limit of materials to transform one thing into another. Painters embraced grisaille, which transferred the hard shine of cameos to the pages of illuminated manuscripts. Painted enamels that assimilated metalwork with paintings began to appear at this time. Metalwork was decorated with designs in dotted chasing that appeared and disappeared according to lighting conditions. In embroidery, the introduction of split stitching made seamless directional change easier and thus enhanced modeling and the description of volumes. The same techniques that in earlier times had been used as a proud assertion of the materiality of images and the distinction among different crafts were now used to trick sensory perception and transform one thing into another: glass into paint, silk into flesh.

This culture of metamorphosis is helpful to put in context the ambiguity of some late medieval representations, like the Frankfurt Paradiesgärtlein (fig. 2.21). The painting depicts the Virgin and Child within a *hortus conclusus* luxuriant with flowers and fruit trees.[96] The Virgin and Child are accompanied by a number of saints: Dorothea to the left picking cherries from a tree, Barbara next to the well, Catherine holding a psalterium for the baby Jesus to play. On the right, St. George sits under a tree next to the archangel Michael. However, none of the saints have halos. Nor do they have visible attributes. Dorothea and Barbara could also be handmaidens picking fruits and fetching water. The

96 The painting is dated to around 1400 and is by an anonymous Rheinish master. See B. Brinkmann and J. Sander, *Deutsche Gemälde vor 1800 in bedeutenden Sammlungen: Illustriertes Gesamtverzeichnis*, ed. G. Holland (Frankfurt, 1999), with further bibliography; H. Keazor, "Manu et Voce: Ikonographische Notizen zum Frankfurter Paradiesgärtlein," in *Opere e giorni: Studi su mille anni d'arte europea; Dedicati a Max Seidel*, ed. K. Bergdol and G. Bonsanti (Venezia, 2001), 231–40.

Virgin herself leafs intently through a big volume, her head decorated with a chapelet, the crown of fresh flowers, common as a gift between lovers. Is this the garden of Eden or a love garden? It is difficult to say and perhaps pointless to try, since both ideas draw upon each other and are based on the same premise: the garden as the deputed place of sensation, where the smell of flowers, the taste of fruits and the sound of water make it possible to contemplate God or fall in love.[97] It is not a matter of choosing between different meanings but rather reconciling them.

The shifting boundaries between sacred and profane are attested by the migration of sacred themes into secular contexts. Emblematic of this phenomenon is the polyvalent nature of Christian symbols like the pelican in its piety, a traditional symbol of Christ's passion, which in Richard of Fournival's *Bestiaire d'amour* becomes a symbol of the power of Love to kill and restore all hopes.[98] This must be the sense of a pelican tearing its flesh represented atop a couple exchanging love promises in a fourteenth-century ivory leaf.[99]

97 For a comprehensive survey of the polyvalent nature of gardens in medieval art see E. Antoine, *Sur la terre comme au ciel: Jardins d'Occident à la fin du Moyen Âge,* exhibition catalogue, Paris, Musée national du Moyen Âge, Thermes de Cluny, 6 Juin–16 Septembre 2002 (Paris, 2002).

98 Richard of Fournival, *Bestiaire*, 30–31.

99 The ivory was part of a recent exhibition at the London dealer Sam Fogg. The pelican appeared also at the top of the fountain dispensing hippocras (a sweet wine) at the wedding of Margaret of York and Charles the Bold of Burgundy in 1468 and is mentioned by Olivier de La Marche, *Mémoires d'Olivier de La Marche*, ed. H. Beaune and J. D'Arbaumont, 4 vols. (Paris, 1883–88), 4:104: "Et devez sçavoir aussi qu'en ladicte court estoit ung pellican moult riche qui par la poitrine jectoit ypocras." Here the Christian theme is reinforced by the wine. On fountains in late medieval courtly culture see K. Oschema, "Liquid Splendour—Table Fountains and Wine-Fountains at the Burgundian Courts," in *Staging the Court of Burgundy: Proceedings of the Conference "The Splendour of Burgundy,"* ed. W. Blockmans, T.-H. Borchert, N. Gabriëls, J. Oosterman, and A. van Oosterwijk (London, 2013), 133–40.

Body and Soul

The blurring of the sacred and profane epitomized by the examples above is emblematic of the religious and philosophical changes that transformed late medieval society. On one hand, the focus on the humanity of Christ resulted in the celebration of sensation to experience his divinity. On the other, the rediscovery of Aristotle prompted a revision of the role of sense perception in intellectual abstraction and spiritual enlightenment. As a result a process of alignment between the sphere of the body and that of the soul began. The existence of miscellanies for lay readership combining a variety of texts ranging from *Chansons de gestes*, to medical disquisitions, to history, to collection of prayers embodies this idea.[100] An exploration of the senses in medieval art, therefore, forces us to consider the theoretical with the experiential, the sacred with the secular, and it must account for the ambivalence that ensued. Sense refinement, sober demeanor, and good looks were the attributes of noble knights and just rulers but also a mark of distinction for bishops and monks. Living sinful rulers exuded the stench of rotten flesh, whereas dead saints smelled of roses. Blindness was not only a physical ailment but also the sign of moral affliction. A fragrant enclosed garden served as the symbol of the Virgin Mary, but equally as the privileged site of gallant encounters. The art of this period responded to the renewed awareness of the physical world with works that materialized sensation to create a multisensory response that spoke to the body and through the body and that was not necessarily intended for spiritual enlightenment alone.[101]

100 This is the case of the already cited manuscripts in the British Library (MS. Harley 273) and Cambridge University Library (G G 1.1).

101 For a discussion of pleasure and beauty in medieval art M. J. Carruthers, *The Experience of Beauty in the Middle Ages* (Oxford, 2013).

I wish to thank Peter Parshall for sharing his wisdom. His comments, insights and suggestions have been very valuable throughout this project. I am also grateful to the anonymous readers for their comments. The research for this article was part of the work leading to the exhibition at the Walters Art Museum (16 October 2016–8 January 2017).

Hearing

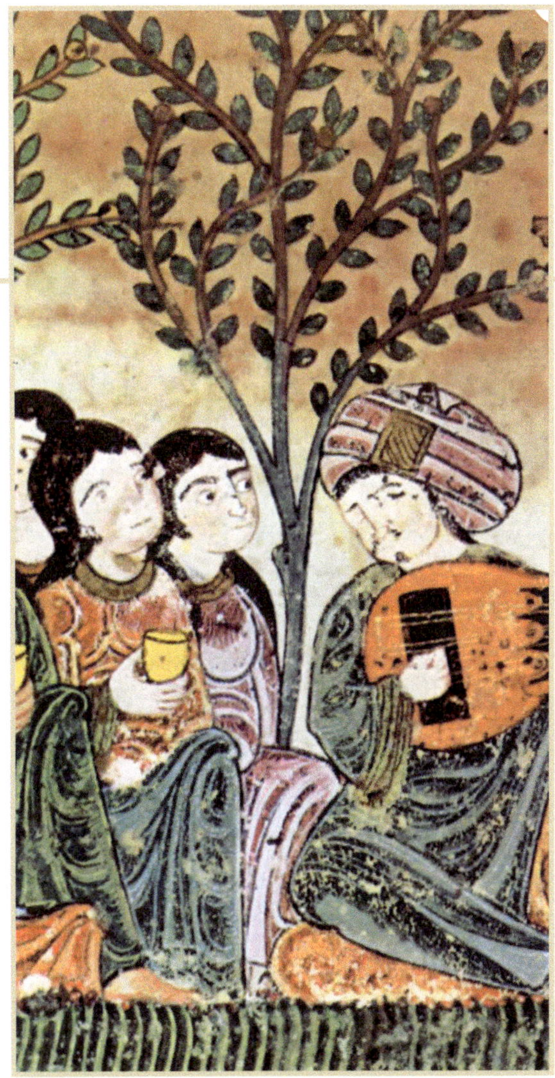

CHAPTER THREE

Perceptions of Sound and Sonic Environments across the Byzantine Acoustic Horizon

AMY PAPALEXANDROU

The Byzantines, like us, were profoundly affected by sound and the psychological dimension engendered by all sonic phenomena. The premodern ear was, after all, the same as our own in terms of its physiology, and despite the substantial increase in overall noise levels since the beginning of the Industrial Age and the gradual mechanization of our soundscapes, we can understand that the auditory sense was a central feature of human experience for the Byzantines just as it is today.[1] As with vision and visuality, a topic of primary importance to Byzantine Studies in recent decades, the importance of sound and hearing as vital signs of the Byzantines have become apparent.[2] And while membership in a world that postdates the Enlightenment and the scientific revolution means that we can hope for little more than partial knowledge of the past, especially concerning the mostly intangible world of sound, it is time to attempt a reconstruction or at least an understanding of whatever aspects of this auditory culture are still accessible, even if only in some small measure. By doing this we may embrace a broader, more engaging, and more textured relationship with the Byzantines. Without the consideration of sound, we have essentially envisioned Byzantine society (to use a modern example) as an old film wherein characters navigate a succession of interesting experiences across an array of scenes—in black and white, and in complete silence. In the process of watching we learn a great deal about them: their actions, their thoughts, and the details of their appearance. We imagine them to speak through inscription-like subtitles. And like the dramatic piano roll in a Charlie Chaplin film, an astounding repertoire of musical accompaniment exists in the form of Byzantine chanted music. But, as of yet we have not dared to flesh out the missing acoustics and render these silent films into talkies, rich with the auditory intensity of stereophonic or even surround sound. The study and reconstruction of this sense offers another platform for analysis, a different bridge for understanding the multiple layers of experience of individuals and groups in Byzantium.

It is, then, instructive to begin with the voice of a notable cleric of the late twelfth century who left us a fascinating account of sounds (and events) as experienced in Thessalonike following the

1 On early mechanization and its effect see especially B. R. Smith, *The Acoustic World of Early Modern England* (Chicago, 1999) and M. McLuhan, *The Gutenberg Galaxy: The Making of Typographic Man* (Toronto, 1962).

2 This has been eloquently discussed in R. S. Nelson, "Descartes's Cow and Other Domestications of the Visual," in *Visuality Before and Beyond the Renaissance*, ed. R. S. Nelson (Cambridge and New York, 2000), 1–21 but especially 1–3 on the many reasons for attending to the visual and, by extension, to the aural/auditory.

Norman sack in 1185. I am speaking of the bishop Eustathios, whose *Capture of Thessalonike* documents and recreates not only the extreme duress of a population in captivity but also the attitudes of captive and captor, the collision of cultural mores, and the vital importance—largely overlooked in scholarly literature—of sound as experienced by individuals of the Eastern Roman Empire.[3] Eustathios's interpretation of events may be biased, but it is nonetheless valuable as an example of the serious and often elaborate attention paid to sound in late antique and Byzantine writings of all kinds. Eustathios informs us that the western invaders forbade the Greeks to sing their hymns in church, and that they (the invaders) would routinely "burst in with the purpose of ruining these sacred sounds, babbling and shrieking in their accustomed fashion, intending to interrupt the progress of the beautiful ritual."[4] Further, Eustathios complains that the Latins "competed with their shouting in opposition to our reading of the holy Gospels, disturbing good order and destroying holy harmony."[5] Sound, according to the bishop, could be used as a weapon. It served as an example, one that created for his readers a sound image with which to reimagine the graphic events of the time. It also underscored the church as an arena wherein the delicate dimension of sound played a crucial role in the lives of ordinary citizens even as it was an element of suspicion and a tool for intimidation in the hands of outsiders.

In what follows, I consider a series of questions that may be unanswerable but potentially worth asking. Is it possible, on some level, to access the vast auditory repertoire of sounds that comprised the soundscape of the Eastern Roman Empire?[6] How were individuals affected by sound, and how did they harness its power? In what ways did they mitigate, modify, or accentuate their environment to accommodate sonic dimensions both real and imagined? How compelling was sound compared to vision? These are difficult questions, of course, because of the obvious barriers. On the one hand sound is so frustratingly ethereal; on the other, there is the thick, impenetrable layer of separation between our own, hyper-mechanized acoustic horizon and the remote and much quieter hubbub of the middle ages.[7] Presumably these obstacles account for the fact that very few components of the Byzantine soundscape have become part of our scholarly dialogue. Exceptions to this are few. There is the chanted music of the church, of course, that traditionally emerges in the literature as the most important category of sound. Of this the

3 Eustathios of Thessalonike, *The Capture of Thessaloniki*, trans. J. R. Melville Jones (Canberra, 1988), the basis of the English translations I have quoted from this work. The aural effects of this work, and the notion therein of "sound pictures," have been briefly commented on by A. F. Stone, "Aurality in the Panegyrics of Eustathios of Thessaloniki," in *Theatron: Rhetorical Culture in Late Antiquity and the Middle Ages*, ed. M. Grünbart (Berlin, 2007), 417–28.

4 Eustathios, *Capture of Thessaloniki*, 134–35, section 121.

5 Ibid., 126–27, section 115.

6 The term "soundscape" was coined by R. M. Schafer in his groundbreaking and still influential study, *The Tuning of the World* (New York, 1977), republished as *The Soundscape: Our Sonic Environment and the Tuning of the World* (Rochester, VT, 1994). My research interests have been focused on issues of sound since 2009, this as a logical offshoot from a related interest in orality. I am grateful for the many enthusiastic responses and suggestions following an initial paper given at the Byzantine Studies Conference in Philadelphia in 2010: A. Papalexandrou, "The Past Is Noise: Architectural Contexts and the Soundways of Byzantium," 36th Annual Byzantine Studies Conference, University of Pennsylvania, Philadelphia, 8–10 October, 2010, *Abstracts of Papers*, 119–20. Likewise I benefited from many stimulating conversations following the delivery of an earlier version of this paper at the Dumbarton Oaks Spring Symposium on the Senses in May 2014.

7 The sources on sound in antiquity, the middle ages and early modernity, many of which I have used and benefited from, have multiplied exponentially in recent years. Important for me have been Smith, *Acoustic World* (n. 1 above); I. Reznikoff, "The Evidence of the Use of Sound Resonance from Palaeolithic to Medieval Times," in *Archaeoacoustics*, ed. C. Scarre and G. Lawson, McDonald Institute for Archaeological Research (Cambridge, 2006), 77–84; M. Bettini, *Voci: Antropologia sonora del mondo antico* (Turin, 2008). For the late antique and Byzantine period the senses in general have gained greater prominence through the work of S. A. Harvey, *Scenting Salvation: Ancient Christianity and the Olfactory Imagination* (Los Angeles, 2006). Her work has done much to place the liturgy within the context of multisensory experience. A number of scholars have alerted us to the overwhelming sensory experience of the great church of Hagia Sophia in Constantinople, most recently N. Schibille, *Hagia Sophia and the Byzantine Aesthetic Experience* (Farnham, Surrey, and Burlington, VT, 2014) with emphasis, however, on the visual and not the auditory aspects of the building. B. Pentcheva has brought us more directly into the sonic realm of the church in "Hagia Sophia and Multisensory Aesthetics," *Gesta* 50, no. 2 (2011): 93–111, utilizing especially the work of a very early pioneer, often forgotten nowadays, W. R. Lethaby, in his fine essay "On Pavements Like the Sea," in *Architecture, Mysticism and Myth* (1892; repr. New York, 2004).

medieval sources are very clear: Byzantine chant was second only to angelic choirs and was considered to be a reflection of the divine order.[8] It was highly regarded by the Byzantines themselves and has been exceedingly well researched in our own time.[9] Issues of orality have also surfaced as an important area of research, especially in the realm of theatra.[10] But what of those sounds that formed part of the average, day-to-day experience of individuals? Are these accessible? And if so, what do they tell us? Can we reconstruct aspects of Byzantine daily life through sound?[11] This opens up the larger conversation on sound—of all kinds, human and nonhuman—that has yet to be fully embraced. While we have produced some interesting sound bites, we lack a rigorous sonic anthropology of the Byzantine world.

The lack of a dedicated scholarly tradition renders a reconstruction of the Byzantine soundscape difficult, but not impossible. We should not underestimate the ability of primary sources to reveal these more obscure elements of the culture. Indeed once we start looking, we begin to discover a roaring river of sources that are poised to open up and expand the possibilities of research. Many individuals recorded their impressions, even if only in fragments, and these informants are worth listening to. In my research I draw from a variety of sources including saints' *vitae*, philosophical and pseudoscientific writings, letters, ekphraseis, inscriptions, historical accounts, divinatory manuals, and so forth.[12] Many sources demonstrate that in all contexts the Byzantines actively attended to hearing as an

8 Literary sources abound. R. Dubowchik, "Singing with the Angels: Foundation Documents as Evidence for Musical Life in Monasteries of the Byzantine Empire," *DOP* 56 (2002): 277–96, offers a most valuable collection of references and explains the underlying spirit and meaning of the angelic topoi as well as clarifying many aspects of the role of liturgical music in Byzantine lives and day to day activities.

9 To name just two from the sea of possibilities: A. Lingas, "From Earth to Heaven: The Changing Musical Soundscape of Byzantine Liturgy," in *Experiencing Byzantium: Papers from the 44th Spring Symposium of the Society for the Promotion of Byzantine Studies*, ed. C. Nesbitt and M. Jackson (Aldershot, 2013), 311–58; J. Raasted, "Byzantine Liturgical Music and Its Meaning for the Byzantine Worshipper," in *Church and People in Byzantium: Society for the Promotion of Byzantine Studies Twentieth Spring Symposium of Byzantine Studies, Manchester*, ed. R. Morris (Birmingham, n.d.), 49–57. See also the next chapter, by Antonopoulos.

10 See the seminal publications of Elizabeth and Michael Jeffreys, conveniently summarized in E. Jeffreys, "Medieval Greek Epic Poetry," in *Medieval Oral Literature*, ed. K. Reichl (Berlin, 2012), 459–84. Interest in theatra and orality is now represented by a bounty of recent work, for example, the collection of studies in Grünbart, *Theatron*. My own thinking about orality, as part of an overall context combining voiced text and architecture, is exemplified in A. Papalexandrou, "Echoes of Orality in the Monumental Inscriptions of Byzantium," in *Art & Text in Byzantine Culture*, ed. L. James (Cambridge, 2007), 161–87.

11 There is much to do regarding sound in the realm of Byzantine material culture and archaeoacoustics. Models will certainly include the stimulating work of C. Witmore, "Vision, Media, Noise and the Percolation of Time: Symmetrical Approaches to the Mediation of the Material World," *Journal of Material Culture* 11 (2006): 267–92. See now also S. Mills, *Auditory Archeology: Understanding Sound and Hearing in the Past* (Walnut Creek, CA, 2014) with emphasis given to the important Neolithic site of Çatal Höyük. Byzantine archaeoacoustics emerge slowly, but the recent work of an interdisciplinary team of archaeologists, art and architectural historians (myself included), musicologists, and acoustic engineers recently involved in measuring and analyzing the acoustic properties of selected Byzantine churches in Greece was promising. Supported by a UCLA OVCR-COR Transdisciplinary Seed Grant, a season of fieldwork in June 2014 allowed us to conduct acoustical testing and document chanted performances in eight churches in Thessalonike. We are grateful to the Ministry of Culture of Greece and Archbishop Anthemos of Thessalonike for permission to undertake this documentary work. Our team members during this time included S. Gerstel, C. Kyriakakis, S. Antonopoulos, J. Donahue, K. Raptis, myself, and a superb cadre of chanters, most notably Demos Papatzalakis and Nektarios Antoniou, who sang for us under the direction of Spiros Antonopoulos. The project is briefly summarized in "Of Bodies and Spirits: Soundscapes of Byzantine Thessaloniki," *Forty-first Annual Byzantine Studies Conference, New York City, October 22–25, 2015, Abstracts of Papers*, 103.

12 Various forms of popular music, such as work songs, lullabies, and lament, remain desiderata. The disappointing lack of evidence from the Byzantine period renders the study of this allusive material difficult at best: R. Beaton, "Modes and Roads: Factors of Change and Continuity in Greek Musical Tradition," *BSA* 75 (1980): 1–11; M. Leiwo and R. P. Pennanen, "Byzantine Secular Music—Fact or Fiction?" *Acta Byzantina Fennica* 8 (1997): 37–51. We are on slightly surer footing for the early period, where John Chrysostom took an anthropological approach. See J. C. B. Petropoulos, "The Church Father as Social Informant: St. John Chrysostom on Folk-Songs," *Studia Patristica* 22, no. 1 (1989): 159–64. Ancient and modern sources are much more accessible thanks to the work of M. Alexiou, *After Antiquity: Greek Language, Myth, and Metaphor* (Ithaca, NY, and London, 2002) and eadem, *The Ritual Lament in Greek Tradition*, rev. D. Yatromanolakis and P. Roilos (Oxford, 2002); and now A. Karanika, *Voices at Work: Women, Performance, and Labor in Ancient Greece* (Baltimore, 2014) on work songs in antiquity. P. Roilos notes Eustathios of Thessalonike's complaints about his colleagues in the twelfth century, for they did not care to report on the everyday, popular songs that we now miss so much: "Oral Literature, Ritual, and the Dialectics of Performance," in *Medieval Oral Literature*, ed. K. Reichl (2012), 225–52.

element of the human condition requiring special consideration. This seems to be true whether we are talking about the creation of performative environments, manifestations of power, the establishment of networks of control, the attention given to scientific phenomena, and so on. And of course it is true at the microlevel of the individual, where sound bears an emotional force that can be overwhelming. The Byzantine appreciation for and reaction to sound is inherently relatable—a common bond, perhaps, across the great divide of time.

As part of my work I have felt it important to recover evidence concerning perceptions of sound from the realm of the common individual as well as the elite. The former is obviously difficult since it is underrepresented in Byzantine literature, and here theoretical models become important to flesh out the hidden possibilities of the more fragmented Byzantine texts. Scholars such as Constance Classen and Mark Smith, whose methodologies for working on the sensorium have been both historical and anthropological, are useful in a general sense for premodern contexts.[13] I have also drawn much inspiration from the historian Richard Cullen Rath's study of Colonial America, especially his emphasis on the power of sound as a medium for earlier societies to structure the world around them.[14] I have found this admittedly unconventional comparison with early America to be in fact a fruitful way to consider and imagine some aspects of the Byzantines and their hearing culture as well as the sonic spaces in which the events of their lives were played out.

The issue of sound's organizing potential in the premodern world raises a potential point of comparison with our own, often visually structured society. In the past, sounds frequently served as identifiers of particular trades or zones of activity within a city or village—the cacophony of the market, the pounding of metal on the forge, the gushing water and slapping of wet clothes at the spring. In the absence of maps, such sounds made it possible to navigate the streets.[15] Bells were supremely successful in structuring societies, and here Alain Corbin's luminous work on the medium of bells in the French countryside inspires a general rethinking of all manmade but often nonhuman sounds and their effect within the larger auditory landscape.[16] Bells signaled the hours of the day, announced the start of circus games, and called for convocation at key moments within the life of a community. Small, usually hammered bells allowed wandering flocks to sonically mark out territory while simultaneously giving each animal its own individual voice.[17] Indeed, according to modern lore, the best shepherd is the one who can identify each one of his goats from the sound of its bell—this while sitting in the coffee house down in the village.[18] The introduction and eventual elevation of large cast bells in the bell tower (*kodonostasion*) after the mid-ninth century but certainly before 1204 meant the establishment of larger sonic boundaries in the land- and cityscape, again a means of defining communities and distinguishing them from neighbors and the wild unknown of the countryside.[19]

13 C. Classen, *Worlds of Sense: Exploring the Senses in History and across Cultures* (London and New York, 1993); eadem, *The Color of Angels: Cosmology, Gender, and the Aesthetic Imagination* (London and New York, 1998); M. M. Smith, *Sensory History* (Oakland, 2007); see also V. Erlmann, *Hearing Cultures: Essays on Sound, Listening and Modernity* (Oxford and New York, 2004).

14 R. C. Rath, *How Early America Sounded* (Ithaca, NY, and London, 2003).

15 Smith, *Acoustic World*, 54–55; D. Garrioch, "Sounds of the City: The Soundscape of Early Medieval European Towns," *Urban History* 30, no. 1 (2003): 5–25.

16 A. Corbin, *Village Bells: Sound & Meaning in the 19th-Century French Countryside* (New York, 1988). In the West, the size of a parish was determined by the distance at which its bells could be heard.

17 A fine, recently excavated example of a hammered animal bell of iron and copper alloy comes from Chersonesos in Ukraine, in this case from an urban setting. See A. Rabinowitz, L. Sedikova, and R. Henneberg, "Daily Life in a Provincial Late Byzantine City: Recent Multidisciplinary Research in the South Region of Tauric Chersonesos (Cherson)," in *Byzanz—das Römerreich im Mittelalter*, part 2.1, ed. F. Daim and J. Drauschke (Vienna, 2005), 453 fig. 28.

18 See the exemplary anthropological study by P. Panopoulos, "Animal Bells as Symbols: Sound and Hearing in a Greek Island Village," *The Journal of the Royal Anthropological Institute* 9, no. 4 (December 2003): 639–56. There is much here to be considered in relationship to the Byzantine material and the polyvalence of bells.

19 The ninth-century bells given by the Venetians to Basil I may or may not have made it to Constantinople, according to E. V. Williams, *The Bells of Russia: History and Technology* (Princeton, 1985), 22. They were certainly installed in towers in the East before the thirteenth century, as is made clear from

Sound was also a key factor in creating networks of behavior. Unstructured noise was bad; structured and directed noise was good. This is nicely pointed out for us in the *Life* of Patriarch Nikephoros I of Constantinople, where its author, Ignatios the Deacon, demonstrates the principle in a classic attractive/aversive comparison between saintly patriarch and evil emperor using sound metaphors. Concerning speech, Nikephoros is said to "tune an elegant lyre," while the emperor Leo the Isaurian "thundered against the faithful in complete madness, like Salmoneus with his oxhides."[20] (Here we are to imagine the mythical king who tried to imitate thunder and lightning by racing his chariot while throwing torches and dragging hides and bronze pans behind him.) Leo's mode of speech, surprising and uncontrolled like thunder, or the din and clang of metal, symbolized his evilness. In a similar way, the booming sound of canon fire and the infamous melée of the Janissaries in the fifteenth century featured drums, trumpets, cymbals, triangles, and bells to disorient and terrorize the inhabitants of Constantinople. By contrast, the donation, in the twelfth century, of two large bells by Isaac Komnenos to his Kosmosoteira monastery at Pherrai, in northeast Greece, marked an event bearing testament to good order rather than deafening chaos. Two large bells were hung high in a tower and, according to the careful specifications of the patron's typikon, were rung loudly on all Sundays and feast days as a sign of comfort and salvific assurance in the afterlife.[21] Monumental sounds such as these were markers of time and territory, but they could also function on a psychological level as deliverers of honor, prestige, health, solemnity, joy, fear, and of course memory.

I want to suggest here that the Byzantines actively attended to the hearing sense as an element of the human condition requiring special consideration in all contexts. In my research I distinguish several categories within sonic studies that are potentially interesting inroads into the Byzantine mindset. There are certainly more that remain to be identified; this is a work in progress. As a starting point, however, I include sound as display; sound as structuring element, especially antiphony; imagined sounds, often discerned through ekphrasis; and nonhuman sounds—a very important category. The Byzantines listened intently to nature sounds, especially animals and birds but also natural phenomena such as thunder.[22] All deserve deeper study. The largest and easiest category to detect is that of sonic environments, including the church, or monumental structures generally, the monastery, especially the refectory (as ultrastructured environment), nature and ruins, and the city. I am addressing the last two categories in a separate publication, so I will focus here on architectural contexts—the monastic environment and the church—since the issue of acoustics within the Byzantine naos has been at the forefront of my research.[23]

The Church of Hagia Sophia

It seems fitting to begin with a brief discussion of the church of Hagia Sophia in Istanbul, since this is the primary building to which acoustic attention has been paid in recent years.[24] It is also perhaps the most difficult church in which to conduct acoustic testing.[25] It is the only specific building I will consider within these pages, not

the monastic typika. See the examples of the Bebaia Elpis and Kosmosoteira monasteries in Dubowchik, "Singing with the Angels" (n. 8 above), 287 n. 40.

20 "Life of the Patriarch Nikephoros I of Constantinople," trans. E. Fisher, in *Byzantine Defenders of Images: Eight Saints' Lives in English Translation*, ed. A.-M. Talbot (Washington, DC, 1998), 128.

21 Dubowchik, "Singing with the Angels," 287; *BMFD* 2:804.

22 The use of thunder sounds as divinatory medium, seen in surviving brontologia, is a topic I am currently researching, a task made easier with the publication of the Etruscan material by J. M. Turfa, *Divining the Etruscan World: The Brontoscopic Calendar and Religious Practice* (Cambridge, 2012).

23 Papalexandrou, "Past Is Noise" (n. 6 above). I have begun to flesh out a theory of sound and sound reception for Byzantium in the course of a number of papers delivered at conferences and public lectures, especially the 44th Spring Symposium of Byzantine Studies (SPBS) at Newcastle in April 2011. I am grateful to the conference organizers, Claire Nesbitt and Mark Jackson, for the opportunity to present my work on "Storied Spaces in the Byzantine Sonic Environment" at this venue.

24 Pentcheva, "Hagia Sophia" (n. 7 above); C. A. Weitze, J. H. Rindel, C. L. Lynge, and A. C. Gade, "The Acoustical History of Hagia Sophia Revived through Computer Simulation," in *Forum Acusticum* (2002), http://www.odeon.dk/pdf/ForumAcusticum2002.pdf (accessed 29 June 2015).

25 It is noteworthy that scientific testing in the building has been confined to nonmusical sounds (balloon pops)

for its accommodation of chant but rather as a building that was created, in the sixth century, to show off the health of the Empire through the majestic sonic events performed there. In this it was a stunning success. Its exquisite marble sheathing, glowing glass mosaics, and shining hard marble columns and capitals all contributed to its grand spectacle of reflection, as Bissera Pentcheva and others before her have eloquently emphasized.[26]

I prefer to begin not with the grand space itself but with one element within the building that is typically overlooked when discussing acoustics: the great ambo—the raised pulpit west of the bema—famously sheathed in silver and rededicated in 563 following the collapse of the first dome in 558.[27] It is useful, I think, to consider the possible acoustic function of components such as large-scale church furniture. Often removed in recent times, these forgotten elements would have played a critical role in the direction and navigation of sound. We know, for example, that monumental ambos addressed sonic as well as visual concerns. The bishop who ascended the marble stairs of the ambo in late antiquity did so for a number of reasons, including safety from swelling crowds and added visibility. But it was especially undertaken to elevate his voice above the masses, and the marble construction of most ambos likely offered additional sound reflection.[28] Given the information from John Chrysostom, who preached in the earlier, wooden-roofed Hagia Sophia in Constantinople, this was an important consideration especially during the homily, when the bishop was forced to compete with a world of ambient sounds, from clapping and singing to coughing, stomping, whispering, and especially audible prayer among the congregation, all within the very large, open space of a wooden-roofed basilica.[29] As described by Sozomen, "So much did the crowd press around him . . . each one struggling to get closer so that by standing near he might hear more accurately what he was saying, that he <Chrystostom> placed himself on the readers' ambo in the midst of all and taught them seated there."[30] Hearing the sermon in this large-scale, open environment must have presented a major challenge to listeners in the pre-Justinianic church.[31]

The ambo in Justinian's sixth-century church of Hagia Sophia was different. It was large and constructed of exquisite, highly reflective silver.[32] We are to imagine it below the dome and slightly to the east—an interesting location, for it places this component at the epicenter of acoustic resonance within the church. While the silver sheathing was certainly designed with visual effect in mind, it would have surely altered the acoustic character of the space below the dome. Singing there, on the ambo, would probably have allowed the voices to spread out with some additional amplification from the reverberation in the church, with the drawback of excessive reverberation time: The words (especially in music) would be more likely to be unintelligible were an utterance to collide with previous echoes still bouncing around the space. Whether the sixth-century engineers intended it or not, the

in accordance with the secular nature of the building. See Pentcheva, "Hagia Sophia," 102.

26 Pentcheva, "Hagia Sophia," Lethaby, "On Pavements" (both n. 7 above).

27 Paul the Silentiary, *Descriptio ambonis*, trans. C. Mango, *Art of the Byzantine Empire, 312–1453, Sources and Documents* (Toronto, 1986), 80–96; S. G. Xydis, "The Chancel Barrier, Solea, and Ambo of Hagia Sophia," *The ArtB* 29, no. 1 (1947): 1–24.

28 Marble columns and screens all have a significant effect on acoustic behavior, as we observed in many instances in the summer of 2014 during acoustic testing in Thessalonike, on which see note 11 above. The marble templon, as well as the later iconostasis, also modified sound effects, perhaps muffling the sounds of feet in the area of the sanctuary. Rath, *How Early America Sounded* (n. 14 above), 98–100.

29 H. F. Stander, "The Clapping of Hands in the Early Church," *Studia Patristica* 26, no. 1 (1993): 75–80; N. Adkin, "A Problem in the Early Church: Noise during Sermon and Lesson," *Mnemosyne,* series 4, 38, no. 1–2 (1985): 161–63. On reading and praying aloud in the early Church see R. F. Taft, "Was the Eucharistic Anaphora Recited Secretly or Aloud? The Ancient Tradition and What Became of It," in *Worship Traditions in Armenia and the Neighboring Christian East*, ed. R. R. Ervine (Crestwood, NY, 2006), 20–27.

30 Sozomen, *Hist. Eccles.* 8.28.7–8, translation adapted from NPNF2 1: 402.

31 Although, as Father Taft has pointed out, many listeners may not have understood much of the sermon in any case, given the lack of education and mix of languages spoken in the capital. See R. Taft, *Through Their Own Eyes: Liturgy as the Byzantines Saw It* (Berkeley, 2006), 82–85. The wooden rafters of the earlier building would probably have helped the acoustics, whereas the speaker/singers in the sixth-century Justinianic building would have had a more reflective space to contend with.

32 Paul the Silentiary, *Descriptio ambonis*; Xydis, "Chancel Barrier."

behavior of this particular region of the church may have been difficult for its users.

Surely this explains the frequent use, throughout the middle ages, of the so-called cavern by chanters in Hagia Sophia. This was the open space immediately underneath the great ambo of the church, within and from which the *psaltoi* often sang. They can be seen, down below the oval of the raised platform, in a number of depictions in later Byzantine manuscripts, a location often attested in literary sources.[33] It was perhaps easier to sing from beneath the ambo, and perhaps also easier for the congregation to hear the singers. It may be that there were certain passages that needed to be more clearly understood, and for these they chose the cavern to minimize the effects of reverberation. By contrast, for the more uplifting passages perhaps the platform of the ambo was used in order to take full advantage of the amplifying power of the acoustics.[34] While the church of Hagia Sophia was, and still is, a spectacularly rich, multisensory environment, it was presumably a difficult one, with acoustic resonance that was big and bold and exceedingly difficult to navigate, especially for chant.

I suspect the design intention of the sixth-century builder-scientists, Isidoros of Miletos but especially Anthemios of Tralles, had more to do with acclamations than it did with chanted song. The great height of the dome and vaults together with the massive, highly reflective surfaces created the perfect storm of noisiness which, when structured, was essential to showing off a healthy state. It placed controlled sound production in a high-level arena of politics and propaganda. It also demonstrated the might of the empire, as the sheer force of the populace, joined together in unison, was expressed.[35] We get some sense of the power of this medium of expression in the event of the ordination of Patriarch Nikephoros I, who in 806 read aloud his profession of faith inside the Great Church. Ignatios the Deacon, the author of his *Life*, tells us: "After divine inspiration accomplished his holy ordination the people cried 'Worthy!' three times in worthy acclamation for this worthy man. <Nikephoros> then ascended the holy vantage point of the <patriarchal> throne, as if it were some extremely lofty peak . . . pronouncing the good <blessing> of the peace upon all the people, and receiving <theirs> in return."[36] The text gives us a sense of the oral dimensions of this service, with its acclamations (and repetition of "worthy!" thrice within the descriptive text) and antiphonal response from the congregation that must have been heard throughout the city. As anyone who has spent time in the Mediterranean knows, a good Saturday night *panegyri* or a wedding reception isn't successful unless you can hear it from at least one village away. The sounds of success need to transcend local boundaries. This was especially true of the church of Hagia Sophia, where the acoustic possibilities were as much a sign of health, wealth, and especially the power and unity of church and state as they were of the spiritual dimensions we typically imagine for this building.

Anthony Kaldellis has recently reevaluated the motives of Anthemios of Tralles, in particular this engineer's involvement with the design project of the Hagia Sophia.[37] He relates his activities in his home workshop where, according to Agathias, he was using steam power to simulate earthquakes, mirrors to simulate lightning, and, most notably, "he contrived to produce the deep, booming sound by the percussion of resonant objects and achieve the effect of loud and terrifying peals of thunder."[38] He was fascinated by sound and its causes, and it may be that Justinian's church provided a unique testing ground for his preoccupation. Perhaps we need to rethink the sonorous possibilities of

33 N. Moran, *Singers in Late Byzantine and Slavonic Painting* (Leiden, 1986), 26–32.

34 I am grateful to Chris Kyriakakis and James Donohue for discussing this matter with me.

35 E. Wellesz, *History of Byzantine Music and Hymnography* (Oxford, 1949), 103–6; Tillyard, "The Acclamations of Emperors in Byzantine Ritual," *BSA* 18 (1911–12): 239–60; M. McCormick, *Eternal Victory: Triumphal Rulership in Late Antiquity, Byzantium, and the Early Medieval West* (Paris, 1986).

36 Trans. from Talbot, *Byzantine Defenders of Images* (n. 20 above), 64.

37 A. Kaldellis, "The Makings of Hagia Sophia and the Last Pagans of Rome," *Journal of Late Antiquity* 6, no. 2 (2013): 347–66. I am grateful to the author for sharing the text with me in advance of its publication.

38 Ibid., 357–58; trans. J. D. Frendo, *Agathias: The Histories* (Berlin and New York, 1975), 5.4 (p. 143).

this important space, where chant was but one component of a much larger and richer program of events.

Monastic Contexts

The church of Hagia Sophia was an exception of mythical proportions. We are again on terra firma in the monastic realm, especially the refectory, where special sounds as well as the lack of sound defined and punctuated time and space. This was a controlled soundscape, within which the refectory became an important locus. It included oral pronouncement, especially biblical readings, in combination with the "silence of the lips" that operated together with the sense of taste as a powerful memory tool.[39] The refectory was surely designed with acoustics in mind: the apse for amplifying pronouncements and especially the readings of saints' lives during meals, the wooden beams below a pitched roof overhead to diminish the reflection of sound.[40] Both would have served to enhance speech, not of the monks as a collective unit but more typically of an individual speaker or reader.

Within the context of mealtime there is the important moment, apparent in many typika, of the tossing of spoons onto plates (in unison) upon completion of the meal.[41] This seems to have been deemed necessary as a means of punctuating the event—as an exclamation point, a stroke of finality. We have something similar in our own culture with the judge's gavel in the courtroom, where one loud blow of the gavel marks the official end of the event: "<Smack!> Court's adjourned!" It not only accentuates but also sonically commemorates the last word of the judge's central authority, and the permission given to make noise and move about. The ninth-century typikon of the Stoudios monastery in Constantinople suggests a hyper-structured world organized by signals each day: a water clock to wake the monk, who sounded the semantron to wake the sleeping or praying community;[42] a psalm on the lips and ring of the bell before the midday meal;[43] a signal for the wine to be poured and another for the food to be served; another for the reading; and finally the tossing of the spoons after the meal. These sonic reminders were important for ordering the days and managing behavior. Imagine the possible chaos without the spoon toss. One might be caught slurping the soup—a natural, earthy sound but perhaps an undesirable one.[44] The typika will certainly prove a copious resource concerning the microcultures built around various aural and oral phenomena in the monastic setting.

Byzantine Sounds and Elite Voices

It is clear that sounds and their perception were thought about and discussed in sophisticated ways within the upper echelons of Byzantine society. A number of individuals stand out for their observations, and it is here that I wish to focus for the remainder of my discussion. In the early years surrounding the period of Iconoclasm it was not uncommon for intellectuals to compare sight and hearing. Discussions typically centered on which of the two was more effective in aiding memory, with hearing often pronounced the loser especially following the reinstatement of images in 843. The patriarch Photios's rousing sermon delivered in 867 in the church of Hagia Sophia, directly below the restored Virgin and Christ child in the apse, is the most famous example. Of that image he said: "The Virgin is holding the Creator in her arms as an infant. . . . the comprehension that comes about through sight is shown in very fact to be far superior to the learning that penetrates through the ears."[45] He was explicit in his belief in the power of images to promote cognition.[46]

39 A.-M. Talbot, "Mealtime in Monasteries: The Culture of the Byzantine Refectory," in *Eat, Drink, and Be Merry (Luke 12:19): Food and Wine in Byzantium: Papers of the 37th Annual Spring Symposium of Byzantine Studies, in Honour of Professor A. A. M. Bryer* (Burlington, VT, 2007), 109–26.

40 A. Orlandos, *Μοναστηριακὴ Ἀρχιτεκτονική* (Athens, 1958), 43–60; S. Popović, "The Trapeza in Cenobitic Monasteries: Architectural and Spiritual Contexts," *DOP* 52 (1998): 292–96.

41 *BMFD* 1:109, 225.

42 Ibid., 1:98.

43 Ibid., 1:112, 225 (Stoudios).

44 Or perhaps this is a modern value judgment? Slurping may have been fully acceptable behavior in the middle ages.

45 *Homily* 17.5, trans. by C. Mango, *The Homilies of Photius, Patriarch of Constantinople* (Cambridge, MA, 1958), 294.

46 This has been discussed by many, myself included: A. Papalexandrou, "The Memory Culture of Byzantium," in *A*

Likewise, vision was deemed more effective in etching itself into the memory. He asked: "Has the mind seen? Has it grasped? Has it visualized? Then it has effortlessly transmitted the forms to the memory."[47] Seeing rather than listening was deemed the better route to God. Of course we should remember that Photios had a bias, which was to promote the Iconophile position. And we should have no illusion: He used sound in its most emphatic rhetorical dimension, in the form of a public address, to convey his message.

Much like Photios, we tend to privilege sight over the other senses, an attitude that is still in evidence for most studies devoted to Byzantine art and culture today.[48] Byzantine intellectuals considered sight to more directly and immediately send signals to the brain and accommodate memory.[49] Modern scholars have often followed suit despite scientific evidence to the contrary.[50] But sound is certainly an equal (if not superior) player when it comes to stirring human emotions. Sound has heft. This is one instance where, in the absence of more detailed information from the Byzantines themselves, it becomes useful to enter the realm of anthropology and consider some elements of our own, admittedly modern but perhaps universal experience of sound.[51] The example of present-day funerals is useful: Vision is a strong component, centered as it is on the icon of the body or its visible container.[52] In recent years in the United States it has become common practice for a photographic image (or images) of the deceased, often blown up to very large scale, to accompany the funeral ceremony. Occasionally there is also a taped recording of a song sung or a speech delivered. While the image of the person is affecting to those present, the sound of the voice devastates. Sound is an emotive force to be reckoned with. The example of music is the most apt and relatable. A certain combination of notes, tones, or cadence—it is different for everyone—goes to our very core. Think, for example, of the almost ritual repetition and inflection of Martin Luther King's vibrato voice in his "I Have a Dream" speech. It is not only the profundity of the message or the underlying tragedies it represents, but also, and especially, the sound of the voice that moves us.

A number of scientific studies aim to show how music, and even the sound of laughter, can lighten psychological burdens.[53] These things were similarly expressed by the statesman and monk Theodore Metochites in the fourteenth century, where he gushed over the antiphonal singing of his fellow monks at the Chora Monastery: "My heart rejoices . . . and every care . . . is dispelled when I stand . . . together with the glorious choristers of God; through you are my ears and mind and all my soul filled with serenity and calm and love; thence have I most precious bliss, and also compunction inducing me to forget this life which carries off without

Companion to Byzantium, ed. L. James (Malden MA, 2010), 108–22. See also R. Nelson, "To Say and to See: Ekphrasis and Vision in Byzantium" in *Visuality Before and Beyond the Renaissance: Seeing as Others Saw*, ed. R. S. Nelson (New York and Cambridge, 2000), 143–68; L. James, "Senses and Sensibility in Byzantium," *Art History* 27, no. 4 (2004): 522–37. The visual element is understood to be the most important because Photios insists on it.

47 Mango, *Homilies of Photius*, Homily 17. On this passage see R. Betancourt, "Why Sight Is Not Touch: Reconsidering the Tactility of Vision in Byzantium," *DOP* 70 (2016): 1–23.

48 On the hegemony of sight see Classen, *Color of Angels* (n. 13 above), 138–39 where she emphasizes "the current climate of hypervisuality" and boldly explores instead the world of the blind. Holistic approaches that integrate hearing into the sensorium can be found in a number of philosophical works dedicated to media or aesthetics. Primary among them are Schafer, *Soundscape* (n. 6 above); M. McLuhan, *The Gutenberg Galaxy*; and W. Welsch, *Undoing Aesthetics*, trans. A. Inkpin (London, CA and New Delhi, 1997), with very strong statements (especially at 157–63) about visual primacy from the time of the ancient Greeks through today.

49 As for example Photios, *Homily* 17.5: "the comprehension that comes about through sight is shown in very fact to be far superior to the learning that penetrates through the ears," trans. Mango.

50 S. Horowitz, *The Universal Sense: How Hearing Shapes the Mind* (London and New York, 2012), 5.

51 See here the fascinating work and "hearing stance" of I. Sykes for eighteenth- and nineteenth-century France and its impact on modern society in *Society, Culture and the Auditory Imagination in Modern France: The Humanity of Hearing* (New York, 2015), especially pp. viii and ix of her preface, where "hearing becomes an anthropological tool for uncovering relational patterns which become set in the landscape to form our modern sound settings."

52 The phrase derives from the work of H. Maguire, *The Icons of Their Bodies: Saints and Their Images in Byzantium* (Princeton, 1996).

53 P. N. Juslin and D. Västfjäll, "Emotional Responses to Music: The Need to Consider Underlying Mechanisms," *Behavioral and Brain Science* 31 (208): 559–621.

ceasing."[54] We have all shared Metochites' experience, where we are utterly transported through sound.

Thessalonike and the Semantron

With this in mind, I turn now to what I take to be one of the few manmade sounds to survive more or less intact from the Eastern Roman Empire. This is the sound of the semantron (or semanterion)—the long wooden board that functions something like a gong and is used primarily as a call to worship.[55] It was (and still is today, especially in the monasteries) held up on the shoulder, or hung on a bracket, and struck repeatedly with a mallet thereby producing a loud but pleasing pattern of wooden or metallic knocks. In Orthodox monasteries today the wood is struck evenly but quickly, the pace building in rapid-fire crescendo and eventually tapering off, typically ending in three (presumably symbolic) blows. I do not know whether the rhythm is a survival, but the instrument itself certainly is, with its utter simplicity of form and the unique sound produced by it. It is best heard live as an authentic sound experience rather than through a recording as a sound artifact. It is quite unique and of interest for a number of reasons. It is part and parcel of the Orthodox experience, yet outside the realm of chant; it takes place outside the sacred space of the church; and it can be categorized as something quasi-architectural. As the monk walks the perimeter of the building striking the wood, he defines a horizon of events that (sonically) exceeds the boundaries of architecture and of the surrounding enclosure walls and yet remains within and part of the monastic complex. Sound reminds and beckons the monks (or nuns) while simultaneously reassuring those outside the walls of constant, dutiful communication with the divine on their behalf.[56] It also presents a sonic barrier that differentiates and separates the monastery from the secular world. And of course it sends heavenward a collective voice of communion and worship. It is an extraordinary sound that holds our imagination and gives us something useful and memorable to think with.

In the late twelfth century, the canonist and churchman Theodore Balsamon was intensely interested in the semantron, so much so that he published a short treatise, *Study Regarding the Three Semanteria Summoning Calls in the Holy Churches of Monasteries*.[57] His primary purpose was to justify the usual method of three semanteria calls (rather than one) to summon the monks to services, and from his discussion we can discern that there had been controversy surrounding the tradition. He explains that his treatise was necessitated by the "clueless individuals" (also called "nonbelievers") who disapproved and derided the multiple soundings of the wooden gongs. These nonbelievers must have been the Norman and Italian invaders of the city of Thessalonike—the very same foreigners decried by the bishop Eustathios in 1185. It is worth recounting here Eustathios's own description of events:

> The Latins also wished to prevent us from using the wooden semantron which is so well adapted to serve as a herald and announce to the people that they should assemble in church. When it was first struck by the Katholike in the late afternoon, the barbarians sprang with drawn swords upon the man who had struck it, at the twinkle of an eye or with the speed of a thunderbolt, and grinding out their usual "Wretch!" to shame us, asked "What is this?" and put a stop to it for the moment. This decision, because of the fear that it caused, went on to affect the rest of those who were accustomed to strike it in this way. But after a few days, when the

54 Translation by J. M. Featherstone, "Metochites's Poems and the Chora," in *The Kariye Camii Reconsidered: Metochites and His Books between the Chora and the Renaissance*, ed. H. Klein, R. Ousterhout, and B. Pitarakis (Istanbul, 2011), 186.

55 On the semantron see W. Smith and S. Cheetham, *A Dictionary of Christian Antiquities*, vol. 2 (Hartford, CT, 1880), 1879; *ODB* 3:1868; L. Allatios, *The Newer Temples of the Greeks*, trans. A. Cutler (University Park, PA, 1969), 41. For modern performances of the semantron, the collection on YouTube provides a variety of popular versions at https://www.youtube.com/watch?v=44gggoAk3XY&list=PL7BC3Vg4ZlS2IbFC9gR8t-WNDekof_F5R (accessed 3 January 2015).

56 R. Morris, *Monks and Laymen in Byzantium, 843–1118* (New York, 1995), 109–10.

57 Translated below, appendix 1. Balsamon's study has been discussed, in brief, in Williams, *Bells of Russia* (n. 19 above), 22.

Feast of the Elevation of the Revered Cross was about to be held on the next day, the priests whose responsibility it was to give the signal ascended to the highest point of the Katholike to make a brief performance of their usual duty, it being impossible to carry it out at any length because any act of worship was likely to give offence. And when they gave an indication with the semantron of the beginning of the feast, there were the barbarians again with their naked swords rushing at them from below, chasing after them and subjecting all those around them to an inquisition in case some plot was there to be uncovered. . . . One question that occurred to us at this time was that we could not understand why they were not suspicious when the great bells aloft in the church of the Myrobletes rang to give the signal for the singing of psalms, when they were so put out by the semantron when it gave the signal at the Metropolitan Church for the holy assembly there.[58]

So, we are made to understand that the Western Christians, and also some Orthodox Christians, were making things difficult (Balsamon says it was "scandal-causing"), including and especially for Orthodox monks, to maintain their rituals and traditions. Here we have an important sonic dimension, recounted by two eyewitnesses, at center stage. It is no wonder that Balsamon addressed the issue so vehemently in his treatise.[59] We have here a wonderful coincidence of opinion—one anecdotal and the other philosophical—from two of the most important thinkers of the late twelfth century. Clearly the unique audio signature of this instrument was of the utmost importance to intellectuals of the time.

From Balsamon's treatise we learn that, to his view, hearing the semantron was deemed essential in city and monastery alike but above all as a means of establishing and regulating order in the monastery. Everything should be on time, announced thrice by the gongs. It is not entirely clear whether he means three instruments or three separate calls on a single instrument, or whether the triad of sounds were sequential or concurrent. Whatever the case, the peals symbolized the Trinity, which Balsamon used to defend the practice within Orthodox theology, delivered in the proper tone and spirit and recalling some aspect of the three daily services. According to him, the semantron spoke very precisely to monastic listeners using sonic vocabulary (perhaps tone and tempo) appropriate to the occasion. It announced not only beginnings but also content and connection—that is, correct associations as determined by the Church. So the monks, he tells us, were summoned to the daily services first by means of the "lesser (or small) semanterion" that had, in his words, a "humbler and darker" tone than that sounded for orthros, and that it functioned essentially as a tool to remind the hearer of the Old Testament foreshadowing ("typos") of the Gospels. Balsamon put it into a context of prefigurations ("eikonismata") of the New Testament and the Passion of Christ. By contrast, the main or "great semanterion" (the second sound) connected the hearer with the Gospel readings and festival books. He does not elaborate on this particular sound except to inform us that this sonic reminder is also used in urban churches to call the faithful. He insists that this practice does not subvert the ecclesiastical order.

Balsamon's third semantron was the bronze one, symbolizing the life of the Church after the Apostles and, he goes on to say, the Last Judgment. We are made to understand straightaway the power and importance of this instrument on many fronts both real and imagined. Again it was a structuring tool, but its special material must have afforded it greater significance through its earthly value, its capacity for greater volume and resonance, and its potential for spiritual connotations. Balsamon attached a crucial memory image: that of the brazen salpinx (the trumpet) that will announce Christ on the Day of Judgment: "for they say that the Lord ascended in jubilation, in the sound of the salpinx. The angels of God will sound the salpinx and the dead will be resurrected, and everyone will be judged according to their deeds."[60] Perhaps it

58 Eustathios, *Capture of Thessaloniki* (n. 3 above), 134–37 (paragraph 122).

59 See appendix 1.

60 The text (see appendix 1 for the context) seems to fuse crucifixion with resurrection here. Compare 1 Thessalonians 4:16.

is not too much of a stretch to attach sound to vision here, as members of the monastic community may have been virtually transported to the dynamic, painted image of the Last Judgment in icons and manuscripts within the space of the church—dramatic and in living color—a noisy netherworld of shouting and thunder overseen by the angel of the Lord sounding the trumpet to wake the dead.[61] Through the semantron, the listening community might have been reminded of these things together with the promise of life after death. Balsamon seems to equate sound with fear, perhaps to invite correct behavior: Listening and obeying the call of the bronze semantron-turned-salpinx leads to salvation. In this way it conveyed a notion of past, present and future, hope and fear, image and sound, all tied up into one dramatic, aural-performative event.

Perhaps Balsamon understood that the regulation of sound could be used to control movement, mood, and thought, and especially that it supported memorywork. Clearly there was a degree of interpretive value placed directly upon differentiated sounds, and the expectation was that the hearer listened carefully and also that he (or she) was cognizant of sound as a dimension of scripture, of the hagiopolitic (Jerusalem) chants, and so forth.[62] This suggests a high level of aural cognition and interpretation among listeners. His treatise presents an intriguing way of reimagining the Byzantine aural experience as one of refined listening and thinking, at least within the monastic environment.

Finally, Balsamon goes on to discuss urban, nonmonastic churches within the city, for which he relates a different custom: the sounding of one great semantron call, which he refers to as the μέγαλον σημαντήριον. Here he gives a rare shout-out to the manual laborers of the city, or as he put it, "those who dig and work the plough," and offers an appreciation, on their behalf, of church music as a "pleasant and proper" experience in their lives.[63] Here there is emphasis more on the Good News than on the Old Testament. That Balsamon felt compelled to justify these things in his writing suggests the inherent importance of the sonic dimension, especially those sounds that affected large communities of laymen and women.

Balsamon's text demonstrates that sound and perceptions of sound were in some cases inherently cultural—in his case a means of distinguishing his own people (the citizens of Thessalonike) from "Latins" (foreigners), whose "brazen-mouthed bell," as he put it, both defined and separated them. (The bell also seems to debase them, in his eyes.) He goes on to relate that their variant tradition of summoning the people to church by means of bells (*kampana*) which they called ἐκ τοῦ κάμπου ("from the field"), was somehow lacking, and that this was due in part to their reliance on psalmody rather than hagiopolitic or Jerusalem chants. He put it, in typically convoluted style, like this: "For they say that just as the field (kampos) presents no obstacle to those willing to walk, so the heavenly resounding of the brazen-mouthed bell spreads to everyone with ease."[64] Is Balsamon referring to the raised height of the bell tower and its acoustic reach, which he may have found as vulgar as the foreigners' speech? This likely stood in contrast to the more earthbound, and to him more relatable, semantron. To Balsamon, unfamiliar sounds may have presented an insurmountable barrier.

Here we return to the nearly contemporary account of Eustathios and his own bitter complaints about the ban placed on the semantron. He and his fellows wondered why the Latins so vehemently forbade the wooden gong but didn't mind the ringing of the bells, even though the latter had been used in Constantinople as a treasonous weapon during the time of Andronikos Komnenos.[65] This reminds us that sound is neither monolithic nor universal. It is allusive and culturally conditioned. This is why the Norman invaders so vehemently forbade the sound of the semantron but readily approved the ringing of bells that, for them, must have signaled

61 A mid-twelfth-century icon from Mt. Sinai (originally from a triptych) bears such a scene, with two angels blowing the salpinx in the lower register, in G. and M. Sotiriou, *Icones du Mont Sinai* (Athens, 1956), 1: pl. 151.

62 On hagiopolitic chants see J. Raasted, ed., *The Hagiopolites: A Byzantine Treatise on Musical Theory,* Cahiers de l'Institut du Moyen-Âge Grec et Latin 45 (Copenhagen, 1983).

63 Appendix 1.

64 Ibid.

65 Eustathios, *Capture of Thessaloniki*, 135–37.

the familiar sound of homeland and a code of communication they recognized. Eustathios painted a picture of tremendous panic among the Normans when the semantron was rung. Such is the power of sound, that it can throw men into fear and confusion even as it unifies others in common purpose. The same was true three hundred years later at the fall of Constantinople, when the collective sounds of the semantra at Hagia Sophia—"four hundred strong" according to the folk tradition—were silenced along with its legendary chorus of "sixty-two bells."[66] From 1453 onward it would be the absence of that sonic power, and the instruments that had produced it, that preserved memory—as sung lament—for those same sounds lost during the four hundred years of Ottoman Turkish domination that were to follow.

Michael Psellos on Acoustics and the "Echo Chamber" of Nikomedeia

In the eleventh century, Michael Psellos published a study devoted specifically to acoustics. This was motivated by his interest in what was known as a "resounding building" (or echo chamber) near his hometown of Nikomedeia, in Bithynia. The local inhabitants there referred to it as *en Nikomedeia Echeion* or more simply as "Sound" (Ἀκοή), and Psellos indicates that it was an attraction that was popular—even famous—in the area. He was curious enough to go and see it, and listen to it for himself, and he came away with personal observations in 103 lines of text.

Today we would call the structure a "whispering gallery," a space usually but not necessarily round, in this case covered by a hemispherical dome. In such a space, a sound in one part of the gallery travels along the base of the dome and can be heard—with absolute clarity—in another part of the space.[67] If you have experienced this quirky acoustic event, you tend to remember it, for it is not only clear but it is often quite loud—louder than you expect—and presents an altogether fascinating and sometimes jarring auditory experience. Psellos thought so too, and he set out to explain the mystery behind its unusual acoustic properties.

Psellos's account is important, not only for his thoughts about architectural design and acoustics but also for his general insights into the history of science and his notions (not necessarily correct) about the human body. He posits axioms and refers to the Hellenistic philosopher Archimedes of Sicily and his burning mirrors; he embarks on a rather long and detailed passage concerning breath, the human voice, thunder, meteorology, and the problems of those who have been "thunderstruck." It is a fascinating and unexpected discussion, one that richly deserves deeper study.

Concerning the Echeion itself, Psellos gives us the general characteristics of the building, emphasizing its small size, low dome, and its unusual echoing effect. He does not know its function. Perhaps it was a ruin—Psellos does not say. As an architectural wonder it seemed to him, initially, more of an acoustical accident than a purposeful design, and in this he was almost certaily correct. Nowadays acousticians refer to such effects as sound creep—a property generally not desired in architectural projects because of its distorting quality. As Psellos continued to write his observations, however, he seems to have changed his mind as he worked through the principles of its structure and rationalized the building in terms of phenomena that could be observed and explained on the basis of a theoretical framework. He weighed the component parts and figured that the "architect" or builder was not specifically trying to create sound effects, but that he knew his trade well. He is at pains to convey that, contrary to popular belief among the locals, there was nothing magical or unexplainable about the building, nor were there hidden devices, such as ceramic tubes deep inside the

66 "And Hagia Sophia, the Great Church, sends signals / It has four hundred semantra and sixty-two bells." C. A. Trypanis, ed., *Penguin Book of Greek Verse*, no. 254.

67 M. Ermann, *Architectural Acoustics Illustrated* (Hoboken, 2015), 110–13. Echo is different from reverberance and is characterized by an unwanted repetition of the initial sound, whereas reverberation is a protraction of sound as it decays over time. T. Cox, *The Sound Book: The Science of the Sonic Wonders of the World* (New York, 2014), 146–77. The space does not have to be domed to display this quirky acoustic attribute, but the most famous examples are domed buildings, for example St. Paul's Cathedral in London and the Hamilton Mausoleum in Scotland.

walls that allowed the sound to travel and emerge stronger.[68] He is measured in his evaluation.

But Psellos is fascinated, and this in itself is fascinating for us. The very idea that a philosopher monk bothered to write on this issue in the eleventh century, that he paid close attention to building design, structure, and the sonic behavior of a given space, and that he took issue with nonelite explanations of the Echeion's resonant vaulting (that it was somehow magical, or supernatural) affirms Psellos's interest in, and elite preoccupation with, sound.

Contemporary enthusiasm for the Echeion and its peculiar echoing effects also may support the notion that the Byzantines learned how to improve their acoustic environment through the use of empirical evidence—cases of success and failure in buildings that must have existed all around them. This would be especially true in the context of church buildings, where domes were often of central importance—visually and symbolically but also sonically. Domes manifest different audio characteristics depending on their overall size, height, and profile, and the texture of their interior wall and vault surfaces.[69] Surely the Byzantines knew this, presumably incorporating the necessary elements or changes in design to improve these significant components of their church buildings. Indeed, Psellos himself seems to suggest this in his treatise when he writes, "art cannot be used to test what occurs naturally; rather, if ever just once what is natural happens successfully, then this one time is compensation enough for all the failed attempts [of art]."

It is unfortunate that the details and function of the renowned Echeion are lost to us. Psellos did not bother with these practical details. What is perhaps most interesting is that he investigated this space in a serious way. He got some essential things wrong (the way the ear perceives sound, for example), but he understood a great deal, especially concerning sound reflection and diffusion, direct and indirect sound, resonance and sound decay, and the importance of symmetry in design for good acoustics. Especially important here, he made it clear that intellectuals of his time were actively discussing acoustic phenomena and its properties. Toward the end of his discussion he revealed that many people "do not accept the explanation according to natural science, but ask that the argument be demonstrated practically." In other words, it is possible that he was asked to prove his point, perhaps by building a model. This may offer evidence for model building as part of the design process in Byzantium, unless Psellos means he was expected to build an actual building—the text is not clear.[70] Of course Psellos did not do this because, as he pointed out, "if I make a similar building, it is not absolutely certain that I will be able to prove the explanandum successfully; rather, there might be aspects of the experiment that would be successful and there might be aspects of the experiment that would be unsuccessful." In other words, it would be difficult to reproduce it, and he understood that sometimes these things are simply a fluke of nature. Also, perhaps, he knew he could not pull it off. In any case Psellos's text on the Echeion is of exceptional importance in establishing a level of learned dialogue about sound, its properties, special sonic environments in Byzantium, and the Byzantine reception of such spaces.

I would like to end with a metaphor coined by Theodore Balsamon in the course of his treatise on the semantron, mentioned only briefly but powerful nonetheless, as a way of contextualizing hearing and sound within the greater Byzantine sensorium. Balsamon imagined a "divine beehive of the Church" that, in his words, "takes up its spiritual struggle by means of the wax of the gospel teachings, the sting that sheds light on the areas of darkness, and through the honey of the

68 Psellos is here clearly referring to "cavity resonators" or "acoustical jars," ceramic tubes or vessels of a type that have been immured in the walls of buildings since antiquity. First commented on by Vitruvius, they appear in many Byzantine churches, especially in corner spaces or pendentives of vaults, where their mouths are sometimes visible. Their effectiveness in increasing sound resonance has been debated: R. Ousterhout, *Master Builders of Byzantium* (Princeton, 2008), 227, 229–30. The question of their efficacy remains unresolved, although new research may bring us closer to an understanding of the problem.

69 Cox, *Sound Book*, 152–55.

70 On model building in Byzantium see C. Maranci, "Building Practice and Cross-Cultural Exchange in Byzantium and Armenia," *JSAH* 62, no. 3 (2003): 294–305. The architect/stonemason Trdat offered a plan for reconstructing part of the dome of Hagia Sophia in Constantinople in 989. This included construction of a model, discussed at 295.

apostolic writings that sweetens the edges of the inhabited world (the Oikoumene)."[71] Perhaps we can add to this the *sound* of the hive—as a naos abuzz with the individual voices and noises that enlivened the spaces and surroundings of the church, and the Byzantine kosmos. These sounds remind us that we cannot merely look at architectural remains to assess sound; we need to repopulate buildings with curious onlookers like Psellos, or people who sang and prayed aloud but also whispered to one another during the course of the liturgy. The metaphor of a beehive, a structure that is both built and inhabited, active and abuzz, rich not only in sound but also smell (beeswax), taste (honey), and touch (the bee sting), is good to hold in mind as we proceed to discover the role of all the senses in Byzantium. In the context of this chapter it reminds us especially of the kinds of utterances, chants, songs, noises—in general the soundways of Byzantium—that existed alongside both the common impulses and extraordinary circumstances of daily life in the middle ages. Their reconstruction is not easy, but the attempt may reward us with a slightly more three-dimensional view of this society and its people.

71 Balsamon, *Study* (appendix 1).

I would like to thank Susan Ashbrook Harvey and Margaret Mullett for the opportunity to participate in the 2014 Dumbarton Oaks symposium on Sense Perception in Byzantium and for graciously including me in the final publication here. I also wish to thank the two anonymous readers whose comments and suggestions expanded aspects of this paper and inspired me to look in new directions and reconsider old notions. I am deeply grateful to Stratis Papaioannou for reading and correcting the two translated texts appended to this article, and to Nassos Papalexandrou for toiling over them in the first place with good humor despite an abundance of convoluted passages. The editorial prowess of Joel Kalvesmaki, in both text and translations, is also much appreciated. Any mistakes and omissions, the latter of which there will surely be many considering the lightning speed at which new sound studies are appearing, remain my own.

APPENDIX 1

Theodore Balsamon, *Study Regarding the Three Semanteria Summoning Calls in the Holy Churches of Monasteries*

Translation: Nassos Papalexandrou,[72] based on the edition in PG 138:1073–76

I see some clueless people who find no time for anything useful, except to tell or hear some new-fangled thing [Acts 17:21], who proclaim that the call through three semanteria for the monks to attend the holy doxologies in churches are vain and scandal-causing. They claim that one [semantron] would be enough for a summons and that in this way the impious that surround us would not scoff or lampoon against the holy Churches of God nor would they compare us to the heathens, nor would the monastic way be ridiculed because, supposedly, they cannot assemble by simply one summoning call. I show with my present study that the announcement of the holy doxologies through three semanteria was conceived neither to cause idle talk among the impious nor to create difficulties for the monks, but for a most important reason rooted in ancient tradition.

The glorifying of our Lord in our Church by day and night follows the prophesy of David, according to which "In the evening, and morning, and noon I will narrate and speak out loud, and the Lord will listen to my voice" (Psalm 54 [55]: 17). From both fulfilled Testaments (namely the New and the Old), and according to the tradition of the holy and god-bearing Fathers it has been decreed that God is glorified first through David's holy cithara, for he says, "I will open my inquiry with the psalter" (Psalm 48 [49]:4) and, after the reading [of the Psalms], the divine beehive of the Church should take up its spiritual struggle by means of the wax of the gospel teachings, the sting that sheds light on the vast areas of darkness, then, through the honey of the apostolic writings that sweetens the ends of the inhabited world, and through the narrations of the life of the martyrs that exalt the incarnation of Christ, our God.

For this reason, for the sake of the six psalms of [David, Christ's] forefather, and for the sake of everything else that is chanted regularly during the matins doxology before the Jerusalem service and whatever is usually chanted during the most divine celebrations and also during the vesperal prayers (before the readings of the Apostle and the Gospel, but also before the *stichera* [i.e., short hymns preceded by Psalmic verses]), the monks are summoned with a small, and somewhat humbler and darker, semanterion; for everything foreshadowed in the Old Testament was a type and a delineation of what was to come.

But for the benefit of the proclamation of the godly voiced Gospels and the reading aloud of all other festival books [namely homilies, the lives of saints, etc.] and, simply, the entire Jerusalem rite, the great semanterion has been found; for the benefit that comes from these things has reached the whole earth and the edges of the inhabited world. And just as these [rites] are performed with piety and with God's sanction, the Lord's people must also be reminded about the coming Judgment, for which we kneel and pray. It is symbolized through the bronze semanterion to remind Christians of that final day [of Judgment]; for it is written that "God ascended in jubilation, the Lord in the sound of the salpinx." The angels of God will sound the salpinx and the dead will be resurrected and everyone will be rewarded according to their deeds.

Now the fact that in the urban catholic churches [the faithful] are summoned not through the fullness of three semanteria but through only one great semanterion, is not a subversion of ecclesiastical order. For the call is for people who do

72 I gratefully acknowledge Stratis Papaioannou for his help in translating this text and the next. With his insights and philological acumen he greatly improved the precision of the translation. I alone am responsible for any errors and omissions.

manual jobs, who dig and work the plough. And it is charitable that they are invited to church at least through the psaltery of the New Testament.

This is the thinking and decisions of those of us who preserve unchanged, with God's grace, the entire ecclesiastical tradition. But the Latins, who have split off badly from us and whose heart is hardened by Satan, even if with words [we] soften them more than mercy, have a different tradition concerning the summoning call of the people to the churches: they use one semantron, I mean the *kampana* [bell] which takes its name from the word *kampos* (i.e., field). For they say that just as the field presents no obstacle to those willing to set out on foot, so the heavenly resounding of the brazen-mouthed bell spreads to everyone with ease. The Latins and Italians do not need many semanteria because they do not use the Jerusalem psalteries but only the cithara of [David].

APPENDIX 2

Michael Psellos, *On the Echeion [Echo Chamber] at Nikomedeia*

Translation: Nassos Papalexandrou, based on *Michaelis Pselli Philosophica Minora* vol. 1, *Opuscula Logica, Physica, Allegorica, Alia*, ed. J. M. Duffy (Stuttgart, 1992), 106–9.

Many marvel at the *Echeion* [Echo Chamber] in Nikomedeia, which is also called Sound (Ἀκοή). This is an enclosed structure with a low roof, which has been carved in a hemispherical shape. This dome is borne by four walls, with distance between them, and where there is a space between the walls, it is loose and free. Now, there are many who think that the resonance (inside the building) is supernatural and cannot be attributed to any [natural] cause. Others hypothesize that there are hidden devices, perhaps some tubes deep inside the walls, through which the sound travels and comes out stronger; they therefore argue that one cannot come up with such an acoustic effect in an echoing building without a device of this or of similar sort.

I saw this small building once, and neither did I marvel at it nor did I count it among the unexplainable things. The echoing of sound is neither the result of magic nor are there any devices hidden in the floor or in the side walls, nor did even he who first constructed this building aim at such sound effects, nor did he aim to produce reverberation and finish the rest of the building accordingly. Rather, without intending what would happen, he created a building for whatever purpose, and it, along with all other usage, simply turned out to be something we now marvel at.

One could explain this echo starting from this point: Our spoken word, which we acquire through learning from hearing, is articulated by means of a natural air. This air is a very thin substance that is channeled—to speak literally—from the lungs through the tube of the lower throat by the trachea. This articulated breathlet flows through thin air and then it is widely and continuously diffused until it vanishes completely. If it runs across bodies of an opposing type, it splinters around them and it does not immediately lose its sound. Still, the voice does not splinter itself when [encountering] all opposing types of bodies. If the room happens to be narrow and its roof rises high up or its distance [from the ground] is not symmetrical, but one part is too low and the other higher than needed, then under the former the voice is compressed and dissipates silently; under the latter, being the opposite, it just spreads and vanishes. If the room is constructed, however, such that the roof is somewhat curved and perimeter distances are symmetrical, then if somebody utters something with a gentle voice, then another who stands on the opposite side and listens to the voice will hear it resounding. And the receiver will think that the echo came to him from the depths of the side he is standing in, yet this is not the case, as the sound originates from the one who voiced it.

All this happens because the ambient air is humid and easily formed, and as such it is, so to speak, inscribed by our articulated voice as if encoded. And receiving the formation of the articulated [sounds], in a continuum, [the air] flows into the hearing of the listener. from there a certain canal conducts it, not leading straight to the membrane [of the tympanum]; the canal is instead crooked so that the breath of the sound does not cause rupture or some other damage, when it falls into the membrane [i.e., the tympanum] suddenly.

This explains also why (to add some supplementary analysis) it is after lightning that we hear thunder. Yes indeed, a cloud first rips apart and then fire comes out [of the cloud]. Now, because the eye protrudes outward and is not concave, it sees what is visible immediately, whereas our hearing faculty receives the sound of thunder with some delay. It thus makes sense that those who have been exposed suddenly to thunder suffer in their membrane and hence they are called "thunderstruck" (ἔμβροντοι).

Returning to what I originally set out to explain, I also have to add the following. I posit, as an axiom, that every small body falling on something else bounces back according to the shape [direction?] of the fall. This may happen either in a straight line, if it is thus released (as happens with leather balls); or along a slanted path, in which case it will bounce back along a slanted path as well. This helps us also understand that our articulated voice, since it too is a formed body, wherever it might fall first, is also audible in a spot diametrically opposite from it (an east spot being opposite from west, south from north). This also is the case in the wondrous building of this discussion. Resonance does not happen between adjoining walls but between those that stand diametrically opposite. Indeed, if there were a secret device built inside the walls, the resonance would not happen between spaces diametrically opposed to each other but in adjacent spaces. In the current arrangement, someone who stands right next to someone speaking will not perceive the articulated sound, whereas someone standing diametrically opposite will sense it much more intensely. Moreover, he will hear not with both ears, but with the one that is placed toward the wall, for the reflected voice does not enter through the ear that faces the middle space but through the one aimed at the wall.

For the refraction of the same voice is double. The first is at the point whence the voice originates; the second precisely at the opposite point, where it pours into the attendant ear. The second echoing is much more resounding, because the voice is strengthened by the well-sounding body of the air between the [originating] tongue and the [receiving] ear. And for all these reasons the tongue might produce opaque sounds but the hearing faculty receives it in greater clarity. To this event the roof contributes, because it is not suspended at great height but, so to speak, attends and does not dilute the sound.

However this may be, one might say that words have the power to rattle the faculty of hearing, yet in reality not be convincing. Just as people request that we demonstrate practically how the slimmest string produces the highest note, by playing the lyre or the psalterion, in this case too many do not accept the explanation according to natural science, but ask that the argument be demonstrated practically. To all those I would respond like this: if I make a similar building, it is not absolutely certain that I will be able to prove the explanandum successfully; rather, there might be aspects of my experiment that would be successful, and other aspects unsuccessful.

For the resonance of the voice does not appear in all structures but only in those that have been designed in such a way that they have symmetry in their component parts *and* their [enclosed] spaces. Everyone familiar with theorems of physics could easily explain the cause of this phenomenon. A successful demonstration of what one has explained is not always possible nor can everyone do it. For the task requires both opportune placement and precise skill in construction and also both appropriate materials and symmetry of height and depth and the other distances through which something hidden in nature can be discovered. Take, for example, Archimedes of Sicily: he knew very well that from symmetrical distances a fire could be ignited from some mirrors that undergo the appropriate preparation and that are arrayed toward the rays of the sun; and indeed he made numerous such constructions that defended the walls of his country, setting fires among the enemies of his fatherland; still, not all of his devices were successful. For it was necessary that the steel he was working with not be excessively concave nor asymetrically bent nor perfectly smooth. Craft is not always capable of perfectly arranging materials in this way. Thus, art cannot be used to test what occurs naturally; rather, if ever just once what is natural happens successfully, then this one time is compensation enough for all the failed attempts [of art].

CHAPTER FOUR

Kalophonia and the Phenomenon of Embellishment in Byzantine Psalmody

SPYRIDON ANTONOPOULOS

Sensory experience in Byzantium, and in particular, the interplay of space, image, and sound in the liturgy, has commanded much scholarly attention in recent years.[1] New interdisciplinary collaborations seek to explore the ceremonial gestalt of public worship in Byzantium, thus providing opportunities to assess how medieval Byzantine chant might have been heard and experienced in its native context—the buildings and divine offices for which it was composed.[2] Hearing and sound occupied a crucial role in the sensorium of Byzantine worship. In particular, musical sound, from the intoned recitation of the Gospel to florid psalmody, functioned as the central sonic pole around which the divine offices orbited. Whereas vision has been widely regarded in Western thought as the highest sense, being the primary "generator of knowledge" and the most trustworthy arbiter of truth,[3] it was hearing that functioned as a primary mechanism for embodied experience in Byzantine worship, encompassing audible theological texts (both intoned and sung) and immersive waves of semantically unintelligible chant alike. This reflects a robust theology of audibility present in Christian sources more generally. The most significant moments in the Gospel narratives feature the aural transmission of truth or knowledge: with the sound of their voices, John the Baptist proclaims the advent of Jesus Christ, the Archangel Gabriel announces the conception to the Virgin Mary, and God the Father bears witness to the theophany at the Jordan River, while the Holy Spirit's visit to the apostles on Pentecost is an equally sonic experience, heralded "with the sound of a violent, rushing wind."[4]

The *melodoi*, the celebrated poet-composers of the Byzantine East who flourished as early as the sixth century and whose output would have a defining impact on the structure of the divine offices of the

1 L. C. Eneix, ed., *Archaeoacoustics: The Archaeology of Sound—Proceedings from the 2014 Conference in Malta* (Myakka City, FL, 2014); W. Woszcyk, "Acoustics of Hagia Sophia: Virtual and Scientific Approach to Humanities and Sacred Space," *Aural Architecture: Music, Acoustics, and Ritual*, https://auralarchitecture.stanford.edu/sites/default/files/onassis_seminar_woszczyk_2014_lt.pdf (accessed 5 June 2015).

2 Two projects whose scope lies at the nexus of these disciplines are Icons of Sound (http://iconsofsound.stanford.edu/), a collaboration including Bissera Pentcheva (Stanford), Jonathan Abel (CCRMA), and Cappella Romana (dir. Alexander Lingas) and Soundscapes of Byzantine Thessaloniki, led by Sharon Gerstel (UCLA) and Chrys Kyriakakis (USC).

3 M. Smith, *Sensing the Past: Seeing, Hearing, Smelling, Tasting, and Touching in History* (Berkeley and Los Angeles, 2007), 6–7, 28–29, 41. See also V. Erlmann, "But What of the Ethnographic Ear? Anthropology, Sound, and the Senses," in *Hearing Cultures: Essays on Sound, Listening, and Modernity* (New York, 2004).

4 Mt. 3:3, Mk.1:3, Jn. 1:23; Lk. 1:28–33; Mt. 3:17; Acts 2:2.

Byzantine Rite, would expound on these aural themes, their poetic exegeses imbuing scriptural accounts with music, as in the climactic phrase of the anonymously transmitted *doxastikon* of the Lauds for the feast of the Dormition: "As they reverently buried you they sang Gabriel's song, crying out: 'Hail, full of grace, Virgin Mother without bridegroom, the Lord is with you.'"[5] In the Gospel passage, Gabriel speaks, but here, he is described as having sung his greeting (μελῳδοῦντες ἀνεβόων), now emulated by the apostles at the Theotokos's burial. The addition of sonic elements occurs as well in the genre of the *kanon*, a type of strophic poem that flourished around the Palestinian monastery of St. Sabas in the seventh and eighth centuries. In the seventh-century kanon of Pascha attributed by tradition to John of Damascus, the hymnographer, while focused largely on light, describes the Resurrection celebration as an overwhelmingly multisensory experience, according special significance to sound and music, as in the second troparion of ode 1:

> Let us purify our senses, and we shall see Christ shining forth, in the unapproachable light of the resurrection, and we shall clearly hear him saying "Rejoice!" as we sing the triumphal song.

On the one hand, the worshippers behold Christ's lightning-like "shining forth" (Χριστὸν ἐξαστράπτοντα), but they also *hear* his resurrectional greeting, an act of auscultation that gives them great pleasure (τρανῶς ἀκουσόμεθα). Furthermore, the lights beheld and the sounds heard are to provoke a joyful, musical response among those performing the kanon who "sing the triumphal song" (ἐπινίκιον ᾄδοντες), a theme invoked several times throughout this kanon and the genre in general.[6]

Around the thirteenth century, a confluence of factors served to heighten the already elevated role of music in Byzantine worship: pictorial representations of anonymous singers, saintly composers, and the hymns themselves appear in monumental paintings, while architectural features evidently designed to enhance acoustical properties enter the churches. In Constantinople's Chora Monastery, a funerary chapel situated to the east of the monastery's main nave features a unique dome and pendentives scheme with Christ as the central figure, flanked by four prolific hymnographers from Byzantium's past—John of Damascus, Kosmas of Maiouma, Joseph the Hymnographer and Theophanes—instead of four evangelists, as is customary. A variation on this theme is found in the Church of the Holy Apostles in Thessalonike. Above the vault connecting the south aisle to the nave, painted next to a typical Nativity scene, is the text of a sticheron from Christmas Vespers, "What shall we offer You, O Christ."[7] Furthermore, in dozens of late Byzantine churches, both in Byzantium and on its periphery, lavishly clad singers are now featured in iconographic schemes, occupying prominent roles in the festivities depicted.[8] These trends seem to reflect a heightened consciousness in the late Byzantine period of the music and sounds that adorned the liturgical services. But perhaps the most significant change of all was in the music itself. Beginning in the thirteenth century, musical manuscripts testify to the emergence of a new species of highly personalized chant, called *kalophonia* by its creators. Kalophonia was an embellished style of psalmody enabled by notational technology that had evolved adequate precision to serve the expressive needs of a cadre of self-consciously authorial composers who flourished during the Palaiologan period. The compositions of these *maistores*[9]

5 Translations of liturgical texts are by Fr. Ephrem Lash, http://www.anastasis.org.uk (now defunct; accessed 2 May 2016, https://web.archive.org/web/20160502141720/http://www.anastasis.org.uk/). Manuscript rubrics are translated by the present author unless otherwise specified.

6 Discussed in D. Krueger, "The Transmission of Liturgical Joy in Byzantine Hymns for Easter," chapter 7 in *Prayer and Worship in Eastern Christianities, 5th to 11th Centuries*, ed. D. Krueger and B. Bitton-Ashkelony (Abingdon and New York, 2016). For a brief discussion and bibliography questioning the attribution of this kanon to John of Damascus, see ibid., 25. I thank the author for sending me a prepublication copy of this essay.

7 S. Gerstel, "Monastic Soundspaces: The Art and Act of Chanting," in *Resounding Images: The Aural and Visual Arts [in Harmony], 800–1500*, ed. S. Boynton and D. J. Reilly (Turnhout, 2015), 135–52.

8 N. K. Moran, *Singers in Late Byzantine and Slavonic Painting* (Leiden, 1986).

9 In late Byzantine sources, the term *maistor* referred to a palace official with musical responsibilities (J. Darrouzès,

were florid, virtuosic, and tended toward abstraction, the proper texts of the divine offices now manipulated to function as objects of meditation, even morphing in some cases into sequences and repetitions of nonsemantic syllables, the famed *kratemata* of the kalophonic idiom.[10]

This study is an attempt to bring the soundscape of worship in Byzantium into relief by focusing on kalophonia in relation to nonkalophonic forms.[11] Specifically, I will analyze two different musical settings of Μάγοι Περσῶν βασιλεῖς (The Magi, Kings of Persia), a festal *sticheron* originally sung after Psalm 50 (LXX) during Christmas Matins of the Sabaïtic Rite. The text is attributed to John the Monk, an eighth-century hymnographer from the desert of Palestine, who in all likelihood would have composed the original tune along with the text, though a few centuries before it would show up in manuscripts notated with chant neumes.[12] The first setting analyzed is the "classical" sticheron, a compact, mostly syllabic chant found in musical collections called *sticheraria* as early as the eleventh century.[13] The second setting is an expansive, kalophonic composition featuring a number of compositional devices that would have demanded a high level of vocal dexterity to execute. The first kalophonic setting of Μάγοι Περσῶν was written in the late thirteenth century by the imperial court musician John Komnenos. Based on concordances I have identified in musical manuscripts and the fourteenth-century *Treatise on Court Titles*, also known as "pseudo-Kodinos," we can now securely argue that this kalophonic composition was composed to adorn the imperial festivities of Christmas day.[14] Komnenos's setting would enjoy a series of embellishments by subsequent composers of the imperial court, yielding multiple layers of artistic manipulation in the form of melodic expansion and contraction, textual rearrangement, and interpolation of ecstatic *teretismata*, the nonsemantic, textual building blocks of the kratemata. Although the ritual settings of the classical sticheron and its kalophonic counterpart differ, a comparison of the two will help to shed light on how these chants might have been heard and experienced in their native contexts.

Of course, cathedral and monastic worship, including their music, were not the only representative soundscapes of medieval Byzantium.[15] A more exhaustive survey of the varied keynotes of Byzantine society—extending beyond music—would be necessary before one might attempt to map a comprehensive theory of aurality in Byzantium. Like any medieval society, Byzantium featured a wide array of preindustrial keynotes, some laden with temporal significance, others serving as markers of space, ethnicity, and social class.[16] The soundscape of Byzantine liturgy itself involved a vast array of nonmusical keynotes, from the wooden *talanton* that regulated life in monasteries, to the ritual movement of clerics and acolytes within large cathedrals, along with any ambient sounds that might infiltrate an ecclesiastical or palatine edifice. Even "silence . . . has a history," arguably of special importance considering the ascendancy

Recherches sur les offikia de l'église byzantine [Paris, 1970], 285, 574), probably the director of both right and left choirs (E. Spyrakou, *Οι χοροί ψαλτών κατά τη βυζαντινή παράδοση* [Athens, 2008], 172).

10 G. Anastasiou, *Τα Κρατήματα στην ψαλτική τέχνη* (Athens, 2005).

11 The term *soundscape* was introduced to the academic vernacular by the composer R. M. Schafer in *The Soundscape: Our Sonic Environment and the Tuning of the World* (Rochester, VT, 1994). See also, A. Lingas, "From Earth to Heaven: The Changing Musical Soundscape of Byzantine Liturgy," in *Experiencing Byzantium: Papers from the 44th Spring Symposium of the SPBS*, ed. M. Jackson and C. Nesbitt (Aldershot, 2013): 311–58.

12 In MS Ambrosianus A 139 this sticheron is attributed to "John," whereas in the nonmusical sources it is often attributed to "John the Monk." See E. Wellesz, *A History of Byzantine Music and Hymnography* (Oxford, 1961), 237.

13 The *sticherarion* is a musical collection containing festal hymns called *stichera*, from the *Menaion* (the fixed cycle), the *Triodion-Pentekostarion* (the movable cycles), and the *Oktoechos* (book of eight modes).

14 See J. Verpeaux, ed., *Pseudo-Kodinos: Traité des offices* (Paris, 1966) and R. Macrides et al., *Pseudo-Kodinos and the Constantinopolitan Court: Offices and Ceremonies* (Farnham and Burlington, VT, 2013).

15 For one view that suggests an imbalance in the attention given to music in sound studies at large, see J. Attali, *Noise: The Political Economy of Music*, trans. B. Maussumi (Minneapolis, 1985), cited in Smith, *Sensing the Past*, 42.

16 One inherently musical keynote that had explicit social meaning in late Byzantium occurred during the *kabalikeuma* (the emperor's "riding out"): the playing of horns signaled to the people that the emperor could be approached by suppliants seeking reparations for an injustice they had suffered (Macrides et al., *Pseudo-Kodinos*, 439).

of a spirituality of "quietude" (ἡσυχία) in late Byzantium.[17] While all these sounds and non-sounds played a role in the composition of the sonic landscape of Byzantium, music was the sonic material at the center of the auditory experience, especially in the context of liturgical worship and imperial ritual. An analysis of changes in musical style by means of this particular case study can provide insight into the impact of embellished music on the listener, revealing how composers of the late Byzantine period manipulated existing material in order to animate texts and enhance the soundscape of Byzantine liturgical offices and imperial ceremonies. This, in turn, enables us to begin to assemble a preliminary framework for assessing the human experience of sound in Byzantium. How was chant heard, and how did chant—both simple and kalophonic—evoke perceptions, memories, and spiritual experiences? Probing these questions may help us assess the ever-changing spirituality and aesthetics of musicians, patrons, and congregations—all active participants in the soundscapes of the Byzantine world.

Orality and Notation in Byzantium

Musical activity in Byzantium encompassed both practical music as well as the theoretical discipline that was one of the four sciences of the quadrivium. Intellectuals of the late Byzantine period wrote extensively on a range of musical subjects, from the cosmology of music to the relationship between ancient Greek and Byzantine ecclesiastical modes,[18] while working musicians played instruments, sung, and composed. Primacy of place belonged to monophonic song, encompassing many vocal genres including church psalmody (i.e., Byzantine chant). Instrumental music, though accorded a secondary position, was still ubiquitous. Instruments such as the lyre, aulos, and pipe organs were found in both domestic and public settings, while brass, percussion, and larger, public organs, such as the one in the Capital's Hippodrome, were utilized during military and civic ceremonies.[19] Instruments feature prominently in descriptions of the *prokypsis* ceremony of Christmas Eve as described in the *Treatise* of pseudo-Kodinos. The playing of trumpets, bugles, clarinets, and kettledrums, marked the exit of the emperor and his retinue from the church following the Divine Liturgy on Christmas Eve, providing a clamorous complement to the *a cappella* chant heard within the church walls during the service.[20] While we have ample evidence describing Byzantine musical instruments, our ability to reconstruct the actual musical form of instrumental musical genres is limited, as virtually no notated instrumental music has survived from the Byzantine period.[21]

On the other hand, we are able to reconstruct the aural profile of Byzantine liturgical offices and some imperial court ceremonies thanks to manuscripts of notated Byzantine chant, which appear first around the ninth to tenth centuries, roughly the same time manuscripts of notated Latin plainchant appear in Western Europe.[22] These "Palaeobyzantine notations" were *adiastematic*, meaning that the neumes transmit information on melodic shape and direction but lack complete pitch specificity, as in the earliest layers of Western plainchant notation. The relatively unspecific nature of Palaeobyzantine notations highlights the indispensable role played by memory and orality in medieval Byzantium. Especially before the emergence of diastematic neumes around the

17 Quotation from J. Parr, "Notes for a More Sensuous History of Twentieth-Century Canada: The Timely, the Tacit, and the Material Body," *Canadian Historical Review* 82 (December 2001): 740, cited in Smith, *Sensing the Past*, 50.

18 See L. Richter, "Antike Überlieferungen in der byzantinischen Musiktheorie," *Acta Musicologica* 70, no. 2 (1998): 133–208, and C. Troelsgård, "Ancient Musical Theory in Byzantine Environments," *CIMAGL* 56 (1988): 228–36.

19 For musical instruments in Byzantium, see N. Maliaras, *Βυζαντινά μουσικά όργανα* (Athens, 2007). See also M. L. West, *Ancient Greek Music* (Oxford, 1992).

20 Verpeaux, *Pseudo-Kodinos*, 189–91. Evidently, by the Palaiologan period organs were no longer featured in imperial ceremonies such as the prokypsis (A. Lingas, "Music," in *Oxford Handbook of Byzantine Studies* ed., E. Jeffreys, J. F. Haldon, and R. Cormack [Oxford, 2008], 928), although there is indirect evidence of the instrument's presence in ceremonial during this period (Macrides et al., *Pseudo-Kodinos*, 441).

21 Lingas, "Music," 928.

22 Ekphonetic notation, used to guide the recitation of the Gospels, Apostles, and Prophecies, is preserved in manuscripts dating from the ninth to the fourteenth centuries (S. Martani, "Das Ekphonetische Notationssystem in den Datierten Evangeliarien des 10. Jahrhunderts," in *Palaeobyzantine Notations*, vol. 3, *Acta of the Congress Held at Hernen Castle, the Netherlands, in March 2001*, ed. G. Wolfram (Leuven, 2004), 27–47.

third quarter of the twelfth century, notation functioned as an aid to memory and most melodies (especially the psalms, kanons, and ordinary chants of the liturgy) would have been learned and performed by ear.[23] Other genres of psalmody would have relied more heavily on notation for their transmission, such as the *stichera idiomela*, a mostly non-melismatic corpus of proper chants interpolated between the psalm verses of Vespers and Orthros (a repertory to which our first example of Μάγοι Περσῶν belongs). These were unique compositions not based on model melodies and, while simple relative to their kalophonic counterparts, they featured brief excursions of melisma, probably on account of the festivity associated with the feasts for which they were composed. Such a repertory would require a consistently notated form to ensure stability in transmission especially since most of these chants were sung only once per year. And in fact, the central repertory of the sticherarion was transmitted with astounding uniformity over the course of the two centuries after the change to diastematic notation.[24] Scribes now had the ability to document the melodic trajectory of a chant with precision, fixing in writing a body of melodies that had been previously transmitted orally. Paradoxically, the very notation that seems to have developed to preserve this mostly syllabic repertory is that which eventually enabled the emergence of a far more florid version of psalmody, the kalophonia.[25]

The Kalophonia

Around the thirteenth century, the musical sources testify to three interrelated phenomena which would have sweeping implications on the soundscape of worship in Byzantium. The first is the development of a more advanced notational technology; the second is the use of this notation to document more precisely not just syllabic chants, but far more elaborate chants that utilized compositional devices not found before; and finally, following these two trends, is the emergence of a cadre of self-consciously authorial composers, or ποιητές, the term that these musicians used to refer to themselves and to their colleagues. Once notation acquired the ability to transmit melodies with more fixity, composers seized the opportunity to elaborate on older forms, which in turn seems to have increased their authority and the status of the chants they authored. Kenneth Levy described this shift in musical creativity as a *grand tournant* that was

> nothing less than a radical recasting of the whole conceptual framework underlying the liturgical chants . . . the change from a conception of Byzantine liturgical *melos* that is traditionally oriented and anonymous, and whose transmission is basically oral, to a new view of it as freshly inspired, precisely written down, personally stylized melody composed in a characteristic idiom by a "name" composer.[26]

Kalophonia, meaning "beautiful sound," is not an anachronistic term: its first appearance is in an early thirteenth-century south Italian manuscript, MS Messina 161, which contains chants that have been called "proto-kalophonic" by some scholars.[27] In its fully developed form, kalophonia is associated with the emergence of a new musical codex, the *Akolouthia*, which contained (mostly) chants for Vespers, Orthros, and the Divine Liturgies according to the "neo-Sabaïtic" liturgical rite.[28] The origins of the Akolouthia

23 Lingas, "From Earth" (n. 11 above), 341.

24 W. O. Strunk, "The Notation of the Chartres Fragment," in *Essays on Music in the Western World* (New York, 1977), 68–111. This repertoire was edited and further standardized by Koukouzeles sometime in the beginning of the fourteenth century (J. Raasted, "Koukouzeles' Revisions of the Sticherarion and Sinai Gr. 1230," in *Laborare Fratres in Unum: Festschrift László Dobszay zum 60. Geburtstag*, ed. J. Szendrei and D. Hiley (Zurich, 1995), 261–77.

25 This layer of notation is referred to as "middle Byzantine" or "round" notation.

26 K. Levy, "Le tournant décisif dans l'histoire de la musique byzantine: 1071–1261," in *Actes de XVe Congrès international d'études byzantines* (Athens, 1979), 474.

27 C. Adsuara, "Remarks on the Structure of Kalophonic Stichera: Working Hypotheses," in *Papers Read at the Cantus Planus Meeting in Sopron, Hungary* (Sopron, 1995); and C. Troelsgård, "Thirteenth-Century Byzantine Melismatic Chant and the Development of the Kalophonic Style," in Wolfram, *Palaeobyzantine Notations*, 67–90.

28 By the fourteenth century, the "neo-Sabaïtic" rite had phased out the prevailing Stoudite practices (already a hybrid of Palestinian and Constantinopolitan liturgy) as well as the archaic Cathedral Rite of Constantinople in the few ecclesiastical establishments where the latter was still practiced. See R. Taft, *The Byzantine Rite: A Short History* (Collegeville, MN, 1992). For the Cathedral Rite of Constantinople, see A. Lingas,

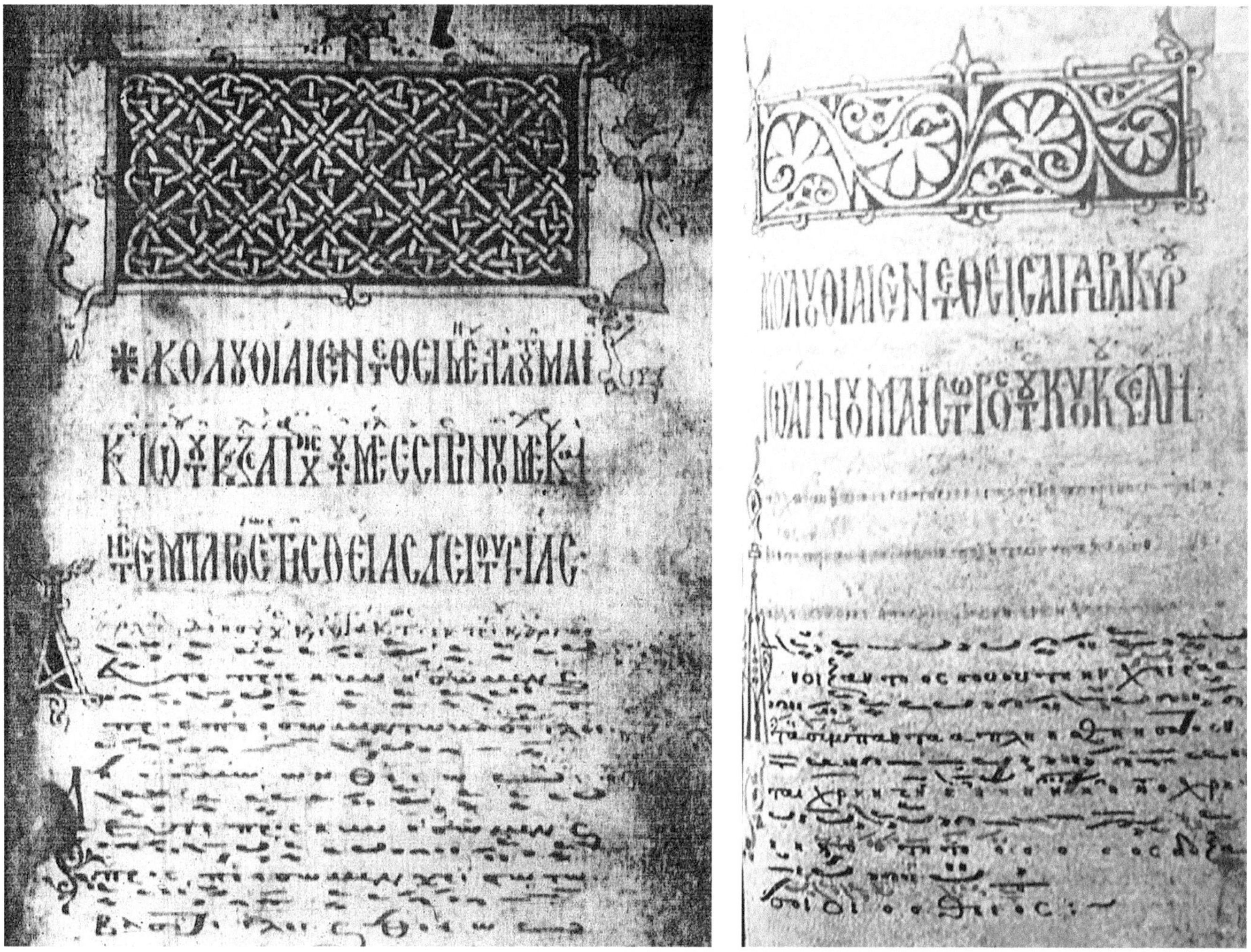

FIG. 4.1. MSS Athens 2458 (left, dated 1336) and Iviron 1120 (right, dated 1458). Left: "The order of services edited by Lord John Koukouzeles the Maistor, from the beginning of Great Vespers through the completion of the Divine Liturgy." Right: "The order of services edited by Lord John Koukouzeles the Maistor." (Courtesy Athens National Library and Iviron Monastery, Mount Athos)

can be traced to the thirteenth century, but the earliest surviving copy that can be precisely dated is MS Athens National Library 2458, copied in 1336. The primary editor of this collection, and the figurehead of the kalophonic idiom according to musicians of the late Byzantine period, is undoubtedly the prolific composer John Koukouzeles (fl. late 13th–mid-14th c.). Evidence for this is seen in the headings of the majority of Akolouthia manuscripts copied in the fourteenth century, a tradition extending to the middle of the fifteenth century, though with less intensity, even after the Akolouthia repertory had been enriched with hundreds of compositions by composers who followed Koukouzeles.[29] For example, the heading of Athens 2458 is nearly identical to that of MS Iviron 1120 (see fig. 4.1), an exemplary Akolouthia copied in 1458 by the last prominent musician of the Byzantine

"Sunday Matins in the Byzantine Cathedral Rite: Music and Liturgy" (PhD diss., University of British Columbia, 1996) and S. Parenti, "The Cathedral Rite of Constantinople: Evolution of a Local Tradition," *OCP* 77 (2011): 451–53.

29 M. Velimirović, "The Prooemiac Psalm of Byzantine Vespers," in *Words and Music: The Scholar's View*, ed. L. Berman (Cambridge, MA, 1972), 317–37.

imperial court, Manuel Chrysaphes (fl. 1440–1470). Thus, Koukouzeles is regarded by musicians of late Byzantium as the primary redactor of the Akolouthia, the representative musical collection of the kalophonic period, establishing him as the champion of this musical style during its acme.

Akolouthiai featured newly composed kalophonic chants alongside older, anonymous repertories, some derived from the Asmatikon and the Psaltikon, others notated for the first time, such as the ordinary psalms of Vespers and Orthros.[30] The older, anonymous chants were often labelled ἀρχαῖον or παλαιόν, while the kalophonic material was introduced with special phrases signaling the new style, as in MS Lavra E 173 (written in 1436), where on folio 31r, after the shorter, anonymous settings of the First Kathisma of Vespers (Psalms 1–3), the scribe and composer David Raidestinos writes the phrase "here begins the kalophonia" to introduce the kalophonic settings of Psalm 2.[31] Similarly, on folio 70r of Iviron 1120, Psalm 2 is introduced with the phrase, "Kalophonic verses of Great Vespers by Lord John Koukouzeles the maistor, plagal fourth mode." These frequently encountered inscriptions suggest that contemporary musicians conceived of kalophonia as a distinctly new art, different from the rest of the chant of the daily and nightly cycle of services.[32] Furthermore, inscriptions in manuscripts of the kalophonic period highlight the elevated status of the kalophonic chants and the relationship of the composers to their compositions. "This is the wonderful ending by the Master" is how the scribe of MS Sinai 1584 (fol. 464), introduces a coda to a kalophonic sticheron composed by Koukouzeles.[33] "I think this composition is the sweetest" is an inscription written by Manuel Chrysaphes in Iviron 1120, to describe a kalophonic composition commissioned by the emperor Constantine XI.[34] Later in the same codex, Chrysaphes writes that a kalophonic setting of Psalm 2:11 is "a composition by the most marvelous teacher among teachers, Lord John Koukouzeles the maistor, [which is] very beautiful."[35] Marginalia describing the aural qualities of specific kalophonic compositions, such as "sweetest," "wonderful," "embellished," "more kalophonic," and so on, abound in the musical manuscripts, differentiating the kalophonia from older forms. Moreover, these marginalia highlight the fact that kalophonia, while not shedding its practical utility as liturgical chant, occupied a special aesthetic class not seen before: music for beauty's sake.

Evidence of kalophonic embellishment is attested to in literary sources as well, although its reception was not always positive. The monastic typikon of Neilos Damalis, written around 1400, offers such a cool assessment, admonishing its singers to avoid "teretismatic odes," which are "more fitting for actors on stage."[36] The notion that music of the wrong type could have a deleterious effect on spirituality dates back at least to fourth-century anchorite proscriptions against singing of hymns.[37] That an opposition to this style of singing existed cannot be doubted; that opposition was endemic is refuted by the abundance of evidence for the flourishing of kalophonic psalmody in not just urban but also monastic environments: the Akolouthiai feature hundreds of chants inspired by and composed for the Athonite all-night vigil (*agrypnia*) and many holy men of this period praised psalmody as a virtuous exercise on the path toward

30 The Asmatikon and the Psaltikon were musical collections from the Rite of the Great Church of Hagia Sophia, featuring music for choir and soloist, respectively.

31 Vespers according to the neo-Sabaïtic usage had as its opening antiphon Psalm 103, after which the verses from the first kathisma of the Psalter were sung (Ps. 1–3). Typically, Akoulouthiai feature kalophonic settings of verses from Psalm 2, interspersed with named kratemata.

32 G. Stathis, "Η ασματική διαφοροποίηση όπως καταγράφεται στον κώδικα EBE 2458 του έτους 1336," in *Χριστιανική Θεσσαλονίκη: Παλαιολόγειος εποχή* (Thessalonike, 1989).

33 Cited in Levy, "Le Tournant," 475.

34 Iviron 1120, fol. 139r; cited also in G. Stathis, "Μανουήλ Χρυσάφης ο λαμπαδάριος," in *Κύκλος ελληνικής μουσικής, βυζαντινοί μελουργοί, Μεγάρου μουσικής Αθηνών* (Athens, 1994–95), 33–45.

35 Iviron 1120, fol. 150r.

36 R. Dubowchik, "Singing with the Angels: Foundation Documents as Evidence for Musical Life in Monasteries of the Byzantine Empire," *DOP* 56 (2002): 294–95.

37 S. Frøyshov, "La reticence à l' hymnographie chez des anachorètes de l' Égypte et du Sinai du 5eme au 8eme siecles," in *L'hymnographie Conférence Saint-Serge, XLVIe Semaine d'études liturgiques, Paris, 29 juin–2 juillet 1999*, ed. J. Claire and A. M. Triacca (Rome, 2000), 229–45. See also A. Louth, *St. John Damascene: Tradition and Originality in Byzantine Theology* (Oxford, 2002), 20–30.

spiritual perfection.[38] In fact, according to his *Vita*, Koukouzeles himself—following a probable stint in the imperial court—became a monk at the monastery of the Great Lavra on Mt. Athos, where he would have overlapped with the champion of the hesychast movement, Gregory Palamas, even perhaps sharing a role as liturgical singers.[39] This connection between Koukouzeles and Palamas is one thread in the compelling web of seemingly related trends percolating in late Byzantium, which has led some scholars to contemplate a connection between kalophonic chant and hesychasm.[40] But, while kalophonia clearly flourished on Mt. Athos, it was also, without question, cultivated in imperial circles, perhaps even originating there. The musicians most associated with this style, Koukouzeles, Xenos Korones, John Kladas, and Manuel Chrysaphes, to name a few, were employed in the imperial court, appearing as titleholders τοῦ εὐαγοῦς βασιλικοῦ κλήρου ("of the sacred and royal clergy") in the musical sources.[41] Furthermore, some of the most elaborate hymns composed at this time, including the kalophonic setting of Μάγοι Περσῶν, were written explicitly for imperial ceremonies. The abundance of kalophonic chant in the sixty or so surviving copies of Akolouthiai from the Byzantine era and the widespread diffusion of the neo-Sabaïtic rite testifies to the fact that this musical style was something radically new, and that it must have been routinely heard by a broad swath of worshippers across a number of churches and monasteries in the empire.[42]

While Koukouzeles was regarded as a founding father of the kalophonic movement by contemporaries and successors alike, it is clear that his activity in the early fourteenth century represented the apex of a tradition which was already well underway by the middle of the thirteenth. This much can be gleaned from Akolouthiai that preserve fully mature kalophonic chants by composers who preceded Koukouzeles, a chronology confirmed in a passage from Manuel Chrysaphes' theoretical treatise. In presenting a defense of his compositional style by means of its (alleged) identity with that of his predecessors, Chrysaphes cites a lineage of composers that begins well before Koukouzeles ("The first composer of *oikoi* was Aneotes and the second was Glykys who imitated Aneotes")[43] yielding the following chronological sequence: Aneotes, John Glykys, Nikephoros Ethikos, Koukouzeles, Xenos Korones, John Kladas, and Manuel Chrysaphes.[44] While Chrysaphes' notion of a two-century-long cadre of insiders in the art of kalophonic composition is to some degree constructed, it cannot be dismissed. This strong sense of collective identity is evident in the headings, rubrics, and ordering of musical manuscripts from this period. It is abundantly clear in the well-known miniature from MS Athos Koutloumousiou 457 (dated by Gregory Stathis to the second half of the fourteenth century), which depicts Koukouzeles and Korones, seated at the feet of their teacher, the thirteenth-century composer John Glykys, holding a staff as he teaches the art of *cheironomia* to his two students.[45] The lineage above is corroborated even more sweepingly by the arrangement of the music in dozens of Akolouthiai, in which compositions within a given genre are typically ordered by relative date of the composer. Taken together, this evidence highlights one of the most remarkable

38 For the development and diffusion of the all-night vigil in the Orthodox world, see M. Arranz, "L'office de la veillée nocturne dans l' Eglise grecque et dans l' Eglise russe," *OCP* 42 (1976): 117–55; 402–25.

39 A. Lingas, "Hesychasm and Psalmody," in *Mount Athos and Byzantine Monasticism*, ed. A. Bryer and M. Cunningham (Aldershot, 1996), 159–60.

40 Ibid., 157, 159.

41 For example, this title appears on fol. 173r of the mid-fifteenth-century MS Iviron 975, describing Manuel Chrysaphes, also the probable scribe of the same codex. G. Stathis, *Τα χειρόγραφα βυζαντινής μουσικής—Άγιον Όρος*, vol. 3 (Athens, 1976), 766.

42 G. Stathis, *Οι αναγραμματισμοί και τα μαθήματα της βυζαντινής μελοποιΐας* (Athens, 1992), 111.

43 D. Conomos, *The Treatise of Manuel Chrysaphes, the Lampadarios* (Vienna, 1985), 44–47. The *oikoi* referred to by Chrysaphes are kalophonic compositions based on verses ("oikoi") from the Akathist Kontakion.

44 Xenos Korones is not mentioned in the passage cited above, but elsewhere in the treatise his place in the chronology—after Koukouzeles and before Chrysaphes—is given (Conomos, *Treatise*, 41).

45 The published miniature is a drawing of an original folio, which no longer survives. According to Gregory Stathis, the original folio was taken from MS Koutloumousiou 457 by Porfirij Uspensky, under whom it was published (*St. Petrov-Hr. Kodov, Old Bulgarian Musical Documents* [Sophia, 1973], 42). See Stathis, *Οι Αναγραμματισμοί*, 126 and Moran, *Singers*, 44.

aspects of this new musical idiom: the emergence and heightened visibility of the figure of composer.[46] Composers of the kalophonic period embellished existing hymns, wrote entirely new settings of ordinary chants, and signed their names in the manuscripts alongside their works, while theorists such as Manuel Chrysaphes refer to specific compositions by name as exemplars to be imitated. All these factors contribute to what has been called the "shift in the status of a given chant from being considered part of the received tradition to becoming a piece of art."[47]

The Classical Sticheron: Μάγοι Περσῶν

The classical sticheron idiomelon Μάγοι Περσῶν provides a baseline against which we can compare later kalophonic compositions. The text of this sticheron is a poetic paraphrase of the Gospel story of the Magi's visit to the newborn Christ child, with a theological postscript juxtaposing the newborn infant and God's timelessness:

> Magi, Kings of Persia, having clearly learned that the heavenly King had been born on earth, drawn by a bright star, arrived in Bethlehem, bringing chosen gifts, gold and incense and myrrh. And falling down they worshipped, for they saw lying in the Cave the Timeless One as a babe.

This hymn first appears with musical notation in sticheraria dated to the eleventh century, and by the third quarter of the twelfth century (1177), it appears in one of the earliest sticheraria written in diastematic neumes, MS Sinai 1218 (fig. 4.2a, lines 6–12). It is transmitted faithfully, as testified to by its appearance in MS Ambrosianus A 139 sup, which was copied in Constantinople in 1342 (fig. 4.2b, lines 8–13). Figure 4.2c provides a transcription of this sticheron into staff notation, based on the later source.[48] Though separated by nearly two centuries, there is only minimal variation between the two manuscripts: the contour of the melody is virtually identical, despite slight embellishments in the Ambrosianus codex not found in earlier sources. The sticheron's melody is mostly syllabic, with a few, brief excursions of melisma. Its vocal range is modest, spanning just over an octave, A to b flat, with cadences on d (the base pitch of plagal first mode), f, and, somewhat uniquely, on B below d (transcribed as a B flat).[49] This is a dignified melody with a regular rhythmic pulse of duple and triple meter featuring a mix of steps and small leaps of thirds and fourths. Interestingly, the brief, melismatic passages do not necessarily correspond to important syllables or words in the text but function as melodic bridges connecting two phrases.

One notable feature of this sticheron is the brief embellishment outlining a perfect fourth (c to f) prior to cadences on B flat on the words ἑλκόμενοι and προσφέροντες. This unique motif is transformed into a thematic element in the later kalophonic embellishments, especially in the lengthy teretismatic passage by Manuel Chrysaphes, who was no doubt paying homage to the original sticheron. Though this chant would have been heard only once a year, its characters (the Magi, the Christ child) and thematic material (the star, the gifts of the Magi, the cave) would have been familiar to both lay and monastic congregations, being derived from the Gospel narrative and expounded in multiple hymns sung throughout Christmas Vespers and Orthros. The chanting of this sticheron would have taken just a few minutes, and its syllabic melody and conservative vocal range would have rendered its text easily intelligible to listeners in a resonant space even with significant reverberation.

46 Miloš Velimirović counts over a hundred names in the early fifteenth-century Akolouthia Athens 2406 (see his "Byzantine Composers in MS. Athens 2406," in *Essays Presented to Egon Wellesz*, ed. J. A. Westrup and E. Wellesz [Oxford, 1966], 7–18).

47 C. Troelsgård, "Tradition and Transformation in Late Byzantine and Post-Byzantine Chant," in *Interaction and Isolation in Late Byzantine Culture, Papers Read at a Colloquium Held at the Swedish Research Institute in Istanbul, 1–5 December 1999*, ed. J. O. Rosenqvist (Stockholm, 2004), 158. The use of the term "independent art works" to describe compositions of the kalophonic period has also been used by Kenneth Levy and Rosemary Dubowchik.

48 I thank John Michael Boyer for typesetting my transcription, which, generally speaking, follows the rhythmic principles laid out in Ioannes Arvanitis's dissertation, "Ο ρυθμός των εκκλησιαστικών μελών μέσα από τη παλαιογραφική έρευνα και την εξήγηση της παλαιάς σημειογραφίας" (PhD diss., Ionian University, 2010).

49 Names of notes follow the Helmholtz pitch system.

FIG. 4.2.
(a) Sticheron Μάγοι Περσῶν, MS Sinai 1218, fol. 74r (dated 1177) (courtesy of the Monastery of St. Catherine on Mt. Sinai); (b) Ambrosianus A 139 sup, fol. 82v (dated 1342) (reproduced with the permission of Monumenta Musicae Byzantinae); (c) transcription of Μάγοι Περσῶν, based on Ambrosianus A 139 sup (transcription: author)

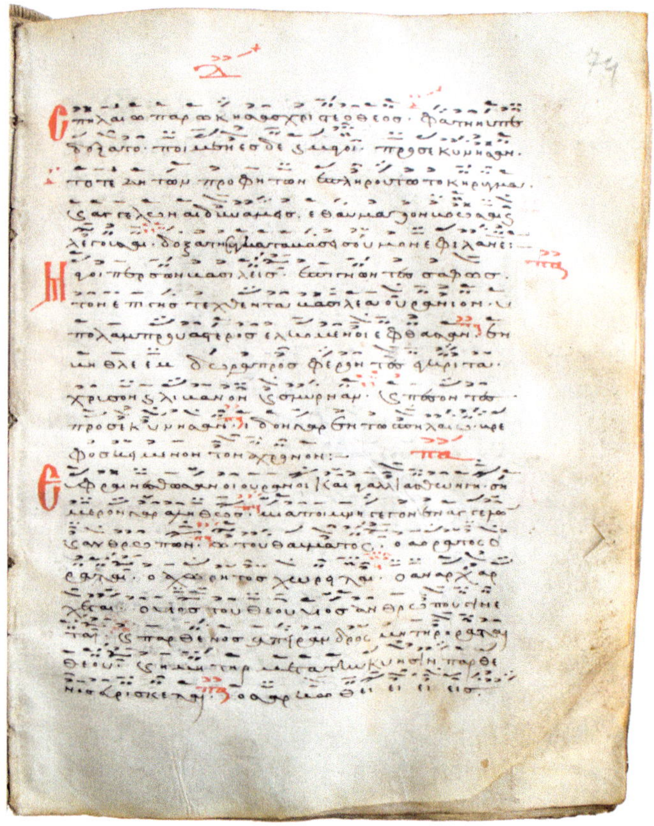
a

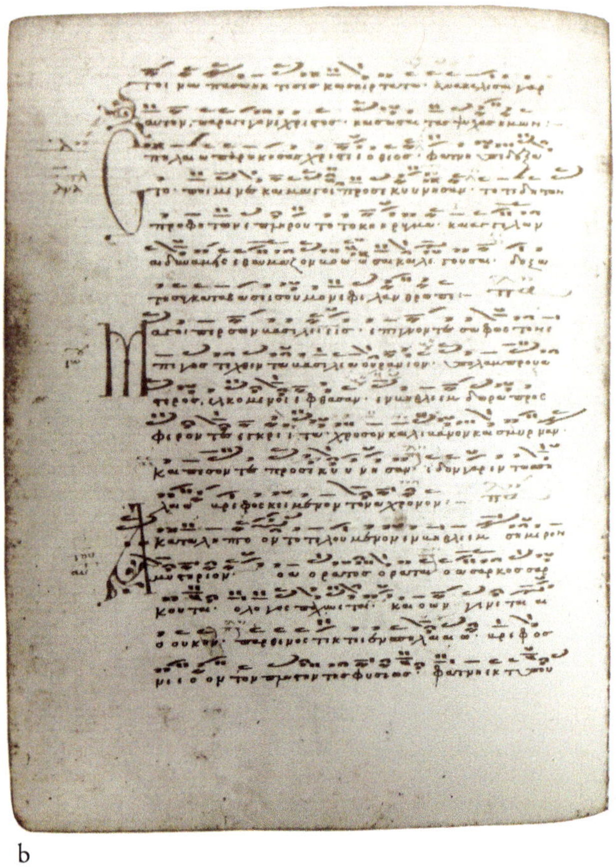
b

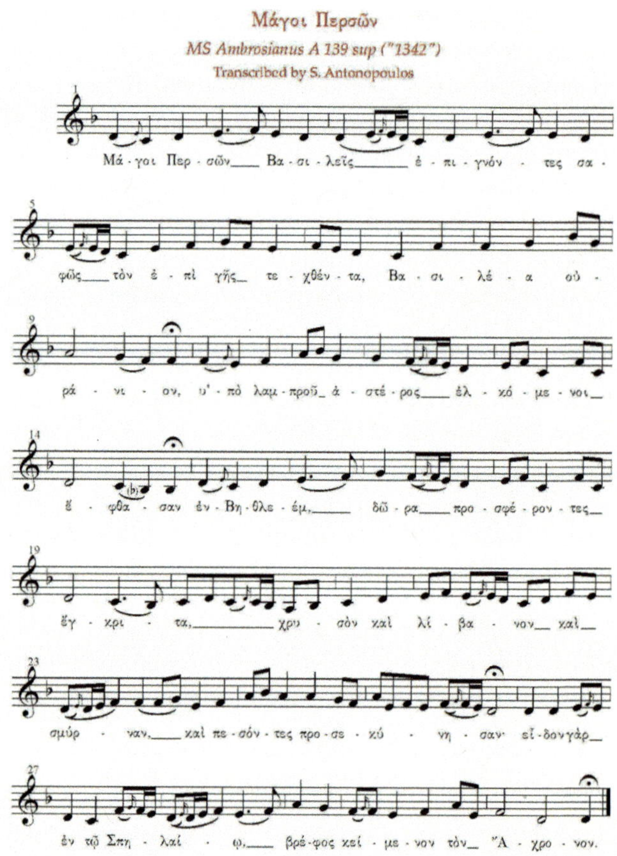

c

The Kalophonic Sticheron Μάγοι Περσῶν

Christmas in the Byzantine Palace

Μάγοι Περσῶν was a hymn ripe for embellishment. Not only was it prescribed to be sung during one of the most festive liturgical periods—the Christmas Orthros—but it also appears in both sources of music and court ceremonial as one of the hallmark musical pieces of the imperial meal on Christmas day, performed by the royal singers in front of the emperor and scores of imperial title holders and foreign dignitaries. Μάγοι Περσῶν is referenced in the fourth book of pseudo-Kodinos, "Concerning the order of the patronal feasts and the customs that apply to those days," which includes a description of the *prokypsis*, a ceremony that featured the emperor elevated on a wooden platform, the prokypsis, accompanied by fantastic visual and aural effects, and repeated imperial acclamations, which served to highlight the allegiance of the courtiers and dignitaries to the emperor and thus affirm his legitimacy.[50] A brief digression detailing the palatine ritual of Christmas as described in pseudo-Kodinos will highlight the centrality of music and imperial singers to these festivities.

The *psaltai*—the corps of imperial singers that would have been directed by the likes of Xenos Korones and Manuel Chrysaphes in their day—appear at the beginning of the observance on the twenty-fourth of December, assembling with other dignitaries before the emperor's first exit out of his private quarters. Decked in purple robes, they greet the emperor with the acclamations of "many years" as he exits and proceeds to venerate the icons in the chapel.[51] An elaborate procession then takes place with the emperor at center, comprising members of the court, including the singers. After various title holders and foreign dignitaries pay homage to the emperor, the hours of Christmas Eve are sung with their accompanying troparia, climaxing at the end of the Ninth Hour with the *protopsaltes'* chanting of the troparion "Today Is Born of a Virgin,"[52] repeated three times and interspersed with the singing of the acclamations and the "many years." After the celebration of the vespers and liturgy of Christmas Eve, the emperor and his retinue exit the palatine church to commence the prokypsis ceremony, arriving before an arrangement of festive banners to a great deal of instrumental clamor. Pseudo-Kodinos states that none of the χαμηλά (soft) instruments were present at the prokypsis, which was an outdoor ceremony, but the players of trumpets (σαλπιγκταί), horn players (βυκινητόρες), drummers (ἀνακαρισταί), and flautists (σουρουλισταί) all sounded, standing in between the festal banners and the royal clergy, and facing the emperor, who had ascended onto the prokypsis.[53] The Varangian guards then make their appearance, standing near the columns of the prokypsis, raising their axes in unison and wishing the emperor "many years" when he finally appears from the height of the prokypsis.[54] The light shining on the emperor, the bright sounds of the instruments, and the festive singing by the choirs, in combination with the emperor's elevated position and his encirclement by the Varangian guards, must have created an awesome visual and aural spectacle for the crowds attending this ceremony.[55]

On the following day, after the celebration of Christmas matins and liturgy in the palatine

50 The prokypsis probably originated in the Komnenian period, replacing the public, grandiose imperial ceremonies of the hippodrome. The first secure use of the term *prokypsis* is during the reign of John III Vatatzes in a group of ceremonial poems written by Nicholas Eirenikos in Nikaia, datable to 1244, although the verb προκύπτω ("to emerge") is used much earlier. See M. J. Jeffreys, "The Comnenian Prokypsis," *Parergon* 5, no. 1 (1987): 40–41. For a more recent discussion of the origins of the prokypsis, see Macrides et al., *Pseudo-Kodinos*, 401–411.

51 An indication of the prevalence of singing in this imperial ceremony is the verb ψάλλειν ("to chant"), which is encountered over twenty times in the treatise's description of Christmas ceremonial, e.g., "Οἱ ψάλται αὐτίκα ψάλλουσι τὸ πολυχρόνιον" in Verpeaux, *Pseudo-Kodinos* (n. 14 above), 190 (4.23).

52 This hymn is modeled poetically and musically after the prototype, Σήμερον κρεμᾶται ἐπὶ ξύλου ("Today He is Hung upon a Tree"), sung at the end of the Ninth Hour of Great Friday.

53 Macridis et al., *Pseudo-Kodinos* (n. 14 above), 440.

54 M. C. Bartusis, *The Late Byzantine Army: Arms and Society, 1204–1453* (Philadelphia, 1992), 282.

55 Nikephoros Gregoras compares the mass of people who attended the Christmas *prokypsis* of John V in 1341, to "rivers that converged." R. Macrides, "Ceremonies and the City: The Court in Fourteenth-Century Constantinople," in *Royal Courts in Dynastic States and Empires: A Global Perspective*, ed. J. Duindam, T. Artan, and İ. Metin Kunt (Leiden, 2011), 234, n. 103.

church, an elaborate imperial banquet takes place. The emperor sits alone at the head table, as was customary, and the breaking of the forty-day fast is blessed by a prayer from the high priest. Various title holders then enter the reception hall and take their positions, after which the singers assemble before the emperor in full regalia. The *Treatise* describes what follows:

> Then the cantors enter in their *epirriptaria* and *kamisia* and chant the idiomelon for this feast, namely, "The Magi Kings of Persia." While they are chanting the emperor sits and refrains from eating for a short time. . . . When they finish their singing and the emperor begins to eat again, the great domestikos approaches the table, going to one end, and summons by name the protopsaltes, the domestikos, the lampadarios, and the maistor. When they come, he gives them plates.[56]

Very few musical performances throughout the year would have had such a distinguished time and audience. The authorial choices made by the maistores in their embellishments of this particular kalophonic sticheron should be considered in light of this ceremony and its participants.

The Kalophonic Sticheron: Sources, Rubrics, and Composers

One of the most elaborate books of kalophonic chant is the ***kalophonic sticherarion***, a type of musical codex containing kalophonic stichera composed for the fixed and movable feasts of the liturgical year.[57] Μάγοι Περσῶν is found in three of the most important kalophonic sticheraria of the fifteenth century and its singing at the meal of the emperor is confirmed in two of these. The first of these three is MS Iviron 975, which was probably written by Manuel Chrysaphes sometime prior to the fall of Constantinople and which contains over 300 kalophonic stichera, including 104 compositions by Koukouzeles and 145 by Chrysaphes. MS Sinai 1234 was written in Venice in 1469 by the Cretan-born intellectual, composer, and later Latin Catholic bishop of Methone, John Plousiadenos. MS Sinai 1251, another probable autograph of Plousiadenos, contains two sections, one written prior to 1469 and one—dedicated almost exclusively to kalophonic stichera by Chrysaphes—written after 1469 and rebound to the first two sections after his death.[58] Although these three codices were written in the mid-fifteenth century, they are valuable witnesses to the kalophonic tradition of the entire period following the Fourth Crusade, as their scribes retrospectively anthologize compositions of "both old and new composers" (παλαιῶν τε καὶ νέων ποιητῶν). As noted above, there are three known kalophonic settings of Μάγοι Περσῶν. Sinai 1234 includes two, the earliest known setting, by Komnenos (although not attributed in this source), followed by an embellishment by Xenos Korones, preceded by the inscription, "another one, more kalophonic" (ἕτερον, καλλιφωνικότερον). Sinai 1251 includes only Xenos Korones' composition. Likewise, Iviron 975 includes one setting, by Manuel Chrysaphes, which is preceded by a revealing inscription on the top of folio 133v (fig. 4.3):

> Another Pentekostarion for this feast [Christmas], a composition by John Komnenos, embellished afterward by Xenos Korones, and then later, unified and embellished a bit by Chrysaphes.[59]

This inscription, written in Chrysaphes' hand, reveals a great deal about the many-layered process of embellishment within the repertory of the kalophonic stichera, but it does not explicitly refer to this composition's place at the meal of the emperor. It is in the Sinai codices where our concordances are to be found. On folio 182v

56 Trans. R. Macrides et al., *Pseudo-Kodinos*, 159, adjusted.

57 The earliest codex that can be called a kalophonic sticherarion is MS Sinai 1311, dated 1356–91 (Dubowchik, "Singing with the Angels" [n. 36 above], 293, attributes this assertion to the unpublished notes of Kenneth Levy).

58 D. Balageorgos, "Οι αποκείμενοι στη βιβλιοθήκη της ιεράς μονής του Σινά αυτόγραφοι κώδικες του Ιωάννου ιερέως του Πλουσιαδηνού," paper read at the First International Conference of the American Society of Byzantine Music Hymnology, Athens, 10–15 September 2007, http://www.asbmh.pitt.edu/page12/Balaogeorgos.pdf (accessed 15 June 2015), 50–51.

59 Ἕτερον πεντηκοστάριον, εἰς τὴν αὐτὴν ἑορτήν, ποιήμα κὺρ Ἰωάννου τοῦ Κομνηνοῦ, ἐκαλλωπίσθη μετὰ παρὰ κὺρ Ξένου τοῦ Κορώνη, ὕστερον δὲ ἡνώθη καὶ ἐκαλλωπίσθη μικρὸν παρὰ τοῦ Χρυσάφου.

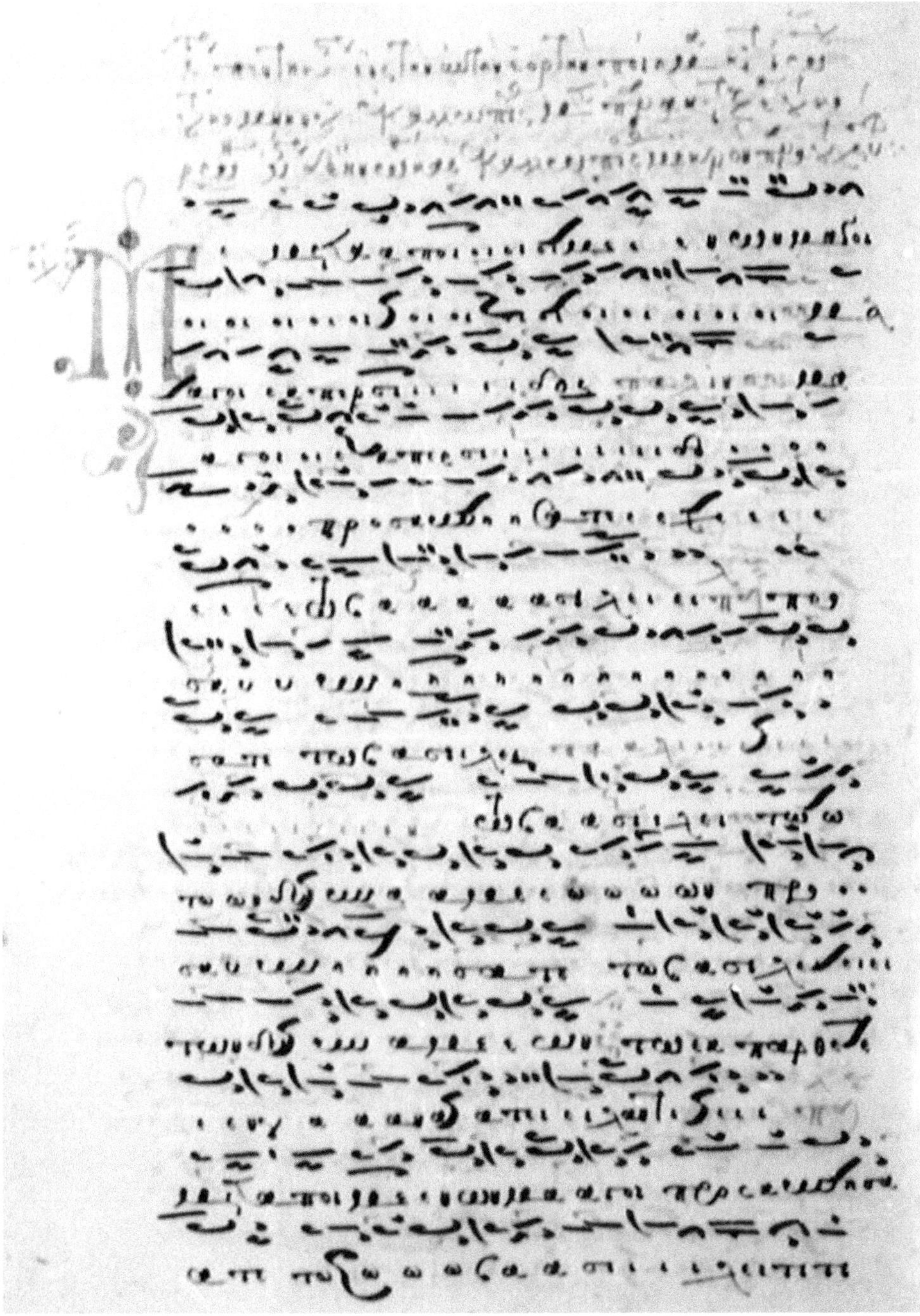

FIG. 4.3.
MS Iviron 975 (mid-15th century), fol. 133v (courtesy of Iviron Monastery, Mount Athos)

of Sinai 1234, Μάγοι Περσῶν is preceded by the text *A Pentekostarion for the Meal of the Emperor.* Virtually the same inscription is found prior to Μάγοι Περσῶν on fol. 115r of Sinai 1251 (figs. 4.4, 4.5).[60] Beyond this, the two Sinai codices are rich with details concerning the celebration of Christmas in the imperial palace. For example, on folio 179v of Sinai 1234, we read, "This is chanted at the prokypsis of the emperor, in mode four," followed by the chant "Christ Who Is Born Is He Who Has Crowned You King." This is followed by rubrics for the performance of the "many years," the singing of which was shared by the soloist (the πρωτοψάλτης) and the people (ὁ λαός). Furthermore, we know that Sinai 1234 corresponds to a period no more than thirty years prior to the time it was written based on imperial

60 Sinai 1234: Πεντηκοστάρϊ εἰς τὸ γεῦμα τοῦ βασιλέως; Sinai 1251: Πεντηκοστάρϊ ψαλόμενον εἰς τὸ γεῦμα τοῦ βασιλέως.

FIG. 4.4. MS Sinai 1234, fol. 182v (courtesy of the Monastery of St. Catherine on Mt. Sinai)

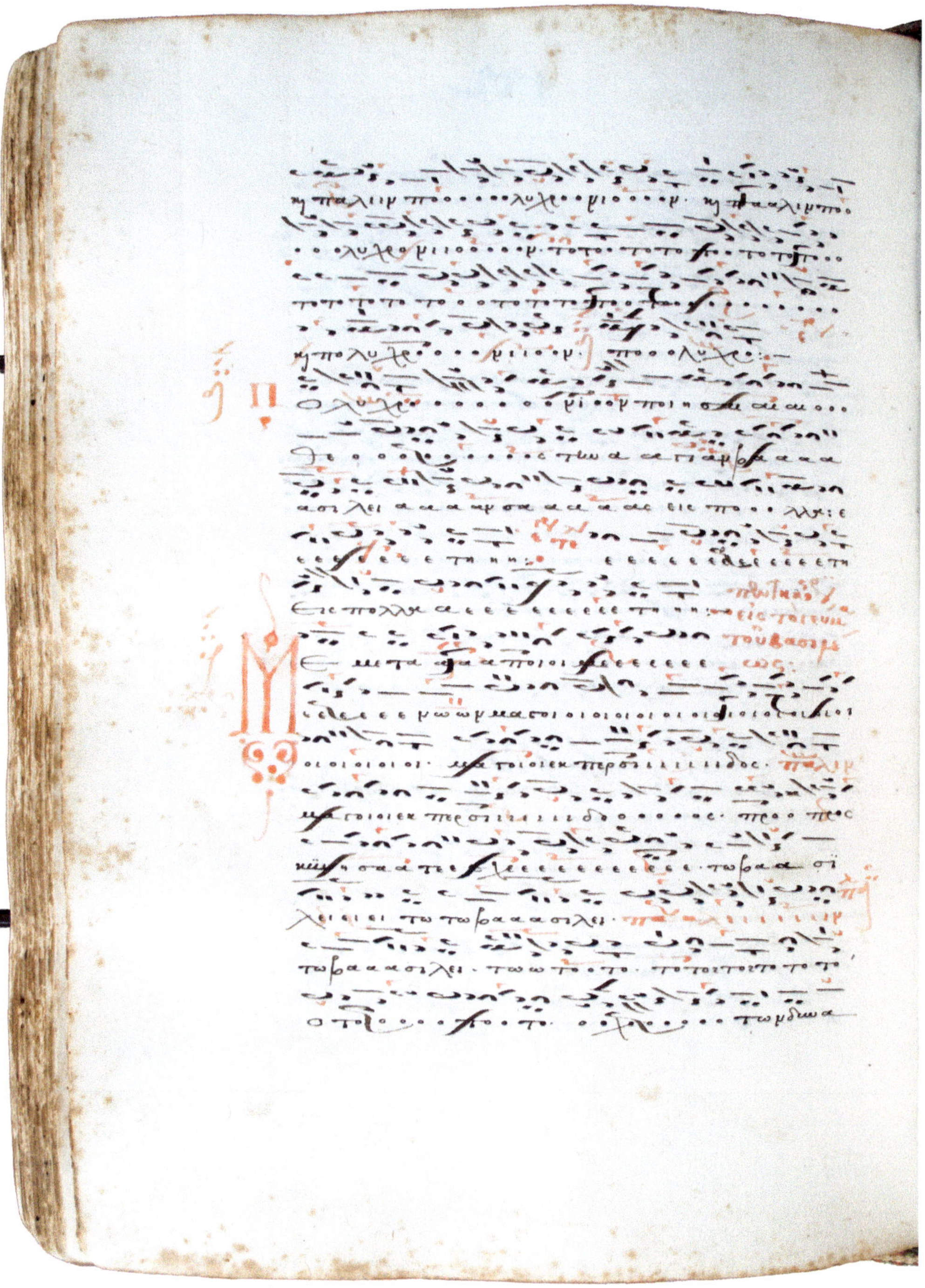

acclamations for the emperor John Palaiologos and his wife, Maria, which are included in this section of the codex.[61]

61 Detailed catalogues of these manuscripts are found in G. Stathis, *Τα χειρόγραφα βυζαντινής μουσικής–Άγιον Όρος*, vol. 3 (Athens, 1993), 759–78 (Iviron 975); D. Balageorgos and F. Kritikou, *Τα χειρόγραφα βυζαντινής μουσικής, Σινά*, vol. 1 (Athens, 2008), 60–97 (Sinai 1234); C. Adsuara, "The

Manuel Chrysaphes' Setting of Μάγοι Περσῶν: Text

The kalophonic sticheron Μάγοι Περσῶν is an *anagrammatismos*, in which the composer

Kalophonic Sticherarion Sinai gr. 1251: Introduction and Indices," *CIMAGL* 65 (1995): 15–58.

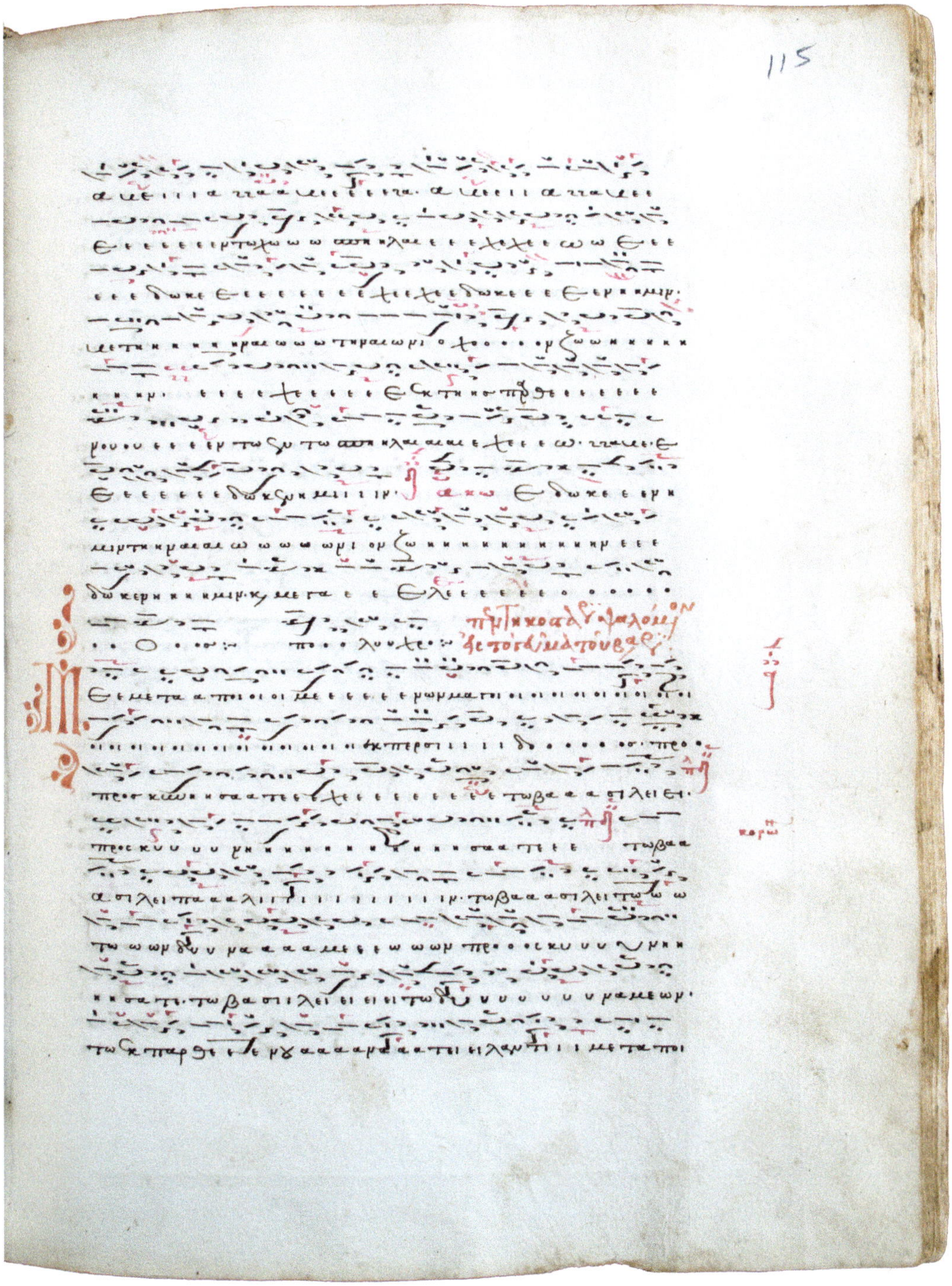

FIG. 4.5. MS Sinai 1251, fol. 115r (courtesy of the Monastery of St. Catherine on Mt. Sinai)

rearranges and repeats words and phrases to cast the original poetic text in an alternate light. All three kalophonic compositions draw from Komnenos's original scheme in which the kalophonic sticheron is actually a mash-up of as many as four hymns from the Christmas period, drawing primarily from Μάγοι Περσῶν, but also taking the incipit from the sticheron from vespers of December 17 and 22, Μὴ στύγναζε Ἰωσήφ ("Do not be downcast, Joseph"), and a phrase lifted from the doxastikon of vespers for the Sunday after Christmas, τὸν ἐκ Παρθένου ἀνατείλαντα ("He who dawned forth from the Virgin"). The original setting by Komnenos concludes with the ubiquitous Christmas quotation of Luke 2:14, "Glory to God in the

TABLE 4.1

ORIGINAL HYMN TEXTS	ANAGRAMMATISMOS BY MANUEL CHRYSAPHES
Μάγοι Περσῶν Βασιλεῖς, ἐπιγνόντες σαφῶς, τὸν ἐπὶ γῆς τεχθέντα, Βασιλέα οὐράνιον, ὑπὸ λαμπροῦ ἀστέρος ἑλκόμενοι, ἔφθασαν ἐν Βηθλεέμ, δῶρα προσφέροντες ἔγκριτα, χρυσὸν καὶ λίβανον καὶ σμύρναν, καὶ πεσόντες **προσεκύνησαν**· εἶδον γὰρ ἐν τῷ Σπηλαίῳ, βρέφος κείμενον τὸν Ἄχρονον. . . . Χριστόν δοξολογοῦμεν, **τὸν ἐκ Παρθένου ἀνατείλαντα**, τὸν καὶ σαρκωθέντα, σῶσαι τὰς ψυχὰς ἡμῶν. **Μὴ στύγναζε Ἰωσήφ**, καθορῶν μου τὴν νηδύν· ὄψει γὰρ **τὸ τικτόμενον** ἐξ ἐμοῦ, καὶ χαρήσῃ, καὶ ὡς Θεὸν **προσκυνήσεις**, ἡ Θεοτόκος ἔλεγε, τῷ ἑαυτῆς μνηστῆρι, μολοῦσα τοῦ τεκεῖν τὸν Χριστόν . . . Δόξα ἐν ὑψίστοις Θεῷ	Μετὰ ποιμένων μάγοι, μάγοι περσίδος – πάλιν – μάγοι ἐκ περσίδος προσκυνήσατε τῷ βασιλεῖ, προσκυνήσατε τῷ βασιλεῖ – πάλιν – τῷ βασιλεῖ τῶν δυνάμεων, προσκυνήσατε τῷ βασιλεῖ τῶν δυνάμεων, τῷ ἐκ Παρθένου ἀνατείλαντι. Μετὰ ποιμένων μάγοι προσκυνήσατε τῷ βασιλεῖ. Τιτιτι . . . τεριριτιτι . . . τιτιριρι . . . τιριρι . . . τιριριρι τερερερε . . . Προσκυνήσατε τῷ βασιλεῖ, τῷ βασιλεῖ τῶν δυνάμεων, προσκυνήσατε τῷ ἐκ Παρθένου ἀνατ είλαντι. Σὺ δὲ Ἰωσὴφ – πάλιν – μηκέτι . . . τιριρι . . . τιτιτι . . . Μηκέτι στύγναζε, ἀλλὰ προσκύνει, ἀλλὰ προσκύνει, ἀλλὰ προσκύνει τὸ τικτόμενον, τῷ ἐκ Παρθένου ἀνατείλαντι Τιριρι . . . τιτιτιτι . . . τερερεριρεμ . . . τιριριρι . . . . Τῷ βασιλεῖ τῶν δυνάμεων ἐκβοῶν:
Magi, Kings of Persia, having clearly learned that the heavenly King had been born on earth, drawn by a bright star, arrived in Bethlehem, bringing chosen gifts, gold and incense and myrrh. And falling down **they worshipped**, for they saw lying in the Cave the Timeless One as a babe. . . . We glorify Christ, **who dawned forth from the Virgin**, and who was crucified, save our souls. "**Do not be downcast, Joseph**, when you see my womb. For you will see what is born of me and you will rejoice and **worship** him as God," said the Mother of God to her own betrothed, as she was about to give birth to Christ . . .	With the shepherds, Magi, Magi from Persia – again – Magi from Persia, worship the King, worship the King – again – worship the King of hosts, worship the King of hosts, who dawned forth from the Virgin. With the shepherds, Magi, worship the King. Tititi . . . terirititi . . . titiriri . . . tiriri . . . tiririri tererere . . . Worship the King, worship the King of hosts, Worship Him who dawned forth from the Virgin. But you, Joseph – again – do not . . . tiriri . . . tititi . . . Do not be downcast, but worship, but worship, but worship the one who is born, who dawned forth from the Virgin. Tiriri . . . titititi . . . terererirem . . . tiriri . . . . [Worship] the King of hosts, crying out:

Highest," whereas the settings of Korones and Chrysaphes do not include this text but are followed by a new composition in the grave mode by Koukouzeles—itself an anagrammatismos of Μάγοι Περσῶν!—with the incipit "Glory to God in the highest." Finally, the composers refer to the subject of their anagrammatismos as the "King of hosts," also ubiquitous in hymns of the Byzantine Rite, a paraphrase of Psalm 67:12. In this way, the composers of the kalophonic period creatively reworked preexisting material to compose veritably original texts. Table 4.1 shows the original texts on the left and the complete anagrammatismos by Chrysaphes on the right.

The text troping employed here must have been particularly salient in the context of an imperial ceremony. Note how manipulated the embellished text is from the original and how the meaning has changed. This is accomplished by rearrangement and then repetition of the phrase μάγοι προσκυνήσατε τῷ βασιλεῖ ("Magi, worship the King"). By changing the verb in the original sticheron, προσεκύνησαν (third-person plural, aorist, indicative, i.e., "they worshipped"), to προσκυνήσατε (second-person plural aorist imperative, i.e., "you, worship!"), and elsewhere by omitting the subject ("Magi," as "Προσκυνήσατε τῷ βασιλεῖ," i.e., "You, worship the King!"), the composer explicitly draws a parallel between Christ and the emperor, shifting the scene from the manger in Bethlehem to the imperial ceremony at which all are present.[62] The command "worship" or

62 The same alteration is applied to προσκυνήσεις ("you will worship") from the text "Do not be downcast, Joseph." In the

"worship the King" is repeated ten times in Chrysaphes' anagrammatismos, and is thus the most prominently intelligible feature of this composition. This kalophonic composition was thus an extension of the imperial acclamations, composed and performed by the elite musicians of the empire, whose performance must have been intended to dazzle the crowds, and thus affirm the legitimacy of the emperor and his family. The musical manuscripts reveal the fact that the directors of the palatine choirs had an abundance of compositional choices, both for the Μάγοι Περσῶν, and for the imperial acclamations which followed. Arguably the most elaborate composition of Μάγοι Περσῶν that survives was that composed by Manuel Chrysaphes, who was in the royal court of the last two emperors of Byzantium.

Manuel Chrysaphes' Setting of Μάγοι Περσῶν: Form and Embellishment

Like so many of his kalophonic stichera, Manuel Chrysaphes' Μάγοι Περσῶν is a model of symmetry. The composition is bipartite, with the first section, Μάγοι Περσῶν, focused on the lower tetrachord of Mode 1, based on d, and the stratospheric second section based on the upper tetrachord, a, a fifth above the first part. Both sections feature important cadences on f between d and a. Within these larger sections, there are three subsections: (1) the opening text, itself divided musically and textually into three smaller sections; (2) a long textless interlude, the kratema, and (3) a recapitulation, with a short text that transitions to the material which follows. Chrysaphes' attention to balance is further exemplified by the fact that his two kratemata are essentially the same length, in terms of both performance time and manuscript lines. The composition takes the following form.

Part I. Μετὰ ποιμένων μάγοι
- A. Prelude and Theme
  - Μετὰ ποιμένων μάγοι / μάγοι ἐκ περσίδος – Πάλιν
  - Μάγοι ἐκ περσίδος / προσκυνήσατε τῷ βασιλεῖ /προσκυνήσατε τῳ βασιλεῖ – Πάλιν
  - τῷ βασιλεῖ τῶν δυνάμεων / προσκυνήσατε τῷ βασιλεῖ τῶν δυνάμεων / τῷ ἐκ Παρθένου ἀνατείλαντι /
  - Μετὰ ποιμένων μάγοι προσκυνήσατε τῷ βασιλεῖ . . . τι . . . τι . . . τι . . .
- B. Kratema
  - Τι . . . ριριρι . . . τι . . . τιριρι . . . τιριρι . . . τιρ ιριρι . . . τερερερερε . . . . τοτοτο ρερε ρερε . . .
- C. Restatement of Theme
  - Προσκυνήσατε τῷ βασιλεῖ / τῷ βασιλεῖ τῶν δυνάμεων / προσκυνήσατε τῷ ἐκ Παρθένου ἀνατείλαντι
  - Intonation bridge: Ανανεανε-ες

Part II. Σὺ δε Ἰωσὴφ
- A. Theme
  - Σὺ δε Ἰωσὴφ – Πάλιν
  - Σὺ δε Ἰωσὴφ, μηκέτι . . . τι . . . τι . . τι . . . τι ριρι . . .
  - Μηκέτι στυγνάζου / ἀλλὰ προσκυνεῖ / ἀλλὰ προσκυνεῖ τὸ τικτόμενον /
  - τῳ ἐκ παρθένου ἀνατείλαντι . . . ρι . . . ριριρι . . .
- B. Kratema
  - Τιριριριρι . . . τερετερεντε . . . κεκεκε . . . ρερ ερερερε . . . .
- C. Coda and Transition
  - τῷ βασιλεῖ τῶν δυνάμεων ἐκβοῶμεν: [Δόξα ἐν ὑψίστοις Θεῷ . . .]

Below, we will point out only a few of the defining musical attributes of this kalophonic sticheron. Aside from the highly manipulated text, the most striking difference between the original sticheron and its kalophonic counterpart is the overall length and vocal range. Figure 4.6 shows graphically the relative lengths (on the horizontal axis) of the kalophonic versions by Komnenos and Chrysaphes in comparison to the classical sticheron, and to one another, and their relative vocal ranges (on the vertical axis). The kalophonic sticheron by Komnenos doubles the original sticheron in length while featuring a wider vocal range (an octave plus a fifth, versus a range of just over an octave). Korones provides an even lengthier exegesis on the Komnenos setting

anagrammatismos, it has been repeatedly manipulated to the imperative, προσκύνει, "worship!"

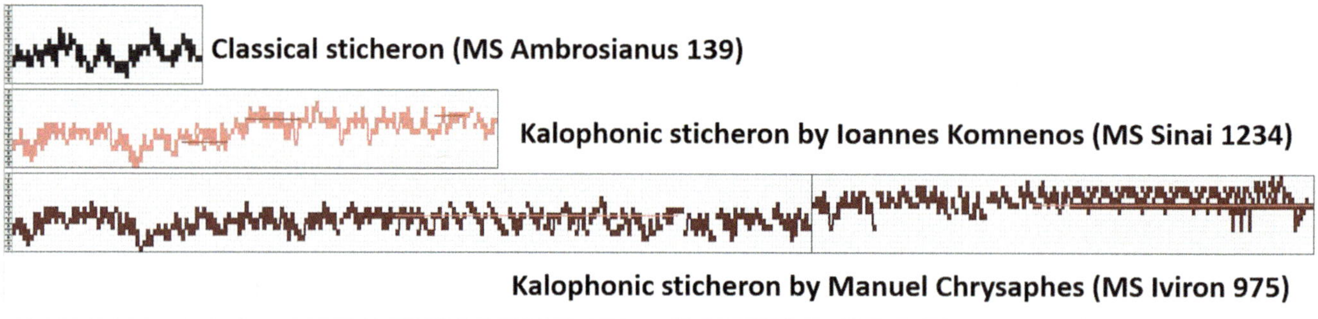

FIG. 4.6. Comparison of the classical sticheron with its kalophonic counterparts (author)

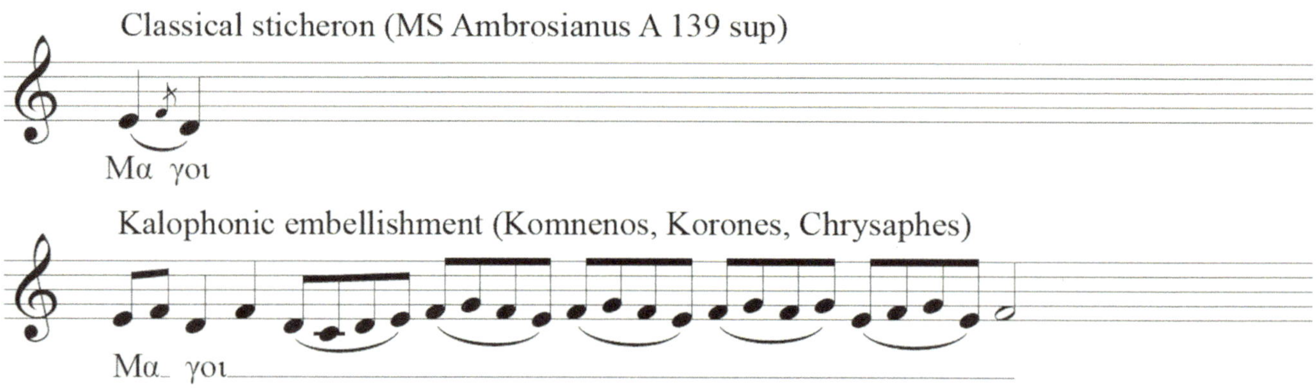

FIG. 4.7. Kalophonic techniques: extension of syllables on melismatic phrases (author)

(not shown in fig. 4.6), but Manuel Chrysaphes' composition is the longest, more than twice as long as Komnenos's kalophonic sticheron, and dwarfing the classical sticheron in length by a factor of at least five.[63] Chrysaphes' composition features a massive range in tessitura of almost two octaves (G–f′). The visualization of the trajectory of these chants at this level is an incomplete but nevertheless useful way of conceptualizing how different the sonic impact of each composition would have been on its listeners.

Moving down a level to the musical mortar of the kalophonic composition, the most important differentiator of the kalophonic idiom is its extremely melismatic nature. Whereas the original sticheron featured 1–2 notes, on average, per syllable of text, the kalophonic stichera feature florid lines, sequences, and vocal turns that average several notes per syllable of text. This occurs throughout the kalophonic settings, but one example will suffice to point out this compositional approach. Figure 4.7 shows the musical setting of *μάγοι* in the classical sticheron (two notes) compared to the lengthy kalophonic melody (25 notes) set to the same word by Komnenos (and followed by Korones and Chrysaphes). Here, a simple two-note descent is transformed into a serpentine elaboration of four segments that cadences on the mediant of plagal first mode, f.

A second example serves to demonstrate difference between the kalophonic settings. This is in the composers' treatment of the word *πάλιν* ("again"), which, along with its counterpart *λέγε* ("say"), constitutes one of the characteristic attributes of the kalophonic idiom. These structural poles, absent from the classical stichera,

63 Viewed independently, this would suggest an inverse relationship between relative wealth and strength of the empire and the degree of artistic embellishment attempted by its composers, a theme worth exploring but surely out of the scope of the present study.

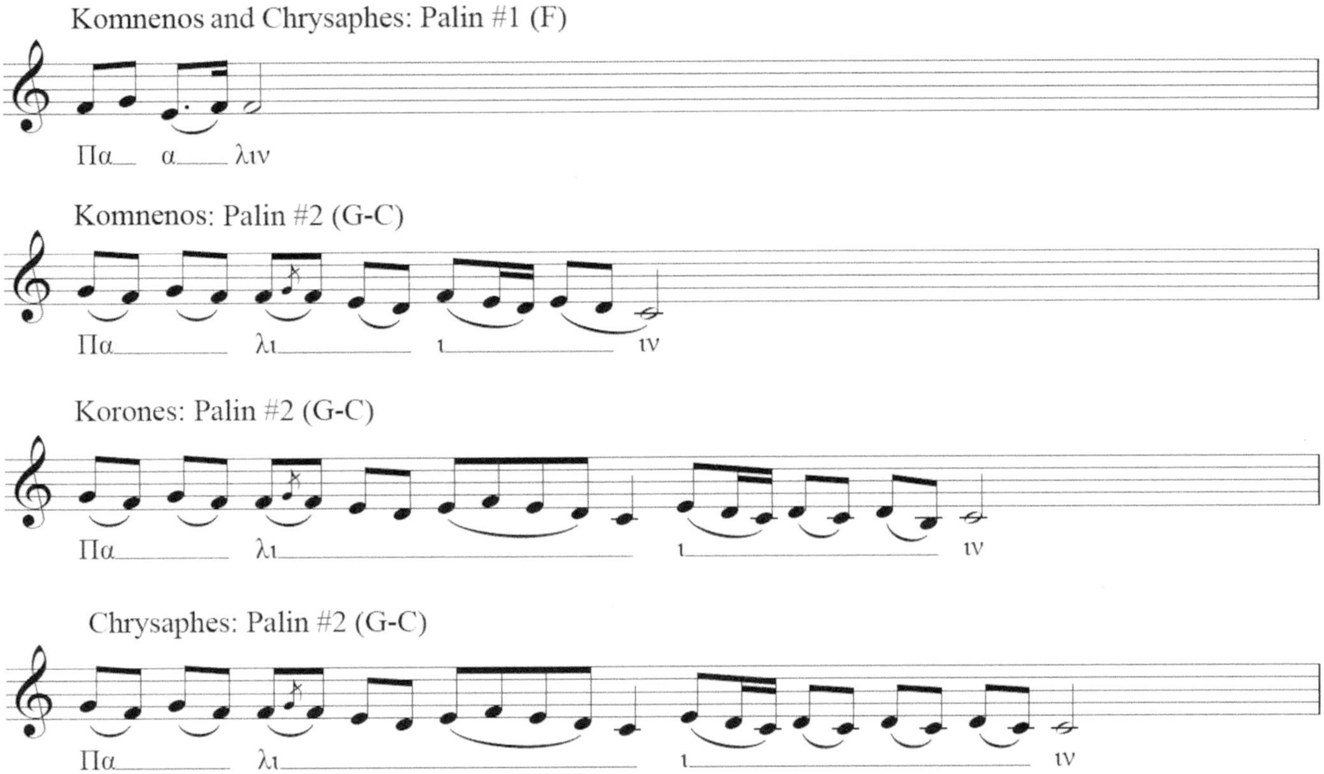

FIG. 4.8. Kalophonic techniques: setting of the structural word *palin* (author)

follow medial cadences, and are followed by a recapitulation of prior material. Written in red, these were sung by soloists who literally exhorted their choirmates to "say it again." There are two instances of this technique shown in figure 4.8. The first is the matter-of-fact interjection found in Komnenos's and Chrysaphes' settings, and the second is a lengthier version found in all three kalophonic settings. The second melody is a florid line descending a fifth from G to C, in which musical tension and resolution are achieved, due to the partial cadence that precedes and the lengthy melisma that follows, suspending time for a moment, until the choir continues with a (usually embellished) repetition of the same text. A recording of the first half of this lengthy kalophonic sticheron allows the listener to appreciate these compositional devices, and the entire kalophonic work, more fully, especially when compared to a recording of the original sticheron.[64]

Manuel Chrysaphes' Setting of Μάγοι Περσῶν: The Kratemata

The most decisive manner in which kalophonic stichera were extended was by inserting teretismata, nonsemantic textual elements, which could function as brief ecstatic outbursts or structural elements with their own formal trajectory. All three kalophonic versions of Μάγοι Περσῶν utilize teretismata, musical interludes that, on the one hand, allowed composers to explore musical ideas not possible when constrained by text, and on the other, functioned as a "vehicle for prodigious singers . . . to practice their virtuoso art."[65] Inserted as brief interludes into the anagrammatismos by Komnenos, the teretismata are spun out into lengthy, structurally distinct sections—veritable kratemata—in the settings by Korones and Chrysaphes. As with the *palin* interjections, Korones and Chrysaphes are closer to one another

64 Both recordings are at http://www.doaks.org/resources/publications/books-in-print/knowing-bodies-passionate-souls.

65 E. Williams, "John Koukouzeles' Reform of Byzantine Chanting for Great Vespers in the Fourteenth Century" (PhD diss., Yale University, 1968), 298.

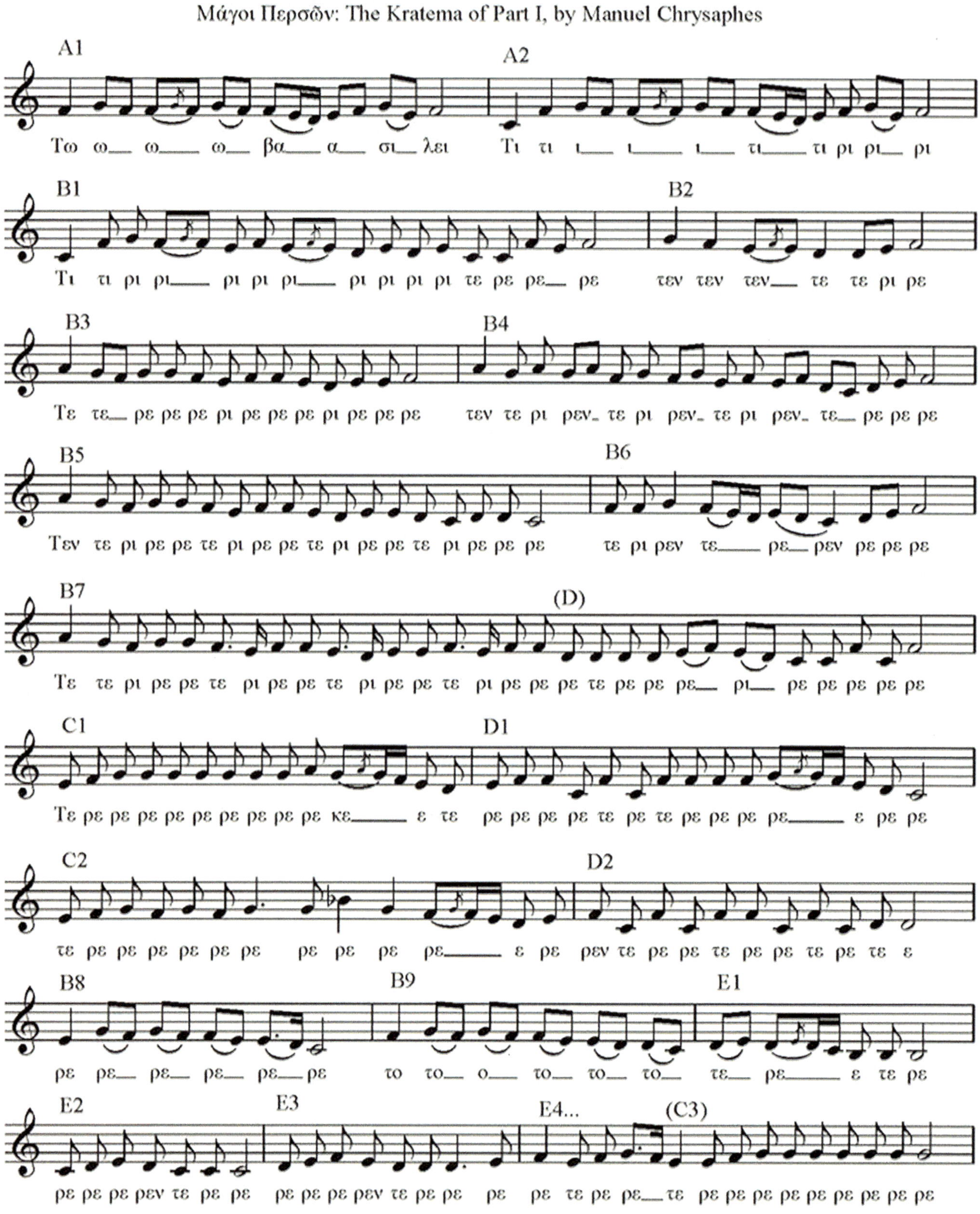

FIG. 4.9. Μάγοι Περσῶν: the kratema of part I, by Manuel Chrysaphes, based on MS Iviron 975 (author)

than they are to Komnenos. It is perhaps for this reason that Chrysaphes wrote that he unified Korones' version and embellished it a little. Many of the structural and melodic ideas in Chrysaphes' kratema were introduced by Korones. But Chrysaphes refined what his predecessor had written, and in doing so, created one of the most deftly crafted kratemata in the repertory.[66]

Figure 4.9 is a transcription of the kratema from part one of Chrysaphes' composition. The first compositional technique employed by Chrysaphes is his seamless transition from text to "nonsense" text. In part A1 of the anagrammatismos, the last syllable of the word βασιλεῖ serves as the springboard for the transition to the kratema. Following the last articulation of βασιλεῖ (fig. 4.9, line 1), the text switches to a phoneme that rhymes, τι, and repeats the same melodic phrase and cadence, in order to mask the transition.[67] The next phrase is the formal beginning of the kratema, comprised of sequences of cascading phrases, first, on the text τιριρι, to ensure a smooth transition, and eventually shifting to other teretismatic elements, such as τεριρεμ, ρερεκε, and τοροpo. Chrysaphes utilizes a minimal palette of melodic material to create an unbelievably varied tapestry, deploying essentially one motif that has five variations (A through E in my transcription, fig. 4.9). This motif consists of a stepwise descent, spanning an interval of a fourth or fifth (or, exceptionally, a sixth), usually followed by a modest ascent, back to the mediant of the mode, f. What engages and delights the listener is Chrysaphes' ability to find a delicate balance between repetition and variety, employing minor variations in rhythm, ornaments, or melodic trajectory within the context of the same motif. The melodic cascades are first relaxed in nature, noodling around f with very balanced treatment of the descending and ascending components of the primary motif. But with each variation the intensity grows, reaching a preliminary climax in line six of the transcription, when the note g is repeated seven times before a cascading descent, immediately answered first by a rather unusual non-stepwise motif of a perfect fourth (c–f) on eighth notes (the "D" theme of the primary motif) and then, by the same cascading descent, which now cadences one step down, on c instead of d. This sequence is echoed in line 7, the melody now ascending to its highest point within the kratema, b flat, before it is answered by the D theme. It is notable that Chrysaphes focuses extensively on this c–f motif as well as utilizing f as a frequent cadential point in both the kratema and the opening section of part one. This may be a direct reference to the original, unembellished sticheron, in which the f is a prominent cadential note. Furthermore, one will remember that in the classical sticheron, the words ἑλκόμενοι and προσφέροντες feature quickly moving, non-stepwise figures, spanning a fourth (c–f). These lines from the classical sticheron are directly quoted in the "D" theme of the kratema in the kalophonic sticheron by Chrysaphes. These concordances lend credence to Chrysaphes' own claim in his treatise that composers of kalophonic stichera adhered to the originals in their compositional techniques, following the original stichera "step by step," even while creating new compositions.[68] It is impossible to know whether this compositional citation would have been perceived, at least consciously, by listeners at the imperial banquet. At all events, the affect achieved by this expertly composed kratema, and the composition as a whole, including its dramatic second kratema—written in the upper range of the vocal register—must have left the crowds in awe, and hopefully for the musicians, won them the approval of their patrons in the imperial court.

Conclusion

The drastically changed context of today's postindustrialized society remains a permanent obstacle, rendering it difficult for the modern scholar to reimagine how sounds were received by the medieval ear,[69] even with surviving accounts of sonic events, information on ritual and spatial

66 The second kratema, not analyzed above due to space constraints, is Chrysaphes' original composition, whereas the first kratema is derived from Korones' version, although with considerable refinement and embellishment. Like the first kratema, Chrysaphes' second creates a densely varied melodic tapestry utilizing just two simple dyads: d′–A and A–D.

67 The same technique is deployed in the kratema of part 2, which blossoms out of the word μηκέτι (i.e., μηκέτι . . . τι τι τι).

68 Conomos, *Treatise* (n. 43 above), 43.

69 Schafer, *Soundscape* (n. 11 above), 71–103.

context, and manuscripts of notated chant.[70] As Mark M. Smith notes, senses are not universal, nor are they transhistorical: sensory experience is imbued with meaning pertinent to the time and culture within which it is experienced.[71] Nevertheless, the analysis of one sticheron and its kalophonic counterpart is a fruitful attempt to slip into the medieval body and contemplate how a sonorous performance of these chants may have been heard and experienced. The reception of a performance of the classical sticheron must have been immediate and direct. Its basic attributes suggest that it was written to function primarily *as chanted text*. On the other hand, a performance of a kalophonic setting of Μάγοι Περσῶν would have enjoyed a more complex reception, where musical elaboration, text, and nontext were all vital components of a larger aesthetic schema.

There is no doubt that the Palaiologan *maestores* believed their compositions to be sonically beautiful masterpieces, and based on their widespread diffusion we must assume that this sentiment was shared by their patrons and many listeners throughout the empire. But beyond composing "art objects" to satiate their creative appetites and to show off their vocal prowess, these composers wrote for their patrons, operating within the context of a highly ritualized, hierarchical society, in which sound, along with sight, played a vital role. The present study has highlighted kalophonic chant's function as an imperially patronized music whose sonic beauty served not only to adorn ritual ceremony but to promote imperial legitimacy. "Dazzling dining" was vital to the process of political legitimization in late antiquity, and it has been argued that the communal chanting of hymns at imperial banquets was a way to express church consent to imperial rule.[72] The kalophonic sticheron Μάγοι Περσῶν is an outstanding example of this phenomenon: a virtuosic composition of considerable length and extraordinary beauty, written by musicians of the Byzantine imperial court, with text that had been manipulated to evoke a double meaning—on the one hand, a celebration of Christ's incarnation, and on the other, an affirmation of the legitimacy of the emperor and his family. The composition by Komnenos and its embellishments by Korones and Chrysaphes were written to stun imperial audiences with florid melismas, meteoric descents and ascents, and expertly crafted kratemata. A comparison of the original sticheron with the kalophonic composition by Chrysaphes demonstrates just how foregrounded melodic elaboration becomes in the kalophonic idiom.

This case study also demonstrates how vital text was to composers for the achievement of their compositional goals. Although the melismatic lines served to delay the delivery of text, intelligibility does not seem to have been compromised, as composers compensated with structural use of repetition and by cloaking dense phrases in ecstatic vocal lines that enhanced rather than obscured meaning. Textual delivery in syllabic genres such as the classical stichera was certainly efficient, akin to the recitatives of Baroque opera, which move the dramatic plot forward in a short time. But, like the dramatic arias of the Baroque period that explore the emotions of a character in great depth, specific moments within the kalophonic stichera were manipulated by composers to stretch time and evoke for listeners a mental "scene" of a particular subject or emotion, by means of florid vocal lines and text repetition. In these moments of stasis, the narrative progression ceases and the listener is drawn in to contemplate an aurally constructed image. In his anagrammatismos for Great Saturday, "I Worship Your Passion" (Μεγαλύνω τὰ πάθη), Koukouzeles' setting of the text "Woe is me, sweetest Jesus" is melismatic but still intelligible: the clarity of this phrase is enhanced by the repetition of text and by plaintive melismas.[73] The music, in combination with

70 Furthermore, the chants investigated above, though written in diastematic notation, still lack vital information on a wide range of performance conventions, demonstrating "the instability of the relationship between a nonlinguistic aural object and its written trace." S. Boynton et al., "Sound Matters," *Speculum* 91 (2016): 999.

71 Smith, *Sensing the Past* (n. 3 above), 3.

72 S. Malmberg, "Dazzling Dining: Banquets as an Expression of Imperial Legitimacy," in *Eat, Drink, and Be Merry (Luke 12:19): Food and Wine in Byzantium: Papers of the 37th Annual Spring Symposium of Byzantine Studies*, ed. A. Bryer et al. (Aldershot, 2007), 75–89.

73 This anagrammatismos has been recorded: Romeiko Ensemble and Cherubic Chorus, *Today, upon the Cross: Byzantine Court Chant and Laments from Good Friday*, CD, DVD, and book (New York, 2011).

the phrase's repetition, serves to create for the listener a static scene of the Virgin Mary weeping at the Cross of Christ, suspended in time and available as an object of contemplation for the listener. In Chrysaphes' composition of the Paschal sticheron, "Come from that scene," (Δεῦτε ἀπὸ θέας), the phrase "receive from us the tidings of joy" is hardly obscured by the melismatic vocal lines to which it is set. Rather, the composer succeeds in momentarily suspending time and depicting in sound the joy of the myrrh-bearing women at the resurrection of Jesus by means of a threefold repetition of the word "receive" (δέχου), and exuberant, florid sequences that ascend to the upper registers.[74] This is exactly the phenomenon at work in Μάγοι Περσῶν under the skilled craftsmanship of Komnenos, Korones, and Chrysaphes. Here, time is suspended for the listeners as they are exhorted, by means of florid vocal lines and repeated phrases such as "worship the King," to meditate on and adore the emperor who sits before them at the imperial banquet.

The suspension of time and space is taken to its extreme in the singing of the kratemata. Being devoid of discursive text and comprising entirely of "nonsense" phonemes, the kratemata occupied a liminal space between the human and the nonhuman, or the material and the immaterial realms.[75] It is well known that the Byzantines conceived of liturgy as a concelebration of the angelic and human orders, a trope found throughout the corpus of Byzantine liturgical commentators from the Cappadocian fathers through Symeon of Thessalonike in the fifteenth century. But, as other scholars have pointed out, the appearance of the wordless kratemata in manuscripts of Byzantine chant corresponds chronologically to the emergence of hesychastic practices on Mt. Athos, Thessalonike, and Constantinople, not to speak of the more general explosion of apophatic mystical literature across the Abrahamic religious traditions around this time.[76] Understood in this context, the devolution of chanted text into repetitions of nonsemantic syllables might be understood as a sonic analogue to hesychastic prayer, where singers and listeners alike could access the ineffable by means of "saying away" the name of God through a kind of textually emancipated, pure music.[77] The kratemata, viewed in this light are not at all devoid of meaning, but rather "encoded with sacred language."[78] Just as the text of the anagrammatismos took on a double meaning in the context of the imperial meal on Christmas day, so too would this "encoded sacred language" of the te-ri-rem bear a multifaceted message. On the one hand, the chanters, as ordained members of the sacred clergy of the church, were enacting a performance of worldess praise to God, an activity sanctioned by scripture and prevalent throughout the cathedrals and monasteries of the late Byzantine period. On the other hand, the kratemata functioned as superhuman praise to the emperor: the singers, having exhausted themselves textually ("Worship the King!"), continued their song in imitation of instruments or other nonhuman sounds, such as the running water or even songbirds, which require no words to produce concordant sound.[79] Thus, the kalophonic stichera feature a striking marriage of text and music, whose cooperation was intended to enhance the sensory experience of listeners, patrons and imperial subjects alike. The sounds were ephemeral, yet the performance had the power to stretch time and space, and thus the ephemeral is undoubtedly material, and of vital importance to the embodied experience of the participants in ritual and worship in late Byzantium.

74 This kalophonic sticheron was recorded by the Psaltikon Ensemble on its album *The Day of Resurrection* (Boston, 2016).

75 The notion of human vs. nonhuman sounds in the medieval period is explored in different ways in the introduction and three essays in Boynton et al., *Sound Matters*, 998–1039.

76 M. A. Sells, *Mystical Languages of Unsaying* (Chicago, 1994).

77 There is not adequate space to explore the possibility that singing a kalophonic kratema induced a physiological response considered beneficial for achieving a state of inner stillness and transcendence.

78 T. Lind, *The Past is Always Present: The Revival of the Byzantine Musical Tradition at Mount Athos* (Lanham, MD, 2012), 183.

79 Indeed, several kratemata by late Byzantine composers such as Koukouzeles, Korones, and Chrysaphes, were named by their creators after their sonic prototypes in the natural environment, such as "river," "wooden plank," "nightingale," and "wild rose," to name a few.

CHAPTER FIVE

Geographies of Silence in Late Antiquity

KIM HAINES-EITZEN

Instead of raw or achieved silence, one finds various moves in the direction of an ever-receding horizon of silence—moves which, by definition, can't ever be fully consummated.

—SUSAN SONTAG, "Aesthetics of Silence"

WHAT BINDS A LANDSCAPE TO THE SENSES AND TO THE IMAGINATION? Or, put differently, what is the affective potential—realized or imagined—of sensory landscapes? More specifically, how does the acoustic signature of a place engage the religious imagination and shape experience? Such questions invite us to consider the role of environmental sounds in religious lore and literature. Ancient and late ancient texts are particularly ripe material: Howling desert wastelands inhabited by terrifying and grotesque demons; paradise, a garden where angels' wings whir and pure light shines; valleys of rattling dry bones, sinews, and skins that breathe with new life; heavens clanging with the sound of war between seven-headed dragons and angels; the Son of Man with a "voice like the sound of many waters" (Rev. 1:15); beasts rising out of the sea, coming to devour the righteous—the religious imaginary is nothing if not sensational. It means to provoke an embodied response and synesthetic experience, to grip an audience by appealing to a rich sensorium, and to shape religious and political identities in manifest and tangible ways; such affects are as much a part of the modern religious imagination as they were in the ancient Mediterranean world, where distinctions between the real and the imagined blurred as dreams, visions, and auditory hallucinations betrayed both fears of the religious "other" and aspirations of communitas. In this sense, the notion of affect as defined by Sara Ahmed is particularly apt: "affect is what sticks, or what sustains or preserves the connection between ideas, values, and objects."[1]

One such object is place itself, for the senses, affect, and religion meet in particular landscapes (real and imaginary) and therefore require us to excavate ideologies of landscapes, environments, topographies, and nature. In doing so, we can attend to the environmental history of sound or, in my case, the history of environmental sounds—an interest that might seem distant from our study of late antiquity and Byzantium.[2] Herein lies the focus of my current research, which seeks to understand how a particular sensory landscape—the desert, or wilderness—functions as an acoustic territory within

1 S. Ahmed, "Happy Objects," in *The Affect Theory Reader*, ed. M. Gregg and G. J. Seigworth (Durham and London, 2010), 29.

2 P. Coates, "The Strange Stillness of the Past: Toward an Environmental History of Sound and Noise," *American Society for Environmental History* 10, no. 4 (2005): 636–65.

the religious imagination of late antiquity.[3] This essay treats one particular aspect of this larger project—namely, the nature of silence within the repertoire of acoustic imagery in late ancient Christian monasticism. That silence is ripe for renewed attention, as evidenced by recent popular interest and by the treatments of Diarmaid MacCulloch and George Prochnik.[4] As we shall see, I resist the notion of silence as absence and instead argue for *hesychia* (stillness, silence) as a state of becoming, one that is never "fully consummated," to use Susan Sontag's phrase.[5]

One of the challenges with studying sound is, of course, its very ephemerality. Sound, in contrast to the visual, "does not sit still to be observed" and "partly because sound is dynamic, Western intellectual traditions show a marked preference for vision as the figure of knowledge. We articulate more effectively the fixed image than the dynamic sound."[6] But, like sight, sound is interwoven with power: "sound cannot be sounding without the use of power."[7] Such a claim can be read in at least two ways: the making of a sound (in its literal auditory sense) requires power or energy; and sound offers a powerful medium (or an instrument of power) in culture. As American historian Mark Smith has argued, "Sounds and their meanings are shaped by the cultural, economic, and political contexts in which they are produced and heard."[8] The intersection of sound and power is particularly apt in the world of the religious imaginary, for sounds (including silence) are both produced by specific techniques and likewise produce a dynamic and effective force in religious ideology and ritual. If, as Carlin Barton has suggested, the ancient eye was both excruciatingly vulnerable and aggressively powerful, so too was the ancient ear; eyes and ears were doors to the soul, orifices through which one might be seduced or saved.[9]

However we might describe sounds, they are also events—located in time and place, defined by specific attributes with varied durations.[10] To consider sounds as events can be understood in concert with the notion of the "soundscape," coined by Murray Shafer in his influential book *The Soundscape: Our Sonic Environment and the Tuning of the World.* As Shafer put it: "A soundscape consists of events *heard* not objects *seen*."[11] As events, though, historical sounds are difficult to reconstruct, although work on mapping acoustic spaces—built environments—is certainly an important piece to the puzzle. Such challenges, however, offer us an opportunity to attend carefully to new approaches. Since my interest is in the environmental sounds represented in late ancient monastic literatures, especially those deriving from Egypt and Sinai, one technique I have begun to employ is field recording in desert landscapes; such recordings are intended to evoke something of the sonic landscapes suggested by our texts—soundbites, if you will, that illustrate but not demonstrate—and, even more, to tune our ears to the landscapes and horizons of our literatures. I encourage readers of this chapter as they peruse my argument also to listen to my recordings of Negev and Judean desert soundscapes at the book's website.[12]

In this essay, I focus on one aspect of the project—namely, how within the vocabulary of sound in late ancient monastic texts, silence occupies a particularly fraught and affectively productive position. Borrowing some language from the field of affect theory—especially its

3 B. LaBelle, *Acoustic Territories: Sound Culture and Everyday Life* (New York and London, 2010).

4 D. MacCulloch, *Silence: A Christian History* (New York, 2013); G. Prochnik, *In Pursuit of Silence: Listening for Meaning in a World of Noise* (New York, 2010).

5 S. Sontag, "Aesthetics of Silence," 4, http://opasquet.fr/dl/texts/Sontag_Aesthetics_of_Silence_2006.pdf (accessed 1 October 2014).

6 A. Evens, *Sound Ideas: Music, Machines, and Experience* (Minneapolis, 2005), ix.

7 W. Ong, *Orality and Literacy: The Technologizing of the Word* (London, 1982), 32.

8 M. M. Smith, *Listening to Nineteenth-Century America* (Chapel Hill and London, 2001), 7.

9 C. Barton, *The Sorrows of the Ancient Romans: The Gladiator and the Monster* (Princeton, 1993).

10 C. O'Callaghan, *Sounds: A Philosophical Theory* (Oxford, 2007), 10–11.

11 M. Schafer, *The Soundscape: Our Sonic Environment and the Tuning of the World* (Rochester, VT, 1994), 8.

12 See http://www.doaks.org/publications/knowing-bodies and https://kimhaineseitzen.wordpress.com/. I recommend highly that readers (listeners) use headphones for the recordings, because many of the details of each soundscape will be missed with the use of speakers. Each figure is associated with a recording, to provide both a visual image of location and an auditory expression of its soundscape.

attention to "in-between-ness," evanescences, resonances, states of becoming—has been helpful. In thinking through the late ancient literature on *hesychia*, a term with a much wider semantic range and dynamic potential, of course, than terms like σιγή and σιωπή (both of which imply silence in the sense of the unsaid, the not-speaking—which is also affectively charged), this language of "becoming"—a language that at once joins incorporeality and atmosphere, evanescences and resonances, with materiality and "what sticks," a language of the shimmer, of a "bloom-space," that "infinity of little affective events"—is to my mind instructive.[13] What strikes me about terms like "evanescence," "resonance," "atmosphere," "shimmer," and "bloom-space" is movement, so I want to bring this in to an understanding of sound and more specifically to a reflection on silence. The practice of hesychia is one that has movement, tension, and anticipation. If for the *Gospel of Thomas*, "the sign of the father in you . . . is movement and repose" (ⲟⲩⲕⲓⲙ and ἀνάπαυσις; §50), for the hesychast literature, hesychia is both movement and repose, kinetic and still. Like a musical rest, which is a pause that has movement and rhythm, tension and stillness, hesychia is a quality of inherent paradox: an active concentration and a moving stillness. In this sense, hesychia is not about absence but a particular kind of sonic movement.

Sound itself, of course, is movement, vibration, waves, and ephemeral shimmers and the terminology used in monastic texts for various sounds implies movement and force, as we shall see. Sound is, above all, "vibrant matter," to use Jane Bennett's phrase.[14] My use of the title "geographies of silence" refers to the relationship of hesychia to place—or, the connections between inner and outer hesychia. After briefly attending to signature sounds—or, sonic imprints—of the desert, I turn to hesychia to explore its position within a desert sensory landscape and the relationship between inner and outer hesychia. My argument is that hesychia, like sound more broadly, is defined paradoxically by stillness and movement, becoming and arrival, solitude and community. It is a term that is translated variously as "stillness," "tranquility," "silence," and "solitude," but I hope to show that none of these English terms quite does justice to the dynamic nature of hesychia that develops over the course of late antiquity.

As an acoustic territory, the desert is an exceptionally rich source of the imagination and experience. "Howling wastelands" is but one characterization and one experience of desert sound, as ancient texts and modern recordings can show. Especially striking are the paradoxes of the desert as an acoustic landscape: profound silence exists alongside descriptions of terrifying noisiness. As the Little Prince put it: "I have always loved the desert. One sits down on a desert sand dune, sees nothing, hears nothing. Yet through the silence something throbs, and gleams."[15] Water, wind, thunder, rain, sand, birds, mammals, reptiles, and sounds of footsteps and voices and singing—the late ancient desert monastic texts are replete with a sonic vocabulary, even if attention to sound is far more infrequent than to the visual and to sight. There is, I think, a late ancient counterpart to Edward Abbey's attention to "native music" in the desert canyons and plateaus of the American Southwest: the sounds of birds, winds, and rivers exist alongside the trope of a silent desert—mysterious and empty, abandoned.[16] We need not resolve such paradoxes of place here.

The most cacophonous late ancient monastic text we have is *The Life of Antony (VA)*, which is dramatically animated by references to the sounds of demons in the desert.[17] As Antony moves ever farther into the wilderness, the sounds of the demons grow more intense—we have a full-on literary display of what Bernie Krause might call "anthropophonies,"

13 M. Gregg and G. J. Seigworth, "An Inventory of Shimmers," in eidem, *Affect Theory Reader*, 15.

14 J. Bennett, *Vibrant Matter: A Political Ecology of Things* (Durham and London, 2010).

15 A. de Saint-Exupéry, *The Little Prince*, trans. R. Howard (San Diego, 2000).

16 E. Abbey, *Desert Solitaire: A Season in the Wilderness* (New York, 1968), 160.

17 In what follows, I depend on the Greek text by G. J. M. Bartelink, *Athanase d'Alexandrie, Vie d'Antoine*, SC 400 (Paris, 2011); for my translations, I have consulted those of R. C. Gregg, *Athanasius: The Life of Antony and the Letter to Marcellinus* (New York, 1980) and T. Vivian and A. N. Athanassikis, *Athanasius of Alexandria, The Life of Antony: The Coptic Life and the Greek Life* (Kalamazoo, 2003).

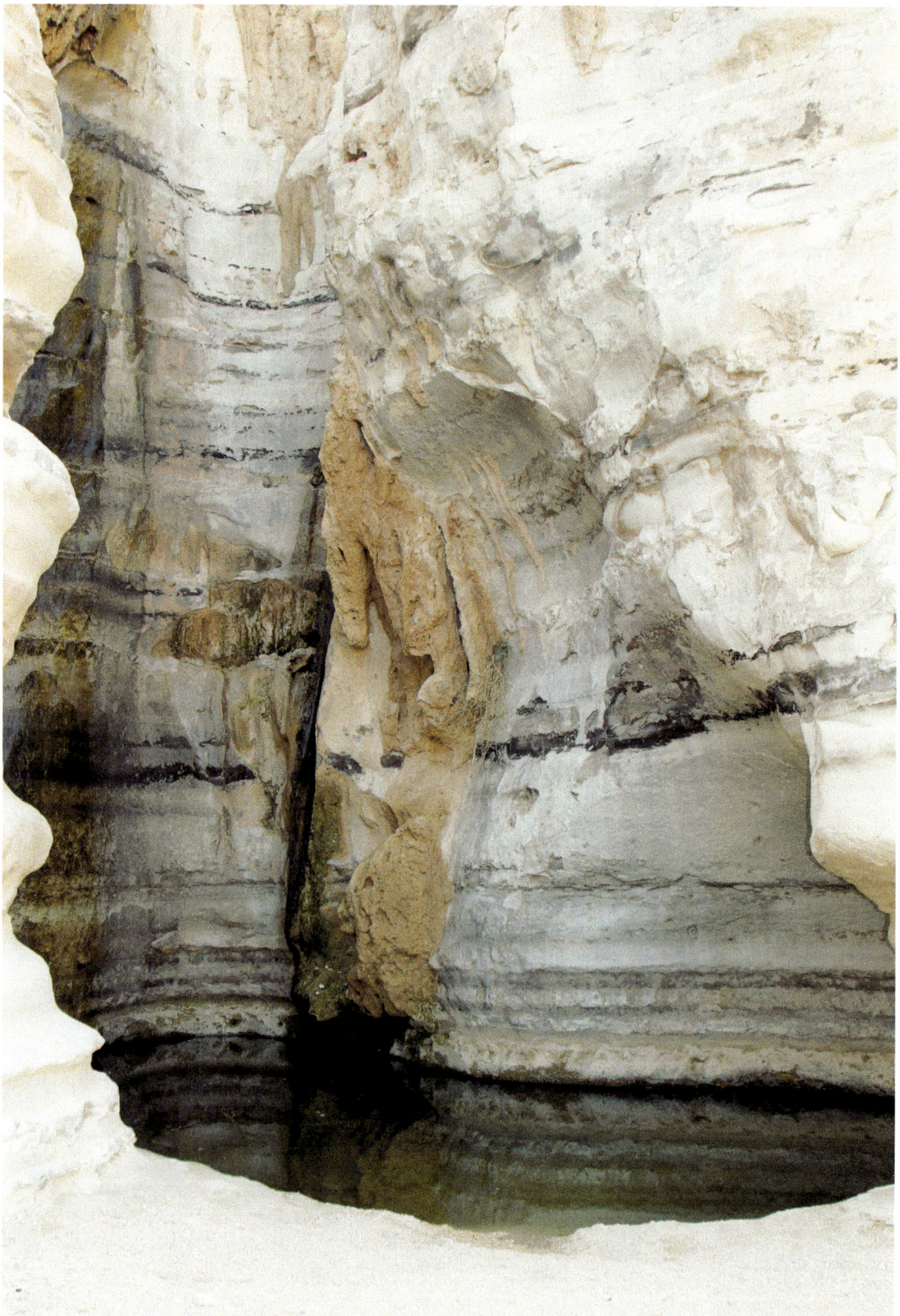

FIG. 5.1. En Aqev, Negev Desert; listen to "Fresh Water Spring in En Aqev," companion recording at http://www.doaks.org/publications/knowing-bodies and https://kimhaineseitzen.wordpress.com/israel-sounds/ (photo: author)

"biophonies," and "geophonies"—human sounds (when the demons sing, chant, quote scripture and when they take on the sounds of mobs), animal sounds (lions, snakes, and so forth), and earth sounds (quakes and thunder):[18]

> Now schemes for working evil come easily to the devil, so when it was nighttime [the demons] made such a crashing noise [κτύπον] that that whole place seemed to be shaken by a quake [σείεσθαι]. The demons, as if breaking through the building's four walls, and seeming to enter through them, were transformed into phantasms of beasts and reptiles. The place [τόπος] immediately was filled with the appearances of lions, bears, leopards, bulls, and serpents, asps, scorpions and wolves, and each of these moved in accordance with its form. The lion roared [ἔβρυχε], wanting to spring at him; the bull seemed intent on goring; the creeping snake did not quite reach him; the onrushing wolf made straight for him—and completely terrible were the ragings of all of these appearances and the sounds of their voices" [Καὶ ὅλως δεινοὶ πάντων ἦσαν ὁμοῦ τῶν φαινομένων οἱ θυμοὶ καὶ τῶν φωνῶν οἱ ψόφοι]. (*VA* 9)

The language here is significant: κτύπον (a crashing noise) is used of thunder that crashes, the rattling of chariots or the clattering sound of horse feet, the sounds of many voices or beating of breasts of mourners; and ψόφοι is used of noise in contrast to both voice and music; the earth's shaking (σείεσθαι) is both sound and its tangible movement as an earthquake. Throughout the text, the demons create an ever increasing cacophony of noise in the otherwise tranquil desert as they hiss like serpents, crash and shake like earthquakes, and sing like monks.[19]

To what extent, however, are such sounds to be relegated solely to the world of the religious imaginary? If there is any question about the "reality" of such sounds, Athanasios resolves them by way of affect and materiality. Anthony's acoustic encounters in the *eremos* are both effective (they transform him over the course of the narrative) and affective (they quite literally hit him):

> The assault and appearance of the evil ones, on the other hand, is something troubling, with crashing and noise and shouting—the sort of disturbance one might expect from tough youths and robbers [Ἡ δὲ τῶν φαύλων ἐπιδρομὴ καὶ φαντασία τεταραγμένη, μετὰ κτύπου καὶ ἤχου καὶ κραυγῆς, οἷα ἂν γένοιτο νεωτέρων ἀπαιδεύτων καὶ λῃστῶν κινήματα]. From this come immediately terror of soul, confusion and disorder of thoughts, dejection, enmity toward ascetics, listlessness, grief, memory of relatives, and fear of death; and finally there is craving for evil, contempt for virtue, and instability of character [Ἐξ ὧν εὐθὺς γίνεται δειλία ψυχῆς, τάραχος καὶ ἀταξία λογισμῶν, κατήφεια, μῖσος πρὸς τοὺς ἀσκητάς, ἀκηδία, λύπη, μνήμη τῶν οἰκείων καὶ φόβος θανάτου· καὶ λοιπὸν ἐπιθυμία κακῶν, ὀλιγωρία πρὸς τὴν ἀρετὴν καὶ τοῦ ἤθους ἀκαταστασία]. (*VA* 36.1–2)

Throughout the *Life* the desert echoes with sound; hissing serpents, roaring lions, crashing rocks and thunder, whistling, singing demons—the desert is anything but silent. Perhaps not surprisingly, in the midst of such noise, there is very little hesychia in this text. The term *hesychia*—and its cognates—is used only twice. The first describes a quality that demons fear in ascetics—other qualities and activities are "fasting, the vigils, the prayers," and so forth (30.2). On the other occasion, it describes how visions of the holy ones come and their affective power:

> For discrimination between the presence of the good and the evil is easy and possible, when God so grants it. A vision of the holy ones is not subject to disturbance [τεταραγμένη], for *he will not quarrel or cry aloud, nor will any one hear his voice* [Mt. 12:19; cf. Isa. 42:2]. But it comes so *hesychos* and gently that immediately joy and delight and courage enter the soul [Καὶ γὰρ τὴν τῶν φαύλων καὶ

18 B. C. Pijanowski et al., "Soundscape Ecology: The Science of Sound in the Landscape," *BioScience* 61, no. 3 (2011): 203–16; see also B. Krause, *The Great Animal Orchestra: Finding the Origins of Music in the World's Wild Places* (New York, 2012).

19 In a striking contrast to the *VA*, the current hegoumen of St. George of Choziba monastery, Father Konstantinos, responded to my recent query about snakes in Wadi Qelt by saying, "only two things are silent in the desert: demons and snakes."

τῶν ἀγαθῶν παρουσίαν εὐχερὲς καὶ δυνατόν ἐστι διαγνῶναι, τοῦ θεοῦ διδόντος οὕτως. Ἡ μὲν τῶν ἁγίων ὀπτασία οὐκ ἔστι τεταραγμένη. "Οὐκ ἐρίσει γάρ, οὔτε κραυγάσει, οὐδὲ ἀκούσει τις τὴν φωνὴν αὐτῶν." Ἡσύχως δὲ καὶ πράως γίνεται οὕτως, ὡς εὐθὺς χαρὰν καὶ ἀγαλλίασιν γίνεσθαι καὶ θάρσος τῇ ψυχῇ.] (*VA* 35.4)

Here the language of disturbance is set in contrast to hesychia, yet both are modes of approach: indeed, what strikes me in the stories of the demons' sounds and the brief uses of *hesychos* is affect, becoming, the angle of arrival: sounds can terrify you and make you listless; visions can bring you joy and delight. Visions and sounds can be disturbances—the very language of troubling tremors, distracting images and sounds, howling winds and terrifying darkness.[20] These are late ancient manifestations of a very modern debate: how are humans shaped by the environment and what are the implications of environmental degradation? Gordon Hempton, known as "The Sound Tracker," has worked to establish something called "one square inch of silence" in Washington state, arguing that to have one square inch of natural environmental acoustic space requires miles upon miles of flight-free and road-free zones.[21] I wonder, too, if we might speak of an "acoustic ecology of belonging" in the late ancient texts and modern literatures: a deep listening to how soundscapes shape identity and affiliations.[22] There are indeed growing literatures—the offspring, perhaps, of writers like Henry David Thoreau, John Muir, Ansel Adams, Mary Austin, Rachel Carson, and Edward Abbey, to name just a few—on the effects of the loss of natural environmental landscapes, including the sonic imprint of these landscapes, and how this loss shapes human emotion and experience.

If Athanasios's *Life of Antony* is a noisy and dissonant text, we can turn to the *Desert Fathers*—in sayings and lives—to find an emergent hesychia that is at once interior and external, two geographies of silence/solitude/stillness that I argue are linked by the qualities of time and movement. In my recent conversation with Father Konstantinos at Choziba, I mentioned to him that I wanted to record the sounds at the monastery and also the natural sounds of Wadi Qelt. His initial response was: there is one thing that recording equipment cannot capture—temperature. Indeed, as anyone who has experienced the acoustic desert knows, when the heat rises to a certain level, the sounds of the birds, frogs, even winds, simply cease and everything goes quiet. Sounds are, indeed, a way of marking time—the use of the wooden sounding board, the semantron, to call the monks to prayers or meals is but one way in which sounds mark time; the morning birdsongs, wind that picks up or dies down, the hush that falls in the heat of the day—such sounds betray time. And sounds are always moving—they are after all vibrations—so perhaps it is unsurprising that hesychia is also constantly moving. A phrase from Wallace Stevens's poem *The Place of the Solitaires* is particularly apt here: "Let the place of the solitaires / be a place of perpetual undulation. . . . There must be no cessation of motion, or of the noise of motion."[23]

The notion of "perpetual undulation" propels us into the sayings of the desert fathers, where we find an ever increasing interest in hesychia. Although I will not rehearse the structure and complexities of the corpus known as the *Apophthegmata patrum*, it is worth recalling that book two of the Systematic Collection is devoted to hesychia. Throughout the corpus, ἡσυχία and ἡσυχάζειν are used nearly one hundred times, most often in the context of describing a qualitative state ("practicing hesychia" or living "in hesychia") of freedom from disturbances.[24] In fact, on several occasions

20 Listen to a night recording of winds in the trees at Nahal Zaror in the Negev Desert at http://www.doaks.org/publications/knowing-bodies and https://kimhaineseitzen.wordpress.com/israel-sounds/: Night winds at Nahal Zaror.

21 See http://soundtracker.com/ (accessed 10 October 2014).

22 I am using the phrase "acoustic ecology of belonging" quite deliberately to combine the field of "acoustic ecology" from the sciences with affect and identity theories, especially Lawrence Grossberg's notion of "ecology of belonging" (see especially "Affect's Future," in Gregg and Seigworth, *Affect Theory Reader*, 325).

23 W. Stevens, "The Place of the Solitaires," in *Collected Poems* (New York, 1990), 60.

24 I have based this rough count on Jean-Claude Guy's edition, which contains a detailed Greek index: *Les Apophtegmes des Pères: collection systématique, chapitres XVII–XXI*, SC 498

hesychia is put in direct contrast to *thoruboi*—disturbances that are both sonic (i.e., noises) and cognitive (i.e., *logismoi*). Take, for example, the (anonymous) elder who says: "The ones who pray to God should make their prayers in peace and hesychia and much tranquility" (ἐν εἰρήνῃ καὶ ἡσυχίᾳ καὶ πολλῇ καταστάσει) and not with "indiscriminate cries" (ἀπρεπέσι κραυγαῖς), like the sick person who courageously maintains self-control during surgery and bears the pain without "noise and disturbance" (θορύβου καὶ ταραχῆς), unlike the one who cries out loudly in pain (*Apoph. pat.* 12.25).

A question that emerges throughout the varied *Apophthegmata* collection is whether hesychia is best practiced in a particular place—namely, is the desert more conducive to the practice of hesychia than the city? Here the tensions between the inner and outer experiences of hesychia seem not fully resolved, for at times there are sayings that seem to suggest that an involvement in commerce, entanglement in a profession, or association with urban life prevents the practice of hesychia (e.g., *Apoph. pat.* 11.64; 20.15) while at other times there is a suggestion that the monk should be able to tend to and to cultivate hesychia in any kind of physical environment. It is to this notion of "cultivation" that I want to turn now.

On several occasions, the *Apophthegmata* use images and metaphors of growing plants and cultivating crops to describe the practice of hesychia. I am especially interested in this language because it illustrates one of my central arguments: *hesychia* implies movement, "vibrant matter," and a state that is constantly in flux. Consider the following:

> An elder said, "In the same way that no plant whatsoever grows up on a well-trodden highway, not even if you sow seed, because the surface is trodden down, so it is with us. Withdraw from all business into hesychia and you will see things growing that you did not know were in you, for you were walking on them." (*Apoph. pat.* 2.33)[25]

It is worth lingering on such a claim, for here we have hesychia as a "bloom-space"—almost literally. Hesychia is something you cultivate, something that grows; it can be walked upon (movement again) and crushed or it can be allowed to bloom and grow, to move and become. If the demons can come at you in the darkness of night and beat you with their sounds, as we find in the *Life of Antony*, hesychia in the sayings of the desert fathers can be cultivated and grown within the solitaire. At times, the *Apophthegmata* tie hesychia even more explicitly to the language of "cultivation": "A brother asked an elder, 'What is the cultivation of the soul so that it brings forth good fruit?' The elder said to him, 'In my opinion, the cultivation of the soul is hesychia with temperance, self-control, bodily mortification, much bodily prayer, and not paying attention to people's errors'" (*Apoph. pat.* 11.124). By drawing the audience toward an image of husbandry, gardening, and harvesting, such sayings emphasize that tending to hesychia is always a moving process, a practice of cultivation—it is, to return to Sontag, "a horizon of silence" that "can't ever be fully consummated."

If "cultivation" implies growth and change, so also do sayings about hesychia that betray a sense of the relationship between sound, time, and movement:

> Abba Antony said, "Just as fish die if they are on dry land for some time, so do monks who loiter outside their cells or waste time with those of the world release themselves from the tension of hesychia. So we should hasten back to the cell (like fish to the sea) lest while loitering outside we forget to keep a watch on the inner (self)." (*Apoph. pat.* 2.1)

(Paris, 2005); in what follows, I depend upon this edition for the Greek text. There are many treatments of the textual and historical complexities of the *Apophthegmata patrum*. An especially helpful introduction and overview can be found in W. Harmless, *Desert Christians: An Introduction to the Literature of Early Monasticism* (Oxford and New York, 2005), 167–273.

25 For the Greek text, see the edition by J.-C. Guy, *Les Apophtegmes des Pères: Collection systématique, chapitres I–IX*, SC 387 (Paris, 1993). In addition, see the Greek text (and also an English translation) in the edition by J. Wortley, *The Anonymous Sayings of the Desert Fathers: A Select Edition and Complete English Translation* (Cambridge, 2013).

Here we find a tension—*tonon*—within hesychia; that tension implies time, movement, energy, and anticipation. The linguistic ties to ancient music theory—especially the acoustic theories of stringed instruments—offer just one way in which this notion of hesychia is tied to sound and silence, to stillness and movement and rhythm. The tension is not about absence, but rather a productive anticipation. Consider, again, a musical rest: here time does not stand still, of course, but continues moving forward; it has a different quality of tension than sounded notes.

Before turning to John Klimakos, it is worth tending to one final passage from the *Apophthegmata*, one that further illuminates this concept of hesychia as movement that I have been exploring. The following saying from Arsenios is instructive:

> Abba Arsenios once came to a place, and there were reeds there blowing in the wind. The elder said to the brothers, "What is this movement?" They said, "Some reeds." Then the old man said to them, "When one who is sitting in hesychia hears the song/voice of the little sparrow, his heart no longer is in hesychia. How much worse it is when you hear the movement/shaking of those reeds." (*Apoph. pat.* 2.8)

There is a lot to unpack here, including the trope of reeds blowing in the wind, which extends at least from ancient Sumerian literary uses of the sounds of reeds to Herodotus's story of Midas seduced by whispering reeds to Jacob of Serug, who, for example, says in his mimra on Symeon the Stylite: "I am Your flute: breathe into me Your Spirit, O Son of God. Let me give forth melodies filled with wonder about this beautiful one. May Your power move me, as wind moves a reed and sings thereby a sweet song in a loud sound. A reed does not have a sound filled with songs. It is shaken by the wind and sounds forth its melodies for its hearers."[26] In the saying of Arsenios, the reeds (and the sound of the sparrow) are a distraction—a disturbance to hesychia. But I want to focus again on one central point—namely, movement. The comparison of birdsong to blowing reeds is a striking one—could it have to do with duration? Time? Volume? Is it a literary trope and nothing more? However we understand this saying, hesychia is again a quality that one cultivates and a quality or disposition that one can cause to bloom much like the wind moves the reeds, like the tension on the strings, say, of a lyre when they are plucked (tonon), it is something that one can grow within.

Thus far I have underplayed the philosophical overtones of this constellation of terms like *hesychia*, disturbances and distractions, winds in the reeds, and birdsongs. A clear exposition of philosophical ideas about hesychia as concentration, as a practice of educational and literary askesis, exists already in Dio Chrysostom's *Oration* 20 (on anachoresis: "retirement, withdrawal"), where he describes the many acoustic distractions of ancient educational settings. The key point I would make briefly is that both Dio and the Desert Fathers are keenly aware that hesychia is both situated within a place (a landscape such as the desert, the streets of Asia Minor, or built urban environments) as well as a quality that is cultivated within oneself through specific techniques. It is not, I believe, a fixed qualitative state, but rather one that is always in flux, always developing, always a "bloom-space."

By way of concluding, I want to turn very briefly to the "bloom" of hesychia in John Klimakos, where we find a much fuller expression and development of "the holy hesychia of body and soul" that in part echoes philosophical attention to *anachoresis* and concentration. A full exploration of hesychia in the writings of John Klimakos is not possible here; Kallistos Ware has highlighted just how integral hesychia is to *The Ladder of Divine Ascent*: "Hesychia is a key word in John's doctrine of prayer, and the step which he devotes to it has proved, with the possible exception of Step 7 on the gift of tears, the most influential in the whole of *The Ladder*. By 'stillness' he means both an outward manner of life—that of the hermit or solitary, living in a cell on his own—and also an inner disposition of continual prayer"; for the hesychast in John Klimakos, Ware argues, "the journey is not outward and physical . . . but inward and spiritual,

26 S. A. Harvey, "Jacob of Serug: Homily on Simeon the Stylite," in *Ascetic Behavior in Greco-Roman Antiquity*, ed. V. Wimbush (Minneapolis, 1990), 15–28.

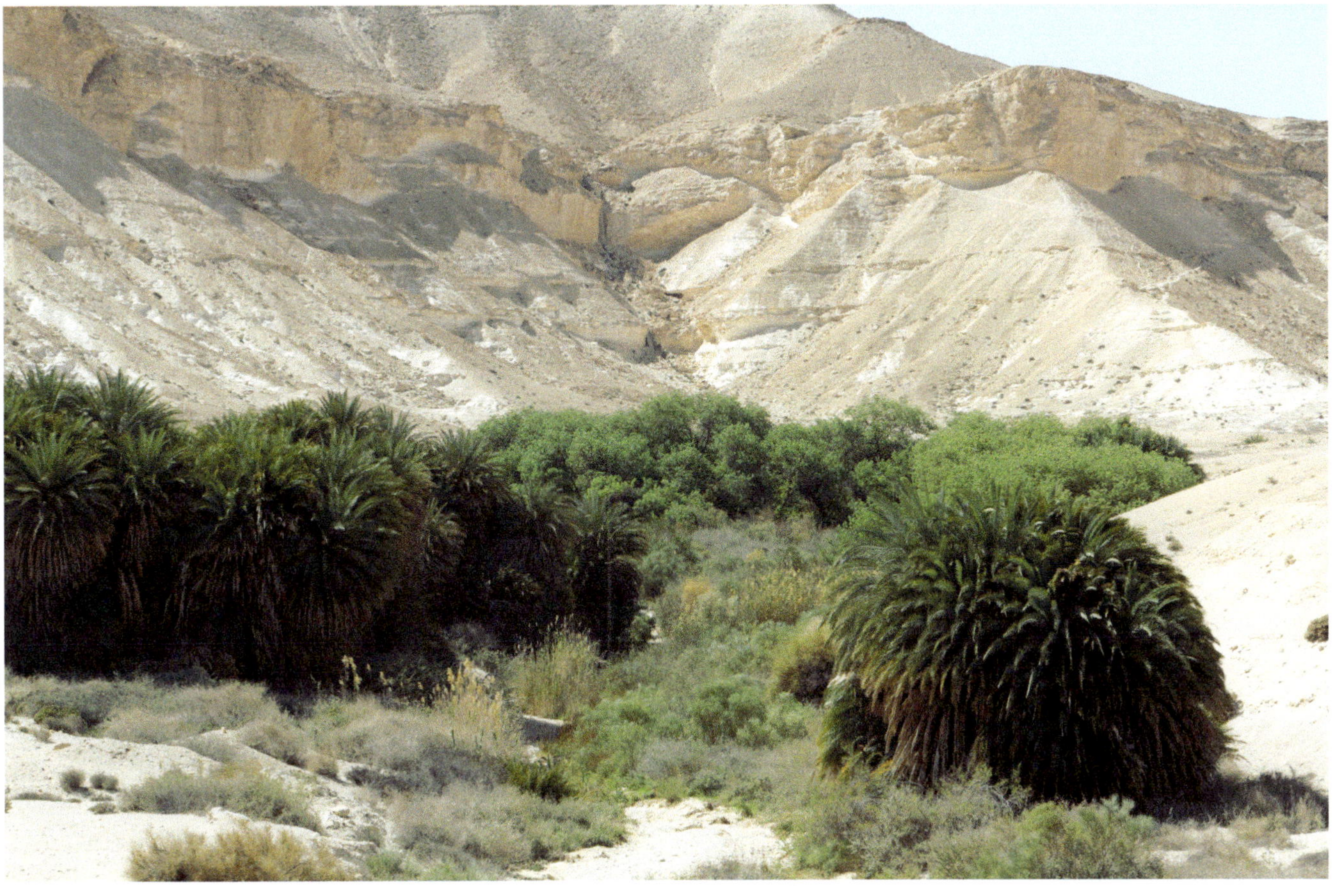

FIG. 5.2. En Shabbib, Negev Desert; listen to "Birds and Wind in the Reeds at En Shabbib," companion recording at http://www.doaks.org/publications/knowing-bodies and https://kimhaineseitzen.wordpress.com/israel-sounds/ (photo: author)

into the sanctuary of the heart."[27] Thus, John Klimakos develops and exceeds the emergent concept of hesychia in the *Apophthegmata* by focusing the attention on its internal qualities. And yet we continue to find hesychia in relationship to a sonic vocabulary of shakes, noise, and disturbances: "The beginning of hesychia is the shaking off of all crashes/noisiness [κτύπον] as something that will shake/disturb the depths of the soul. The end is when one is not afraid of disturbances [θορύβουν]" (*Ladder* 27.402).[28] Terms like κτύπος, σείεσθαι, ταράσσοντες, and θόρυβοι—the affective language of sound: sound crashes, disturbs, and shakes you—it, quite literally, can hit you with its force and motion. Hesychia blooms most fully when one is not shaken by such sounds. As John Chryssavgis has put it: "When hesychia has reached the depths of the heart, the latter becomes immune to demonic intrusions."[29]

For John Klimakos, hesychia is near the culmination of the ladder of divine assent and the depths of the ascetic project: "He who has achieved hesychia has arrived at the very center of the mysteries, but he would never have reached these depths if he had not first seen and heard the sound of the waves and of the evil spirits, if he had not even been splashed by those waters. Paul confirms this. If he had not been caught up into Paradise as into hesychia, he would never

27 See K. Ware, "Introduction" in *John Climacus: The Ladder of Divine Ascent*, trans. C. Luibheid and N. Russell (Mahwah, NJ, 1982), 50 and 51.

28 For the Greek text, see PG 88:1097; for an English translation: Luibheid and Russell, *John Climacus*.

29 J. Chryssavgis, *John Climacus: From the Egyptian Desert to the Sinaite Mountain* (Aldershot, 2004), 89.

have heard the unspeakable words. The ear of the *hesychast* will hear wonders from God. Hence the words of the all-wise Job: 'Will not my ear receive amazing things from Him?' (Job 4:12)" (*Ladder* 22.405–406).

There is a lot to say about this passage: one reaches the depth of the mysteries, the hesychia, only by first hearing the sounds—literally the disturbances—of crashing waves and evil spirits; hesychia is likened to a thing of motion—the waves. By being caught up—grabbed—into paradise "as in hesychia," the hesychast then hears the "unspeakable words"—ἄρρητα ῥήματα. Then the ear of the hesychast will hear wonders just as Job did. The metaphor of disturbing waves—both their treachery for those crossing the seas as well as their sonic qualities—have a long literary history by the time of John, one that we cannot fully unpack here. If the *Apophthegmata* draw in significant ways upon the metaphor of cultivating fruit, one of John Klimakos's preferred metaphors is the language of the sea, of ships and seafarers, as we see above and at many points throughout *The Ladder*: he writes, for example, of "sailing the tides of spirituality," "harbors of salvation," and "shipwrecks"; the differences between "sailors and helmsmen" and the "sea and the harbor"; the "deep calm" that emerges after "stormy seas"; and "ships with good navigators come safely to port" (respectively, *Ladder* 2.19; 4.10–11; 4.59; 16.9)—John uses each of these metaphors to speak to the practice of hesychia, and the monastic life and purpose more broadly. The frequent use of such metaphors has led scholars to speculate about John's personal background; for my purposes here, the language he chooses speaks above all to the ways in which landscapes (and seascapes) can dynamically animate and evoke a sense of rhythm, movement, and the "perpetual undulation" that is essential to hesychia.[30]

In countless ways and through diverse images and metaphors, the late ancient literature on desert monasticism betrays a growing interest in hesychia—it seems at times to be a notion of "silence" or "quietude" and at other times an "inner tranquility." But in striking contrast to the connotations of "stillness," hesychia is dynamic, always moving, and ripe for cultivation. In this sense it is a kind of sound in itself: it shares the quality of vibration with sound as some of the most effective metaphors used to articulate the meaning of hesychia are those that evoke movement (the wind in the reeds, the waves of the sea, and the strings on a musical instrument). Although I take issue with anthropologist Tim Ingold's stance against the materiality of sound, I agree with him that sound is a "phenomenon of experience": "Sound, like breath," he writes, "is experienced as a movement of coming and going, inspiration and expiration.... It is like setting sail, launching the body into sound like a boat on the waves or, perhaps more appropriately, like a kite in the sky."[31] Even at our distance in time and geography, if we listen carefully to the desert monastic literature we can catch the barest shimmer, a whir of wings and tinkling birdsong, the windy reeds, and the distant crash of the desert.

30 In my book *Acoustic Encounters in the Late Ancient Desert* (in progress), I explore more fully the range of "sea metaphors" used by John Klimakos and also his wide array of other ecological, geological, and biological metaphors, all of which suggest an inextricable link between landscapes, the environmental world, and monastic practice. On the speculation of some scholars about John's background, see Ware, "Introduction," 3.

31 T. Ingold, *Being Alive: Essays on Movement, Knowledge, and Description* (London and New York, 2011), 139.

I am grateful to Susan Ashbrook Harvey and Margaret Mullett for the invitation to participate in the stimulating symposium, and to the anonymous readers of this essay for their helpful queries and suggestions.

Smell

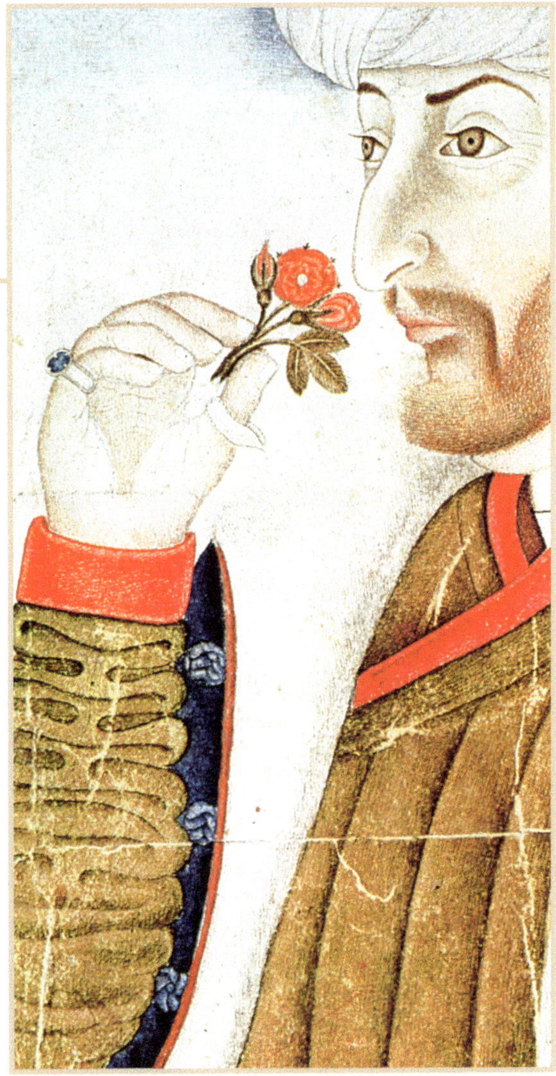

CHAPTER SIX

Scent, Sound, and the Senses in Islamic Gardens of al-Andalus

D. FAIRCHILD RUGGLES

In thinking of Islamic gardens, what springs to mind is often a visual image of a cultivated place visited or seen in photographs. Historically, Islamic gardens *were* beautiful to look at, but they were more than mere pictures. They were rich sensory environments that offered the pleasing sight of shape, color, and texture; the tactile sensation of the refreshing spray of water; the olfactory sensation of sweet and pungent smells; and sounds, celebrated in poetry and painting, where a raven's caw or a nightingale's song can still be heard.

Al-Andalus, the Muslim-ruled kingdom on the Iberian peninsula (under Umayyad rule 755–1031, and thereafter under the rule of various other Muslim dynasties until 1492), was celebrated by geographers and chroniclers for its fertile land and abundant gardens, which included many fragrant plants. For the most part, they paid attention to the landscape's productivity, mentioning the great variety of trees and plants, often listing them by name and praising their exceptional quality. Aḥmad al-Rāzī (flourished second half of the tenth century) wrote: "A perpetual spring reigns over all of al-Andalus, this being the reason why most of the fruits of the earth grow in all seasons, and the crops succeed one another without interruption."[1] The verdant landscape was admired for its beauty, as in the description by al-Shaqundī (d. 1231–32) of Cordoba's Guadalquivir riverbank of orchards and cultivations "which enliven the eyes of the spectators, and have the most brilliant effect."[2] But when he praised the roses of Cordoba, which grew naturally on a hill outside of the city and contributed to a robust market in rose petals, he was interested mainly in their economic value, assessing them in terms of weight and price.[3]

Cordoba's roses had value for the perfume industry, as did other plants cultivated there. Most of the plants and trees in the *Kitāb al-filāḥa* (Book of Agriculture) of the botanist Ibn Baṣṣāl (d. 1105) were grown for food, spices, or textile fiber, but there were many that were prized primarily for their visual beauty and aromatics, such as the rose, jasmine, lupine, viola, stock, oleander, and four varieties

1 Adapted from al-Maqqarī, *The History of the Mohammedan Dynasties in Spain*, trans. P. de Gayangos, 2 vols. (London, 1840), 1:18. The work translates the first half of the *Nafḥ al-ṭīb* by the great maghrebi historian al-Maqqarī (1577–1632). He wrote his historical and literary compendium of al-Andalus in the early seventeenth century in Cairo, but because he quoted so extensively from much earlier and often eyewitness sources like ʿIsa Ibn Aḥmad al-Rāzī and the twelfth-century historian and geographer Ibn Ghālib, his history is invaluable.

2 Al-Maqqarī, *History*, 1:42.

3 Ibid., 1:41.

FIG. 6.1.
Dioscorides, *De materia medica*, Byzantine copy on vellum, ca. 930–70, in Greek with Arabic gloss, Morgan MS. M.652, fol. 142v (photo: Morgan Library)

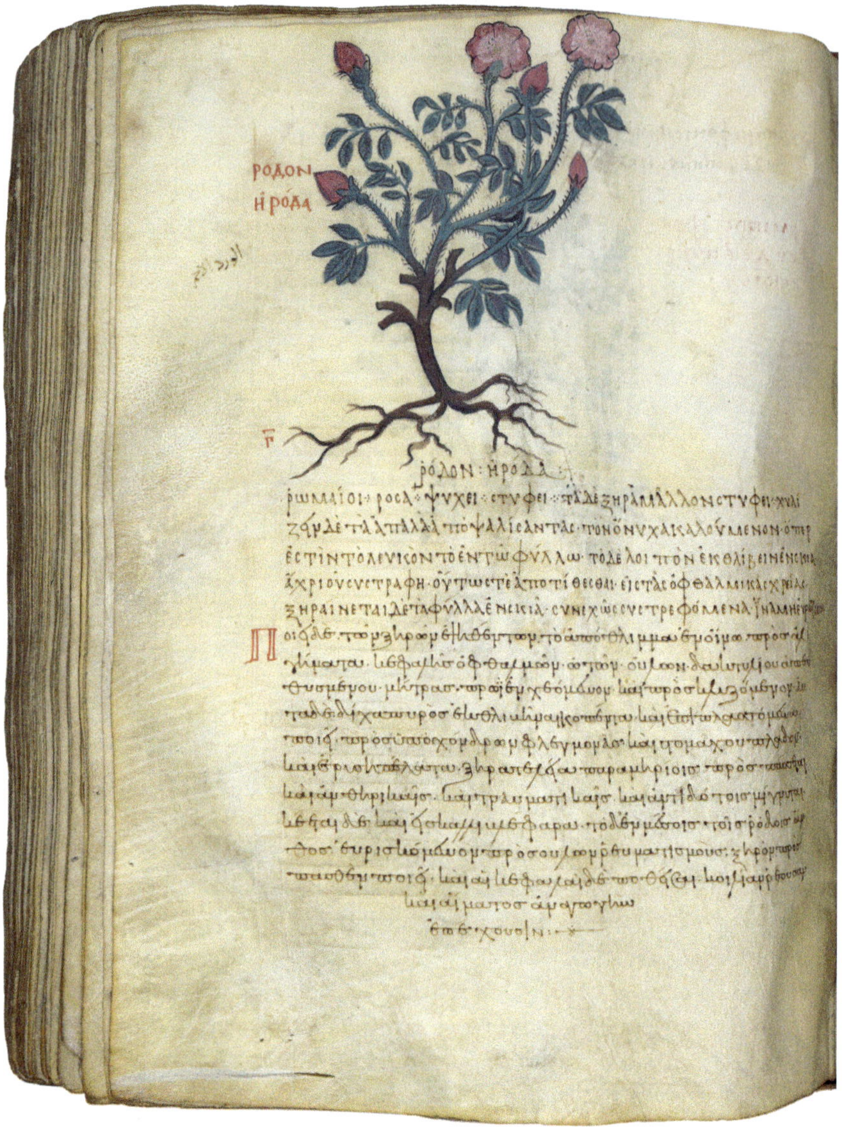

of narcissus.[4] Ibn Baṣṣāl's work is invaluable for having been based almost entirely on observation and experience, as distinguished from other scientists in al-Andalus who wrote about farming, botany, and pharmacology by glossing or adapting older texts (including classical sources) for use in the new environment. Although illustrated exemplars of Andalusian agronomic and botanical texts do not survive, it is likely that some had images, following the model of Dioscorides' *De materia medica* (written 78 CE), of which a Greek copy as well as translated versions circulated in al-Andalus from the tenth century onward. Judging from the surviving manuscripts, there were many illustrated medieval copies of *De materia medica* in Greek and Arabic (fig. 6.1). Such treatises tell us what kinds of plants were grown in the garden, but they were largely utilitarian, explaining the root structure, stalk, foliage, flower, and bud and habits of each plant in order to facilitate identification and cultivation. Likewise, when the historian and geographer Ibn Ghālib (d. 1175–76) wrote that al-Andalus had 25 different sources of perfume in plants such as spikenard, clove, gillyflower,

4 Ibn Baṣṣāl, *Libro de Agricultura*, ed. and trans. J. M. Millás Vallicrosa and M. Aziman (Tetuan, 1955). Ibn Baṣṣāl's plant list is compiled and analyzed in J. E. Hernández Bermejo and E. García Sánchez, "Economic Botany and Ethnobotany in Al-Andalus (Iberian Peninsula: Tenth–Fifteenth Centuries), an Unknown Heritage of Mankind," *Economic Botany* 52 (1998): 15–26.

sandalwood, cinnamon, and saffron, he emphasized consumption over aesthetic appreciation.[5] In sum, while the botanical treatises, farm manuals, and geographical descriptions produced in al-Andalus reveal a great deal about the kinds of aromatic flowers and herbs grown on the Iberian peninsula and their utility for making perfume, they don't divulge much about the human experience of smelling those scents. For that, we must rely on the historians and poets (categories that were not mutually exclusive).

When al-Shaqundī described the environment around Murcia, he defined beauty not only in visual terms but also in terms of its effect on the ears and nose: "[T]he music of the waterwheels on its banks, the charming melody of the singing birds, the sweet perfumes exhaled by the flowers, are indeed beauties which baffle all description."[6] Poets specifically extolled the fragrance of flowers. The eleventh-century ruler of Seville—an accomplished poet—wrote about the scent of the lotus:

> Oh see you not the joyful lotus' freshness,
> And the perfume of its center, sweetly fragrant.[7]

The Cordoban poet Ibn Zaydūn (1003–1070) wrote about the scent of waterlilies:

> In the bright sun, red buds light up the rose bushes
> making the morning brighter still.
> Fragrant breaths come from the pome of the waterlilies,
> sleepyheads with eyes half-opened by dawn.[8]

These sensory delights were often enjoyed together with music, food, and drink as in verses by the eleventh-century Andalusian poet and geographer, Abū ʿUbayd al-Bakrī:

> Oh friends, I'm thrilled with the desire to drink,
> And to inhale the fragrance of myrtles and violets:
> Let's go and listen to songs and music.[9]

What were those heady scents that inspired the poets? The flowers lived at most a few seasons—perhaps only a few hours—and we cannot experience today the encounters they offered to those who enjoyed them in the moment. Their fleeting effects pose an obstacle for contemporary historians who wish to understand the sensory experiences of the past, and indeed for anyone wishing to fix the exterior world in a manner that can be codified and communicated.[10]

The early Muslim philosophers understood this fugitive effect and consequently ranked sensory perception lower than the intellect with its capacity for pure abstraction. Al-Kindī, writing in the first half of the ninth century, made a distinction between two forms of perception. The first was intellectual knowledge acquired through reason, and the second was knowledge acquired through the senses. He asserted that while intellectual knowledge deals with the abstract ("essential nature") and is therefore reliably constant, sensory perception relies on actualities ("the sensible") that are particular, embodied, and thus unstable. For this reason, he regarded intellectual knowledge as vastly superior to sensory knowledge.[11]

Similarly, Avicenna (Ibn Sīnā, 980–1037) wrote:

> It should be known that the intellect's apprehension of the intelligible is stronger than the sense's apprehension of the sensible.

5 He wrote that the few ingredients that could not be found naturally growing there—namely aloe and camphor—were imported from India. Al-Maqqarī, *History*, 1:88.

6 Ibid., 1:68–69.

7 Abū al-Qāsim Muḥammad Ibn ʿAbbād, translated in A. R. Nykl, *Hispano-Arabic Poetry and Its Relations with the Old Provençal Troubadours* (Baltimore, 1946), 128.

8 Ibn Zaydūn's poem remembered a love affair at the palace of Madīnat al-Zahrā'. It was recorded in Ibn Khāqān, *Qalā'id*, and translated in E. García Gómez, *Poemas Arábigoandaluces*, 5th ed. (Madrid, 1971), 104.

9 Abū ʿUbayd al-Bakrī of Huelva (d. 1094) translated in Nykl, *Hispano-Arabic Poetry*, 195–96; also in R. P. A. Dozy, *Recherches sur l'histoire et la literature*, 2 vols., 3rd ed. (Amsterdam, 1965), 1:263.

10 M. M. Smith, *Sensing the Past: Seeing, Hearing, Smelling, Tasting, and Touching in History* (Berkeley and Los Angeles, 2007), 121.

11 *Al-Kindi's Metaphysics: A Translation of Yaʿqūb ibn Isḥāq al-Kindī's Treatise "On First Philosophy" (fī al-Falsafah al-Ūlā)*, trans. and comm. A. L. Ivry (Albany, 1974), 61–62.

> [This is] because it—I mean, the Intellect—conceives and apprehends the permanent, universal thing; unites with it, becoming in some manner identical with it; and apprehends it in its internality, not its outward [aspects]. This is not the case with the senses [in relation to] the sensible object. Thus, the enjoyment which necessarily obtains for us when we intellectually apprehend a suitable thing is above the enjoyment that obtains for us by our sensing a suitable thing.[12]

In the early Islamic world, the senses were not directly associated with beauty, which in any case was not well defined by a theory of aesthetics. To the extent that the philosophers discussed beauty at all, it was with respect to poetry and the physical appearance of people and things, in which symmetry and repetition (which lent themselves to abstraction, the "essential nature" of intellectual knowledge) were regarded as positive attributes.[13]

Those philosophers were wary of the materiality of the world, because of both its particularity and the subjectivity of its reception: in al-Kindī's words, "All sensibles . . . are always material, and the sensible is always body and in a body."[14] The modern historian, in contrast, delights in the world's materiality since it is through that materiality that the objects of the past—including words written on vellum, paper, and stone—survive, but encounters the same unreliability with respect to how those objects were received through the senses of vision, hearing, smelling, tasting, and touching. Lacking access to the historical sensory experience of the now absent body, modern scholars must rely on the words of poets.

Among the senses that the garden stimulated, the most fleeting was that of smell. Scent is elusive—it must be experienced in the moment—and yet smell is a primal way of experiencing the world around us. We breathe in and out more than twenty-three thousand times a day, and the air carries odors, whether we want them or not.[15] Indeed, they invade the body, because with each inhaled breath, scents enter our nasal passages and lungs. The catalyst may be "out there," but it quickly becomes part of the subjective sensate self. It has been argued that smell *only* exists as a subjective experience that occurs because the nose and brain can detect them. Thus Avery Gilbert writes, "Odors are perceptions, not things in the world. The fact that a molecule of phenylethyl alcohol smells like rose is a function of our brain, not a property of the molecule."[16]

This is utterly different from vision, for which we have to open the eyes to see, and therefore can elect to close them. In Andalusian architecture, vision is emblematized by the mirador, a place for seeing that can take the form of a window, balcony, or pavilion, often overlooking a garden or landscape. My own interest in Islamic gardens began with the premise that the garden was a spatial field in which architecture served to position the viewer and thus create the positions of subject-viewer and object-view. I looked at visuality in the Alhambra Palace (13th–14th-century Granada) and noted how many of its pavilions and halls offered views to interior courtyards as well as the distant landscape of Granada. I proceeded to explain how one chamber in particular, the exquisitely ornamented Lindaraja Mirador, had a large open window with a view that treated the far landscape as a picture (figs. 6.2–6.4). There was a real landscape beyond the window frame (which, like a picture frame, delimited the visual field as a finite rectangle), but when the sultan and steward of that landscape—who inhabited the Alhambra and ruled the territory around it—stepped into the hall and looked through the window, it was also an *idea* about landscape that was suddenly called into being. At that moment, the landscape became a designated view, the sultan became the viewer, and to drive the point home, the poem

12 Avicenna, *The Metaphysics of Healing*, parallel English-Arabic text, trans. M. Marmura (Provo, 2005), 298 (8.7 [17]).

13 S. Kahwaji, "ʿIlm al-Djamāl," *EI*², 3:1134–35.

14 *Al-Kindi's Metaphysics*, 61.

15 K. Barrett, S. Boitano, S. Barman, and H. Brooks, *Ganong's Review of Medical Physiology*, 24th ed. (New York, 2012), chapter 34, "Respiratory Physiology: Mechanics of Respiration," http://accessmedicine.mhmedical.com.proxy2.library.illinois.edu/content.aspx?bookid=393&sectionid=39736782 (accessed 6 September 2016).

16 A. Gilbert, *What the Nose Knows: The Science of Scent in Everyday Life* (New York, 2008), 25.

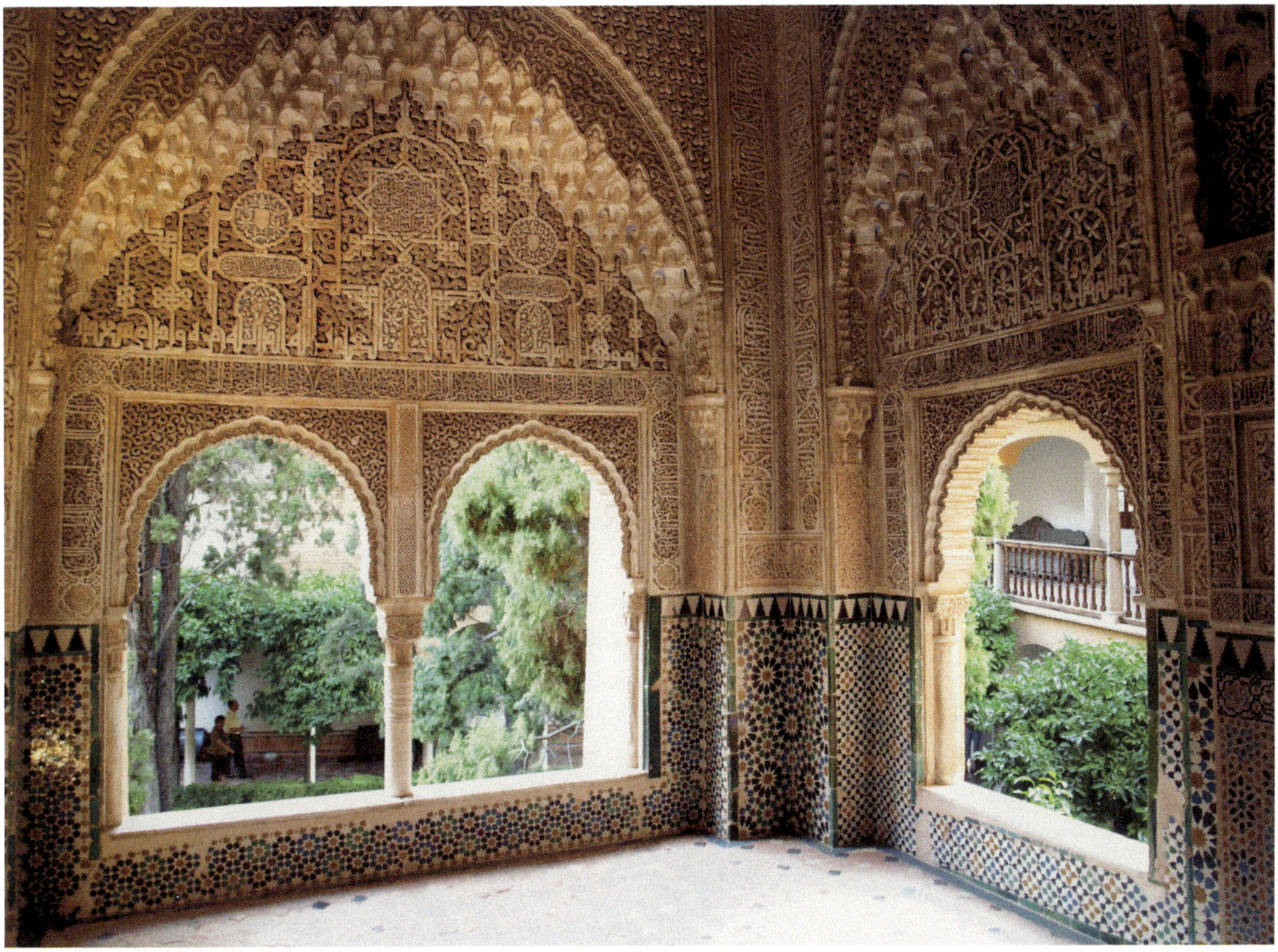

FIG. 6.2. Alhambra, Lindaraja Mirador, facing north (photo: courtesy Ivonne Wallace-Fuentes)

encircling the window anthropomorphized the mirador to describe the viewer and the view:[17]

> In this garden I am an eye filled with delight
> and the pupil of this eye is, truly, our lord, [Sultan] Muhammad [V] . . .
> In me he looks from his caliphal throne
> toward the capital of his entire kingdom. . . .

Vision has the dual ability to reach out to the exterior world and yet hold it at a distance, seen as it is through the window frame that separates not only "here" from "there," but self from all else. It is that external world that becomes the object, the object being that thing that is not me. In contrast, to inhale a scent is *not* an encounter with a distant object seen from afar, but rather an intimate experience of the sensate body.[18] For this reason, scent may have been one of the most powerful experiences that the garden offered. It provoked consciousness of the body in an environment here and now. Moreover, because the garden was not static but changed with the heat of the sun, the rain's moisture, and the maturity of the plants, it beckoned again and again, each experience slightly different from the previous one.

Beyond mere bodily pleasure, scent had a moral dimension as well. Nina Ergin has explored

17 D. F. Ruggles, *Gardens, Landscape, and Vision in the Palaces of Islamic Spain* (University Park, PA, 2000), 163–208; eadem, "The Eye of Sovereignty: Poetry and Vision in the Alhambra's Lindaraja Mirador," *Gesta* 36, no. 2 (1997): 180–89.

18 This comparison between vision and smell is a summarized from eadem, "Listening to Islamic Gardens and Landscapes," in *Music, Sound, and Architecture in Islam*, ed. M. Frishkopf and F. Spinetti (Austin, forthcoming). On the intimacy of smell, see H. Lefebvre, *The Production of Space*, trans. D. Nicholson-Smith (Oxford, 1991), 197.

FIG. 6.3.
Alhambra, plan of the Lions Palace (plan: author)

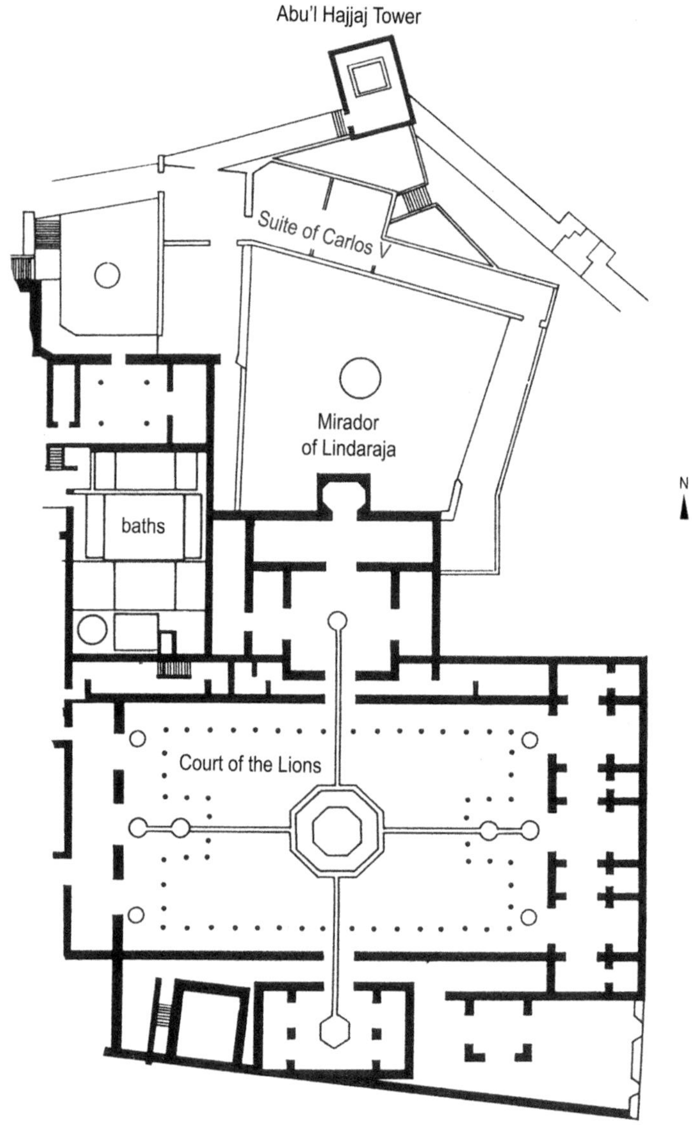

the pious attitude toward scent as recorded in the *hadith*: paradise is described as having sweet-smelling soil, its water scented as musk, and the *houris* themselves as having "light and pleasant scent." In paradise the newly arrived are sprinkled with musk and perfume, their braziers burn fragrant aloewood, and even their sweat has the scent of musk.[19] The Prophet himself is said to have smelled of ambergris and musk.[20] To evoke paradise and to forge a connection to the Prophet, and perhaps also influenced by the Christian tradition of placing oil lamps and incense burners in places of prayer and religious ritual, mosques and tombs were often scented, the purifying incense paid

19 N. Ergin, "The Fragrance of the Divine: Ottoman Incense Burners and Their Context," *ArtB*, 96, no. 1 (2014): 70–97; see 72, citing the hadith of Bukhārī, *The Translation of the Meanings of Sahih al-Bukhari*, trans. M. M. Khan (Lahore, 1983), book 8, no. 345 and book 54, nos. 468 and 469, available from the University of Southern California and the Center for Muslim-Jewish Engagement (CMJE) compendium of religious texts, http://www.usc.edu/org/cmje/religious-texts/hadith (accessed 23 May 2016). See also T. L. Henrick and N. Ergin, "A Shared Culture of Heavenly Fragrance: A Comparison of Late Byzantine and Ottoman Incense Burners and Censing Practices in Religious Contexts," *DOP* 69 (2015): 331–54.

20 Ergin, "Fragrance," 72, citing Sahih Muslim, *Being Traditions of the Sayings of the Prophet Muhammad as Narrated by His Companions and Compiled under the Title al-Jami' us-Sahih*, trans. A. H. Siddiqi, 4 vols. (Lahore, 1971–75), book 30, nos. 5759 and 5760; Sahih al-Bukhari, book 26, no. 611, and book 56, nos. 573, 761. Both hadith collections are available from the CMJE (see prev. note).

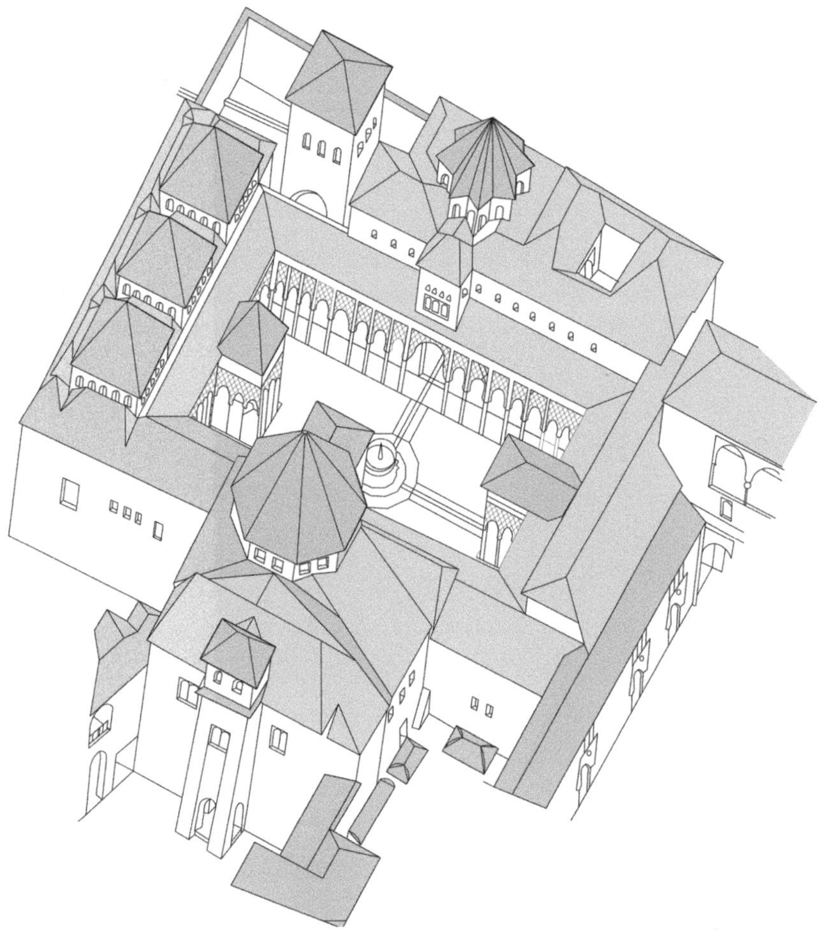

FIG. 6.4.
Axonometric view of the Court of the Lions (plan: M. Guragain)

by endowment.[21] Yet scent could also lead one astray from the path of moral righteousness. Ergin explains that perfume was forbidden during the hajj (pilgrimage) and during periods of mourning, and that whereas the souls of believers were said to smell sweet, unbelievers smelled foul.[22]

Our ability today to understand the sensations of the past relies on reenactments in which we hope that the scent of a modern rose captures that of the rose blooming a thousand years ago. Yet, such reenactments are doomed to failure because, despite extraordinary modern scholarship in the field of botanical history, we do not have the exact plants and cannot recreate the precise environmental conditions of the past. With the exception of the Great Mosque of Cordoba, where the courtyard seems to have been continuously planted with some variety of fruit trees since the early ninth century (and more likely from the mosque's foundation in 786), the historic Islamic gardens of al-Andalus are gone.[23] Madīnat al-Zahrā᾿ (built 936) and the other great palaces that garlanded the city of Cordoba are now dusty archaeological sites with little or no pretense of botanical accuracy: the only flowers are those planted to please the modern eye and alleviate the monotony of the stone walls and pavements. The few descriptions of how an Andalusi garden estate should be planted are very much in the vein of instructional advice, and none describe the sensory effect of those plantings or the experience of being in a fragrant garden.[24]

21 "Masdjid," *EI*², 6:666. On the Christian tradition see S. A. Harvey, *Scenting Salvation: Ancient Christianity and the Olfactory Imagination* (Berkeley and Los Angeles, 2006), and B. Caseau, "The Senses in Religion: Liturgy, Devotion, and Deprivation," in *A Cultural History of the Senses in the Middle Ages, 500–1450*, ed. R. Newhauser (New York, 2014), 89–110.

22 Ergin, "Fragrance," 72.

23 D. F. Ruggles, *Islamic Gardens and Landscapes* (Philadelphia, 2008), 90–96.

24 These are translated and discussed in Ruggles, *Gardens, Landscape, and Vision*, 25–27.

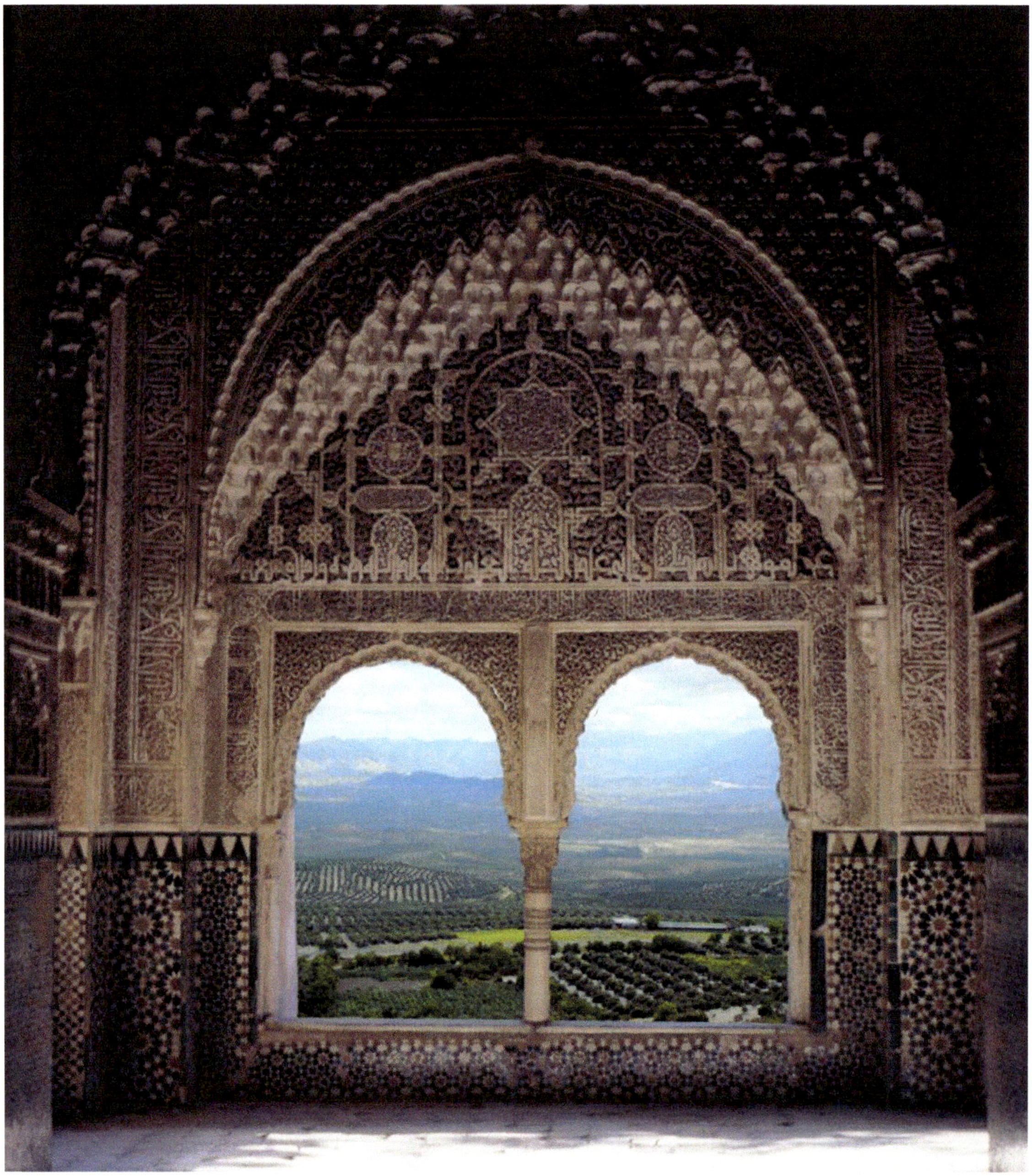

FIG. 6.5. Alhambra, Lindaraja Mirador with digitally corrected view showing panorama (photo: author)

Sound is similarly ephemeral, yet we know quite a bit about the sonic environment of the Alhambra Palace. In its reception halls, poetry was performed aloud, and those select compositions that most pleased the sultan were honored by being inscribed on the palace walls. The result is that the Alhambra, like few other palaces, can be read like a book. In some cases, the poetry seems to have been composed with the future architectural location already in the poet's mind. In the Lindaraja Mirador, the window is enframed by the poem by Ibn Zamrak (1333–soon after 1393) that begins "In this garden, I am an eye." The garden to which the poem refers is outside the window in the courtyard below, but the view extended from the window across the gardened courtyard to the cultivated landscape in the distance. The view was only partially

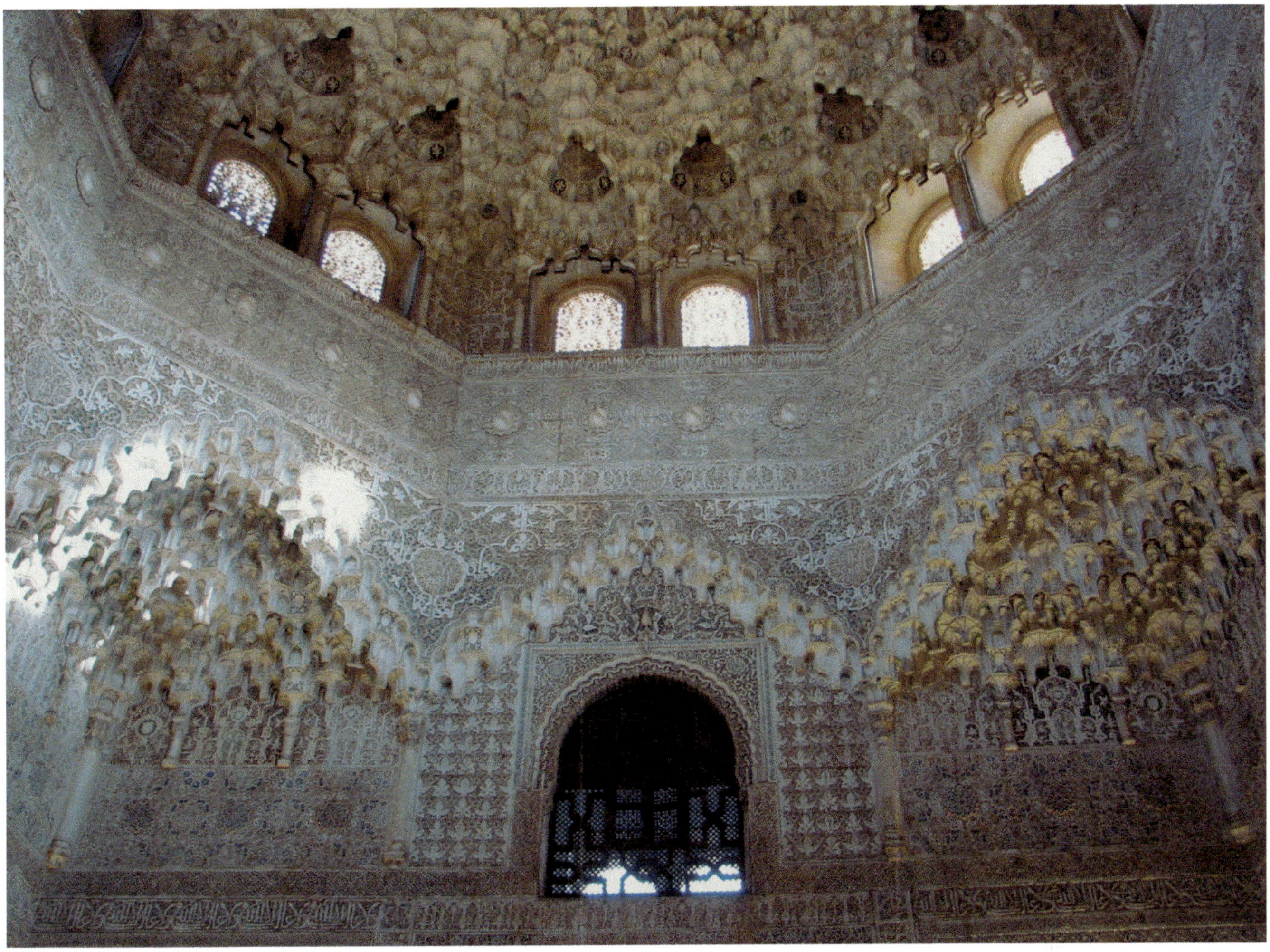

FIG. 6.6.
Hall of the Two Sisters, muqarnas dome and upper story window (photo: author)

impeded by the Abū'l Ḥajjāj tower on the far side of the courtyard, until the walls were heightened in the sixteenth century, whereupon the view was altogether blocked (fig. 6.5; cf. fig. 6.2).[25] The poetic inscription that is physically and visually present in this elegant hall is a visual trace of an actual sonic performance from the fourteenth century, and it is but one of many such architecturally attuned inscriptions.[26]

We also know about the acoustical resonance of the Alhambra's spaces, such as the Hall of the Two Sisters and the Hall of the Abencerrajes on either side of the Court of the Lions (fig. 6.6). Both chambers had high balconies or interior windows where musicians could sit unseen and play for the assembly below, the sound resonating from the extraordinarily elaborate *muqarnas* domes overhead to the heavy marble slab floors below. The curved cellular construction of a muqarnas dome and its miniature squinches provides a multifaceted surface for the reflection of sounds. At the same time, because the entire surface of plaster cells is an illusory membrane that is suspended from a wooden armature attached to the hall's walls and ceiling, the empty space between that membrane and the building is like the body of a drum, magnifying sound. The dome is a visually dazzling work of architecture, which is how it is invariably treated by historians and architectural historians, but it had an impact that was more than optical.

A representation of the senses that is literary and imagined rather than actual occurs

25 Ruggles, "Eye of Sovereignty," 180–89; L. Torres Bálbas, *Arte almohade: Arte nazarí; Arte mudéjar*, Ars Hispaniae 4 (Madrid, 1949), 117.

26 The poems are transcribed in J. M. Puertas Vílchez, *Reading the Alhambra* (Granada, 2010). See also O. Bush, "'When My Beholder Ponders': Poetic Epigraphy in the Alhambra," *Artibus Asiae* 66, no. 2 (2006): 55–67.

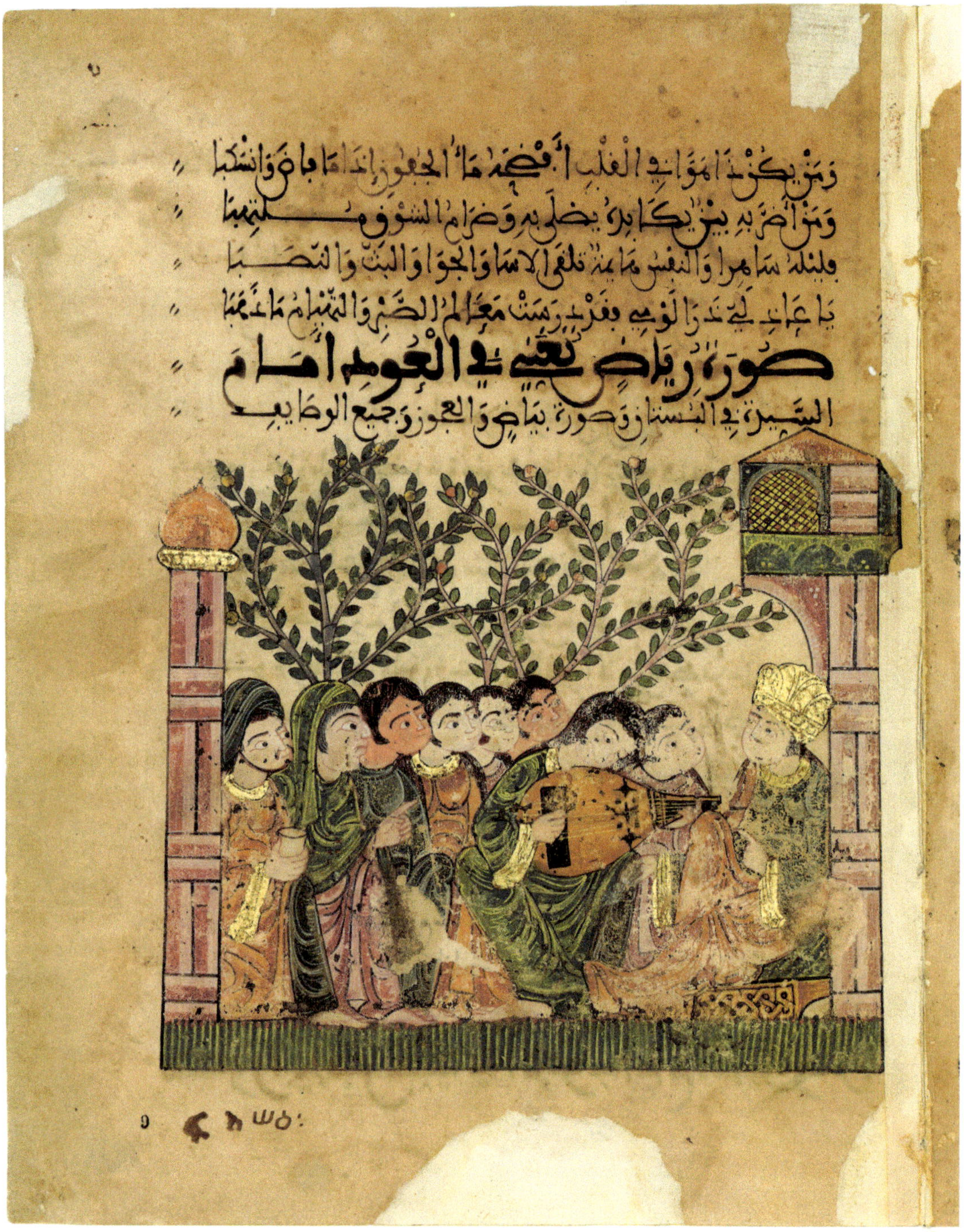

FIG. 6.7. *Bayāḍ wa Riyāḍ*, A Garden Party, Biblioteca Apostolica Vaticana, MS. ar. 368, fol. 9r (photo: Biblioteca Apostolica Vaticana)

in an illustrated manuscript of the *Bayāḍ wa Riyāḍ*, from thirteenth- or fourteenth-century al-Andalus.[27] The story tells of a secret love between a young man named Bayāḍ and a slave girl named Riyāḍ with many scenes set within walled gardens. In the early illustrations, the assembled handmaidens and slave girls drink

27 The Spanish version published by A. R. Nykl, *Historia de los Amores de Bayad wa Riyad* (New York, 1941) can now be replaced by the lively and highly readable translation of C. Robinson, *Medieval Andalusian Courtly Culture in the Mediterranean* (London, 2007). The codicological analysis and conclusions of the latter, however, have been critiqued by A. D'Ottone, "Il manoscritto Vaticano arabo 368, Hadit Bayad wa Riyad: Il codice, il testo, le immagini," *Rivista di Storia della Miniatura* 14 (2010): 55–70. I have written about the manuscript's pictured soundscapes in Ruggles, "Listening" (n. 18 above).

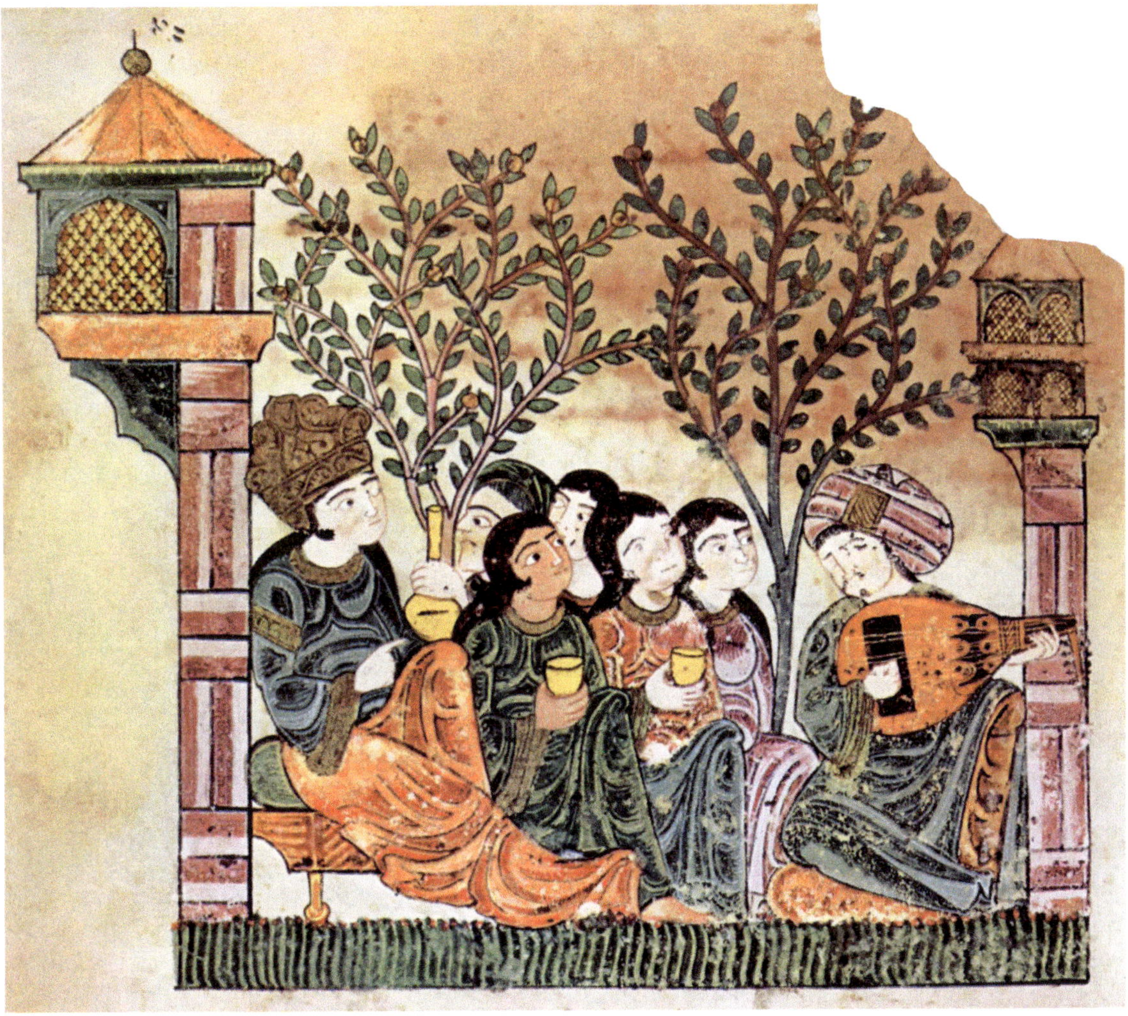

FIG. 6.8.
Bayāḍ wa Riyāḍ, Bayad Plays the Lute, Biblioteca Apostolica Vaticana, MS. ar. 368, fol. 10r (photo: Bridgeman images)

from golden cups in the shade of leafy trees, gathered at the feet of the hostess with the golden headdress who sits on a raised stool (fig. 6.7). Also attending the gathering is Bayāḍ, who, having already glimpsed the lovely Riyāḍ from afar (as likewise she had seen him by climbing a tree to look over the wall), had engaged a go-between to arrange for him to attend the gathering so as to see his beloved up close. Unfortunately, Riyāḍ has already been claimed by the father of the hostess, who, like Bayāḍ, has been attracted by her wafting perfume and her comeliness—"like a star shining in the blackness of the night."[28] Unlike Bayāḍ, the older man actually owns the slave girl.

When Bayāḍ arrives at the garden party, the slave girls are singing plaintive love songs to the accompaniment of the lute, each ballad provoking the hostess to cry for more. Eventually the young man begins to sing, after which he confesses his attraction for Riyāḍ (fig. 6.8). Soon, it becomes a back-and-forth of songs sung by Riyāḍ and Bayāḍ to each other. Toward the end, Bayāḍ sings a song describing Riyāḍ that ends with the verse:

> Beauty is resplendent in the rays which shine
> from her forehead,
> And from her wafts a breeze of camphor and
> musk.
> She deprived me of the forces of my patience
> and I do not hope
> For remedy for my love in this world, if it
> come not from her.[29]

28 Robinson, *Medieval Andalusian Courtly Culture*, 18 (folio 2r).

29 Ibid., 34 (folio 11v).

By now the mistress has discerned the situation and, while initially sympathetic to the plight of the two lovers (perhaps as a result of having just heard a great many songs about romantic longing), she loses her patience, exclaiming to Riyāḍ: "[My] father has asked me to give you to him, but I couldn't bring myself to do that, but by God, now I'll sell you in the market for nothing!"[30] There follow weeks of sorrow, the separated lovers moaning about their plight, exchanging letters, starving themselves to the point of swooning, and yet recovering to compose poems about their tortured hearts. Because the manuscript's final pages have been lost, we do not know precisely how the story ends, although the hostess seems finally to be working on behalf of the lovers.

The manuscript not only provides the illustrations depicting the musical soirees and meetings of the various characters, it also contains the lyrics to the songs. It is significant that approximately a third of the extant text occurs in the form of song, twenty-five of them in the garden. Yet they are songs that we cannot hear, only see.

The *Bayāḍ wa Riyāḍ* is unique as the only such fully illustrated manuscript to survive from the Islamic West. It bears clear eastern influences and its illustrations conform to pan-Islamic types, in which two figures in conversation face each other or in which parties are held in landscape settings, with music and other evocations of sound such as creaking waterwheels, flowing fountains, and birds.[31] The garden scenes make a direct appeal to the sense of taste, indicated by wine cups and trays of food, to vision through the brilliant color of the flowers, and to hearing through the prominence of the lute. Moreover the sensory experience is controlled by the surrounding high walls that place people in close contact with the garden. The poet and philosopher Ibn Ḥazm (994–1064) knew well the phenomenon of sensory proximity, commenting, "The senses of taste and touch . . . perceive objects only through contact, and hearing and smell apprehend them only if they are close by."[32] The same enclosure that provides an envelope for containing scent, for putting the nose and hands close to fragrant blooms and aromatic foliage, also serves to keep urban stench away. The garden rejects the urban cacophony of the bustling bazaar and the grunts and odors of barnyard animals, instead inviting the pleasing sound of birdsong, fountains (which gently mask other sounds), and sometimes ladies strumming the lute.

We can read all of this from the text and images of the *Bayāḍ wa Riyāḍ*, and can extrapolate additional information about the sensory appeal of gardens from what we know about other Andalusian sites such as Madīnat al-Zahrāʾ and the Alhambra. But while we may project ourselves into the image and imagine ourselves drinking wine in a garden with pleasant music, we cannot actually smell what the characters smelled, taste what they tasted, or hear what they heard. The poetry, music, and banquets were all ephemeral performances that last only through the medium of surrogate images and words. We do not actually know *how* poetry was declaimed or precisely *what* the musical performances sounded like; even if we read aloud the lyrics in the *Bayāḍ wa Riyāḍ* manuscript, we do not know the tunes to which they were sung.

In like manner, although we can easily see things that activate the sense of smell, we cannot experience the actual historic aroma. While scientists today can record a molecular formula using a gas chromatograph and recreate it to produce a precise scent, in the medieval world that could not be done. Similarly, today we can make precisely constructed artificial molecules that smell like vanilla without actually being derived from the very expensive vanilla pod, but these were unknown five hundred years ago.[33] The experience of smell depended on the reiteration

30 Ibid., 35 (folio 12r).

31 G. Levi Della Vida, review of *Al-Iklīl (al-juz' al-thāmin)* by Al-Ḥasan ibn-Aḥmad al-Hamdānī, ed. N. A. Faris, and *Historia de los amores de Bayāḍ y Riyāḍ: Una chantefable oriental en estilo persa* (Vat. Ar. 368), trans. A. R. Nykl, in *Journal of the American Oriental Society* 61, no. 4 (December 1941): 303–5; S. Khemir, entry 82 in J. D. Dodds, ed., *Al-Andalus: The Arts of Islamic Spain* (New York, 1992), 312–13; D'Ottone, "Il manoscritto Vaticano arabo 368," 55–70.

32 Ibn Ḥazm, *The Ring of the Dove: A Treatise on the Art and Practice of Arab Love*, my adaptation from the translation of A. J. Arberry (London, 1994), 70.

33 L. Turin, *The Secret of Scent: Adventures in Perfume and the Science of Smell* (New York, 2006), 38–40 on gas chromatography, 46–47 on vanillin, and passim.

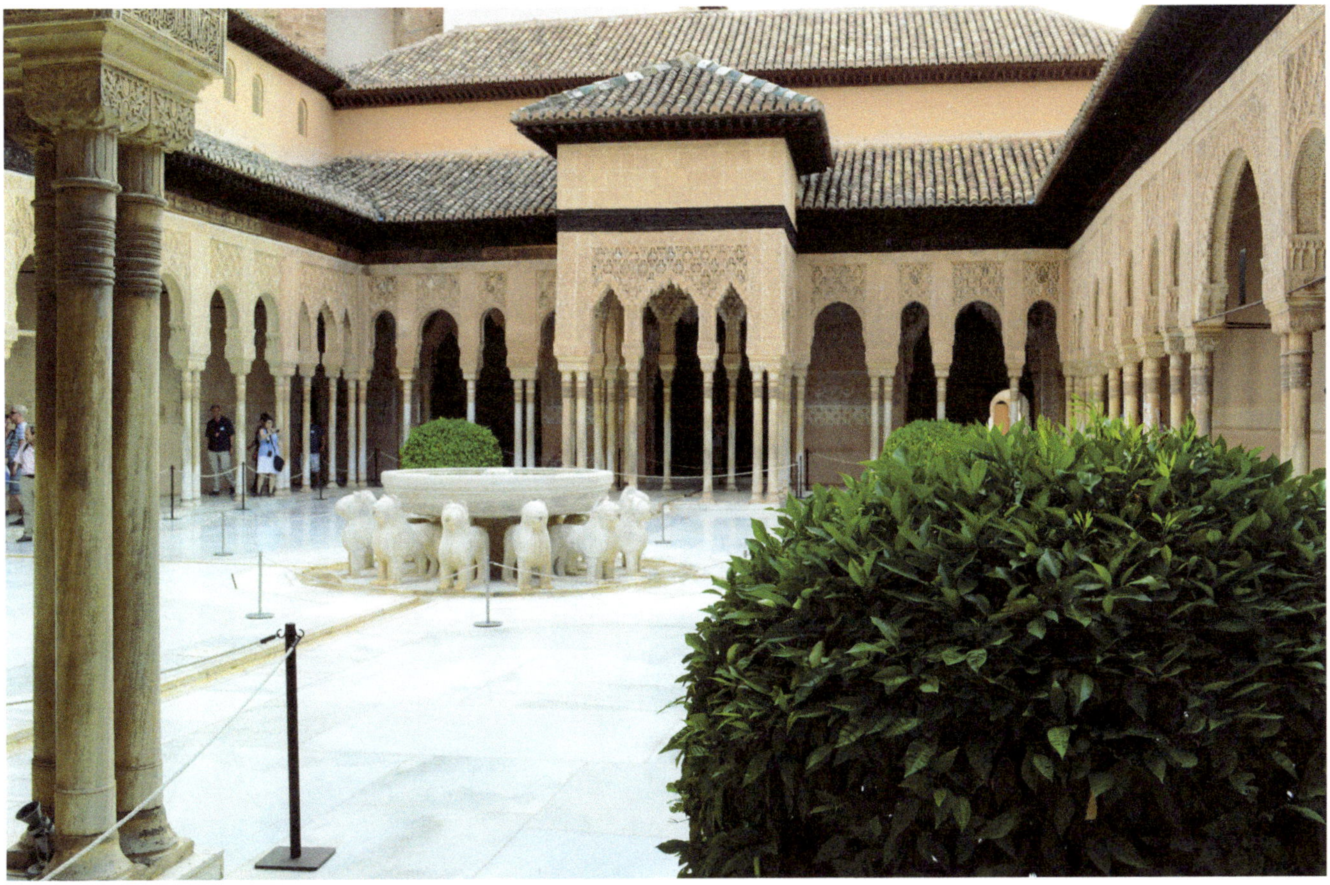

FIG. 6.9.
Alhambra, Court of the Lions, courtyard view (photo: author)

of an ephemeral effect that occurred at the site of the body, and it had to be captured in the moment—which is part of the pleasure—and yet for the same reason, remains elusive.

Of course, like smell, vision is also an embodied experience. How can twenty-first-century eyes accurately assess what the fourteenth-century sultan saw when he looked at the Alhambra's Lindaraja Mirador or Court of the Lions (fig. 6.9)? The act of looking at the Alhambra is in many ways a performance of viewing again and again, each time from a different temporal stance. The difference is that the palace walls are enduring. The stucco and stone that the sultan himself touched still remain for the most part, whereas the musicians and gardeners packed up their lutes and shovels and left long ago. The problem is not only in the act of human sensation but also in the thing to which we wish to apply that sense. Very simply, both the flower and the nose are short-lived.

In addition to the ephemerality of smell and the subjective, thus variable, response to it of the human nose and brain, smell poses other challenges to the historian. In the body's nervous system, the eyes pass information into the analytical, logical part of the brain (the cerebrum), while smell and taste go directly into the older, inner, and more primitive area of the brain (the limbic system) that governs emotions and memory (fig. 6.10). The eyes are thus connected to the intellectual functions, which lead us to associate vision with intelligence. In contrast, the power of smell and taste (which is closely related to smell because in tasting we engage in a "reverse sniff" that allows the nose to supplement the sense of taste) is that they bypass the logical brain; they seem to control us instead of we them.[34] Things not thought of in years can be suddenly and vividly recalled through the whiff

34 Gilbert calls this "retronasal olfaction," *What the Nose Knows* (n. 16 above), 92, citing H. Finck, "The Gastronomic Value of Odours," *Contemporary Review* 50 (1886): 680–95.

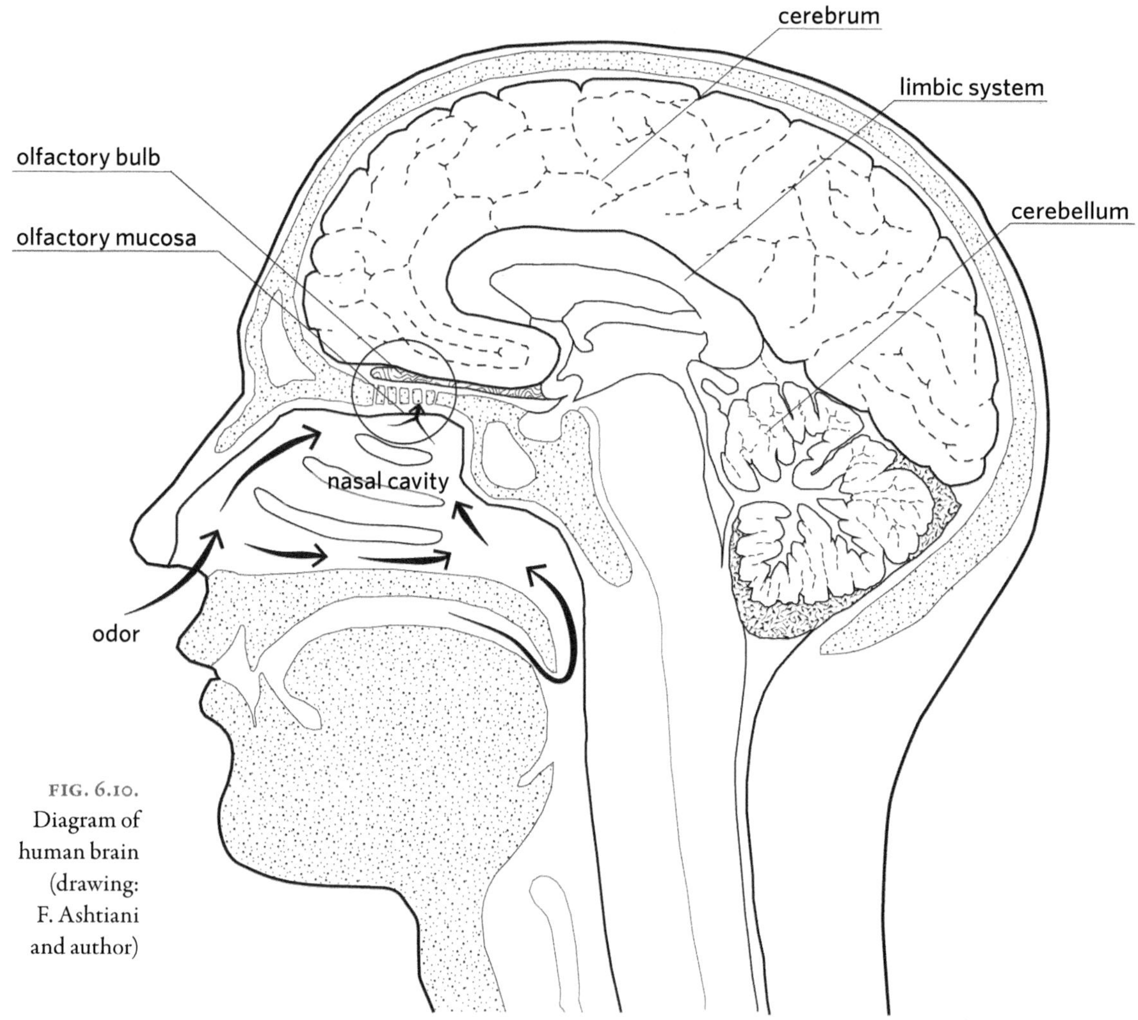

FIG. 6.10. Diagram of human brain (drawing: F. Ashtiani and author)

of an aroma. The scientist Trygg Engen says that smell memory is "impervious to time" and that, unlike other forms of sensory memory which diminish with the passing of time or the layering of subsequent experiences, smell memory has "the ability to reinstate the past and to ignore subsequent odor experiences not associated with the formative event."[35]

This suggests that the most profound power of smell may lie not in its ability to trigger memories, but in its uniqueness. The perfume scientist Luca Turin writes that each odor is specific and that no two different molecular compounds or perfume blends will ever smell alike: "There are no exact equivalents in smell, you have to hit the tiny nail smack on the head or you'll miss it by miles. That's why the event is rare, and that's why we notice it."[36] Thus smell is utterly specific, and yet vague, in that we lack adequate vocabulary to categorize it. This is a problem for scholars trained to think in terms of textual and visual representation, which is predicated on synonymous relationships in which, say, a precisely drawn square reproduces the geometrical properties of a crystalline formation. Smell does not do this: it can approximate through association but cannot reproduce precise qualities of something other than itself.

Gardens are replete with semiotic potential—from Islam's garden of Paradise to the Christian *hortus conclusus*—and yet their fleeting scents are hard to describe. Scent can be allusive (think of how cinnamon may conjure up the idea of

35 T. Engen, *Odor Sensation and Memory* (New York, 1991), 81.

36 Turin, *Secret of Scent*, 14.

cooking and thus the home kitchen) but it lacks the rich connotative and denotative properties of visual symbols. Historians and poets may praise a garden for its "fragrant breaths," but they rarely say much else, simply because it is exceedingly difficult, and maybe impossible, to go further than, "it smells like" or "it reminds me of."[37] The problem is not in their ability to create rich imagery, but in the available means for analyzing scent because, until the invention of the modern gas chromatograph in 1955, there was no way to objectively record scent. Instead, a desired perfume was made by manufacturing it from the same ingredients again and again, and it was analyzed by associating one aroma with other aromas (hence the categories of citrus, spicy, musky, etc.). Although a scent can prompt memory of the past, the act of smelling is a performance occurring in present time. To smell a rose, the words and images from Dioscorides are not enough: one must smell an actual rose, or a distillation of that rose. As for the vocabulary for describing that experience of sniffing the rose, it is much poorer than the vocabulary for vision because smell lives in the wrong cranial neighborhood.

I have been arguing that there are several things that complicate the analysis of smell. The first is that both the sources of smell and the bodily sensations were emphemeral: not only do we lack the flower that the historical subject sniffed, we lack that subject's olfactory palette. Just as the social constructedness of vision produces what art historians call the "period eye," so too did the Ottoman sultan Mehmet Fatih's experience of smelling a rose depend on his tolerance for and appreciation of a scent that was as much learned as natural (fig. 6.11).[38] Both the scent and the sensory body are absent. This image of a man engaged in smelling points to the second impediment in the analysis of smell: representation. While gas chromatography has permitted the precise measurement, documentation, and thus reproduction of aromatic molecules, this is an entirely modern phenomenon. Therefore, in our pursuit of historical olfactory sensations, we are compelled to return to the visual evidence that shows scent through pictorial representation of its production and effect.

In considering the usefulness of visual evidence, I am not talking about the classic representational strategies that objectify architecture and landscape: ground plan, elevation, axonometric reconstruction, and situated view (as provided in figs. 6.3–6.5). Those classic visualizations propose, in a strangely self-fulfilling manner, that the garden is an entirely optical experience and can therefore be represented adequately by pictures, as indeed they were from the sixteenth century onward in Europe and from the seventeenth century onward in Iran and India, where gardens offered dramatic vistas that could be seen from a single standpoint. However, in al-Andalus, from the eighth through the fifteenth centuries, such representational techniques were unknown, and experience mattered more than perspectival focus. As the twelfth-century agricultural manual of Ibn Luyūn advised—"in the center of the garden let there be a pavilion in which to sit"—the garden was designed around the central presence of its occupant with all the flowers, evergreen trees, climbing vines, fruit trees, climbing roses, and myrtles arrayed in relation to that central point and surrounding walls.[39] Rather than plants subordinated to a scheme in which the principal design requirement is visual, the design of Andalusian gardens was built entirely around both plants whose needs for shade, water, and trellising were clearly spelled out, and an occupant who sat in a pavilion covered with fragrant roses "with vistas on all sides" and "of such a form that no one approaching could overhear the conversation within."[40] In such a space, seeing, smelling, and hearing all matter.

They matter, and yet we do not have access to them. To understand such gardens, where

37 Scientists are not entirely sure *why* scents resemble each other. The fact that we perceive them to smell alike is not due to similarity in the structure and composition of the molecules (Gilbert, *What the Nose Knows*, 22).

38 M. Baxandall, *Painting and Experience in Fifteenth-Century Italy: A Primer in the Social History of Pictorial Style* (Oxford, 1972). With respect to odor specifically, Alain Corbin discusses the historically changing "threshold of olfactory tolerance" and changing expectations regarding desirable and undesirable odors (*The Foul and the Fragrant* [New York, 1986], 58 and 71–74).

39 Ibn Luyūn, *Tratado de agricultura* (Arabic), ed. and trans. J. Eguaras Ibánez (Granada, 1975), 171–75; trans. J. Dickie, "The Islamic Garden in Spain," in *The Islamic Garden*, ed. E. MacDougall and R. Ettinghausen (Washington, DC, 1976), 94.

40 Ibid.

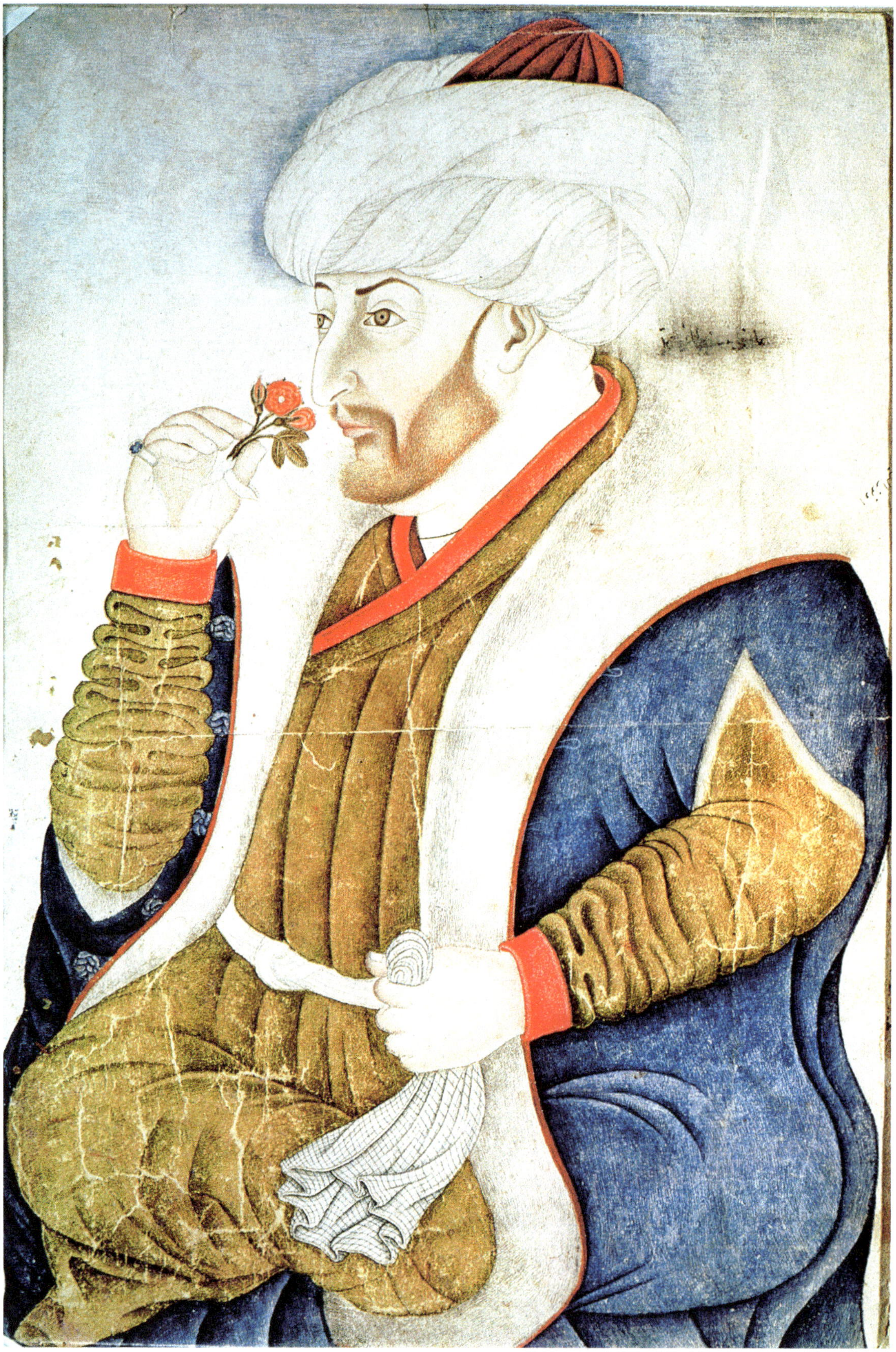

FIG. 6.11. Portrait of the Ottoman sultan Mehmet Fatih smelling a rose, by Sinan Bey, late 15th century, Topkapi Palace Museum, MS. Hazine 2153, fol. 10a (photo: Bridgeman images)

we can no longer hear the conversation or smell the flowers, our best recourse is to enlist the visual, not as an instrument for objectification in which the image stands in for the garden as a whole, but as a tool to capture the echoes of other important sensory ways of knowing the historical world. To understand Islamic gardens in all their sensory splendor, we must understand that while the eye may have to substitute for all the other senses, it is forever incomplete. We want the entire sensate body, even if we cannot have it.

The ill-fated lovers Bayāḍ and Riyāḍ knew this well. For Bayāḍ, it was not enough merely to see his beloved from a distance: he wished to sit inside the walled garden with her, to sing to her, and pass her the wine cup. History tells us little else about them. But I can imagine that as the comely Riyāḍ strummed the lute and sang of her passion, the infatuated young man may have leaned past the other women, toward the object of his desire in hopes of inhaling the "breeze of camphor and musk" that was her "wafting perfume." For Bayāḍ and Riyāḍ, seeing was not enough.

CHAPTER SEVEN

The Smell of Time

Olfactory Associations with the Past in Premodern Greece

FELIPE ROJAS AND VALERIA SERGUEENKOVA

What did the past smell like in the past? This question may seem bizarre. Most of us today approach antiquity primarily through our eyes: we read about it in books and look at it in museums. Few of us would attempt to smell the past, or even think that olfactory engagements with antiquity are possible. Smells are furtive and fleeting, the opposite of the visible and tangible remains that we usually associate with former times; smells are also notoriously difficult to pin down with words (simile is almost inevitable: things smell like x or y);[1] moreover, smells defy taxonomy and elude the archive. And yet, at least at the level of the individual, smells spur memory and the imagination, often inciting instant, vivid recollection.

This paper considers evidence from premodern Greece that shows that many individuals and communities were attuned to olfactory cues as a means of accessing the remote past. Our principal area of expertise is classical antiquity and most of our examples date from the Roman period; however, we venture into the Byzantine and Ottoman worlds to probe analogous situations in which smells triggered historical reflection. Our study cases are varied: a captive archbishop in twelfth-century Thessalonike was moved by the stench of human feces to make diachronic analogies between his captors, present-day savages from the Latin west, and their primitive counterparts from Greek antiquity; an erudite traveler in Roman Greece was told of the peculiar odors of primeval beasts and men in the local landscape; those odors, in turn, enabled small communities to claim very deep antiquity; an Ottoman visitor in seventeenth-century Athens communed with Plato "the Divine" after inhaling exotic aromas in mysterious caves near the Acropolis. Throughout we make two basic claims: that smells sometimes functioned as indices of specific historical and mythical events and that, when they did so, smells tightened social bonds among individuals and within groups.

Our investigation matters for several reasons. The first and most obvious is that the hegemony of sight has had a huge impact on our own scholarly construction of the past, and because—despite recent exciting incursions into the cultural significance of olfaction in the ancient world[2]—smell

1 A. Jasper and N. Wagner ("Notes on Scent," *Cabinet* 32 [2008–9]: 36–42) provide an entertaining discussion of the classificatory challenges posed by smells.

2 For the Greek and Roman periods now see the essays in M. Bradley, ed., *Smell and the Ancient Senses* (Oxford and New York, 2014). Notable contributions dealing with early Christianity include B. Caseau, "Euōdia: The Use and Meaning of Fragrances in the Ancient World and Their Christianization (100–900 AD)" (PhD diss., Princeton University, 1994) and the outstanding S. A. Harvey, *Scenting Salvation: Ancient Christianity and the Olfactory Imagination* (Berkeley, 2006), both relying almost exclusively on texts. From further afield, see J. McHugh, *Sandalwood and Carrion: Smell in Indian Religion and Culture* (New York, 2012) on smell and religion in the premodern Indian subcontinent, and in pre-Columbian Mesoamerica the section entitled "Classic Maya Smell"

remains arguably the least explored of the western senses among scholars of antiquity.[3] As a result of the general tyranny of the eyes in western epistemology, the classical Mediterranean in particular has often been imagined—even by scholars studying smell—as a largely mental, if not exclusively literary realm.[4] While much of the evidence examined in this chapter is textual, we are not interested primarily in rhetoric and metaphor, or in ancient discourse and theories about perception. Instead, we ground smells and the texts that speak of them in a material matrix.[5] This permits us to investigate literal rather than literary smells, and to elucidate the cultural significance of olfactory cues for specific communities and individuals. As the archaeologist Yannis Hamilakis has argued, greater attention to the senses—including the sense of smell—forces us to become more aware of the vitality of matter and of embodied experiences in the past.[6] Second, in recent years, scholars have demonstrated that the western sensorium is, at least partly, a cultural construct, and that there are and have been people whose own hierarchy and taxonomy of the senses differ radically from our own.[7] To imagine the past by smelling is counterintuitive and surprising, and yet, some people in premodern Greece were convinced that smells did in fact provide compelling proof of what had happened in the past. Our study of when and why those people exercised their nostrils to access antiquity is thus intended as a contribution to the history of the historical imagination.

Brute Stench

During the Norman siege of Thessalonike in 1185, invaders took over the archbishop's residence, allowing a group of Greek refugees to occupy the garden.[8] For archbishop Eustathios, this was a paradoxical inversion: civilized Hellenes braving the elements in the garden while barbarians enjoyed the comforts of the palace. The archbishop's firsthand description of the events captures the pathetic situation: even the well-tended plants fell victim to the savagery of the Norman hooligans. The height of the invaders' savagery came when the invaders approached Eustathios and his group, exposed their rumps, and began defecating in front of the refugees—an unambiguous embodied lesson in the new dynamics of power in Thessalonike. According to Eustathios, Norman feces flowed like water (the result of the laxative effect of the

in *The Memory of Bones: Body, Being, and Experience Among the Classic Maya*, ed. S. D. Houston, D. Stuart, and K. Taube (Austin, 2006), 141–52. For a stimulating article that uses primarily archaeological evidence to explore bad smells across millennia, see L. Bartosiewicz, "'There's Something Rotten in the State . . .': Bad Smells in Antiquity," *European Journal of Archaeology* 6, no. 2 (2003): 175–95.

3 A frequent complaint among scholars of ancient smells is the overvaluation of sight at the expense of other senses; see, e.g., Harvey, *Scenting Salvation*, 3–4, McHugh, *Sandalwood*, 9, and Bradley, "Introduction," 2 and 8.

4 S. Lilja, *The Treatment of Odours in the Poetry of Antiquity* (Helsinki, 1972) is an example of earlier work on the significance of smell in classical antiquity with an exclusively literary focus; similarly, C. Classen, D. Howes, and A. Synnott, *Aroma: The Cultural History of Smell* (London and New York, 1994) devote one chapter to the aromas of antiquity—basically a short survey of ancient literary passages; see also, G. Squillace, *Il profumo nel mondo antico: Con la prima traduzione italiana del «Sugli odori» di Teofrasto* (Florence, 2010), which focuses on perfume in textual sources. Other scholars interested in ancient perfumes and spices have been more sensitive to material evidence, see, e.g., P. Fauré, *Parfums et aromates de l'Antiquité* (Paris, 1987) and A. Verbanck-Piérard, N. Massar, and D. Frère, *Parfums de l'antiquité: La rose et l'encens en méditerranée* ([Morlanwelz], 2008).

5 Scholars working in different disciplines have advocated for careful attention to the material matrix of smell: Houston, Stuart, and Taube, *Memory of Bones*, 141–52; A. Barbara and A. Perliss, *Invisible Architecture: Experiencing Places through the Sense of Smell* (Milan, 2006); McHugh, *Sandalwood*.

6 Y. Hamilakis, *Archaeology and the Senses: Human Experience, Memory, and Affect* (Cambridge, 2014) calls attention to the connection between what he terms "indigenous archaeologies" (i.e., engagements with antiquities at the hands of local communities) and "the archaeology of the senses" (i.e., an approach to the past that is multisensory and affective); he sets both indigenous archaeologies and the archaeology of the senses in sharp opposition to western-style institutionalized archaeology (though see ibid., 63–64) and argues for a fundamental recalibration of archaeological methodology; a favorite example of his highlights the olfactory experience of antiquity (ibid., 35–41).

7 See, for example, C. Classen, "Other Ways to Wisdom: Learning through the Senses across Cultures." *International Review of Education / Internationale Zeitschrift für Erziehungswissenschaft / Revue Internationale de l'Education* 45, nos. 3–4 (1999): 269–80.

8 Eustathios of Thessalonike, *The Capture of Thessaloniki*, trans. J. R. Melville Jones (Canberra, 1988), 110–13 (§96); on this passage, see I. Nilsson, "Nature Controlled by Artistry: The Poetics of the Literary Garden in Byzantium," in *Byzantine Gardens and Beyond*, ed. H. Bodin and R. Hedlund, Acta Universitatis Upsaliensis, Studia Byzantina Upsaliensia 13 (Uppsala, 2013), 15–17, who called our attention to Eustathios.

grapes the Latins had consumed), provoking disgust and outrage among the helpless Greeks:

> [M]y companions, who were nauseated, as might be expected, by this abominable behaviour, were ready to burst with rage and were inflamed with the desire to drive them away ignominiously—these Ozolians, if we may give them the ancient Greek name. But we restrained them from doing so, because in our judgment those who roll in the mire with sinners may expect to acquire the same odours.[9]

The coprological spectacle incited a comparison across time and space: the Normans that Eustathios had before his eyes (and nose) were essentially living Ozolians, the proverbially primitive people of ancient Ozolian (or western) Lokris. The name "Ozolian" seemed related to the verb ὄζειν, meaning "to smell"; it had been the recurrent subject of discussion among many classical authors Eustathios knew well.[10] Stink in Thessalonike triggered a diachronic analogy with moral and intellectual implications. Eustathios was fond of finding links between present and past.[11] What is particularly interesting about this account—apart from the shocking behavior of the Normans—is that smell moved the archbishop to remember classical discussions about the curious name of an obscure Greek region and its people. Those explanations attributed the smell of Ozolian Lokris either to a mythical pollution or to the primitive customs of locals (for details, see next section). By suggesting that the Normans were like the Ozolians and thus that the ancient Ozolians smelled like shit, Eustathios was highlighting his own extensive classical learning, and also participating in a long intellectual tradition that stretched back many centuries.

The fetid smell of the Normans' excretions also strengthened social bonds among the Greek refugees; the brute stench brought them together in the face of the Norman invaders. Eustathios was thus a member of at least two olfactory communities: that of the men in the garden smelling the Normans' stool, and that of Greek men of letters from classical antiquity. This double engagement, whereby smell incited reflection about the past and defined social and cultural groups, is not exceptional and is at the heart of our investigation. Other people elsewhere and at other times have also smelled the past, and have come together as a community by doing so.

Stinky Debates

By equating Normans and Ozolians, Eustathios was participating in a discussion whose origins dated back at least to the Hellenistic period. In antiquity, the strange name Ozolian invited etymologizing.[12] The geographer Strabo, the antiquarian Plutarch, the traveler Pausanias, and other ancient authors were intrigued by the origins of this appellation, which seemed to many to mean "smelly" or "stinky." In addition to linguistic speculation, actual sensory stimuli offered the possibility of probing the origins of the term—for in Ozolian Lokris people could still smell the traces of remote historical and mythical events.

While traveling through ancient Phokis (fig. 7.1), Pausanias came to Lokris and recorded various explanations concerning the divergent etymologies of "Ozolian":

> The land of the Ozolian Lokrians, as they are called, adjoins Phokis in the direction of Kirrha. I have heard different explanations of the surname of these Lokrians, all of which I will set down. When Orestheus, son of Deukalion, reigned in the land, a bitch of his littered a stick instead of a puppy. Orestheus

9 Eustathios, *Capture of Thessaloniki*, 113 (§96), trans. Melville-Jones.

10 Eustathios was familiar with Strabo (9.4.7–8) and perhaps also with Plutarch, *Quaestiones Graecae* 294f–295a (discussed below). Homeric scholia preserve variants of the main interpretations of the name Ozolian: see *scholia vetera* D *ad Iliadem* 2.527 and compare Eustathios's remarks in his commentary on *Iliad* 2.235 as well as on Dionysios Periegetes' *Description of the Earth* 426. A version of one of the classical explanations is also recorded in the Byzantine lexicographical tradition, see *Etymologicum Magnum* and *Etymologicum Symeonis*, s.v. βδόλος.

11 A. Kazhdan, *Studies on Byzantine Literature of the Eleventh and Twelfth Centuries* (Cambridge, 1984), 184.

12 On the many etymologies and their possible motivations, see L. Lerat, *Les Locriens de l'ouest*, Bibliothèque des Écoles françaises d'Athènes et de Rome 176 (Paris, 1952), 3–4, 7, with references to earlier discussions.

FIG. 7.1. Greece, showing main ancient sites discussed in text (map: J. Wallrodt)

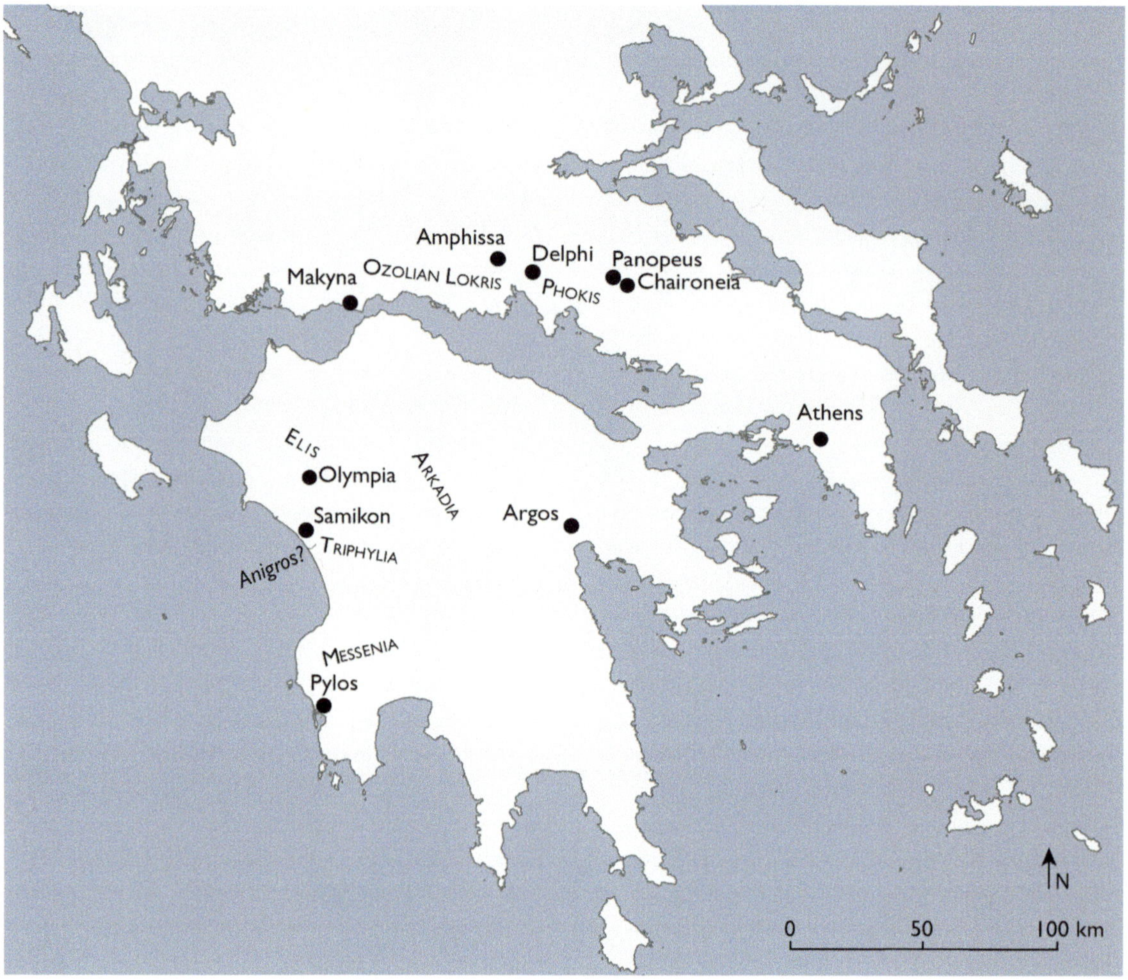

buried the stick, but when spring came round, a vine, they say, grew out of the stick, and from the branches of the stick the people got their name. Others think that while [the centaur] Nessos was acting as ferryman on the Euenos he was wounded by Herakles, but not killed outright, and that he escaped to this country, and when he died his body rotted unburied and tainted the atmosphere with its noisome smell. The third explanation is that the exhalations and even the water of a certain river were fetid; while a fourth is that asphodel grows in plenty, and when it is in flower. . . .[13] by the smell. It is also said that the first inhabitants were aborigines, and that, not knowing as yet how to weave garments, they made themselves coverings of untanned skins of wild beasts as a protection against the cold, turning the shaggy side out for the sake of appearance. So their skin must have stunk like the hides.[14]

As these explanations make clear, by the second century CE, the connection of the name Ozolian with olfaction was less controversial than the exact causes of the smell (or smells) behind the toponym. Plutarch, who wrote slightly before Pausanias and was familiar with the region,[15] knew of this debate:

> Some say that the Lokrians are called Ozolian because of Nessos, others because of the serpent Python. The monsters were cast

13 The text has an unfortunate lacuna.

14 Pausanias (10.38.1–3), translated by J. G. Frazer, ed., *Pausanias's* Description of Greece, 6 vols. (1898; repr. London, 1913), slightly modified.

15 Plutarch was born in Chaironeia and spent many years of his life as a priest in Delphi.

out by the sea and then rotted in the land of the Lokrians. According to some others, the people in this country smell bad because they wear the skins of sheep and goats and spend their time with herds of goats. Some, however, claim that, on the contrary, this is a country of many flowers and its name comes from its wonderful smell. One of these is Archytas of Amphissa, who writes: "Lovely Makyna wreathed with grape clusters and smelling of perfume."[16]

Pausanias's and Plutarch's testimonies give a sense of the disagreements among those who cared about the origins of the name "Ozolian." But who disagreed and what was at stake? Plutarch and Pausanias were both erudite antiquarians who lived at a time of intense interest in the past when control over abstruse details of local history was a matter of cultural prestige. And yet, although intellectual one-upmanship might have driven some, for others the motivations and the stakes were not solely academic. Thus, we can also detect factions along geographic lines, opposing explanations being favored by locals, on the one hand, and foreigners, on the other.

Ozolian Lokris had been considered a cultural backwater for centuries—as Thucydides observed already in the fifth century BCE, and as Strabo implied in the time of the emperor Augustus, pointing out that the Ozolians were neglected by Homer and mentioned by few others.[17] Plutarch and Pausanias were part of discussions that had been going on for hundreds of years. In the third century BCE learned outsiders such as the historian Myrsilos of Methymna and the paradoxographer Antigonos of Karystos had already explained the term "Ozolian" by making reference to the stench of Nessos's decomposing carcass; furthermore, they had argued that the rot had contaminated a nearby local river on Mt. Taphi(ass)os, which they etymologized as meaning "the tomb" (τάφος).[18] By contrast, at about the same time, Archytas of Amphissa had highlighted a positive connection between the ethnonym and "smelling of perfume" Makyna, a town near Mt. Taphi(ass)os. Local pride seems to have motivated at least some ancient interpretations. The divide between locals and foreigners is especially interesting if we consider that locals would probably have been accustomed to most of the smells in their territory—whatever they were—whereas foreigners would be disturbed, or at least struck by them. In this regard, it is worth remembering that the Ozolian Lokrians never referred to themselves as Ozolian ("smelly"), but only as Western Lokrians.[19]

Whatever the true origin of "Ozolian," most people associated the name with smell; in fact, by the Byzantine period that seems to have been the only etymology available. The idiosyncratic odor of Ozolian Lokris could have been produced by local flora or mineral springs;[20] whatever the cause, these smells incited those who perceived them to pick sides, as it were, and become part of olfactory communities with divergent memory horizons. The choice between centaur and python, or sulphur and asphodel had more than merely scholarly repercussions because the various historical or mythical narratives explained also who the Lokrians were with respect to others past and present. The nose could thus be witness to a site's (and a people's) cultural significance. Since smells were inherent in the landscape, whole networks of features, not just single olfactory cues, were affected by the conflicting explanations; the importance and antiquity of mountains, rivers, flowers, trees, and most of all people, were all at stake.

A second example may clarify the stakes in ancient debates about smells. If Ozolian Lokris

16 Plutarch, *Quaestiones Graecae* 294F–295A; authors' trans.

17 Thucydides 1.5.3; Strabo 9.4.7.

18 *FGrH* 477 F6 = Antigonos of Karystos, *Historiae Mirabiles* 3rd c. BCE; see also Homeric scholia cited above in note 10 and Strabo (9.4.7–8), who gives the alternative name of the mountain and mentions the "tomb(s) of Nessos and the other centaurs."

19 As pointed out by Lerat, *Les Locriens de l'ouest*, 7, who further argues that the profusion of etymologies was a result of the opacity of the name and assumes local patriotism to be the motive for Archytas's poem.

20 Edward Dodwell, an Irish classicist who traveled to Greece in the first decade of the 19th century, proposed a connection with the *Euphorbia peplus*, or milkweed, which "gives peculiar sour smell to the whole country while in bloom" and "according to the locals occasions bad air" (E. Dodwell, M. Ferdinando, and S. Pomardi, *A Classical and Topographical Tour through Greece, during the Years 1801, 1805, and 1806* [London, 1819], 131); he recorded the plant's name as *galaxidi*, with the meaning "sour milk," and thought it to be the namesake of modern Galaxidi (ancient Oianthia) in southern Phokis.

was not a celebrated land, Panopeus, a small community in neighboring Phokis, had a modicum of fame. In Greek epic "famous Panopeus"[21] was a city of kings and mythical heroes such as Epeios (builder of the Trojan horse) and Tityos (whose liver and heart were forever eaten out by two vultures in the underworld).[22] The town was situated on an important pilgrimage route along the Sacred Way from Athens to Delphi. Pausanias was fully aware of the town's literary fame; precisely for this reason, he was underwhelmed when he visited the place in the second century CE:[23]

> It is twenty furlongs from Chaironeia to Panopeus, a city of Phokis, if city it can be called that has no government offices, no gymnasium, no theater, no marketplace, no water conducted to a fountain, and where the people live in hovels, just like highland shanties, perched on the edge of a ravine. Yet its territory is marked off by boundaries from that of its neighbors, and it even sends members to the Phokian assembly.

Guided by locals, Pausanias could still make out the material traces of the Homeric past: "the perimeter of the ancient city" (10.4.2)—surely the remains of the monumental fortifications which are conspicuous to this day—and a mound that was thought to be the tomb of Tityos (10.4.5). As far as Pausanias was concerned, and in spite of those massive ruins, Panopeus was just a little town, not a *polis*. And yet, the locals were eager to remember their Homeric past and claim present significance in the region and in Greece at large. They did so in an agonistic spirit, emphasizing highly localized identities that distinguished the Panopeans from other nearby communities as well as from Delphi.[24] Unlike in Ozolian Lokris, where locals and foreigners argued about the nature of the smell that gave the region its peculiar name, in Panopeus it was the local inhabitants who argued among themselves about their town's antiquity. From the account of Pausanias, it is clear that disagreement arose about what must have been the most precious object in town:

> At Panopeus there is beside the road a small building of unburned brick, and in it is an image of Pentelic marble, which some say is Asklepios and others Prometheus. In proof of the latter view they produce evidence. At the edge of the ravine lie two stones, each big enough to load a cart. Their color is that of clay, not an earthy clay, but such as you would find in a ravine or a sandy torrent; and they smell very like the flesh of a man. They say that these stones are remains of the clay out of which the whole race of man was molded by Prometheus.[25]

Smell was thus of central importance in Panopeus. The strange stones in the ravine, whatever the exact nature of their odor, offered proof to some locals that their shantytown had been the birthplace of humanity.[26] Indeed, many of our ancient examples involve communities that were perceived by outsiders as insignificant and marginal. Locals there seem to be eager to incorporate smells in debates about antiquity that elsewhere revolve around tangible and visible remains. Was the smell of the Panopean clay comparable to a *xoanon*—one of the archaic wooden statues prized by Pausanias and his contemporaries for their antiquity—or to the giant bones of prehistoric creatures often treasured as the remnants of monsters? What is beyond doubt is that in Roman Greece smell incited the historical imagination.

Monumentalizing Olfaction

Smells were not superficial aspects of the landscape, but co-substantial with it. People could invoke mythical or historical narratives to call attention to local odors, as happened in Ozolian

21 *Iliad* 17.307; cf. 2.520. On Panopeus (also known as Phanoteus), see J. McInerney, *The Folds of Parnassos: Land and Ethnicity in Ancient Phokis* (Austin, 1999), 295–96 with further references and index, s.v. "Panopeus."

22 *Iliad* 23.665; *Odyssey* 11.576–581.

23 Pausanias 10.4.1, trans. Frazer, slightly modified.

24 McInerney, *Folds*, 128, highlights their efforts to distinguish themselves from the "Phokian commonwealth" and in particular from Delphi.

25 Pausanias 10.4.4, trans. Frazer, slightly modified.

26 The early modern traveler William Gell mentioned stones by a brook in Panopeus that emit odor upon rubbing; nobody else has ever found them. W. Gell, *The Itinerary of Greece: Containing One Hundred Routes in Attica, Boeotia, Phokis, Lokris, and Thessaly* (London, 1819), 201.

Lokris and Panopeus; sometimes those narratives could be further enhanced by physical interventions that framed a landscape's sensorial relevance. Our next examples involve Roman-period architectural features that were made to highlight olfactory hotspots.

In the region known as Triphylia, on the Western coast of the Peloponnese, lies Samikon; on its acropolis are the ruins of a classical fortification as well as other conspicuous prehistoric remains. In antiquity the foul-smelling Anigros River formed seasonal pools of stagnant water near the town before discharging into the sea. Although the site has changed much since the Roman period, there are still caves with sulphuric springs overlooking this marshy landscape.[27] According to Strabo and Pausanias, people disagreed about the causes of the stench of the Anigros.[28] Strabo identified the cave spring and stagnant water as the source of the odor, while Pausanias believed that the river's waters were contaminated by a peculiar soil near its head further inland in Arkadia.[29] These authors also reported alternative explanations according to which the Anigros bore the olfactory traces of mythical pollution. One version derived the stench from the monstrous Hydra, whose poisonous blood Herakles had applied to arrows with which he wounded a centaur—some said Chiron, others Pylenor. Whoever it had been, the centaur had allegedly washed his wound in the waters of the Anigros, and thus the river stank, charged with the stench of at least two mythical monsters. Others connected the foul smell to the seer Melampos of Pylos, who had tossed into the Anigros the medical potion he used to purify the daughters of King Proitos.[30]

Pausanias also reported that the waters near the mouth of the river healed leprosy and other skin diseases. After praying and making a dedication in the cave of the local river nymphs, the sick would wash in the foul-smelling water, swim across the swampy river, and come out cured.[31] For the locals, who stood to benefit directly from the popularity of a healing spot in their territory, the story relating the stench to the remnants of Melampos's remedy would have provided a welcome aetiology for their bleak landscape: a deserted swampland and river with toxic fish.[32]

As at Ozolian Lokris and Panopeus, the stories about the cause of the smell of the Anigros should be understood in a larger cultural context. Samikon too was relatively obscure in the Roman period and there had long been disagreements about political and civic allegiances in the region of Triphylia.[33] The myths associated with the smell of the river reflect some of these divisions: Herakles was most readily associated with Olympia, while Melampos would have been associated with Argos. Furthermore, both Strabo and Pausanias frame their accounts of this site as part of an exercise of Homeric exegesis. Locals pointed out landmarks quoting the *Iliad*, while learned visitors passed judgment on whether those identifications should be accepted or rejected. Pausanias's account hints at how both elements, regional politics and Homeric learning, were intertwined:

> None of the Messenians or Eleans could point out to me with certainty the ruins of Arene. The subject is one on which those who choose to do so may indulge in a variety of conjectures. The most plausible account seemed to me to be that in ancient times and in the heroic age Samikon was called Arene. Those

27 On Samikon and its surroundings see H. L. Bisbee, "Samikon," *Hesperia* 6 (1937): 525–38; this landscape had become a permanent lagoon by the early 19th century CE, see W. M. Leake, *Travels in the Morea* (London, 1830), 1:53–54, 61–66 and idem, *Peloponnesiaca: A Supplement to Travels on the Moréa* (London, 1846): 108, reporting on lumps of yellow sulphur in one cave and local superstition about sailing near it. According to Frazer's note on Pausanias's description of this place (3:479), the caves "emit foul mephitic vapours and inflammable gas."

28 The exact location of the Anigros is not known.

29 Strabo 8.3.19; Pausanias 5.5.9–11.

30 The daughters of Proitos were variously afflicted in the many versions of this story; a disgusting skin condition was part of their punishment according to the oldest version (Hesiod, fragments 132–33 M.-W.).

31 Pausanias 5.5.11; cf. Strabo 8.3.19.

32 Both Strabo (8.3.19) and Pausanias (5.5.8) mention the inedible fish of the Anigros.

33 On the internal dynamics of Triphylia in the Classical and Hellenistic periods see T. H. Nielsen, "Triphylia: An Experiment in Ethnic Construction and Political Organisation," in *Yet More Studies in the Ancient Greek Polis*, ed. idem (Stuttgart, 1997), 129–62.

who gave this explanation quoted the verses in the *Iliad*:

> There is a river Minyeïos falling into the sea
> Fast by Arene.

These ruins are very near to the Anigros. And though it may be questioned whether Samikon was once called Arene, the Arkadians are agreed that the ancient name of the river Anigros was Minyeïos.[34]

Manmade structures were thus also part of the networks of landscape features that were affected by explanations about the origins of a local smell. These structures included prehistoric monumental remains around Samikon, as well as more recent buildings. According to J. G. Frazer, who witnessed patients bathing at one of the caves by the Anigros in the late nineteenth century, "in antiquity the caves were approached by a stone causeway, of which there are remains in front of the caves."[35] It appears therefore that the people of the region had built a bridge for the pilgrims to access the smelly sanctuary.[36] The landscape of Samikon with its ruins, smells, and Homeric references was thus designed to function as a pilgrimage destination.

When thinking about the foul-smelling Anigros, Pausanias also remembered the landscape of his native Anatolia: "I am persuaded that the odd smell of the Anigros is caused by the soil through which the water rises, just as the same cause operates in the case of the waters inland from Ionia, the exhalation of which is poisonous to man."[37]

Pausanias here is referring to the thermal springs at Nysa on the Maeander and Phrygian Hierapolis. In the Roman period, those pilgrimage sites owed their renown to peculiar geothermal phenomena, including hot springs and caves out of which noxious gases emanated. While a stone causeway was built specifically for pilgrims to access the healing cave by the Anigros, in several cities in western Anatolia the process of institutionalization of local olfactory hotspots was taken much further. Discussion of those sites would take us far beyond the scope of this chapter, but it is worth noting that by the first century CE, a cave at Hierapolis which exhaled odorless lethal vapors was lavishly monumentalized.[38] Pilgrims were not allowed to go into this cave; instead a sensational ritual involving controlled asphyxiation was performed for their benefit: animals (including birds and cattle) were driven into the cave to their deaths, while eunuch priests entered the cave and emerged unscathed.[39] Unlike the old but humble communities in Greece which we have examined in this paper, Roman-period Hierapolis was thriving—but it was a boom town with a relatively shallow past when compared to those of nearby cities such as Sardis or Ephesos. What Hierapolis lacked in historical credentials, the city compensated for by monumentalizing a cave with mysterious gases that could be associated with remote historical and mythical events, including the slaying of a dragon.[40] In this new urban landscape the embodied experience of a lethal vapor spectacularly verified the city's claim to historical and mythical importance. In the same way, though much humbler in scale and with much more modest resources, the community near the Anigros caves highlighted a foul smell in a landscape of ruins and natural landmarks charged with healing potential, mythical memories, and political meaning.

Sniffing Plato

We began with a Byzantine case of a smell triggering reflection about antiquity, and we end with an Ottoman one. In the mid-seventeenth century CE, the renowned Ottoman traveler Evliya Çelebi visited Athens and described the once-great city in his *Seyâhatnâme* or *Book of Travels*.[41]

34 Pausanias 5.6.2–3, trans. Frazer, slightly modified.

35 Frazer, *Pausanius's* Description, 3:479.

36 Bisbee, "Samikon," 525, n. 1 mentions "submerged buildings."

37 Pausanias 5.5.9, trans. Frazer, slightly modified.

38 F. D'Andria, "Il Ploutonion a Hierapolis di Frigia," *Istanbuler Mitteilungen* 63 (2013): 157–217.

39 Strabo 13.4.14 and Dio Cassius 68.27.3.

40 On the lasting relevance of dragons in Hierapolis see I. Rutherford, "Trouble in Snake Town: Interpreting an Oracle from Hierapolis-Pamukkale," in *Severan Culture*, ed. S. Swain, S. J. Harrison, and J. Elsner (Cambridge and New York, 2007), 449–57.

41 There is no complete English translation of the *Seyâhatnâme*, but see the selections in R. Dankoff and S. Kim, *An Ottoman Traveller: Selections from the Book of Travels of Evliya Celebi* (London, 2010), including much of his account

Evliya prefaced his account with the claim that Athens had been the home of seven thousand philosophers and physicians, who sought an antidote for death and devised cures for many diseases. To Evliya the city appeared laden with unmistakable material vestiges of its former intellectual grandeur. Some of Athens' most "dazzling" monuments, including the famous "Tower of the Winds" and the "Friday Mosque in the Walled City" (i.e., the Parthenon),[42] deserved extended reflection, partly because Evliya associated them specifically with Plato "the divine." Athens offered remains that were not only visible and tangible, but also—remarkably—olfactible. The traces of Plato and other ancient Greek luminaries that Evliya knew had once roamed its streets were accessible through the nose:

> At the bottom of the cliff that looms over (!) this Athens castle are caves with all sorts of domes and palaces and hermit's cells. All the ancient sages—Aristotle, Hippocrates, Socrates, Pythagoras the Monotheist, Galen, Feylekos [Philip], Feylesof ["Philosopher"], Ptolemy, Mihan (?), Michael, and Plato—had cells in these caves. If you go inside them your brain will be perfumed by the fragrance of nutmeg, cubeb, cinnamon, long pepper, ginger, aloes, pellitory and cardamon. Since some of these cavemen practised alchemy, you can also smell sulphur and mercury and arsenic.[43]

This is an enigmatic passage, but we can reimagine the Ottoman traveler's experience through a combination of archaeological and literary evidence. Though Evliya may have visited many caves in Athens, those mentioned here appear to be specifically the caves at the foot of the Acropolis. Among them are those once sacred to Apollo, Pan, Zeus, and Aglauros (daughter of King Kekrops) as well as the cave directly above the top row of seats at the theater of Dionysos, which in the fourth century BCE was incorporated into the monument of Thrasyllos.[44] Many of these caves became Christian chapels in the Byzantine period—including the one monumentalized by Thrasyllos, which was transformed eventually into the church of Panagia (Khryso)spiliotissa.[45] The antiquarian traveler Richard Chandler described seeing the inside of that cave chapel, "covered in holy portraits" and "filled with smoke of incense" in the late eighteenth century.[46] More recent testimonies describe it as a healing site for women who would bring their sick children and leave votive candles that were as tall as their infants.[47] At another cave, in or near the Panathenaic stadium, the early nineteenth-century British traveler John Cam Hobhouse saw pieces of colorful cloth, glass, and food offerings left by women who practiced nocturnal magical healing.[48] Evliya seems to have visited some of these cave chapels, but failed (or neglected) to recognize them as churches filled with Orthodox Christian paraphernalia.[49]

What did he think those caves were? In Athens, as elsewhere in Greece, Evliya would have

of Athens (278–93). K. Kreiser, ed., *Evliya Çelebi's Book of Travels: Land and People of the Ottoman Empire in the Seventeenth Century* (Leiden and New York, 1988–), includes extended selections in English or German translation.

42 On Evliya's accounts of the "Tower of the Winds" and the "Friday Mosque in the Walled City," see Dankoff and Kim, *Ottoman Traveller*, 288–91 and 281–86; on the latter, see also D. G. Wright, "Evliya Visits the Acropolis," http://surprisedbytime.blogspot.com/2010/01/evliya-visits-acropolis.html (accessed 24 May 2016), and M. Beard, *The Parthenon* (London, 2002), 71–76, who calls Evliya's account "the most interesting description of the Parthenon in this [i.e., Ottoman] period (arguably in any period)."

43 Dankoff and Kim, *Ottoman Travellers*, 290. The "(!)" seems to indicate that Evliya's description of the location is unintelligible.

44 On these caves, see J. M. Hurwit, *The Athenian Acropolis: History, Mythology, and Archaeology from the Neolithic Era to the Present* (Cambridge, 1999), index, s.v. "caves."

45 See M. Bires, "Ἡ Παναγία Σπηλιώτισσα στὴν Ἀκρόπολη Ἀθηνῶν," in *Ἐκκλησίες στὴν Ἑλλάδα μετὰ τὴν Ἅλωση* (Athens, 1979), 195–96; K. Bires, *Τα αττικά του Εβλιά Τσελεμπή: Αι Αθήναι και τα περίχωρά των κατά τον 17ον αιώνα* (Athens, 1959), 51, n. 83 associated this cave with the passage under discussion.

46 R. Chandler, *Travels in Greece or an Account of a Tour Made at the Expence of the Society of Dilettanti* (Oxford, 1776), 63.

47 On the custom see Linda Theodorou's blog: http://churchesingreece.blogspot.com/2013/11/athens-classical-monuments-and.html (accessed 24 May 2016); on other rituals in this cave, see J. Freely, *Strolling through Athens: Fourteen Unforgettable Walks through Europe's Oldest City*, 2nd ed. (London and New York, 2004), 41–42.

48 J. C. Hobhouse, *A Journey through Albania, and Other Provinces of Turkey in Europe and Asia, to Constantinople, during the Years 1809 and 1810* (London, 1813), 325.

49 R. Dankoff, *An Ottoman Mentality: The World of Evliya Çelebi*, Ottoman Empire and Its Heritage 31 (Leiden and Boston, 2004), 52 points out that despite frequent visits, Evliya was neither interested nor particularly knowledgeable about churches.

been shown around by local guides, who pointed out notable landmarks and provided lively details.[50] We can get a sense of what Athenian guides told someone like Evliya from references by Constantinopolitan visitors to the city in the late Byzantine period (11th–12th c.).[51] Some of their stories also appear in two Greek manuscripts, written just after the fall of Constantinople: *The Theaters and Schools of Athens* and *On Attica* (known also, respectively, as the *Vienna Anonymous* and the *Paris Anonymous*).[52] Those texts suggests that the classical past, and, in particular, the classical past as projected onto material remains of various dates, was shown off proudly to distinguished visitors, both Christian and Muslim. So, for instance, the so-called Tower of the Winds, which Evliya called "Plato's pavilion," was "Socrates' School" according to the two anonymous manuscripts from Vienna and Paris.[53]

We do not know whether smells played a role in the stories the Athenian guides told about local ruins, but we do know that Evliya was unusually attuned to smells: fruits, baths, eggs, bat-droppings, flowers, walls, and the inside of the pyramid of Cheops are a few of the objects and places that drew his nose's attention during his travels.[54] It is thus not surprising that Evliya went beyond mere associations between Athenian ruins and famous ancient Greek philosophers, that he felt his "brain was perfumed" with the traces of philosophical and alchemical genius. By smelling the classical past he connected directly to the famous minds of Greek antiquity. In fact, Evliya was part of a learned Sufi tradition that associated specific smells with the godliness of Muslim saints. The aromas that he sensed in the caves of the Acropolis confirmed to him that the city had truly been the "abode of sages" (*dâr-ı medîneti'l-hukema ve'l-kudemâ*) who, moreover, had a place of honor in his intellectual and spiritual world.[55]

Smells abounded in Ottoman Athens as they abound today in any city; some places, like the caves at the foot of the Acropolis, were more interesting or intriguing to the nose than others. Those places attracted Evliya's attention, because he belonged to a culture in which divinity and divinely granted wisdom were often associated with fine aromas.[56] Whatever Evliya smelled in the caves of the Acropolis not only confirmed, but also brought to life in an embodied and immediate fashion local stories according to which the city had been the haunt of Plato "the Divine" and that the caves were the laboratories of ancient philosophers, alchemists, and physicians. Smell allowed Evliya to be part of an imagined olfactory community of enlightened minds stretching back several millennia and it also confirmed—at least to Evliya himself—that "this humble servant" was indeed a pious Sufi and a *derviş* (or mystical seeker) on a godly mission.[57]

Conclusions

We have made two basic claims: that smells sometimes functioned as indices of specific events in the past, and that they helped to strengthen

50 Although Evliya does not mention guides in this passage, he regularly does elsewhere, e.g., the priests leading him in the Davelis cave in Mt. Pendeli near Athens; see N. Cheiladakes, trans., *Ταξίδι στην Ελλάδα: Εβλιά Τσελεμπή* (Athens, 1991), 189–90.

51 On Byzantine interest in classical antiquity, and a forceful critique of the Western European claim of being the true heir of Athens, see A. Kaldellis, *The Christian Parthenon: Classicism and Pilgrimage in Byzantine Athens* (Cambridge and New York, 2009), 178–95.

52 Texts in C. Wachsmuth, *Die Stadt Athen im Alterthum*, vol. 1 (Leipzig, 1874), 731–44; see his comments on popular traditions about Athenian antiquities on pp. 56–62. On the *Vienna Anonymous* as a possible "*vade mecum* for the Turkish sultan" see W. Miller, *The Latins in the Levant: A History of Frankish Greece (1204–1566)* (New York, 1908), 441; cf. K. M. Setton, *Catalan Domination of Athens, 1311–1388* (Cambridge, MA, 1948), 236 for a very cautious suggestion about a connection to the visit of sultan Mehmet II to Athens in 1458.

53 Wachsmuth, *Die Stadt Athen*, 743 with n. 2 (*Vienna Anonymous* 2) and p. 731 (*Paris Anonymous*).

54 Smell is also key in his account of the dream in which the Prophet compels him to travel; as he kisses the hands of the Prophet and his companions, Evliya relates: "Some of their hands smelled of musk, some of ambergris, some of hyacinths, some of roses, some of sweet basil, some of violets, some of carnations. But the scent of the Prophet was of blooming saffron rose" (Dankoff and Kim, *Ottoman Traveller*, 6).

55 Quote from ibid., 279. On Evliya's interest in the smells of saints, see M. van Bruinessen and H. Boeschoten, *Evliya Çelebi in Dıyarbekır: The Relevant Section of the Seyahatname*, vol. 1 in Kreiser, *Evliya Çelebi's Book* (n. 41 above), 224–25, n. 156. On the importance of incense in the Ottoman world, see N. Ergin, "The Fragrance of the Divine: Ottoman Incense Burners and Their Context," *ArtB* 96 (2014): 70–97.

56 Ibid.

57 Dankoff, *Ottoman Mentality*, 117–22.

social bonds within imagined communities.[58] The variant interpretations of a smell, such as the fetor of human excrement, aromatic asphodel, or "the fragrance of nutmeg, cubeb, cinnamon, long pepper, ginger, aloes, pellitory and cardamom" served to define one's place in the world as well as in history. Why could olfaction serve this purpose? Because identifying the cause of a smell often required giving it moral and social valuation, which in turn reified cultural division lines. For the contemporaries of Plutarch and Pausanias, olfactory associations with the past had social repercussions as well: to identify a rotten centaur, flowers, or clay as the cause of a specific smell was to align oneself with others who thought or had thought likewise.

We have drawn our main examples from Roman Greece, but we have also tried to point to analogous Byzantine and Ottoman cases. In 1982, the French historian Alain Corbin wrote what is arguably the most influential cultural history of smell, *The Foul and the Fragrant*, a meticulous analysis of how olfactory cues helped encode social distinctions in eighteenth- and nineteenth-century France.[59] Ever since its publication, historians, anthropologists, and sociologists have noted the importance of smell in the construction of identity, especially among different groups inhabiting the same city or territory. As we have tried to show here, these olfactory communities have a diachronic as well as a synchronic dimension.[60] Smells brought people together by prompting them to zoom in on distinct memory horizons. By smelling, a Byzantine archbishop defied the brutality of military occupation and confirmed that he was part of a venerable intellectual tradition; the inhabitants of a little town with prehistoric ruins in Phokis proudly verified that their town had indeed been the cradle of mankind; and the great Ottoman traveler Evliya Çelebi really communed across millennia with Plato "the Divine."

Finally, our ideas about a monolithic Western sensorium in which, ever since Plato and Aristotle, eyesight has reigned supreme over hearing, and those two over more "primitive" senses such as touch, taste and smell, ignores alternative hierarchies of the senses within western traditions. The investigation of these "alternative sensorial frameworks," as Hamilakis calls them, is important because it can illuminate noncanonical, but widespread, ancient (and modern) history making practices.

58 On the notion of an imagined community, see B. Anderson, *Imagined Communities: Reflections on the Origin and Spread of Nationalism* (1983; rev. London and New York, 2006).

59 A. Corbin, *The Foul and the Fragrant: Odor and the French Social Imagination* (Cambridge, MA, 1988), esp. 142–61 (originally published as *Le miasme et la jonquille: L'odorat et l'imaginaire social XVIIIe–XIXe siècles*, Collection historique [Paris, 1982]). Classen, Howes, and Synnott, *Aroma* (n. 4 above), 2 speak of odors as "essential cues in social bonding."

60 For one such diachronic community, whose reach stretched into the future as well as into the past, see Harvey's analysis (*Scenting Salvation* [n. 2 above], 46–56) of how the smells of martyrs helped encode the paradisiacal prospect of the heavenly life to come in early Christianity.

We thank Sue Alcock, Mark Bradley, John Cherry, and Elif Özgen for their comments on earlier drafts of this chapter.

CHAPTER EIGHT

FRAGRANT MATTER

The Work of Holy Oil

SUSAN ASHBROOK HARVEY

HOLY OIL PRESENTS THE HISTORIAN WITH A RICH ENTRY INTO THE Byzantine sensorium. Its usage and meanings tell us much about Byzantine sensory culture and further, Byzantine cosmology. At the same time, holy oil raises and complicates sensation as a category of critical analysis. Revered in its fragrance, yet oil was more than its scent. Its fragrance was also material substance, its availability and usage somehow mercifully abundant, engaging the full sensory palate of embodiment. In its varied aspects, holy oil exemplified the Byzantine conception of an ordered cosmos in which human and divine domains intersected in terms sensorily grasped and experienced. Human–divine relation could be, and was, materially encountered and corporeally demonstrated in life-giving terms, concretely evidenced by the senses, both here and in eternity. Holy oil was a constant indicator of this view.

In this essay, I explore holy oil as a material, olfactory component of Byzantine culture. I use the term "holy oil," as did the Byzantines, in its most capacious sense: fragrant oil with divine qualities, whether activated by ritual consecration or by miraculous agency. I begin with a brief survey of the evidence for the use of holy oil, then turn to holy oil as a rhetorically constituted agent, that is, a substance whose affects and powers were articulated textually. With these distinctions as frame, the final portion of my essay will consider holy oil in its later Byzantine presentation as emblematic of Byzantine religion more broadly. What did holy oil do, how and why? And how were the senses essential to that work?

Habits of Piety: Fragrance and Oil

The religious use of fragrant oil was ubiquitous in early Byzantine culture, in continuity with ancient, pan-Mediterranean customs. A wide variety of bodily practices and social habits made such usage part of daily life. At base was the presupposition that scented oils or lotions were effective agents for hygiene and health practices. Aromatic products were used in the household to clean, disinfect, repair, and polish; to protect from bugs, rodents, mold, rot, or disease; and to adorn with fresh, sweet, healthy air. In medicine, scented oils soothed rashes, burns, or inflammation; cleaned and disinfected wounds or bites; restored dried, damaged skin; cleansed and healed internal organs. In all such uses, the olfactory component of the oil or lotion or ointment was as crucial an active agent as the viscosity of the substance containing it. Smell as well as tactile application was necessary for the substance to be effective.[1]

1 Important surveys are now available in M. Bradley, ed., *Smell and the Ancient Senses* (London, 2015); J. P. Toner, ed., *A Cultural History of the Senses in Antiquity* (London, 2014); B. Caseau, "Parfum et guérison dans le christianisme ancient et byzantin: Des

Religious uses of holy oil were rooted in these practical habits, acknowledging scented oil as a basic tool for producing and maintaining healthy life, whether in spaces, objects, or bodies. Once applied, its substance penetrated deep below surfaces or skin into interiors; its lingering fragrance provided indication of its efficacy. Ritual anointing for religious purposes carried cultural references to practical uses, actively marked by their sensory components.[2]

The Bible provided a further source for religious usage that bolstered cultural expectations, offering a rich array of memories regarding sacred perfumed ointments. Various terms—μύρον, ἔλαιον, χρῖσμα—were used for the unction that consecrated priests, kings, prophets, altars and temples; Christ himself was the Χριστός, God's chosen Anointed One.[3] In the New Testament, Jesus was anointed on his feet with perfumed ointment by the Sinful Woman in Luke 7:36–50; and on his head in Matthew 26:6–13, by a woman of Bethany in anticipation of his burial. In Mark 6:13 and James 5:14, oil was used to anoint the sick.[4] Such biblical passages lent the resonance of sacred narrative to Christian ritual use, providing analogy, typology, and explication for how and why perfumed ointment could be a sacramental agent.

In early Byzantine rites, holy oil was used to anoint the baptized, ritually reconcile heretics, anoint the sick, consecrate baptismal waters, and consecrate altars.[5] Its penetrating qualities and its lingering fragrance marked divine presence and participation. The Byzantines affirmed such presence—of God, of Christ, of the Holy Spirit—by citing Song of Songs 1:3, "And the smell of thine ointments [ὀσμὴ μύρων σου] is better than all spices [τὰ ἀρώματα]: thy name is ointment [μύρον] poured forth."[6] These biblical passages were widely familiar in Byzantine society, reflected in hymns, prayers, homilies, and hagiographies, as well as in ascetic or monastic literature and in intellectual culture. Their uses were dependent neither on literacy, per se, nor on liturgical context, but rather on familiar cultural habit. While different terms for holy oil continued to be used, myrrh and myron became the most common in Byzantine religious texts, often used interchangeably.[7]

Holy oil as a religious substance thus drew on a complex of inherited cultural associations, medicinal, hygienic, and biblical. Used liturgically, holy oil gained ritual definition as a sacred substance, and ritual agency as an efficacious one.[8] Plentiful in its mundane uses, fragrant oil

huiles parfumés des médicins au *myron* des saints byzantins," in *Les pères de l'église face à la science médicale de leur temps*, ed. V. Boudon-Millot and B. Pouderon (Paris, 2004), 141–91; M. Roch, *L'intelligence d'un sens: Odeurs miraculeuses et odorat dans l'Occident du haut Moyen Âge (Ve–VIIIe siècles* (Tournhout, 2009); S. A. Harvey, *Scenting Salvation: Ancient Christianity and the Olfactory Imagination* (Berkeley, 2006); D. A. Green, *The Aroma of Righteousness: Scent and Seduction in Rabbinic Life and Literature* (University Park, PA, 2011); C. Classen, D. Howes, and A. Synnott, *Aroma: The Cultural History of Smell* (New York, 1994), esp. 13–50. On the matters of materiality and touch, I am especially influenced by P. C. Miller, *The Corporeal Imagination: Signifying the Holy in Late Ancient Christianity* (Philadelphia, 2009); V. Marinis, "Piety, Barbarism, and the Senses in Byzantium," in *Sensational Religion: Sensory Cultures in Material Practice*, ed. S. M. Promey (New Haven, 2014), 321–40; C. W. Bynum, *Christian Materiality: An Essay on Religion in Late Medieval Europe* (New York, 2011).

2 For the ubiquity of oil as an ancient Mediterranean habit, in addition to the above bibliography, see S. Dalley, "Anointing in Ancient Mesopotamia," and A. Bowie, "Oil in Ancient Greece and Rome," both in *The Oil of Gladness: Anointing in the Christian Tradition*, ed. M. Dudley and G. Rowell (London, 1993), 19–25, 26–34, respectively.

3 J. R. Porter, "Oil in the Old Testament," in Dudley and Rowell, *Oil of Gladness*, 35–45.

4 J. John, "Oil in the New Testament," in Dudley and Rowell, *Oil of Gladness*, 46–76.

5 S. Parenti, "Anointing the Sick in the First Four Centuries," and idem, "Care and Anointing of the Sick in the East," both in *Handbook for Liturgical Studies: Sacraments and Sacramentals*, vol. 4, ed. A. Chupungco (Collegeville, MN, 2000), 155–60, 161–70, respectively; J. Halliburton, "Anointing in the Early Church," in Dudley and Rowell, *Oil of Gladness*, 77–91. See the entries in G. W. H. Lampe, *A Patristic Greek Lexicon* (Oxford, 1961): s.vv. ἔλαιον, μύρον, χρῖσις and χρῖσμα.

6 Song of Songs 1:3–4, trans. from *The Septuagint with Apocrypha: Greek and English*, L. C. L. Brenton (repr. Hendrickson 1986), 830.

7 Technically, the terms σμύρνα or μύρρα referred to the spice of myrrh, often used in funerary practices. In turn, μύρον had the base meaning of fragrant perfume. In early Christianity, myron was already used to refer to the substance miraculously exuded by martyrs' relics. It is not hard to see how the two became conflated, especially in the context of miraculous substances produced by relics, or later, by icons (for which, see below). For myron as the substance from relics, in addition to its other wide usage, see Lampe, *Patristic Greek Lexicon*, 889–90.

8 Fundamental here is C. Bell, *Ritual Theory, Ritual Practice* (Oxford, 1992). For the study of liturgy, a particularly useful collection is P. Bradshaw and J. Melloh, *Foundations in Ritual Studies: A Reader for Students of Christian Worship* (Grand Rapids, MI, 2007).

easily became abundant in its religious applications. Absolute consistency emerged neither in terminology, nor in sacramental elaborations.[9] Holy oils of different kinds, blessed by various means, proliferated throughout ancient Christianity.

The fourth century marked a distinct and broad "material turn" in the Mediterranean world, whereby the body and physical experience took on new, strikingly positive valuation in religious thought and practice. Materiality, sensation, and sensory awareness gained heightened attention as the physical realm was explored for its capacity to provide religious knowledge; and to display virtue and vice, or divine presence, negative or positive, in human bodily experience. The change was evident, for example, in the Neoplatonic practice of theurgy, or in the exuberant décor of Jewish synagogues and Rabbinic exegesis.[10] For Christians, this shift accompanied their legalization in the Roman Empire and subsequent rise in political, social, and economic power. Rather than perceiving a hostile physical world, Christians began to express and perform a piety that understood the world as revelatory of its Maker. Christian uses of holy oil demonstrated such a shift in clear terms.

Early Christian literature referenced the use of oil, ritually sanctified by prayer, for blessing, consecration, and healing. During the fourth century, a changed emphasis appears in textual references to holy oil, with specific attention to its fragrance or sweet scent. Earlier texts mentioned the importance of anointing as an action.[11] Now, for example, the catechetical homilies of Cyril of Jerusalem, John Chrysostom, Ambrose of Milan, and Theodore of Mopsuestia all discussed the significance of baptismal anointment as an olfactory event, one in which the smell was an important component of the ritual process.[12] Unbaptized catechumens were anointed with olive oil. But the newly baptized were immediately evident by the fragrance they exuded, now anointed with perfumed chrism.[13] In the sixth century, pseudo-Dionysios the Areopagite described a complicated rite of consecration for holy myron. His account is notable not only for its ritual detail but also for its scrupulous attention to the olfactory qualities, affect, and meanings of the perfumed ointment.[14]

In accordance with this material turn, during the early Byzantine era the presence and usage of holy oil in Christian piety multiplied exponentially. Fragrant oil poured forth in abundance from the tombs and relics of martyrs. Caskets for the holy dead contained holes, through which

9 R. Taft, "Unction," *ODB* 3:2142, insists on the importance of distinguishing different liturgical rites for holy oil one from another. Yet, as Parenti, "Anointing of the Sick," points out, third- and fourth-century sources are not clear in their distinctions, whether between charistmatic anointing from that which would now be considered sacramental (i.e., oil blessed by a holy man as opposed to that blessed by an ordained official); nor is it clear whether the same oil was used for different rites. The proliferation of ritual prescriptions not only in Greek and Latin, but also in Coptic, Syriac, Armenian, and other ancient Christian languages serves to demonstrate the impossibility of consistency or exclusivity in either terminology or liturgical practice. Parenti, "Anointing the Sick" and idem, "Care and Anointing," have good bibliographies for both primary and secondary sources.

10 This cultural shift has been treated at length, for example, in S. A. Harvey, "The Senses in Religion: Piety, Critique, Competition," in Toner, *Cultural History*, 91–114; Harvey, *Scenting Salvation*; Miller, *Corporeal Imagination*; and Green, *Aroma of Righteousness*. See also the important new work on sight by R. Neis, *The Sense of Sight in Rabbinic Culture: Jewish Ways of Seeing in Late Antiquity* (Cambridge, 2013).

11 Parenti, "Anointing the Sick"; Halliburton, "Anointing in the Early Church."

12 Cyril of Jerusalem, *Procatechesis* 1, *Mystagogical Lectures* 2.3, 3, 13, 14, ed. A. Piédagnel and P. Paris, *Cyrille de Jérusalem, Catéchèses mystagogiques*, SC 126 (Paris, 1966); Ambrose of Milan, *Sacraments*, 1, 2.4, ed. B. Botte, *Ambroise de Milan, Des Sacrements: Des Mystères, Explication du symbole*, SC 25 bis (Paris, 1994); Theodore of Mopsuestia, *Cat. Hom.* 13, 14, 15, ed. R. Tonneau and R. Devresse, *Les Homélies Catéchétiques de Théodore de Mopsueste*, Studi e Testi 145 (Città del Vaticano, 1949); John Chrysostom, *Baptismal Instructions*, 2, 4, 6, 10, for which see the commentary and discussion in P. W. Harkins, *John Chrysostom, Baptismal Instructions*, Ancient Christian Writers 31 (New York, 1963). For detailed discussion of these sources, see below, nn. 13, 16.

13 E. Yarnold, *The Awe-Inspiring Rites of Initiation: The Origins of the* RCIA, 2nd ed. (Collegeville, MN, 1994), provides an excellent overview of these sources and relevant scholarship. Harvey, *Scenting Salvation*, 65–83, discusses the shift in attention to sensory elements in detail. S. P. Brock, "Anointing in the Syriac Tradition," in Dudley and Rowell, *Oil of Gladness*, 92–100, points out the lack of consistency in terminology and practice. The differences between Syriac tradition and the Greek and Latin sources are notable. See, e.g., S. P. Brock, *The Holy Spirit in the Syrian Baptismal Tradition*, Syrian Churches Series 9, 2nd ed. (Poona, 1998); B. Varghese, *Les onctions baptismales dans la tradition syrienne,* CSCO 512, Subs. 82 (Louvain, 1989).

14 Pseudo-Dionysios, *Ecclesiastical Hierarchy*, 2.4, trans. C. Luibheid, *Pseudo-Dionysius: The Complete Works* (New York, 1987), 224–32. See Harvey, *Scenting Salvation*, 136–41.

oil was poured and collected, rendered powerful as an agent of blessing or healing by its tactile encounter with sacred bones.[15] In the late fourth century, John Chrysostom admonished his congregation in Antioch to visit the tombs of the martyrs. There they should grip the coffin, reverence the bones, and lavishly anoint themselves with the oil:

> Embrace the coffin, nail yourself to the chest. Not just the martyrs' bones, but even their tombs and chests brim with a great deal of blessing. Take holy oil and anoint your whole body—your tongue, your lips, your neck, your eyes—and you'll never fall into the shipwreck of drunkenness. For through its pleasant smell the oil reminds you of the martyrs' contests, and bridles and restrains all wantonness in considerable patience, and overcomes the diseases of the soul.[16]

In Chrysostom's rendering, the oil *as substance* physically linked the body of the martyr to the body of the faithful, at the same time physically linking sacred place (the holy tomb) to worldly space (one's ordinary life), and holy power to mundane bodies. But its efficacy lay further in the lingering effects of its fragrance. Carrying its scent on the skin, absorbed into one's body, or in small containers (*enkolpia*), the faithful Christian carried a constant reminder of the martyr as exemplar of virtue. The fragrance worked to discipline body and thoughts, guiding the Christian to virtuous conduct. Myron, then, provided means and method for Christian self-awareness, the fashioning of Christian subjectivity. It was an agent for moral formation and moral psychology, accompanying the Christian on a daily basis.

In jars and flasks, Christians collected blessed fragrant oil from churches or shrines, from priests or holy men or women. Ampullae for the oil were imprinted with images of the saint or the place from which it came. Of the numerous surviving examples, images such as St. Menas or St. Thecla or the church of the Anastasis in Jerusalem are common. These containers were made of clay, glass, or metal, elaborately or simply decorated. They could be small enough to wear on the body, whether for blessing or protection or simply in devotion.[17] The incised image of the saint or shrine designated the holy source of the oil. That source was specific, locatable, and emplaced.[18] At the same time, the holy power of the saint or site was transferable by means of the blessed substance carried in the container. Its fragrance accompanied the bearer in the terms Chrysostom had exhorted, as a continual presence and reminder.

Holy oil was characterized by its abundance: one did not need to be wealthy or powerful to receive it or its benefits. Religious and governmental authorities used myron to mark religious festivals or political ceremonies or civic celebrations; the faithful took it home for anointing their households, fields, the sick, the distressed, or the hopeful.[19] Oil was mixed with dust, pebbles, or bones to make a fragrant and potent balm, carried in amulets, enkolpia, or personal reliquaries such as pectoral crosses that could be worn or privately venerated.[20] In Syriac such balm was called *hnanā*, blessed and offered by the likes of Symeon the Stylite to service the needs of the faithful.[21]

15 D. Krueger, "The Religion of Relics in Late Antiquity and Byzantium," in *Treasure of Heaven: Saints, Relics and Devotion in Medieval Europe*, ed. M. Bagnoli, H. A. Klein, C. G. Mann, and J. Robinson (Baltimore, 2010), 5–18; Harvey, *Scenting Salvation*, 90, 272 n. 184.

16 John Chrysostom, *Homily on the Martyrs*, trans. W. Mayer and P. Allen, *John Chrysostom* (New York, 2000), 93–97 at 96.

17 G. Frank, "From Antioch to Arles: Lay Devotion in Context," in *Cambridge History of Christianity*, vol. 2, *Constantine to 600*, ed. A. Casiday and F. Norris (Cambridge, 2007), 531–47; G. Vikan, *Early Byzantine Pilgrimage Art*, rev. ed. (Washington, DC, 2010); B. V. Pentcheva, *The Sensual Icon: Space, Ritual, and the Senses in Byzantium* (University Park, PA, 2010), 17–44. For the analogous collection of sacred dirt, see also M. Duncan-Flowers, "A Pilgrim's Ampulla from the Shrine of St. John the evangelist at Ephesus," in *The Blessings of Pilgrimage*, ed. R. Ousterhout (Urbana and Chicago, 1990), 125–39.

18 For the Holy Land, see now J.-P. Sodini, "La terre des semelles: Images pieuses ramenées par les pèlerins des Lieux saints [Terre sainte, Martyria d'Orient]," *Journal des Savants* (January–June 2011): 77–140.

19 Caseau, "Parfum et guérison" (n. 1 above); Harvey, *Scenting Salvation*, 83–90.

20 B. Pitarakis, "Objects of Devotion and Protection," in *A People's History of Christianity*, ed. D. Janz, vol. 3: *Byzantine Christianity*, ed. D. Krueger (Minneapolis, 2006), 164–81.

21 For *hnanā* see, e.g., *The Syriac Life of Simeon the Stylite*, trans. R. Doran in *The Lives of Simeon Stylites* (Kalamazoo,

As in John Chrysostom's admonition, holy oil linked places, spaces, and persons, across worldly and divine domains, by means of fragrant materiality. Its efficacy, for the Byzantines, lay in its use as a tactile, concrete channel by which the divine was active and present in human life.

Hence the line between holy oil as a product humanly produced and one divinely generated was easily crossed. Ritual provided means to make oil "special": myron or chrism was oil consecrated by priests or other holy figures.[22] That is, it was ritually marked by ritual agents in a ritual process that activated potency.[23] But for the Byzantines, such a ritual process was ultimately a conduit for divine activity. It signified divine action that might be otherwise available through divine initiative. By the middle Byzantine period, holy unction had acquired precise canonical instructions regarding composition, preparation, and dispensing.[24] Such specificity lent weight to broader uses. The ritual efficacy of fragrant oil, whether sacramentally blessed or blessed by virtue of its source or use, engaged the ritual authority of formally consecrated oil.

But already in the sixth century, one need not pour oil over the bones of martyrs or saints to produce sanctified fragrant substance. Instead, sweet-scented oil streamed from the bodies and relics of saints. Thus John Klimakos described the burial of the monk Menas, who had lived fifty-nine years at the monastery of St. Catherine on Mt. Sinai:

> Three days after the death of this saintly monk, when we had finished with the customary rites, the place where he lay was suddenly filled with a great fragrance. We were allowed by the superior to open the coffin in which he lay, and when this was done we had a sight of what seemed like two streams of myrrh flowing from his venerable feet. The teacher said to all of us: "Look, the sweat of his labors has been offered up as myrrh to God, and has been truly accepted."[25]

The sanctity of the monk was marked by olfactory transformation.[26] Mortal smells had defined the monk, both alive and dead: the sweat of his earthly labors and the odor of his decay as a corpse. These now changed into the intense fragrance of holiness, the odor of sanctity. Scent announced the transformation and heralded its meaning. Opening the coffin, the monks saw this transformation in substance: scented moisture that poured forth abundantly from the dead man's body. This was the myrrh, the holy myron, of divine grace.

Holy oil was substance. One could see it, touch it, carry it, and clearly smell it. Its sweet fragrance denoted its divine source, or the participation of the divine in its function; its abundance evidenced God's abundant mercy. People expected it and received it in just such terms. In the sixth-century *Life of St. Matrona*, the saint found herself in the eastern Empire when the head of John the Baptist was discovered. Bishops, clergy, laity, and monastics flooded to assemble a liturgical procession to bring the head into the church. The relic and its significance were indisputably evidenced by a sudden flood of myron:

> As proof to the assembled throng and confirmation of the discovery, fragrant oil gushed forth from <the head>, and all were drawing it off for themselves as a blessing. [Matrona] also came forward to draw off <the fragrant oil>; and having drawn it, she became distributor thereof, involuntarily. For the throng would not cede her an exit: cut off in their midst she was forced to distribute to all

1992), 123, 124, 141, 142; John of Ephesus, *Lives of the Eastern Saints*, ch. 4, trans. E. W. Brooks, PO 17 (Paris, 1923), 64–67.

22 See, e.g., E. Lanne, "La benediction de l'huile," and G. Wagner, "La consecration du myron," both in *Les bénéditions et les sacramentaux dans la liturgie conferences Saint-Serge XXXIVe Semaine d'Études Liturgiques Paris, 23–26 juin 1987*, ed. A. M. Triacca and A. Pistoia (Rome, 1988), 165–80, 285–94, respectively.

23 Bell, *Ritual Theory, Ritual Practice* (n. 8 above), 197–223; J. Z. Smith, "The Domestication of Sacrifice," reprinted in *Relating Religion: Essays in the Study of Religion* (Chicago, 2004), 145–59.

24 *ODB* 1:107 "Anointing" (M. McCormack), 3:2142 "Unction" (R. Taft).

25 John Klimakos, *The Ladder of Divine Ascent*, "Step Four: On Obedience," trans. C. Luibheid and N. Russell (New York, 1982), at p. 102.

26 On the literary tradition of olfaction for marking transformation, see M. Teló, "Aristophanes, Cratinus and the Smell of Comedy," in *Synaethesia and the Ancient Senses*, ed. S. Butler and A. Purves (Durham, 2013), 53–69.

of them as they all cried out to her: "Dispense to all, O servant of Christ!"[27]

In the *Life of Theodore of Sykeon*, it was not relics but icons that shed forth fragrant moisture—termed dew or myrrh in the text.[28] Himself one who encountered miraculous myrrh, Theodore in turn cured and healed others by the generous use of sweet-scented holy oil.[29]

In post-Iconoclastic Byzantium, myron became a hallmark of Byzantine faith, streaming miraculously and generously from relics and icons alike.[30] Its appearance was notable for an array of saints. St. Demetrios and St. Theodora in Thessalonike, St. Nicholas at Myra, St. Mary the Younger at Vizye, and St. Nikon of Sparta all had shrines to which the faithful flocked to receive the precious and fragrant substance that flowed from their bodies and places of burial.[31] In the thirteenth century, John Staurakios, an administrator of the church in Thessalonike, described the scene at the shrine of St. Demetrios, where an elaborate system of piping supplied myron to pilgrims and devotees: "Men, women, and children extract the myron with their hands and straws and anoint their eyes, mouths, and ears with it along with their chests and their entire bodies. . . . All ages and nations are endlessly being anointed with the myron of the martyr and, in particular, women ceaselessly anoint their eyes and chest, and their breasts and arms."[32]

Holy oil—abundant, fragrant, and potent—poured through the devotional lives of Byzantine Christians. We know this from the copious material evidence that indicates its prevalence in religious uses personal and collective, and from numerous textual references to its use.[33] Textual references are sometimes descriptive, sometimes imaginative, and sometimes prescriptive. But they are invariably interpretive. If, for the Byzantines, holy oil was a substance to smell and touch, for the historian it is a material significantly discursive in constitution.

Habits of Rhetoric

Without question, when it comes to the senses, the historian must rely heavily on texts. Material evidence tells us a great deal about practices, including indications of prevalence, varieties of provenance, availability of participation, and material markers of signification. But how to understand "what the Byzantines thought" depends in large degree on access to their own words. Scholarship on the senses has been significantly shaped and enriched by anthropologists who have instructed us on the variability of culturally constructed meanings.[34] Still, texts

27 "The Life of St. Matrona of Perge," sec. 12, trans. J. Featherstone and C. Mango, in *Holy Women of Byzantium: Ten Saints' Lives in English Translation*, ed. A.-M. Talbot (Washington, DC, 1996), 13–64, at 31 (square brackets mark my insertions; angeled, Featherstone and Mango's). Compare sec. 38, at p. 53: "[the feast of St. Lawrence] is a great one and is celebrated gloriously, fragrant oil from his holy relics being distributed on this day to the honor and glory of his martyrdom."

28 *The Life of St. Theodore Sykeon* 108, trans. E. Dawes and N. H. Baynes, *Three Byzantine Saints* (Oxford, 1977), 87–192, at 160; ch. 8, p. 91 for the icon of Christ shedding drops of dew.

29 *The Life of St. Theodore Sykeon* 81, 85, 87–88, 102, 112 (trans. pp. 144, 147, 147–48, 156, 161).

30 This is a mode of piety still vibrant among Orthodox Christians today. Icons purported to weep fragrant tears or to exude fragrant dew or myrrh have drawn huge crowds at Orthodox churches in North America in recent years. These are not necessarily old icons, but include some recently made, including prints. A myrrh-streaming icon from Hawaii was officially recognized by the Russian Orthodox Church in 2008, and has toured North American parishes extensively: http://www.orthodoxhawaii.org/icons.html (accessed 15 November 2016). St. Nicholas Albanian Orthodox Church and St. George Antiochian Orthodox Church, both in Chicago, IL, have received much popular attention in recent years for icons weeping fragrant tears, again with official, episcopal recognition. See, for example, http://www.antiochian.org/Orthodox_Church_Who_What_Where_Why/Why_Do_Icons_Weep.htm. (Both websites accessed 2 October 2015.)

31 C. Bakirtzis, "Pilgrimage to Thessalonike: The Tomb of St. Demetrios," *DOP* 56 (2002): 175–72; J. Skedros, *Saint Demetrios of Thessaloniki: Civic Patron and Divine Protector 4th–7th Centuries, CE* (Harrisburg, 1999); B. Pitarakis, "New Evidence on Lead Flasks and Devotional Patterns: From Crusader Jerusalem to Byzantium," in *Byzantine Religious Culture: Studies in Honor of Alice-Mary Talbot*, ed. D. Sullivan, E. Fisher, and E. Papaioannou (Leiden, 2012), 239–59.

32 Cited in J. Skedros, "Shrines, Festivals, and the 'Undistinguished Mob,'" in Krueger, *Byzantine Christianity* (n. 20 above), 81–102, at 94.

33 See Krueger, *Byzantine Christianity*, especially: Skedros, "Shrines"; S. E. J. Gerstel, "Layperson in Church," 103–23; N. Constas, "Death and Dying in Byzantium," 124–45; C. Barber, "Icons, Prayer, and Vision in the Eleventh Century," 149–63; Pitarakis, "Objects of Devotion and Protection"; A.-M. Talbot "Devotional Life of Laywomen," 201–20. The volume contains much useful information for the study of the senses.

34 The problem is vexed—see the previous chapter, by F. Rojas and V. Sergueenkova. The issue has been pressed perhaps most

provide crucial access to how people understood their own practices, and what made cultural meanings distinct from physiological processes. Much of what historians are trying to grasp through work on the senses, ironically, relies on what texts have to say. In order to assess the citations I have already quoted, for example, we must consider senses as textually constituted; or, sensory rhetoric as a discursive strategy.

About words in texts, we must ask: *when* are sensory details mentioned, and *why*? These are rhetorical choices, strategies of an author or editor. Sensory details are important in particular places and not others; they serve rhetorical functions. Sensory details often carry valuation because they point to practices (myron, incense); the sensory experience they reference is one that carries significance of association within a given culture, and for the Byzantines, within their given religious culture(s).

But the ubiquity of bodily sensations in daily life necessitates a certain textual *inattention* to sensory awareness. Quite often, the absence of sensory detail is simply because the sensory elements of the account were taken for granted, so that the writer thought them unnecessary to point out. It is a *rhetorical* move to draw attention to sensations. They are highlighted for a purpose, each time. Those purposes point to shared assumptions, shared valuation, shared contexts: of culture, society, and religion. When Byzantine authors discuss holy oil with reference to its texture and scent, then, we must ask what is being articulated, and why.

Consider, again, the case of Theodore of Sykeon. In the seventh-century *Life of Theodore of Sykeon*, the saint provides blessed oil to anoint the sick or afflicted, all of whom are subsequently healed.[35] Holy oil in this text is presented as an instrumental substance, the usage of which would be habitual and familiar to the reader. Anointment with oil blessed by a holy ascetic was a practice Byzantines knew well as a standard therapy for cures. The scent of the oil is not mentioned in these passages, which instead speak of the oil as the substance used therapeutically, with anointing as the method. These passages are textually framed by the saint's own encounters with miraculous ointment. At the age of twelve, suffering from bubonic plague, Theodore was cured by "drops of dew" that dripped from an icon of Christ.[36] Later, during his ascetic career, amid the numerous healings he performed, many with oil, the following is recounted:

> Then [Theodore] entered the venerable church of the all-holy Virgin Mary, the Mother of God, where the God-given myrrh flows, and stretched out his arms, and standing thus in the shape of a cross, he prayed and steadfastly gazed at the miraculous "Icon of the myrrh" opposite him. By divine working, the myrrh gathered into a bubble and then rained down plentifully upon his eyes and anointed his whole face so that all who saw witnessed this divine testimony said, "Verily he is a worthy servant of God."[37]

In the case of this hagiography, Theodore's capacity to generate divine agency in the oil he blessed for his suppliants was demonstration of his own sanctity. To underscore the point, the author provides this additional account of the saint himself as one miraculously and generously anointed with myron. The literary account is tightly framed with ritual indicators: the event takes place in a church; the saint takes up the stance of cruciform prayer directly facing the icon. Within the designated authority of ecclesiastical space, in ritual stance (the shape of the cross) and ritual act (prayer), directly facing the ritual presence of Mary in the icon, the saint provokes a potent indicator of divine approval and divine mercy. Myron bubbles up and rains down upon Theodore. The word itself—myron or myrrh—requires an intrinsic quality of fragrance. Yet the

creatively by Y. Hamilakis, *Archaeology and the Senses: Human Experience, Memory, and Affect* (Cambridge, 2013), for which see also the review by F. Rojas, *AJA Online* 119, no. 4 (2015): http://www.ajaonline.org/online-review-book/2503 (accessed 25 August 2016). See, among others, the theoretical and methodological challenges posed in M. Jenner, "Follow Your Nose? Smell, Smelling and Their Histories," *American Historical Review* 116 (2011): 335–51; or, from the anthropological side by D. Howes, ed., *Empire of the Senses: The Sensual Culture Reader* (Oxford, 2005); idem, *Sensual Relations: Engaging the Senses in Culture and Social* Theory (Ann Arbor, 2003).

35 *The Life of St. Theodore Sykeon* 81, 85, 87, 88, 102, 112.

36 *The Life of St. Theodore Sykeon* 8 (p. 91).

37 *The Life of St. Theodore Sykeon* 108 (p. 160).

text in no way emphasizes the olfactory dimensions of the episode. Instead, the account evokes divine agency known through materiality and visual witness. The myron as substance is abundant, enough to anoint Theodore's face "plentifully." It provides measure of the saint's capacity to work miracles among the faithful in God's stead. The author does not need to emphasize olfaction. Its presence pervades the account.

Holy oil in the *Life of Theodore of Sykeon* provided the author an effective image because it indexed a common set of cultural significations. Byzantine authors participated in an inherited, deeply embedded cultural rhetoric of the senses that marked the pan-Mediterranean world long before and long after Byzantium's own expressions of it.[38] Consider another example of holy oil, from the sixth-century *Life of Daniel the Stylite*. One day the saint's power caused a demon to leave a possessed boy. "As the demon came out, he created such a stench that all the crowds present could not endure the stench and had to cover their noses." The boy lay unconscious on the ground, his father beating his breast in agony. Daniel called for the boy to be given holy oil to drink. "And as the boy drank, vomiting came upon him and he brought up black clotted blood." At once the boy stood up, healed and healthy.[39]

Here again, holy oil effects the cure. But the smells emphasized by the author are not those of the oil. Rather, the text lingers on the stench of the demon and the unpleasant therapeutic indicators of vomit and black blood, details which carry intrinsically visceral olfactory associations. These details rhetorically evoke emotions of disgust and horror. They serve to intensify the terrifying nature of the episode, casting it as a literal encounter between death and life. Here, as in the *Life of Theodore of Sykeon*, smells are an assumed aspect of the event; they are part of what makes the literary portrayal effective for the reader. Yet, they need not have been elaborated for the reader to understand their presence and role in the event recounted. The fragrance of the holy oil was not highlighted, but rather evoked by the contrasting stench of demon, vomit, and blood in the story. In Theodore of Sykeon, the saint is miraculously anointed with myrrh and becomes himself a source of healing. In Daniel the Stylite, the foulness of demons and death provide the measure of the holy oil's contrasting power of life.

For the Byzantines, as for other Mediterranean peoples, sensory rhetoric drew on cultural codes that used binaries to mark cosmic order. Sweet fragrance indicated health, well-being, saints, miracles, and divine presence; stench marked illness, decay, demons, heretics, Satan, and death. Invisible, immaterial, but concretely sensed, smells crossed and delineated visible and invisible terrains, as human and divine domains intersected and permeated one another.[40]

Materiality itself could mark the same binary: substance could indicate potent, life-giving strength, or the wasting decay of mortality. What oil or ointment provided for myron or chrism was a substance through which olfactory agency worked. Divine presence was encountered through the fragrance of holy oil; divine power was active through its application. Sacred oil—whether humanly made and consecrated (in *Daniel the Stylite*), or divinely generated (*Theodore of Sykeon*)—was a singularly effective channel between divine and human actors. For the Byzantines, the interplay between divine and human domains was rendered concrete in holy oil as a fragrant substance of immense potency. Their awareness of its power was cultivated through practices that regularly employed scented holy oil, and through rhetoric that continually engaged its efficacy.

Not surprisingly, smell and oil could be combined in binary opposition to myron. The

38 Harvey, *Scenting Salvation*; Classen, Howes, and Synnot, *Aroma* (n. 1 above); Toner, *Cultural History* (n. 1 above); R. G. Newhauser, *A Cultural History of the Senses in the Middle Ages* (London, 2014); A. Zohar and E. Lev, "Trends in the Use of Perfumes and Incense in the Near East after the Muslim Conquest," in *Perfumery and Ritual in Asia*, ed. D. Jung, special issue of *Journal of the Royal Asiatic Society* 23, no. 1 (2013): 11–30; B. Grami, "Perfumery Plant Materials as Reflected in Early Persian Poetry," in ibid., 39–52; T. L. Hedrick and N. Ergin, "A Shared Culture of Heavenly Fragrance: A Comparison of Late Byzantine and Ottoman Incense Burners and Censing Practices in Religious Contexts," *DOP* 69 (2016): 331–54; N. Ergin, "The Fragrance of the Divine: Ottoman Incense Burners in Context," *ArtB* 96, no. 1 (2014); A. al-Azmeh, "A Rhetoric for the Senses: A Consideration of Muslim Paradise Narratives," *Journal of Arabic Literature* 26 (1995): 215–31.

39 *The Life of St. Daniel the Stylite* 33, trans. Dawes and Baynes, *Three Byzantine Saints*, 7–84, at 26.

40 Harvey, *Scenting Salvation*, 11–56.

tenth-century hagiographical novel *The Life of Andrew the Fool* included a story of the magician Vigrinos, who nearly brought the destruction of a pious wife when she employed his services to correct the behavior of her unfaithful husband.[41] In the account, Vigrinos worked his sorcery with a ritual involving oil and an oil lamp set before the household icons. His magic worked, but the woman began to suffer heinous nightmares. In dreams and subsequently in consultation with the saint, Vigrinos was revealed for his true identity. The oil in his lamp was urine, the icons were anointed with excrement; his ritual was the nefarious inversion of holy sacrament.[42] The logic of the story requires its foil in the notion of fragrant holy oil, effective, powerful, and life-giving: a fragrant substance starkly absent from this episode.

Binaries provide order; they work to sustain systems of virtue and vice. But their simplicity as classifications limits their usefulness in the face of the messiness of life. Indeed, Mediterranean cultures complicated and destabilized sensory binaries by their most basic habits of practice: medicine and hygiene. In these contexts, unpleasant substances like sulphur, urine, or dung were often utilized as potent cleansing or healing agents.[43] These malodorous materials had a bodily counterpart in the holy ascetic, whose self-mortifications yielded a body that displayed the inversion of basic sensory cultural codes. Symeon the Stylite stank from the gangrenous wound on his thigh so badly that his own disciples could not bear to approach him without incense and covered noses.[44] After two years buried in a cave, Theodore of Sykeon came out "covered in sores and pus, his hair [matted with] an indescribable number of worms lodged in it; his bones were all but through the flesh and the stench was such that no one could stand near him."[45] These two, like other saints, embodied mortality at its most gruesome manifestation. Yet they were repeatedly effective and generous sources of healing for the sick, of food and water in times of famine or drought, of abundant crops, and of social justice, comfort, and mercy.[46] Their malodorous ascetic practices yielded life-giving results for the larger community.

Similar descriptions characterized the portrayal of the raising of Lazarus in Byzantine homilies and hymns. His disintegrating, worm-infested, stinking corpse grew fragrant, vibrant, and whole as Jesus summoned him forth from the dead.[47] For the Byzantine liturgical calendar, the raising of Lazarus was the start of Holy Week, the celebration of Christ's own passion and resurrection. The Raising of Lazarus was the type, the Resurrection of Christ its cosmic fulfillment of a promise now offered to all mortal beings. Olfactorily dense materiality supplied the imagery celebrated in liturgical splendor.

Sensory rhetoric invariably elicited emotion and heightened affect. It did so by tying emotion to physical experience. Such rhetoric could be an effective strategy for moral formation and moral coding. As in the accounts of Daniel the Stylite healing the possessed youth or Vigrinos the magician, negative sensory rhetoric inherently reinforced the power of its binary opposite. In the descriptions of Symeon the Stylite's gangrene or Theodore of Sykeon's putridity, or

41 The episode is quoted at length and discussed in G. Calofonos, "The Magician Vigrinos and His Victim: A Case of Magic from the *Life of St. Andrew the Fool*," in *Greek Magic: Ancient, Medieval and Modern*, ed. J. C. B. Petropoulos (London, 2008), 64–71.

42 An excellent consideration of this episode in terms of materiality is offered in Marinis, "Piety" (n. 1 above).

43 Toner, *Cultural History* (n. 1 above); Newhauser, *Cultural History* (n. 38 above).

44 Symeon's battle with gangrene was reported in all three of his hagiographies: Theodoret of Cyrrhus, *History of the Monks of Syria*, ch. 26.23; Antonios's Life, sec. 17; and the anonymous Syriac Life, secc. 48–53. All are conveniently collected in Doran, *Lives of Simeon Stylites* (n. 21 above).

45 *The Life of St. Theodore of Sykeon* 20 (trans. p. 101, adapted).

46 On holy stench, see Harvey, *Scenting Salvation* (n. 1 above), 201–21. Mark Bradley, "Foul Bodies in Ancient Rome," in Bradley, ed., *Smell and the Ancient Senses* (n. 1 above), 133–45, discusses foul and fetid bodies with respect to order and matter out of place. On the connection between extreme asceticism and social justice, also S. A. Harvey, "Foreword," in Doran, *Lives of Simeon Stylites*, 7–12.

47 E.g., M. Cunningham, "Basil of Seleucia's Homily on Lazarus: A New Edition (BHG 2225)," *AB* 102, nos. 1–2 (1986): 161–84; Romanos the Melodist, "On the Raising of Lazarus I," "On the Raising of Lazarus II," trans. M. Carpenter, *Kontakia of Romanos, Byzantine Melodist*, vol. 1, *On the Person of Christ* (Columbia, MO, 1970), 137–56. In Byzantine iconography, the scene is often depicted with bystanders covering their noses. See, for example, discussion of the scene in M. Acheimastou-Potanianou, ed., *Holy Image, Holy Space: Icons and Frescoes from Greece* (Athens, 1988), 195 for pl. 33.

in recounting the raising of Lazarus, sensory rhetoric shook people out of complacency; it heightened the saint as an agent of power over mortality, suffering, and death. Rhetorics of disgust invariably carry moral valence.[48] Olfaction and tactility in such literary passages contributed to the larger sensorium in which fragrant holy oil participated. Sensory rhetoric of various kinds strengthened the discursive construction of fragrant holy oil as a vibrant instrument in Byzantine culture.

Oil at Work

For the Byzantines, holy oil was about relationality. Through substance and fragrance, it physically established direct relation between human and divine domains, between sacred and mundane locations, between persons holy or ordinary. I turn now to two texts that rely on the use and imagery of holy oil in particularly instructive ways: the historically grounded late ninth-century *Life of St. Theodora of Thessalonike*, and the tenth-century hagiographical novel *The Life of St. Basil the Younger*. Important in each case is a significant awareness of the interplay between practice and rhetoric in passages involving holy oil.

In *The Life of St. Theodora of Thessalonike*, fragrant substances began to appear after the saint's death, as soon as Theodora's body was laid in state by her fellow nuns.[49]

> Thus the blessed Theodora was laid out for burial, with her face full of wrinkles because of old age; but suddenly her face appeared to be shining, so that those who were watching closely thought, on account of its beauty, that it was emitting rays. And there also appeared on her face beads of perspiration, which emitted a divine sweet fragrance, and her venerable and angelic face was seen to smile. So much grace of such a sort did the divine power instill in her body.[50]

Nine days later, amid an air of miraculous healings already begun, the lamp hanging above Theodora's tomb began to burn brilliantly despite its oil having run low. Suddenly, the lamp began to gush forth streams of oil, overflowing noiselessly but copiously.

> And they all witnessed that astonishing and great miracle, how the sweet-scented oil flowed in streams from the lamp onto the earth, and anointing themselves with it in faith they returned home glorifying and praising God. And they were forced to place a vessel beneath the lamp to catch the overflowing oil.
>
> And from that moment until now <the lamp> has kept burning and never runs out <of oil>. And sometimes it gushes forth oil abundantly and overflows onto the ground, <as if> issued from an unseen vein, or rather from divine blessing. And may it never run out <of oil>. . . . so that her oil may proclaim with wordless voice her compassion for those who suffer.[51]

Nuns and townspeople, rich and poor, began to flock to the tomb, anointing themselves and others with her oil. Sick and demon-possessed were healed. Soon, an icon was painted of Theodora. Hanging in the tomb, it, too, began to stream with myrrh in such quantities that a lead receptacle was set up to catch the fragrant oil and distribute it to the suppliants who came, for anointing or drinking or carrying to others who could not come in person. Whether from lamp or icon, Theodora's myron healed and soothed, gaining great reputation.[52]

In a subsequent account of the translation of her relics by a certain cleric named Gregory, miraculous myron increased. When the nuns

48 W. I. Miller, *The Anatomy of Disgust* (Cambridge, MA, 1997); R. A. Kaster, *Emotion, Restraint, and Community in Ancient Rome* (Oxford, 2005), 104–33.

49 Trans. Alice-Mary Talbot, in eadem, *Holy Women of Byzantium* (n. 27 above), 159–237. It seems that this cult competed with the better-known cult of St. Demetrios, also in Thessalonike and also expressed with an elaborate cult of miraculous holy oil. But there is no direct evidence for how people understood the close proximity of the two cult shrines. See the discussions in ibid., 202 n. 217; 215 n. 271. Explicit evidence for miraculous holy oil at the shrine of St. Demetrios may in fact have been considerably later, in the twelfth century: see C. Bakirtzis, "Byzantine Ampullae from Thessaloniki," in Ousterhout, *Blessings of Pilgrimage* (n. 17 above), 140–50.

50 *The Life of St. Theodora of Thessalonike* 43 (p. 201).

51 *The Life of St. Theodora of Thessalonike* 47–48 (p. 205).

52 *The Life of St. Theodora of Thessalonike* 48–61.

prepared Theodora's body to move it to a new grave, her relics also began to issue sweet-smelling myrrh through a small hole in her casket. The fragrance was so strong that it awakened neighbors as the body was being moved. Theodora's oil was now thrice-holy:

> That same day fragrant oil began to pour forth in streams from the aforementioned hole in the sarcophagus, in every way indistinguishable from and similar to the <oil> from the lamp and the icon; and it flooded the entire floor of the church. And God has granted that up to this day it gushes forth on each occasion through the intercessions of the blessed <Theodora> to heal us in body and soul.[53]

And thus the healings continued, with myron abundantly pouring from lamp, icon, and the saint's own body. Throughout the account and the subsequent narrative of the translation, the author highlights the sweet fragrance of the oil or myrrh, repeatedly citing the fragrance itself as an agent working separately and in tandem with the myron. Fragrance announced the oil's appearance, adorned its quantities, summoned people from afar, and marked the healings as the oil was ingested or anointed. The fragrance was underscored further by episodes in which the myron was used for particularly foul illnesses. A young man long possessed by a grievous demon was brought to the shrine and repeatedly anointed with the lamp oil, while his mother shouted Theodora's name. Finally, one of the nuns had a vision of Theodora cleaning excrement from the man's mouth with her right finger. Sure enough, his healing quickly followed.[54] Later, a smallpox epidemic afflicted the region. The cleric Gregory presents agonized descriptions of the illness, its "unspeakable putrefaction," its stinking pustules "exud[ing] streams of purulent serious discharge," the "foul stench" of the sick, and the anguish of all. Here the healings were long and painful. Yet the sweet smelling oil from the Theodora's shrine did its work, pitting fragrance against stench, soothing oil against ruptured sores, and ultimately, life against death.[55]

The *Life of St. Theodora of Thessalonike* is notable for its emphasis on a local cult, with active involvement by Theodora's family members, the nuns of her convent, local clergy, and townspeople, as the cult focused on her body and tomb gained traction. The accounts are rife with local attestations, stories, dreams, and associations. The chapters focused on the cult are awash not only with reports of the copious myron that gushed from lamp, icon, and relics; but further, of piety enacted through practices that engaged the myron. People drank, anointed, collected, carried, venerated, told, and heard about the fragrant oils from her tomb. Miracles took place at the tomb, in the town, or in nearby households. Domestic spaces are as frequently cited as scenes for the miracles as the tomb itself. Neither the town or city as a civic space, nor a church or cathedral as an ecclesiastical one, feature strongly in this extensive text. Theodora becomes a people's saint, her fragrant oil abundantly and freely available to all, without political, clerical, or monetary mediation.

The pragmatic (albeit wondrous) narrative provided about the myrrh-streaming relics and objects of Theodora's cult has a counterpart in the elaborately constructed mid-tenth-century *Life of St. Basil the Younger*.[56] In this hagiographic confection, sensory practices and imagery both human and divine adorn the text at every turn. Physical and moral conditions are described with detailed sensory rhetoric, heavily freighted with moralistic overtones and a fearsome apocalypticism. The narrative is presented through different voices: Gregory the principal narrator, Basil himself, a devoted woman named Theodora, and a variety of heavenly and demonic figures. Locations lurch between ordinary life at home, and vast, incredible journeys through purgatory, heaven, and hell. Both the saint's heavenly abode and God's paradise are described

53 Gregory the Cleric, *Narrative about the Translation of the Venerable Relics of Our Blessed Mother Theodora* 9, in Talbot, *Holy Women*, 218–37, at 225. (This narrative is directly appended to the "Life of St. Theodora of Thessalonike" in Talbot, *Holy Women*, as in the manuscript.)

54 *The Life of St. Theodora of Thessalonike* 51 (pp. 208–9).

55 Gregory the Cleric, *Narrative of the Translation* 16–18 (pp. 231–34).

56 *The Life of Saint Basil the Younger*, trans. D. F. Sullivan, A.-M. Talbot, and S. McGrath, DOS 45 (Washington, DC, 2014).

at length, as are the torments of the damned; celestial liturgy, above all, is celebrated in splendid terms. Life and afterlife interflow. Fitting to such a literary production, sensory descriptions are constant, thick, and densely wrought.

In this extravagant text, olfaction is often engaged, both in this life and in the next. On earth, perfumed holy oils attend devotional practices;[57] in heaven, fragrant oil called "the oil of mercy" is stored in a vast spread of jars, counted and kept for use as God commands, whether to cleanse and purify the repentant or to reward the pious.[58] Sickness, heresy, and sin alike are presented with olfactory and visual indicators that befoul the reader's mind with scenes of stinking, repulsive filth. In turn, Basil's miracles, or the heavenly abodes of the saved, or God's enthroned glory, are all articulated with imagery of sweet scents, wondrous flowers, breathtaking perfumes, fragrant dew, and sumptuous olfactory delights.

Frequently in this text fragrance and oil converge. When the pious Theodora is shown Basil's heavenly home, for example, angels poured the heavenly oil of mercy on her head until she was "completely covered with oil and filled with mercy and spiritual fragrance."[59] At the celestial liturgy celebrated by the Lord in all his splendor "[I]mmortal noetic dew poured into the hearts of the hallowed ones from the springs of the All-Holy Spirit. . . . When the time for communion drew near, the Lord distributed to them the spiritual and divine manna of His own divine life and gave them to drink from the noetic and spiritual perfumed oil of His divinity."[60]

The *Life of St. Theodora of Thessalonike* and the *Life of St. Basil the Younger* are texts deeply immersed in the sensory culture of Byzantine piety. They are especially evocative of the prominence and prevalence of a devotion to fragrant oil in Byzantine religious usage. Where the Theodora narratives provide a window into concrete local practices, the Basil extravaganza engages the Byzantine imaginary that provided vibrancy and even urgency to the qualities of those practices. Both are texts with extensive olfactory descriptions; both repeatedly render their fragrances, mystical scents, and overwhelming perfumes in the materiality of oil. Pouring, collecting, anointing, applying, rubbing, exuding, drinking: time and again, oil renders the fragrances palpable and transferable.

In such texts, we are shown precisely how fragrant holy oil was both a practice and a rhetoric. It brought together the social habits of medicine and hygiene, even as it drew on imagery resonant with moral coding rendered through biblical cadences. Health, healing, life and afterlife, earth and heaven—and certainly a vividly imagined hell—are domains engaged and affirmed in social practical terms by such narratives and by the ritual practices they represented.

Oil and Life

From the perspective of the Byzantine theologian, the work of the senses was established in the most basic of sacraments: baptism and Eucharist. In just such terms did Nicholas Kabasilas speak of the significance of olfaction and materiality in his fourteenth-century treatise *The Life of Christ*.[61] In this work, Kabasilas exhorts that what the body learns and knows now in its physical, mortal life provides instruction regarding the life to come. In the most fundamental terms, Kabasilas insists, bodily experience offers as much knowledge as we can have prior to eternal life. The senses provide the epistemological foundation for the faithful's understanding of salvation and indeed, their knowledge of God. Pale though the foreshadowing may be, yet it is sure.

> The life in Christ originates in this [present] life and arises from it. It is perfected, however, in the life to come. . . . But if the life to come were to admit those who lack the faculties and senses necessary for it, it would avail nothing for their happiness, but they would be dead and miserable living in that blessed and immortal world. The reason is that the light would appear and the sun shine with its pure rays with no eye having been formed to

57 E.g., *The Life of Saint Basil the Younger* 1.34.

58 E.g., *The Life of Saint Basil the Younger* 1.55, 2.11.

59 *The Life of Saint Basil the Younger* 2.11 (at p. 209).

60 *The Life of Saint Basil the Younger* 5.126 (p. 661).

61 Nicholas Cabasilas, *The Life of Christ*, trans. C. J. de Catanzaro (Crestwood, NY, 1974).

> see it. The Spirit's fragrance would be abundantly diffused and pervading all, but one would not know it without already having the sense of smell... it is this [present] life which is the workshop for all these things.[62]

Thus, Kabasilas argues, one must use temporal reality as a school in which to learn what awaits. This is not because bodily, sensory life provides an analogy for the life to come, or even a type. Rather, it is because our very sensory reality is already drawing in something of God's reality. "[T]hat future life is, as it were, infused into this present life and mingled with it. For us too that Sun has graciously risen, the heavenly fragrance has been poured forth into the malodorous places, and the Bread of angels has been given even to men."[63]

What enables this to happen, Kabasilas writes, and what enables the faithful believer to obtain such knowledge, is the effect of the sacraments on the human body. Baptism is the formative birth for the Christian in Kabasilas's presentation. It brings forth a body shaped and empowered for perception in this full sense. Anointed with holy oil, it is divinely infused with dynamic life; it is prepared, then, to be nourished and sustained by the bread of life. Kabasilas is precise on this process. Baptism is birth, Eucharist is food. By means of smell and taste, quite literally, Christ renders the human body his own and protects its sacramental formation.

> He Himself occupies the entrances of life. He appropriates the organs by which we introduce air and food to aid the life of the body, and through them He enters our souls; through the former He comes as chrism and a sweet odour, through the latter as food. We breathe Him, He becomes food for us. Thus, as He blends and mingles Himself with us throughout, He makes us His own body and He becomes for us what a head is for the members of a body.[64]

In this treatise, Kabasilas analyzes baptismal anointment in detail. He examines the qualities of olfaction and viscosity with scrupulous care; he recounts their effects meticulously, on both the exterior body and its interior organs.[65] Lacing his account with copious biblical citations, Kabasilas interweaves ritual procedure, physiological affect, and theological doctrine. Each of these aspects becomes a mirror for the others. Repeatedly, he reminds his reader that once the body has been sacramentally fashioned, sensory experience and sensory knowledge are the sources of true belief. All bodily sensation becomes receptive to divine interaction.

In the case of holy oil, Kabasilas points out, fragrance and oil are combined in order for the faithful to understand how Christ can be both divine and human in two distinct but united natures. The faithful experience holy oil as sweet scent poured out, and as ointment rubbed into their flesh; they smell it and they touch it. This double sensory encounter Kabasilas offers as a paradigm for the incarnation: "so chrism represents Christ as the point of contact between both natures; there could be no point of contact were they still separate."[66] Holy oil is, in fact, both its fragrance and its substance, inseparably, just as Christ is God and man. Kabasilas insists that because human and divine joined in Christ at the incarnation, so, too, does holy oil provide the faithful with the meeting point between the human and the divine. It materially joins the one to the other. Its fragrance marks that work.

Kabasilas concludes with a vivid image of anointment with holy oil as the action by which Christ "infuses Himself into us and mingles Himself with us." The human person is transformed, as if a drop of water were added into "an immense sea of ointment." That ointment renders the faithful not only sweet-smelling like perfume, but wholly and utterly into fragrance itself, scent and substance: "'for we are the sweet savor of Christ' (2 Corinthians 2:14)."[67]

For the Byzantines, fragrant oil proved to be an especially powerful indicator of human–divine

62 Kabasilas, *Life of Christ* 1.1 (pp. 43–44).

63 Kabasilas, *Life of Christ* 1.2 (p. 45).

64 Kabasilas, *Life of Christ* 1.11 (p. 62).

65 Esp. Kabasilas, *Life of Christ* 2.2, 2.8.

66 Kabasilas, *Life of Christ* 3.2, p. 105.

67 Kabasilas, *Life of Christ* 4.6, p. 123.

relation as a concrete, materially evident aspect of human existence. In myron or myrrh, the Byzantines found repeatedly generous affirmation of divine presence, no matter their political or social circumstances. They perceived a reality intimately sensed, cognitively realized, and physically known. In holy oil they smelled and absorbed divine presence in materially restorative terms.

Familiar habits of practice and familiar conventions of rhetoric provided the Byzantines with tools by which to navigate a complex, unstable universe. As Nicholas Kabasilas explained, sensation could open awareness of order in the present physical domain, as well as revealing a cosmology far greater than immediate physical reality might indicate. Sensory experience lifted the body out of the merely physical or mortal into an existence engaging other domains—divine, demonic, heavenly, eternal. Holy oil combined fragrance, substance, and abundance. Practice elicited sensation; sensation declared meaning.

I am grateful to the Senior Fellows in Byzantine Studies at Dumbarton Oaks for encouraging me to do this essay, and especially to Margaret Mullett. I am grateful further to Michael Maas, Gabriel Radle, and the anonymous readers for helpful guidance; and to Abby Linn, Evan Strouss, and Gabriella Reyes for their research and editorial assistance. Remaining problems, of course, are my own.

Taste

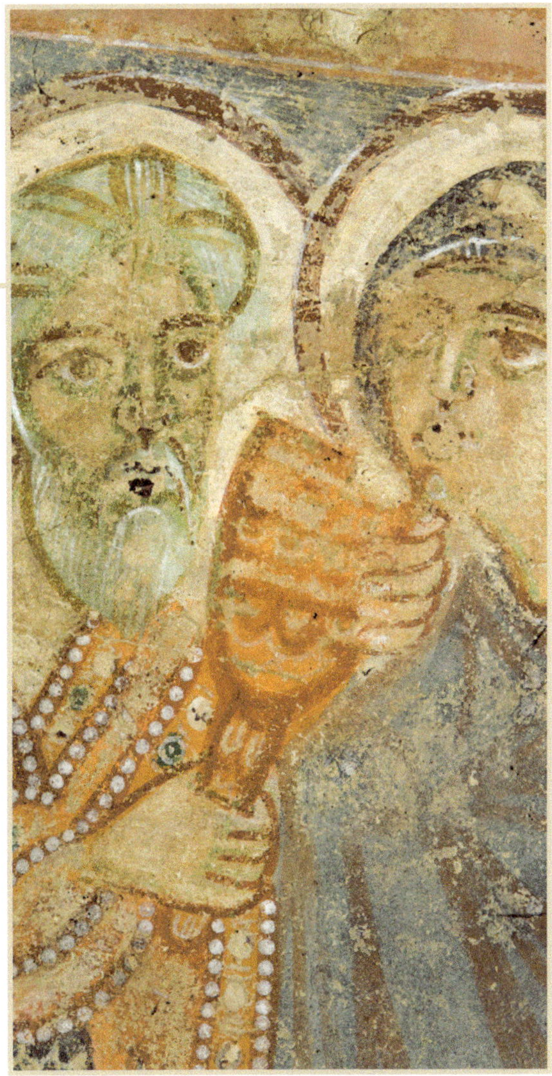

CHAPTER NINE

Struggling with Romanos's Dagger of Taste

THOMAS ARENTZEN

When the world was first created, God told Adam to eat, according to Romanos the Melode (d. ca. 560). God says:

> —Enjoy . . . everything I have given you,
> for in your enjoyment of it I will be satisfied.
> If you observe my commandment,
> I will guard your enjoyment.[1]

In this hymn *On Fasting*, the poet reflects an idea found in the Book of Genesis (Gen 2:16), an idea that is central to Christian understanding of the human condition: nourishment is created and provided by God. It is good and natural to eat the fruits of God's creation. Although fasting and abstaining from certain food complicates this simple picture, eating is a fundamental bodily function, and tasting belongs to the basic sensual features of embodied human experience from the very beginning. Human transgression was initially a disobedient offence in the realm of taste.

At the same time gustation usually occupies the lower stratum of ancient taxonomies of sense perception. As opposed to the more distanced and reflective vision, for instance, taste presupposes proximity to its object. Ancient thinkers, therefore, generally regarded it as inferior or primitive.[2] As Carolyn Korsmeyer points out: "Taste is early placed on the margins of the perceptual means by which knowledge is achieved; its indulgence must be avoided in the development of moral character; and it perceives neither objects of beauty nor works of art."[3] Elite Roman writers tended to treat eating and food in a depreciative manner because of its close connection to coarse corporeal needs.[4]

These philosophical views do not reflect late ancient skepticism toward gustation as such. People enjoyed food, and the literature of antiquity and late antiquity is not devoid of meals.[5] Athenaeus of Naucratis's *Deipnosophists* reads as a praise of assorted tastes and good wine. In literature, eating is usually endowed with a surplus of meaning, and it often involves more than sensory pleasure and satisfaction of hunger; it contributes to the characterization of the eater.

1 Romanos, *Hymn* 51.6.5–8, "Κατατρύφα," γὰρ ἔλεγε, "πάντων ὧν κεχάρισμαι, / τῇ τρυφῇ γάρ σου τῇ τούτων ἀρεσθήσομαι· / ἐὰν φυλάξῃς τὴν ἐντολήν μου, / φυλάξω σε τρυφῶντα." Two critical editions of the Romanos corpus are current among scholars: P. Maas and C. A. Trypanis, eds., *Sancti Romani Melodi cantica: Cantica genuina* (Oxford, 1963) and J. Grosdidier de Matons, ed., *Romanos le Mélode: Hymnes I–V*, SC 99, 110, 114, 128, 283 (Paris, 1964–81). I cite the former. Unless otherwise noted, the translations are my own.

2 R. Jütte, *A History of the Senses: From Antiquity to Cyberspace*, trans. J. Lynn (Cambridge, 2005), 61–71.

3 C. Korsmeyer, *Making Sense of Taste: Food & Philosophy* (Ithaca, NY, and London, 1999), 11–37; quote from 11.

4 E. Gowers, *The Loaded Table: Representations of Food in Roman Literature* (Oxford, 1993), 2–5.

5 Ibid.

How did tasting and eating signify in the increasingly hegemonic Christian worldview of late ancient Constantinople? This article explores the works of a poet who addressed and created models for the urban Christian public, as he engaged subterranean ingestion in grotesque characterizations and human longing for gustatory sensations. Romanos the Melode's writing assumes sensual desire to be a vital impetus in religious realms; his characters long to see, yearn to touch, or crave a kiss.[6] As flavors intersect with rich patterns of gustatory expectations and excitement, the longing of the characters is meant to arouse a similar longing in the listener. In Romanos's poetry the reader meets a God who can exclaim about his relation to his people:

> —I brought [them] water from a rock in a waterless place.
> In addition to this, I provided them ungrudgingly
> with quail, for I am
> *the heavenly bread of incorruption.*[7]

Tasting and eating draw away from the margins of perception and become vital parts of the human appreciation of the world.

Romanos was the most outstanding liturgical poet of this era, and he composed long semi-liturgical songs, often called *kontakia*, for the Constantinopolitan rite.[8] Posterity regarded his opus as supernaturally inspired; when the legend attempts to explain how he acquired his talent, it tells a story of digestion: One Christmas eve in Constantinople the Virgin Mary appeared to the young Romanos and gave him a roll of papyrus to eat. He swallowed it, and immediately started to sing his most famous hymn.[9] Eating transformed him and turned him into a divinely gifted voice.[10] The spirit of inspiration has been replaced by the textual matter of ingestion.

In Romanos's own poetry, tasting starts in Paradise and ends up intersecting with the Cross. At acute points, as at the edge of a dagger, savors appear. The *dagger* is a metaphor that Romanos himself uses: *On Fasting* lets God describe the one tree whose fruits Adam and Eve must not eat:

> —While the nature of the tree is not bad,
> the partaking in it will be
> a cause of harm for you, for it has
> a hidden whetstone of thoughts and a dagger of taste;
> so if you eat from it,
> *you throw away forgiveness and eternal life.*[11]

The imagery is no less startling than puzzling. The dagger obviously connotes danger, and yet one is left wondering how the sharpening of thoughts may produce a sharp taste. And how can flavor be a weapon? The connection with fasting is clear from the context—the whole hymn concerns the observance of Lent—and it suggests that although tasting and eating are God-pleasing activities, they are also potentially dangerous. A dagger is a tool that cuts through and brings about transformation, and tasting converges with several forms of metamorphosis in this poetry; when a change of fate occurs, there is very often eating involved.

6 See, e.g., G. Frank, "Dialogue and Deliberation: The Sensory Self in the Hymns of Romanos the Melodist," in *Religion and the Self in Antiquity*, ed. D. Brakke (Bloomington, 2005), 163–79; eadem, "Sensing Ascension in Early Byzantium," in *Experiencing Byzantium: Papers from the 44th Spring Symposium of Byzantine Studies, Newcastle and Durham, April 2011*, ed. C. Nesbitt and M. Jackson (Farnham and Burlington, VT, 2013), 305–9.

7 Romanos, *Hymn* 13.17.7–10 (*On the Multiplication of the Loaves*), ἐκ πέτρας δὲ ἐξήγαγον τὸ ὕδωρ ἐν ἀνύδρῳ· / πρὸς ἐπὶ τούτοις ὀρτυγομήτραν / παρεσχόμην ἀφθόνως αὐτοῖς ὡς ὑπάρχων / *ἄρτος ἀφθαρσίας ἐπουράνιος*. Trans. E. Lash, *St. Romanos the Melodist: On the Life of Christ: Kontakia* (San Francisco, 1995), 95.

8 For a general introduction to the corpus, see J. Grosdidier de Matons, *Romanos le Mélode et les origines de la poésie religieuse à Byzance* (Paris, 1977) and S. Gador-Whyte, *Theology and Poetry in Early Byzantium: The Kontakia of Romanos the Melodist* (Cambridge, 2017); for a recent treatment of Romanos and the Christian self, see D. Krueger, *Liturgical Subjects: Christian Ritual, Biblical Narrative, and the Formation of the Self in Byzantium* (Philadelphia, 2014), 29–65.

9 For the legend and other biographical sources, see Grosdidier de Matons, *Romanos le Mélode*, 159–98.

10 For the Marian implications, see T. Arentzen, *The Virgin in Song: Mary and the Poetry of Romanos the Melodist* (Philadelphia, 2017).

11 Romanos, *Hymn* 51.7.5–10, ἡ οὐσία τοῦ ξύλου γὰρ ἔστι μὲν οὐκ ἄχρηστος, / ἡ δὲ τούτου μετουσία σοὶ γενήσεται / βλάβης αἰτία, ἔχει γὰρ τοῦτο / ἀκόνην λογισμῶν ἐγκεκρυμμένην καὶ γεύσεως μάχαιραν· / ἂν φάγῃς οὖν ἐκ τούτου, / *ἀποβάλλεις τὴν [ἄφεσιν καὶ] ζωὴν τὴν αἰώνιον.*

Overeating in the Underworld

For an overture we shall turn to the underworld. In the subterranean regions of Romanos's world, grotesque dramas are played out.[12] While decent humans are expected to fast and be temperate, the species of the underworld show the reader the opposite way. In a kontakion on the Resurrection, for instance, the personified Hades complains:

> —I lament myself, the way I have been mocked,
> and this alone was not sufficient shame for me, but I am also being ridiculed;
> a glutton who eats everything they call me, those who have escaped me,
> and with such words they provoke me, saying, "Why do you gape beyond measure?
> Why do you stuff your throat, and for what, again and again, you insatiable and greedy one?
> Why do you rush for food, upsetting your stomach?[13]

Hades feels misjudged and misunderstood. As the reader learns, however, the accusations are not entirely groundless. There is much to be critical about in the way he eats.

Earlier Roman writers had displayed grotesque behavior in order to ridicule. The historian Suetonius, for instance, described how Emperor Vitellius—who "delighted in inflicting death and torture on anyone whatsoever and for any cause whatever"[14]—enjoyed a most overweening platter:

> he mingled the livers of pike, the brains of pheasants and peacocks, the tongues of flamingoes and the milt of lampreys, brought by his captains and triremes from the whole empire, from Parthia to the Spanish strait. Being besides a man of an appetite that was not only boundless, but also regardless of time or decency, he could never refrain, even when he was sacrificing or making a journey, from snatching bits of meat and cakes amid the altars, almost from the very fire, and devouring them on the spot; and in the cookshops along the road, viands smoking hot or even those left over from the day before and partly consumed.[15]

Obviously, this description relates as much to his imperial rule as to his palate. Nevertheless, it shows in a most outstanding way how invested with meaning ingestion might be and how eating habits could be used to characterize people. Vitellius's body knows no limits.

Overeating involves more than an occasion for mockery. "In the act of eating," Mikhail Bakhtin contends, "the body transgresses . . . its own limits: it swallows, devours, rends the world apart, is enriched and grows at the world's expense."[16] In the grotesque we encounter bodies that undergo change, bodies that destabilize.[17] Eating subverts distinctions between entities and brings about radical transmutations. This transgressional and transformative aspect of consumption is exploited by Romanos in his characterizations of death and destruction. What David Williams calls "the figure of the monstrous hell-mouth" in Christian tradition is often connected to the Anglo-Saxon iconography of mediaeval times.[18] Romanos's example, however,

12 For another presentation of these corners of Romanos's world, see G. Frank, "Christ's Decent to the Underworld in Ancient Ritual and Legend," in *Apocalyptic Thought in Early Christianity*, ed. R. Daly (Grand Rapids, 2009), 211–26; for a recent narrative analysis of one of the underworld kontakia, see U. H. Eriksen, "The Poet in the Pulpit: Drama and Rhetoric in the Kontakion 'On the Victory of the Cross' by Romanos Melodos," *Transfiguration: Nordic Journal of Religion and the Arts* (2010): 103–23.

13 Romanos, *Hymn* 25.4.1–6, "ἐμαυτὸν θρηνῳδῶ πῶς ἐχλευάσθην· / καὶ οὐκ ἤρκεσε τοῦτο μόνον εἰς αἰσχύνην μου, ἀλλ' ὅτι καὶ ἐμπαίζομαι· / λίχνον γὰρ καὶ παμφάγον οἱ φυγόντες με καλοῦσι με / καὶ ῥήμασι τοιούτοις παροξύνουσι με λέγοντες· 'τί γὰρ χαίνεις ὑπέρμετρα; / τί τῷ λαιμῷ σου ἐνωθεῖς ἢ τί δήποτε ὡς δήποτε, ἀκόρεστε, ἄπληστε; / τί ἠπείχθης πρὸς ἔδεσμα ταράσσων τὴν γαστέρα σου;'"

14 Suetonius, *Vitellius* 14.1. Trans. from Suetonius, *The Lives of the Caesars*, vol. 2, trans. J. C. Rolfe, Loeb 38 (Cambridge, MA, 1914).

15 Suetonius, *Vitellius* 13.2–3.

16 M. Bakhtin, *Rabelais and His World*, trans. H. Iswolsky (Cambridge, 1968), 281.

17 Ibid., 26–27.

18 D. Williams, *Deformed Discourse: The Function of the Monster in Mediaeval Thought and Literature* (Exeter, 1996),

shows that this way of portraying Hades appears in a different cultural milieu much earlier in Christian history.

We can be pretty sure that Romanos wrote his songs about Death and the Devil and Hades for the latter part of Lent. As the faithful approach Easter they observe a strict diet with little or at times no food. A certain amount of hunger—or at least craving for food—must have afflicted Romanos's audience. Into this craving congregation he hurls his subterranean dialogues, which comprise dramas designed to ridicule the powers of destruction. These poems strive to make people quite literally laugh in the face of death.

In the Resurrection kontakion quoted above, Hades eventually loses control over his stomach. This is when the major transformation takes place: Christ is about to resurrect; Hades' engorgement has gone too far. He has gulped down another body—from Calvary—and his haste has made his digestion turn on him. Frustration overwhelms him as he exclaims:

> —A sweet-tasting flower became a spurge to me
> And my whole throat was irritated by the taste, and I disgorged those that I had held.[19]

Christ appears as a sweet flower, and the image of the grotesque monster swallowing the lovely flower makes for quite a contrast. Yet the flower becomes a poisonous spurge in Hades' throat. Spurge or euphorbia is a plant that has been used as purgative agent in traditional medicine. In other words, Hades eats everything he sees, and eventually he stumbles over something he should not have touched; it makes him vomit—drastically. Or, according to another Resurrection hymn, he swallows the bait and is caught:

> Hades takes Christ like any of the earthborn;
> he swallows like a bait the heavenly bread,
> and gets wounded by the hook of divinity.
> With a tormented voice Hades cried out:
> —I am pierced in the stomach; the one I am swallowing I do not digest;
> for me what I ate became strange eating.[20]

In both cases, as in other Byzantine stories of grotesque healing and salvation, some form of tool opens up the body.[21] The dead are all released from Hades' belly, and the untasteful scene transforms his monstrous figure into an empty shell, not unlike a balloon pricked by a needle. In the next stanza Hades lies naked on the ground, derided. Christ, on the other hand, surrounds himself with servants who appear as bees around a honeycomb. Christ (the honeycomb) stands at the center of a honey-image, which highlights his sweetness in contrast to the embittered Hades. Eventually, the bees bind Hades up and make fun of him.

Another variation on the resurrection-by-vomit theme appears in the kontakion *On the Raising of Lazarus I*. Hades does not feel well; he complains to his friend and servant Thanatos:

> —Do not bring me food, for I cannot digest it;
> you put wrapped corpses in front of me, and gulping them down I immediately vomit;
> I cheer and grab them when they are buried, but I cannot hold them when they are decaying.[22]

Thanatos replies, annoyed and sarcastic:

> —Discuss that with that belly of yours, which you have not yet fully stuffed!
> I have worn myself out bringing you food, and yet you did not say: "I am full!"
> but you became stretched out like the sea, receiving rivers of dead

143; see even pp. 144–45. The motif is common in post-Byzantine iconography as well.

19 Romanos, *Hymn* 25.6.3–4, τὸ ἄνθος τὸ γλυκάζον ἐμοὶ γέγονε τιθύμαλλος, / καὶ ὅλος μου ὁ φάρυγξ ἐπικράνθη ἐκ τῆς γεύσεως, καὶ οὓς εἶχον ἀπέπτυσα·

20 Romanos, *Hymn* 26.7.2–7, δέχεται ὁ Ἅιδης [τὸν] Χριστὸν ὡς ἕκαστον τῶν γηγενῶν· / καταπίνει ὡς δέλος τὸν οὐράνιον ἄρτον, / τιτρώσκεται ἀγκίστρῳ θεότητος. / [ὁ] Ἅιδης δὲ ὀδυνηρὰς ἀνεβόησε φωνάς· / "Κεντῶμαι τὴν κοιλίαν· ὃν κατέπιον οὐ πέπτω· / ξένην μοι βρῶσιν παρέσχεν ὅ<ν> ἔφαγον·"

21 For examples, see S. Constantinou, "Grotesque Bodies in Hagiographical Tales: The Monstrous and the Uncanny in Byzantine Collections of Miracle Stories," *DOP* 64 (2010): 43–54.

22 Romanos, *Hymn* 14.9.3–5, μὴ φέρε μοι τροφήν· οὐ πέπτω γὰρ αὐτήν· / προσάγεις μοι δεδεμένους νεκροὺς καὶ καταπίνων εὐθέως ἐμῶ· / χαίρω καὶ αἴρω θαπτομένους, οὐ κατέχω δὲ φθειρομένους·

and never did you reach satiety.[23]
. . . .
The life of mortals has always seemed like
water to you;
hence you have opened wide and never
stopped gulping them down;
be satisfied, now, so you don't multiply
yourself.[24]

Thanatos's harsh words hurt Hades and he weeps over himself. At the same time he witnesses what happens to Lazarus's body, the very body which he has recently eaten. In an instance of bizarre gastric introspection he sees the disintegrated limbs of the dead body within himself. These putrefying parts, like an army of dead meat, are now mobilizing; they are in the process of being joined together again. Hades says:

—I see the limbs of Lazarus, those that
corruption dissolved,
are expecting to rise again; they are
practicing to reassemble,
for they creep like ants now after the
worms withdrew
and the stench left them.[25]

Death is overeating, Romanos says; vehement consumption belongs to the decaying forces of the underworld. Hades disgusts the reader as he stuffs himself with all sorts of bodies. Unhealthy eating brings about an unfortunate transmutation, and Hades is transformed into a weak and pathetic figure, a victim of his own eating, of the dagger of taste. Fasting, on the other hand, involves controlling one's appetite.

Grotesque eating happens among the living too. An aboveground vomiter is Herod Antipas. At his birthday banquet the saturated party guests around the table enjoyed themselves and stuffed themselves. It was the ill-fated feast known from Mark 6.14–29. All of a sudden, in the middle of the boggled crowd,

the head of the Faster [i.e., John the
Forerunner]
was served up as food
. . . and bitter lament was mixed with the
laughter
when the platter with the head of the Baptist
appeared to them all.[26]

When the request to behead John was uttered to Herod, he tasted the wicked demand, Romanos says, a demand metaphorically called the "bitter weed of evil root":[27]

Herod, when he tasted it, did not spit it out,
but held it within;
since he did not reject it, he spewed
bloodshed
and vomited forth the chopping of the godly
Forerunner.[28]

The actions of the gluttonous devour the faster. This banquet shows the listener beyond much doubt how an unrestrained appetite slaughters fasting and leads to murder. The congregation's digestion is supposed to take part in the opposite side of the metamorphosis, the fasting side. Since in the season of Lent engorgement relates to death, fasting comes to signify participation in the human transformation from death into life.

Between Sweet and Bitter

Sensing is not merely a physiological act, but also a cultural one, as we learn to sense in certain ways.[29] Late ancient people were partly attentive to other

23 Romanos, *Hymn* 14.10.4–7, νουθέτησον τὴν γαστέρα τὴν σήν, ἣν οὐκ ἐχόρτασας ἕως τοῦ νῦν· / καὶ γὰρ ἀπέκαμόν σοι φέρων, καὶ οὐκ εἶπας λοιπόν· 'ἀρκεῖ μοι', / ἀλλ' ἡπλώθης ὡς ἡ θάλασσα ποταμοὺς τελευτώντων δεχόμενος / καὶ μηδέποτε κόρον λαμβάνων·

24 Romanos, *Hymn* 14.11.1–3, Ὕδωρ σοι ἔδοξεν ἡ ζωὴ τῶν βροτῶν πάντοτε· / ὅθεν ἐπλάτυνας καὶ οὐκ ἐπαύσω ἀεὶ καταπίνων [αὐτούς]· / ἀρκέσθητι οὐκοῦν μὴ πληθύνῃς σαυτῷ.

25 Romanos, *Hymn* 14.12.4–7, τὰ μέλη γὰρ τοῦ Λαζάρου ὁρῶ, ἅπερ διέλυσε πρὶν ἡ φθορά, / ὡς προσδοκῶντα ἀναστῆναι· μελετᾷ γὰρ συναθροισθῆναι, / ὅτι ἕρπουσιν ὡς μύρμηκες, ἐπειδὴ ἀνεχώρησαν σκώληκες, / καὶ ἀφῆκεν αὐτὰ δυσοσμία·

26 Romanos, *Hymn* 38.1.2–6, ἡ κεφαλὴ <ἡ> τοῦ νηστεύοντος / παρετέθη ὥσπερ ἔδεσμα· . . . καὶ τῷ γέλωτι ἐκράθη πικρὸς ὀδυρμός, / ὅτι τὴν κάραν τοῦ βαπτιστοῦ πίναξ φέρων / ἐπὶ τῶν πάντων εἰσῆλθεν.

27 Romanos, *Hymn* 38.17.2, ῥίζης κακῆς πικρὸν ζιζάνιον.

28 Romanos, *Hymn* 38.17.4–6, ἧς γευσάμενος Ἡρώδης οὐκ ἀπέπτυσεν, ἀλλ' ἔσχεν ἔνδον ἑαυτοῦ· / ὅθεν μὴ πέμψας τοῦτο ἠρεύξατο φόνον / καὶ τὴν τοῦ θείου προδρόμου ἤμεσε τομήν.

29 See, e.g., C. Classen, "Foundations for an Anthropology of the Senses," *International Social Science Journal* 153 (1997): 401–12.

flavors than we are, and in other ways. The second-century physician Galen suggests tasting the patient's sweat in order to give a proper diagnosis;[30] the taste would in other words tell truths hidden to sight and other senses. The fourth-century physiologist and philosopher Nemesios—who was bishop in Romanos's hometown Emesa—distinguishes between eight separate tastes.[31] He notes, "At least in the case of dried figs, raisins and dates one quality, sweetness, is dominant, but taste distinguishes the difference between the kinds."[32] To him the palette of flavors consists of a complex muddle of nuances. Romanos is less concerned with nuances. He teaches his listeners attentiveness toward the tastes of sweet and bitter. These two tastes of qualities are invested with distinct symbolic value where the former implies goodness and the latter some form of wickedness.

Like other late ancient authors, Romanos may use bitter taste as a bad omen. In his kontakion *On Baptism* he recapitulates how the prophet Elisha once healed and transformed a spring of bad water in Jericho. The best-known version of this story is found in 4 Kingdoms (2 Kings) 2:19–22, where the author tells of a spring that yields infertility and bad crops. This Old Testament version does not, in any explicit way, speak of drinking or tasting the water. To Romanos, however, the spring's lack of fertile powers cannot be witnessed only in the fields; it is something that meets the tongue:

> The source of a very evil stream was once
> healed
> by Elisha, the very wise prophet;
> the taste of the waters made women barren
> as they caught the disease of childlessness.[33]

Romanos does not describe the flavor here. The text seems to imply that the taste will be fresh and healthy after Elisha's healing, but it is not particularly explicit on that point. It is more explicit about the baptismal connection. The whole kontakion is about baptism, and the transformation of the water serves to forebode transformations in the font. Tasting Elisha's water meant fertility and life, and, by extention, tasting the baptismal water means life to the candidate. Tasting does not need to imply actual experiencing of its flavor, but it does mean—more or less metaphorically—to experience the water. And Romanos returns to the taste of baptismal water elsewhere too. In *On Peter's Denial*, the poet exclaims to the newly baptized:

> cry to the Creator, you newly enlisted,
> since you taste the sweet and good source of
> the font.[34]

We may wonder whether the baptismal water would actually inspire any immediate sensations in people's mouths—would the candidates have tasted the water as they descended? Perhaps they did, but more importantly this relates to the figurative use of taste language. Any dictionary will tell us that sweet and bitter—in Greek as well as in English—often function metaphorically. We all know a sweet girl or a bitter old man, but we do not have to taste them in order to know this. As Emily Gowers has observed, "Eating was linguistically ubiquitous" in the ancient world.[35] Hence separating metaphor from matter may be easier said than done, and perhaps it should not always be done. Romanos seems to be playing with the ambigiously figurative language—as if aware that deep down all language speaks metaphorically. In his world the distinction between figurative sensuality and concrete senses is blurred, and so, ultimately, a sweet person may actually taste sweet. The baptismal candidates have been changed, and the baptismal water has become the life-giving spring of which they have drunk; they can, as it were, sense the change by the sweetness of the water. Mark Smith shows, in his *Sensing the Past*, how a modern *E. coli* contamination of a water source led people to doubt their own tongues or negotiate the reliability of

30 Galen, *On the Preservation of Health* 4.4 (6.251 K).

31 Nemesios, *On the Nature of Man* 9.66.10–11.

32 Nemesios, *On the Nature of Man* 9.67.2–3, trans. by R. W. Sharples and P. J. van der Eijk (Liverpool, 2008), 115.

33 Romanos, *Hymn* 53.8.1–4, Ναμάτων κακίστων πηγή ποτε ἰάθη / ὑπὸ Ἐλισσαίου τοῦ σοφωτάτου προφήτου· / ἐστείρου γὰρ τὰ γύναια ἡ τῶν ὑδάτων γεῦσις / νόσον ἀτεκνίας παρεχόμενα·

34 Romanos, *Hymn* 18.23.1–2, τῷ πλάστῃ βοήσατε, ὑμεῖς οἱ νεόλεκτοι, / ἐπειδὴ τῆς κολυμβήθρας ἀπογεύεσθε γλυκείας πηγῆς καὶ ἀγαθῆς· Trans. Lash, *St. Romanos*, 251.

35 Gowers, *Loaded Table*, 8.

gustatory knowledge.[36] Romanos seeks to instill such reliability; good waters do taste sweet, and bad waters tend toward bitter.

Paradise comprises a favorite source of taste language for the Melode as well as for other Christian authors. Already in the Genesis text, the tasting of the fruit plays an important role. Romanos holds that everything *there*, in the Garden, initially tasted good; as we have seen, God tells Adam explicitly to appreciate its fruits. The world is good and healthy and its harvest is to be enjoyed. Tastes reflect the true nature of phenomena. But things were not entirely uncomplicated in Paradise; a big transformation was imminent. The Devil was about to interfere, and Romanos introduces the dagger.

In the kontakion *On Fasting*, Romanos shows how Adam and Eve were fooled by the Devil in Paradise. The poet does not want the fruit of the forbidden tree to taste bitter, since it is after all created by God and is not in itself an evil tree.[37] Theologians tend to emphasize that fasting means abstaining from certain foods—not because the food itself is evil, but because asceticism consists of struggle with desire. Romanos shows us Adam and Eve, like the congregation, in the middle of a fast.[38] The forbidden tree is the food they should abstain from. He informs us that the very nature of the tree is harmless and that it does taste good.[39] The enjoyment of its savor, however, is forbidden by God. Since Romanos wants to avoid equivocality in the taste itself, he locates the snare of ambiguity in the serpent's words: "In his fatal speech the enemy mixed a sweet taste."[40] Flavors do not per se deceive, but when they are mixed and manipulated, telling sweet from bitter becomes complicated. This is also an instance where metaphors and sensuality intertwine; conceptual and sensual realms turn inseparable. The serpent mixes his cunning words with the sweet fruit, creating a deadly concoction which belongs neither to the verbal nor the sensorial world exclusively.

In an Easter dialogue between the Devil and his companion Hades, a similar mixture of tastes appears. The former bemoans what happened with the Cross, the event that radically altered their existence. He tries to comprehend the incident and communicates his painful insights in a rather complex web of taste language in a hymn which has been called *On the Victory of the Cross*:

> —We grafted to [the Tree] bitter shoots.
> We did not transform the sweetness in it.[41]
>
> —Did not the Master, by the tree he showed
>   to Moses,
> which once sweetened the water at Mara,
> teach what it was and what its root?
> . . . .
> all things have been made pleasant, but we
>   have been embittered.
> From our root, a Cross has blossomed
> that was cast into the earth which became
>   sweet.[42]

The tree of the Cross commutes between good and bad in the same way as the tree in Paradise; its nature is inherently good, but then again it is not just good. Sweetness functions as a metaphor, but also as a reference to the sweet fruits of paradisiacal trees and sweet waters.

The problem of taste ambiguity Romanos solves in a different way here: bitterness has simply been grafted into a sweet tree. The tree itself is left sweet and good, while its daggers are attached by Hades and the Devil. Its fruit, the sweetening of the earth, may be unambiguously explained in tangible language of sweet taste.

The passage also allows Romanos another detour into Old Testament waters in order to

36 M. M. Smith, *Sensing the Past: Seeing, Hearing, Smelling, Tasting, and Touching in History* (Berkeley and Los Angeles, 2007), 90–91.

37 Romanos, *Hymn* 51.7.

38 According to the manuscript (Patmiacus 213 fol. 19r) this is a hymn for the Wednesday of the second week of Lent; Grosdidier de Matons, *Hymnes I*, 70.

39 Romanos, *Hymn* 51.7 cf. 17.

40 Romanos, *Hymn* 51.12.1, Ῥήματι οὖν θανατηφόρῳ γλυκεῖαν ὁ ἐχθρὸς συγκατέμιξε γεῦσιν.

41 Romanos, *Hymn* 22.12.7–8, στελέχη πικρὰ ἐγκεντρίσαντες αὐτῷ / τὸν ἐν αὐτῷ γλυκασμὸν οὐ μετεποιήσαμεν. Trans. Lash, *St. Romanos*, 160.

42 Romanos, *Hymn* 22.15.1–3, 6–8, Ἆρα ὅπερ ἔδειξε τῷ Μωϋσῇ ὁ δεσπότης / ξύλον ὃ ἐγλύκανε ποτὲ τὸ ὕδωρ εἰς Μέρραν, / ἐδίδαξε τί ἦν καὶ τίνος ἡ ῥίζα; . . . ἰδοὺ γὰρ τὰ πάντα ἡδύνθη, ἡμεῖς δὲ παρεπικράνθημεν· / ἐκ ῥίζης ἡμῶν ἀνεβλάστησε σταυρός, / ὃς ἐνεβλήθη τῇ γῇ καὶ γλυκεῖα γέγονεν· Trans. Lash, *St. Romanos*, 162.

explain the change: The miracle recounted in Exodus 15:23–25, where Moses makes bitter water drinkable, follows the same pattern as that of Elisha: bitterness gives way to sweetness as the prophet intercedes. The transformation does not involve only taste; the story implies a metamorphosis of the water's nature. This miracle points to the metamorphic sweetening of the earth by the Cross. There is an inherent sweetness in Christ's tree which the Devil and Hades have been unable to alter. What may have appeared evil to those who only taste the buds turns out to be sweet on the inside. It is not so much a question of gustatory deception, but somehow the Devil has been able to coat certain sweet things with a layer of bitterness, to graft certain bitter shoots into a sweet tree. The flavor can indeed deceive, just as it did Adam and Eve once, but the problem is not human sense perception; Romanos reveals no fundamental skepticism toward sensual perception. The problem consists of a devilish manipulation with the phenomena of this world, a weaving together of good and bad. This sweet and sour brew confuses people.

In the hymns sweet and bitter surpass the arbitrary metaphor and converge with sensory experience, and yet the sensory experience of taste does not respond to the modern culinary search for aesthetic pleasure or Nemesios's nuanced taste pallet. Romanos's sweet and bitter are woven into a web of values more akin to Galen's diagnostic technique. Taste becomes important as a means to evaluate the quality of phenomena. If the quality of a phenomenon changes, its flavor alters. What is ontologically good, healthy, or even divine, usually reveals its goodness by a sweet taste. Evil or unhealthy things, on the other hand, taste bitter. In this way he is able to infuse sacramental life with expectations of gustatory tangibility. Tastes, like other sensual experiences, may help the characters of the kontakia—and consequently its audience—to understand the quality of what they encounter.

The Anticipation of Tastes: Savoring the Virgin

Tastes can also be an object of sensual longing, an immense—and at times dangerous—force. After the serpent had spent stanzas trying to tempt Eve to try the fruit in *On Fasting*, he finally managed to convince her, and the desire to taste overwhelmed her. Romanos writes:

> When she herself saw the tree as beautiful
> and pleasant, Eve
> was aflame and pressed herself with
> expectations toward the taste.[43]

Tasty fruit arouses desire, and thus savor can be a dangerous weapon. Some fruits are not to be eaten. Only stanzas earlier the audience has heard about the taste dagger. Eve's movement here emerges almost like a suicide; she throws herself toward its edge. And as Eve and Adam lose their self-control, surrendering to their gustatory temptation, they are crippled.[44]

The poet, of course, tries to instill in his audience the opposite movement, a longing for what is good and healthy. An entire kontakion is, for instance, dedicated to the Samaritan woman and her thirst for living water.[45] Another example is the Virgin Mary and her breast milk in the hymn *On the Nativity I*, the song which Romanos allegedly sang after he had eaten the Virgin's roll.

The anonymous *Akathistos* hymn calls Mary a "beautiful *kourotrophos* [i.e. nurse] of virgins,"[46] but Romanos is among the first Christian writers to characterize the Virgin more broadly as nursing.[47] In *On the Nativity I*, she becomes

43 Romanos, *Hymn* 51.15.1–2.

44 Romanos, *Hymn* 51.20.

45 Romanos, *Hymn* 9.

46 *Akathistos* 19.16, καλὴ κουροτρόφε παρθένων. My translation. For an introduction to the *kourotrophoi* and their cult, see T. H. Price, *Kourotrophos: Cults and Representations of the Greek Nursing Deities* (Leiden, 1978).

47 For a more developed exposition of the theme of Marian nursing in Romanos, see Arentzen, *Virgin in Song*, ch. 3; for the general theme of nourishment from the Virgin, see M. B. Cunningham, "Divine Banquet: The Theotokos as a Source of Spiritual Nourishment," in *Eat, Drink, and Be Merry (Luke 12:19)—Food and Wine in Byzantium. Papers of the 37th Annual Spring Symposium of Byzantine Studies, in Honour of Professor A. A. M. Bryer*, ed. L. Brubaker and K. Linardou (Aldershot, 2007), 235–44. The *galaktotrophousa* motif in early Christian literature has not been sufficiently studied. Studies that focus primarily on the visual representation include E. Bolman, "The Enigmatic Coptic Galaktotrophousa and the Cult of the Virgin Mary in Egypt," in *Images of the Mother of God: Perceptions of the Theotokos in Byzantium*, ed. M. Vassilaki (Aldershot, 2005), 13–22; A. Cutler, "The Cult of the Galaktotrophousa in Byzantium and Italy," *JÖB* 37 (1987): 335–50; L. Langener,

"mother and nurse for a fatherless son," as the Magi remark.[48] But the question is if she does not even turn into a breast-feeder for the whole congregation? Elsewhere Romanos calls her the "mother and nurse of our life."[49]

The poet opens *On the Nativity I* by presenting the Bethlehem cave as a Marian space, paralleling the inner cavity of the Virgin with that of the Earth:

> The Virgin today gives birth to the Transcendent One,
> and Earth offers the cave to the Unapproachable One;[50]

Inside this cave the listener is about to discover the abundance of sensual delights, a foretaste of Paradise, in connection with the Marian body:

> we have found hidden delight; come, let us receive
> the [joys] of Paradise within the cave;
> . . . .
> *there* has been found an undug well
> from which David once longed to drink;
> *there* a virgin giving birth to a baby
> has quenched at once Adam's and David's thirst.[51]

The language of a new Paradise runs through Romanos's entire corpus. Whether the imagery converges with the Virgin's body, as in this example, or with the Tree of the Cross, the expectation of sweet Edenic fruits and the anticipated sensation of its flavors lurk always in the undergrowth of the narration. In this instance, the grotto not only houses the Virgin but is also, so to say, flavored by her. The stanza invites the audience into the womb of the earth, where the Virgin Mary and the pleasures of Paradise intersect, where human thirst meets what Mary has to give.

The central imagery in the stanza is the undug well of the Marian cave, a well from which David has desired to drink and which now quenches his thirst. A well (φρέαρ) is naturally something that the thirsty long for; hence Athenaeus of Naucratis, for instance, uses the word metaphorically for something from which to drink, like a cup or a glass.[52] The connection with breast milk is not obvious, and it may not have been to Romanos's contemporaries either, but there is a striking parallel in Ephrem the Syrian, who opens his *Hymn 11 on Paradise* by comparing the air of Paradise to a mother's breast:

> The air of Paradise
> is a fountain of delight
> from which Adam sucked
> when he was young;
> its very breath, like a mother's breast,
> gave him nourishment in his childhood.[53]

I am not arguing for any direct connection between the two poems, but perhaps the fact that the Ephrem tradition—to which Romanos in some sense adheres[54]—is able to think of the air of Paradise as a mother's breast opens up for the possibility that Romanos's stanza did evoke mammary ideas? After all, Romanos's text says that she has quenched the thirst of David and Adam.

Romanos casts his listeners as eager to see and take part in the luxuries of paradise, as yearning, like David and Adam. These two forefathers are filled with desire specified as *thirst*. The well of the Marian cave stands against the thirst of

---

Isis lactans—Maria lactans: Untersuchungen zur koptischen Ikonographie (Altenberge, 1996); L. Mirković, "Die nährende Gottesmutter (Galaktotrophusa)," *SBN* 6, no. 2 (1940): 297–304; V. Tran Tam Tinh, *Isis Lactans: Corpus des monuments greco-romains d'Isis allaitant Harpocrate* (Leiden, 1973).

48 Romanos, *Hymn* 1.4.8, ἀπάτορος υἱοῦ ἐγένου μήτηρ καὶ τροφός.

49 Romanos, *Hymn* 36.1.2, μητέρα καὶ τροφὸν τῆς ζωῆς ἡμῶν; cf. also the refrain of his *Nativity of the Virgin*: τὴν θεοτόκον καὶ τροφὸν τῆς ζωῆς ἡμῶν.

50 Romanos, *Hymn* 1.Pro.1–2, Ἡ παρθένος σήμερον τὸν ὑπερούσιον τίκτει, / καὶ ἡ γῆ τὸ σπήλαιον τῷ ἀπροσίτῳ προσάγει·

51 Romanos, *Hymn* 1.1.2–8, τὴν τρυφὴν ἐν κρυφῇ ηὕραμεν, δεῦτε λάβωμεν / τὰ τοῦ παραδείσου ἐντὸς τοῦ σπηλαίου· / . . . / ἐκεῖ ηὑρέθη φρέαρ ἀνόρυκτον, / οὗ πιεῖν Δαβὶδ πρὶν ἐπεθύμησεν· / ἐκεῖ παρθένος τεκοῦσα βρέφος / τὴν δίψαν ἔπαυσεν εὐθὺς τὴν τοῦ Ἀδὰμ καὶ τοῦ Δαβίδ· Trans. Lash, *St. Romanos*, 3, with slight modifications.

52 Athenaeus of Naucratis, *Deipnosophists* 5.18.33, πίνει ἐξ ἀργυροῦ φρέατος.

53 Ephrem, *Hymns on Paradise* 11.1. Trans. from *St. Ephrem the Syrian: Hymns on Paradise*, trans. S. P. Brock (Crestwood, 1990), 154.

54 This is not to say that there has to be direct literary dependence as argued by e.g. W. L. Petersen, *The Diatessaron and Ephrem Syrus as Sources of Romanos the Melodist* (Leuven, 1985), but the Ephremic, or at least Syriac, influence on Romanos is well established among moderns scholars.

David and Adam and the congregation, and the one who quenches the thirst is no one but the Virgin, who has given birth. Her body opens as a treasury of sensual pleasure. To drink from her implies participation in salvific transformation.

The poet has given his audience the cue to thirst for the quenching Virgin. And he has exclaimed: "come, let us receive!" Having been invited in with his or her thirsting self, the listener is led into the more dramatic stanza two. The flip side of the image of thirsting appears in Mary's monologue to her Child:

> contemplating him the Mother said:
> —Tell me, my Child, how were you sown in me or how planted in me?
> I see you, my flesh and blood, and I am amazed
> that I give suck and am not married;[55]

The poet has evoked thirst; the audience is ready to drink. And precisely then the Virgin introduces herself as a miraculous milk-giver. When the metaphors of wells and thirst are flipped, the other side shows a virgin breastfeeding. She speaks *to* her child, but she speaks *about* herself, her own body; the focus is not on his sucking, but her breastfeeding. She gives suck, and the listener cannot be entirely sure whether the receiver is the divine child or thirsty congregation. The text rather tempts the latter to think of itself as the receivers of her milk. How the milk may taste is not revealed to us, but the first stanza gives a clear indication that the cave hides pleasant fluids.

At the end of the same kontakion, Mary speaks again. Once more she appears as a provider, not only to the characters in the narrative, but even to its audience. She turns to the Christ Child in prayer, yet as before she speaks about herself rather than about him:

> —I am not simply your Mother, compassionate Savior;
> I do not suckle the provider of milk without reason,
> but for all I implore you.
> . . . .
> [My entire race] looks to me, those who were cast out
> of the Paradise of pleasure, for I bring them back
> to let them sense everything through me.[56]

The nursing Mother reopens Paradise and makes it perceptible, palpable. By juxtaposing the suckling and the delightful Garden the text summons the listener to associate the two phenomena. Romanos teaches his audience to anticipate bodily sensations, to long and yearn for it. Like Christ, Mary has a paradisiacal body. The listeners are exhorted to imagine her with their taste buds and their thirst, to recognize the flavor of an idyllic garden in the landscape of Christ and Mary's bodies.

Tasting the Sacrifice

From the Virgin's body, we turn to Christ's. The Eucharist itself almost defines the word *transformation* in a liturgical Christian context. It involves most profoundly eating, drinking, and tasting.

On the way to the Cross, Jesus describes his own sweetness in *On Mary at the Cross*. Approaching the Crucifixion together with his Mother, he explains in imagery how he, the Divine Logos, was translated into human flesh in her. He says of himself:

> [I,] the Sweet One came down from heaven like manna,
> not onto Mount Sinai, but into your belly,
> for within it I was curdled, as David foretold.
> Consider the "cheese-filled mountain," Revered One;
> I am, for being Logos in you I became flesh.[57]

55 Romanos, *Hymn* 1.2.3–6, ὃν κατανοοῦσα φησὶν ἡ τεκοῦσα· / "Εἰπέ μοι, τέκνον, πῶς ἐνεσπάρης μοι ἢ πῶς ἐνεφύης μοι; / ὁρῶ σε, σπλάγχνον, καὶ καταπλήττομαι, / ὅτι γαλουχῶ καὶ οὐ νενύμφευμαι·" Trans. Lash, *St. Romanos*, 3, with slight moderations.

56 Romanos, *Hymn* 1.23.1–3, 7–9, "Οὐχ ἁπλῶς γὰρ εἰμι μήτηρ σου, σῶτερ εὔσπλαγχνε· / οὐκ εἰκῇ γαλουχῶ τὸν χορηγὸν τοῦ γάλακτος· / ἀλλὰ ὑπὲρ πάντων ἐγὼ δυσωπῶ σε· . . . ἐμὲ ὁρῶσιν οἱ ἐκβληθέντες / τοῦ παραδείσου τῆς τρυφῆς, ὅτι ἐπιστρέφω αὐτοὺς / λαβεῖν αἴσθησιν πάντων δι' ἐμοῦ." Trans. Lash, *St. Romanos*, 11–12, with slight moderations.

57 Romanos, *Hymn* 19.6.2–6, ὁ γλυκὺς οὐρανόθεν νῦν κατῆλθον ὡς τὸ μάννα, / οὐκ ἐν ὄρει τῷ Σινᾷ, ἀλλ' ἐν γαστρί σου. / ἔνδοθεν γὰρ ταύτης ἐτυρώθην, ὡς Δαυὶδ προανεφώνει· / τὸ τετυρωμένον ὄρος νόησον, σεμνή, / ἐγὼ γὰρ ὑπάρχω, ὅτι λόγος ὢν ἐν σοὶ σὰρξ ἐγενόμην·

The curdling here is an ancient metaphor of conception which goes back to Aristotle—and possibly further.[58] It imagines the semen to curdle female fluidity into flesh the way rennet curdles milk into cheese. For the present purpose, however, the gynecology of Incarnation is of lesser concern. What one may observe in the passage is how Christ's account of the event seems to start from the Eucharistic experience: Through the liturgical meal Romanos's audience *knows* Christ first and foremost as taste. He is the sweet-tasting one, and his *kenosis* reminiscent of the sweet manna that fed the people of old. In the Eucharist, divine sacrifice converges with human tasting. And as Christ approaches the sacrifice in this kontakion, the poet carefully—yet subtly—brings the taste of the mystical table to mind.[59] The Eucharistic bread and the Old Testament manna merge into one sweet sensation. Indirectly Romanos appeals to the congregation to recognize the Christ that they have tasted—and is going to taste. It is as if the poem fuses the Incarnation and the Eucharistic transformation into a single movement, a movement that leads to a gustatory sensation. There is no tongue in the passage, but there is a language of cheese curdling (τυρόω), which faintly connotes the edible, and there is sweetness and there is manna.

Additionally, there is the strange notion that this sweet stuff goes into the Virgin's belly. It means that she becomes pregnant, of course, but the ambiguity of the poet's language seems almost to suggest that she *ate* the Logos. Anyone who had not heard the reference to the Virgin might well have interpreted the entire stanza as a reflection on the reception of the Eucharist. For to say that he, the Sweet One, entered the belly like manna suggests a parallel between eating Christ's body sacramentally and conceiving him into a womb. The audience that heard this intersection of sweet flavors and bodies anticipated partaking in the Eucharistic body.[60]

The most important point in relation to taste and transformation, however, is the poet's insistence on continuity. We remember how prophets changed the nature of bad water so it ended up tasting good. Here, with Christ, a substantial transformation has taken place, and yet the taste is the same. In other words, the Christological conviction that the divine Logos became man without a deprivation of divinity is expressed in the language of taste: sweetness was there before and after the descent; this sweetness may be tasted by the communicant in the liturgy.

A much more explicit reference to the taste of the Eucharist appears in the kontakion *On the Wedding at Cana*. Sorrow turns into joy when Christ turns water into wine. "Let the whole crowd and the groom himself enjoy it," says Christ, "for I have miraculously given cheerfulness to all."[61] And the poet explains that this was exactly what happened—and is going to happen—everyone is taking part in this tasty and joyful meal:

> The whole crowd enjoyed themselves, as they
> found the taste marvelous.
> At the moment we all delight in the supper
> in the church
> for wine changes into Christ's blood
> and we drink it/him with holy cheerfulness.[62]

Romanos suggests a direct correlation between the transformation in the Eucharist and the transformation in Cana. On the other hand, he is not able to make it into a complete parallel. Christ transformed water into wine so a new and better flavor appeared, but the transformation of wine into Christ's blood does not alter the taste

58 See Aristotle, *Generation of Animals* 1.20; Romanos refers to a cryptic verse in Psalm 67.16 (LXX); for the Christian use of this "curdling mountain," see E. Lash, "Mary in Eastern Church Literature," in *Mary in Doctrine and Devotion*, ed. A. Stockpoole (Dublin, 1990), 70–71.

59 It should be noted that liturgical eating in the Byzantine church was not restricted to the Eucharistic bread. Naturally, *antidoron* was distributed, but the more prosperous might also bring such foods as cheese, fruits, and olives that would be distributed among the poor; see, e.g., B. Caseau, "Experiencing the Sacred," in Nesbitt and Jackson, *Experiencing Byzantium*, 74–75.

60 For the liturgical context of the kontakia, see A. Lingas, "The Liturgical Place of the Kontakion in Constantinople," in *Liturgy, Architecture and Art of the Byzantine World: Papers of the XVIIIth International Byzantine Congress (Moscow, 8–15 August 1991) and Other Essays Dedicated to the Memory of Fr. John Meyendorff*, ed. C. C. Akentiev (St. Petersburg, 1995), 50–57.

61 Romanos, *Hymn* 7.19.7–8, ἀπολαυέτω πᾶσα ἡ [πλ]ηθὺς καὶ ὁ νυμφίος αὐτός· / παραδόξως γὰρ πᾶσιν ἔδ[ω]κα τὴν εὐφροσύνην.

62 Romanos, *Hymn* 7.20.2–5, εὐφράνθη ἅπαν τὸ πλῆθος θαυμασίαν τὴν γεῦσιν αὐτοῦ ἡγησάμενοι· / ἄρτι δὲ ἐν τῷ δείπνῳ τῷ ἐν τῇ ἐκκλησίᾳ ἀπολαύομεν ἅπαντες· / εἰς αἷμα γὰρ Χριστοῦ μεταβάλλεται οἶνος, / καὶ πίνομεν αὐτὸν εὐφροσύνῃ ἁγίᾳ.

or its sweetness. Hence the stanza does not mention the taste of the ecclesistical supper.

In the kontakion *On the Prodigal Son,* Romanos turns the scene of his homecoming party into a sacrificial gathering and a mystical banquet. The father in the story represents God the Father, says Romanos, while the Prodigal Son represents Romanos's audience. The Son of God, on the other hand, is represented by a calf. The Father presides over the banquet and inaugurates the meal, saying:

> —Sacrifice this calf
> and, to all who are worthy of my supper, give to eat
> the spotless calf, pure in any way,
> fattened from the unsown earth which he fashioned!
> Give them a precious drink,
> blood and water which spring from his side for those who believe!
> Eat this then all of you always,
> . . . .
> for he offers himself as all-holy food![63]

From the sacrificial calf the reclining participants at the banquet receive blood to drink. Interestingly, the participants are even able to handle snakes without being hurt, as in certain ancient sacrificial orgies.[64]

The banquet now takes on transhistorical dimensions:

> As the whole company of the invited were supping
> and as all were celebrating, they sang a godly hymn.
> The Father, first of those present, began the ceremonies.
> "Taste," he said, "and see that I am Christ."
> Then after this the psalmist,
> striking the lyre, cries with sweetest voice,
> "Quickly bring
> undefiled sacrifice that has been blessed
> to the all-holy altar.
> Bring a calf with thanksgiving."
> And after him Paul cried out,
> "Our paschal lamb has now been sacrificed, Jesus Christ,
> *the Master and Lord of the ages.*"[65]

Saintly members of the divine household are present as the Father slaughters the calf. He cries out: "Taste and see that I am Christ [Χριστός]!" In the Biblical Psalm 33 (34):9 the singer exclaims "Taste and see that the Lord is good [χρηστός]," but Romanos ingeniously substitutes the phonetically identical iota for eta, rendering the Father gustatorily identical with the Son.[66] In this sacrifice the sacrificed and the sacrificer come to taste the same. Romanos translates the Eucharistic experience, to which the whole hymn alludes, into a gustatory encounter with the Father. In other words, the extraordinary banquet contributes to the blurring of a distinction between Trinitarian persons in the realm of taste. They are gustatorily speaking *homoousios.* In this stanza, the refrain—elsewhere denoting the Father—refers to the Son, the calf. Narratively speaking, the Father invites the Prodigal (the listeners) to lie next to him and enjoy the sacrificial

63 Romanos, *Hymn* 49.9.1–11, "θύσατε τοῦτον τὸν μόσχον / καὶ δότε πᾶσι τρώγειν τοῖς τοῦ δείπνου μου ἀξίοις / τὸν ἄσπιλον μόσχον, τὸν καθαρὸν κατὰ πάντα, / τὸν σιτευθέντα ἐξ ἀσπόρου γῆς ἥσπερ ἔπλασε· / δότε δὲ πρὸς τούτοις τίμιον πόμα, / αἷμά τε καὶ ὕδωρ τὸ ἐκ τῆς πλευρᾶς τῆς αὐτοῦ πηγάζον τοῖς πιστεύουσι· / πάντες οὖν πάντοτε φάγετε τοῦτον· / . . . / εἰς ἔδεσμα γὰρ πρόκειται πανάγιον." Trans. Lash, *St. Romanos*, 105.

64 Romanos, *Hymn* 49.7. Both Clement of Alexandria, *Hortatory Address to the Greeks* 2.12.2 and Arnobius of Sicca, *Against the Pagans* 5.19 attest to the notion that Bacchanalias involved snake handling; how common this was in reality is of lesser importance to the present argument.

65 Romanos, *Hymn* 49.10, Τῶν κεκλημένων πᾶς λοιπὸν ὁ θίασος ὡς ἐδείπνει, / καὶ πάντες εὐφρανθέντες ἐμελῴδουν θεῖον ὕμνον, / ὁ πατὴρ μὲν πρῶτος κατήρξατο τῶν παρόντων· / "Γεύσασθε," λέγων, "καὶ ἴδετε ὅτι Χριστός εἰμι." / εἶτα μετὰ τοῦτο ὁ ψαλμολόγος / κρούων τὴν κιθάραν κράζει ἡδυτάτῃ φωνῇ· "Σπουδαίως προσαγάγετε / θύματα ἄχραντα, ηὐλογημένα / πρὸς τὸ πανάγιον θυσιαστήριον· / ἀνοίσατε μόσχον μετ᾽ εὐχαριστίας·" / καὶ μετ᾽ αὐτὸν δὲ βοᾷ ὁ Παῦλος· / "Τὸ πάσχα τὸ ἡμέτερον ἐτύθη νῦν Ἰησοῦς ὁ Χριστός, / *ὁ τῶν αἰώνων δεσπότης καὶ κύριος.*" Trans. Lash, *St. Romanos*, 105–6, with minor adjustments.

66 To the listener, who only hears the text, the phrase is, of course, ambiguous anyway.

meal[67] and "eat with delight."[68] Yet, eventually it is not his son in the story, but the sacrificed virgin calf,[69] which appears as indistinguishable from him. And the Father, who presents the divine Son as food,[70] virtually turns edible himself. As banquet customs demanded, the guests contributed with their acclamation and others entertained with music.[71]

More references to sacramental forms of tasting emerge at the Cross. In one of the subterranean dialogues between Hades and the Devil the former seeks to convince the latter of the gravity of what has just happened in the Crucifixion. He points to the Tree of the Cross and says:

> —Behold, that Tree, which you call dry and barren,
> bears fruit; a thief tasted it
> and has become heir to the good things of Eden.[72]

At the very end of his life, the thief gets to experience the taste of transformation as the Tree of the Cross has turned into a Tree of Life. His tasting mimics Adam and Eve's tasting of old, but the transformative movement goes from bad to good. As Lent turns into Easter he gets to eat the sweet fruit. The good taste leads to the tasteful things of Eden. Tasting the fruit of the Cross the thief comes to take part in greater fruit. The words follow a sacramental logic: momentary tasting opens up to a whole world of Paradisiacal delights.

A similar thing happens to a group of beggars who have gathered underneath the Cross; they long to taste its fruit:

> beneath [the Tree of the Cross] have sheltered
> and will nest in its branches
> thieves, murderers, and publicans and harlots, that they may reap
> sweet fruit from the supposedly arid.[73]

A motley crew has assembled around the Tree to enjoy it; all kinds of people long for sweet tastes and crave them. These characters are sinners—they yearn fervently for the fruits of Salvation. When Romanos wants to create literary models for his congregation, he habitually uses typical sinners like these from the holy stories rather than Christ and his Mother, and this is a typical instance of Romanos writing his own congregation into the holy stories: They are all gathered around waiting for the sweet fruit of Christ's sacrifice, the Eucharistic meal.

The harlot has her own kontakion, so we may conveniently turn to her to get a more detailed idea of how longing for Jesus overtakes her. As Patricia Cox Miller has noted about other Christian "harlots," she is not really a prostitute, but a lustful woman.[74] For Romanos's heroine it all starts when she sees "Christ's words like sweet drops of fragrance raining down everywhere"[75] and "the fragrance of Christ's table breathed gently [on her]."[76] After this relatively sober and sensual opening, things get more intense; the scents turn her on, and she falls wildly in love with Jesus and is stricken with desire. Owing to

67 Romanos, *Hymn* 49.2. In the sixth century, reclining was still the normal banquet posture, while sitting indicated humility or deviance; see S. Malmberg, "Dazzling Dining: Banquets as an Expression of Imperial Legitimacy," in Brubaker and Linardou, *Eat, Drink, and Be Merry*, 83, 87–88; see also J. Vroom, "The Changing Dining Habits at Christ's Table," 193–95 in the same volume.

68 Romanos, *Hymn* 49.8.10, φαγόντες ἐπευφρανθῶμεν.

69 Romanos, *Hymn* 49.8.2.

70 Romanos, *Hymn* 49.9.11.

71 For the issue of acclamation, religious chanting, and music at imperial banquets, see Malmberg, "Dazzling Dining," 86–87.

72 Romanos, *Hymn* 22.5.6–8, ἰδοὺ γὰρ τὸ ξύλον ἐκεῖνο, ὃ λέγεις ξηρὸν καὶ ἄκαρπον, / βλαστάνει καρπόν, οὗ γευσάμενος λῃστὴς / τῶν ἀγαθῶν τῆς Ἐδὲμ κληρονόμος γέγονεν. Trans. Lash, *St. Romanos*, 157.

73 Romanos, *Hymn* 22.16.4–7, οὗ ὑποκάτω κατεσκήνωσαν / καὶ ἐπὶ κλάδοις τούτου ἐννοσσεύουσι / λῃσταὶ φονευταὶ καὶ τελῶναι καὶ πόρναι, ἵνα τρυγήσωσι / καρπὸν γλυκασμοῦ ἀπὸ τοῦ δῆθεν ξηροῦ. Trans. Lash, *St. Romanos*, 162.

74 P. C. Miller, "Is There a Harlot in This Text? Hagiography and the Grotesque," *Journal of Medieval and Early Modern Studies* 33, no. 3 (2003): 429.

75 Romanos, *Hymn* 10.1.1–2, Τὰ ῥήματα τοῦ Χριστοῦ καθάπερ ἀρώματα / ῥαινόμενα πανταχοῦ. Trans. Lash, *St. Romanos*, 77. For a discussion of scent language in this kontakion, see S. A. Harvey, *Scenting Salvation: Ancient Christianity and the Olfactory Imagination* (Berkeley, 2006), 152–55.

76 Romanos, *Hymn* 10.3.1, Ὑπέπνευσεν ἡ ὀσμὴ τῆς τραπέζης τοῦ Χριστοῦ. Trans. Lash, *St. Romanos*, 78.

her undisciplined behavior, people think she is drunk.[77] When she approaches Christ's table, she reveals her swollen appetite:

> And so with greedy haste she reaches the
> table,
> and leaving the crumbs that were beneath it,
> she took the bread.
> Hungrier than the woman of Canaan earlier,
> she satisfied her empty soul.[78]

It may perhaps surprise us that this kontakion, too, was written for the final days of the Lenten period, namely for Holy Wednesday. Would someone so greedy, so sensually involved with Christ's physical body, really do as part of a Lenten service? And not only was the hymn performed during the service, but Romanos presents her—explicitly—as a model for his congregated audience. It is, of course, the Eucharist that the harlot hungers so passionately for, and Holy Wednesday precedes Maundy Thursday, the day of the Last Supper. Her appetite may be as socially questionable as her profession, but Romanos describes her as starving for Christ's food and for intimacy with his body. In other words, she turns away from other foods and other bodies in order to be with this one, to reap his sweet fruit. Fasting does not mean to forsake one's appetite, but to direct it toward the body of Christ. The congregation should learn to long for the Sweet One as intensely as she did.

77 Romanos, *Hymn* 10.8.5.

78 Romanos, *Hymn* 10.3.5–8, διὰ τοῦτο λίχνῳ δρόμῳ φθάνει αὐτήν, / καὶ λιποῦσα τὰ ψιχία τὰ ὑπ' αὐτὴν τὸν ἄρτον ἦρε· / τῆς πάλαι Χαναντίδος πλεῖον πεινάσασα, / ψυχὴν κενὴν ἐχόρτασεν. Trans. Lash, *St. Romanos*, 78.

Conclusion

This exposé started with what the poet calls "strange eating"[79] and ended where the Divine Logos coagulated into sweet bread. Romanos's songs teach devotees to experience the Christian Gospel with the tongue. The Eucharist contributes to a reshaping of familiar stories in ways that give priority to tasting and leads the listeners toward eucharistically flavored epistemologies. While ancient philosophical traditions may have favored vision over taste and touch, the liturgical tradition of Justinianic Constantinople involves even the less reflective segments of human sensation.

The Eucharist is a gustatory event, and so the Cross is a gustatory event. Eating is nothing innocent in Romanos. Christians should ensure that they use their mouths and tongues in appropriate ways, lest they be longing fervently for flavors that are sweet and bitter at the same time. Tasting such dangerous mixtures may lead to meals that hide pointed blades.

Savors are not just cosmetic. Eating means corporeal comprehension and participation in the transformative processes of Christian life. Teaching the audience to anticipate and enjoy the taste of this life means training them to long for transformation: bread, water, and wine changed into tangibles of divine intervention. As death is converted into life, the bitterness of everyday troubles is transfigured into sweet delight among the fruits of the Garden. For the Logos turns into flesh, flesh turns into bread, bodies turn into corpses, and corpses turn into bodies. These are the processes we eat, says Romanos. This is the sweet taste of salvation.

79 Romanos, *Hymn* 26.7.7, ξένην . . . βρῶσιν.

CHAPTER TEN

Monks Baking Bread and Salting Fish

An Archaeology of Early Monastic Ascetic Taste

DARLENE L. BROOKS HEDSTROM

Good taste is both tempting and dangerous. Tasting good things leads directly to desire and pleasure; thus taste paves the way to gluttony—the most dangerous of the eight thoughts outlined by Evagrios of Pontos.[1] Taste could be good when it was linked to spiritual eating, especially the Eucharist. The allegory of eating the delicacy of Christ's body and blood fostered one's thirst and desire after God. Desiring God's nourishment was far more appropriate than a desire for earthly delights. Medicine could be bitter, wine could be sour, tears could be sweet, and just a drop of olive oil could transform a monastic meal into a feast.[2] Tasting good food and drink could be intoxicating. When Aristotle describes taste in the *Nicomachean Ethics* 3.10, he articulates the uniqueness of taste as an individualized sense, for one's preference, for good food or drink varied, and thus taste is the lowest of the senses.[3] Unlike the other senses, taste is personal and "cannot be shared."[4] It would not be until the eighteenth century that Edmund Burke and others would dramatically modify our perception of taste from a base, physiological desire to an expression of refined, intellectual engagement and aesthetical appreciation of things within the world and not just within the body.[5] Therefore, to consider taste in Byzantium means we must begin with a more somatic or corporeal view of taste. In particular, examining how monastic communities experienced the world through taste can offer a sensorial history of daily monastic living that was in many ways very personalized and reflected the individual temptations and needs that appear throughout early Byzantine monastic literature.

For Byzantium, taste could be linked directly to the dangers of gluttony but also to the delights of heaven.[6] The ultimate sensorial taste came with the eating of the Eucharistic meal as one consumed the body and blood through a multisensory interaction with bread and wine including sight, touch,

1 Although gluttony is a central theme in Christian approaches to food, gluttony was well recognized as a problem in earlier Greek and Roman sources. For example, gluttony is at the heart of Petronius's satirical study of feasting in the *Banquet of Trimalchio*.

2 Honey or sweet tears appear frequently in monastic literature. See *Life of Shenoute* 12; trans. D. Bell, *Life of Shenoute* (Kalamazoo, 1983). The current study is limited to the relationship between taste and food. I recognize there is a great deal to be learned from other avenues for taste involving beverages and medicine.

3 Aristotle, *Nicomachean Ethics* 3.10; trans. *Nicomachean Ethics*, trans. T. Irwin, 2nd ed. (Indianapolis, 1999), 81.

4 P. P. Ferguson, "The Senses of Taste," *American Historical Review* 116, no. 2 (2011): 371–84, at 371.

5 E. Burke, *Burke's Philosophical Inquiry into the Origin of Our Ideas of the Sublime and Beautiful: With an Introductory Discourse concerning Taste* (Baltimore, 1833), 13.

6 I. Anagnostakes, ed., *Flavours and Delights: Tastes and Pleasures of Ancient and Byzantine Cuisine* (Athens, 2013).

and taste in a fully interoceptorial experience.[7] Although this meal offered the greatest joy, the greatest challenge came with daily meals in which the desire for food and satiation led to an array of challenges. The love of food reflected a love of and reliance on the body—a body that could experience the delights of apples and well-cooked game, to the pleasure of digesting the milk of heaven.[8] The letters of Barsanouphios and John of Gaza document monastic struggles with proper behavior at the monastic dining table for it was here that one could observe and compare the eating habits, tastes, and preferences of others. In *Letter* 546, monks were told to give thanks to God for their food "so that through your thanksgiving he might be able to liberate you from the [spiritual] warfare of the stomach."[9]

For nonmonastics, food could be consumed in a variety of cooked and uncooked forms; for monastics the dietary array was much more limited and restricted by fasting regulations.[10] Ancient philosophers and doctors, who all expressed grave concern about the dangers of wet and rich food, helped shape early Christian and later Byzantine attitudes toward food and its connection with sexual activity.[11] A love for food, they asserted, fueled a love for sex and luxury. As the quintessential sense linked to a highly personalized predilection for overindulgence, taste could undermine the spiritual progress of monastics if they were given dangerous foods and beverages.[12] Eating and drinking were essential for life, but the reliance upon sustenance was a constant reminder of the frailty of the human body and a shared fate with animals. As a result, it was even more fundamental that monks become more like animals in eating only what was absolutely necessary for the body's survival and not let one's taste, or preference, dictate what the body consumed. Positive associations with food consumption were linked to the Eucharist for here was one area in which eating and a multisensorial experience were essential to allow individuals to be fed from the divine table.[13]

The denial of the pleasure of food and the limitation of eating brought about an overall devaluation of food in general, according to Antony Eastmond and Liz James. Their analysis of Byzantine opinions about gluttony and obesity led them to conclude that in the afterworld food had little importance.[14] Once a monk died to earthly ties and became one of the angels, his body was no longer tied to the base needs that made him human. The most successful monks, as explained by hagiographers, maintained a minimal diet of bread and water, followed with several periods of total abstinence from any food.[15] The only food that one needed was the spiritual food found in being with God. Until death released monastics from the daily battle against their tastes, it was clear that monastic communities needed continual guidance in coping with the very real challenges of food consumption.

7 H. Hunter-Crawley, "Embodying the Divine: The Sensational Experience of the Sixth-Century Eucharist," in *Making Sense of the Past*, ed. J. Day (Carbondale, IL, 2013), 160–76.

8 *Kyrillos von Skythopolis*, ed. E. Schwartz, TU 49.2 (Leipzig, 1939).

9 *Letter* 546. Barsanouphios and John of Gaza, *Correspondance*, ed. F. Neyt and P. de Angelis-Noah, trans. L. Regnault, SC 426–27, 450–51, 468 (Paris, 1997–2002); J. Chryssavgis, *Barsanuphius and John: Letters*, 2 vols., Fathers of the Church (Washington, DC, 2007).

10 I. Anagnostakis, "'The Raw and the Cooked': Ways of Cooking and Serving Food in Byzantium," in *Flavours and Delights*, 175–81.

11 A. Rousselle, *Porneia: De la maîtrise du corps à la privation sensorielle, IIe–IVe siècles de l'ère chrétienne* (Paris, 1983); T. Shaw, *The Burden of the Flesh: Fasting and Sexuality in Early Christianity* (Minneapolis, 1998); C. W. Bynum, *Holy Feast and Holy Fast: The Religious Significance of Food to Medieval Women* (Berkeley, 1987).

12 S. E. Hill, *Eating to Excess: The Meaning of Gluttony and the Fat Body in the Ancient World* (Santa Barbara, 2011); V. Grimm, "The Good Things That Lay at Hand: Tastes of Ancient Greece and Rome," in *Food: The History of Taste*, ed. P. Freedman (Berkeley, 2007), 63–97.

13 See B. Caseau, "Experiencing the Sacred," in *Experiencing Byzantium: Papers from the 44th Spring Symposium of Byzantine Studies, Newcastle and Durham, April 2011*, ed. C. Nesbitt and M. Jackson (Surrey, 2013), 59–78; G. Frank, "L'eucharistie et la mémoire sensorielle selon Jean Chrysostome," in *Pratiques de l'eucharistie dans les Églises d'Orient et d'Occident (Antiquité et Moyen Âge)*, ed. N. Bériou, B. Caseau, and D. Rigaux (Paris, 2009), 765–78.

14 They write: "It is perhaps unsurprising that with all this loathing of gluttony, abuse of fatness and emphasis on vomit and regurgitation at the end of the world, there seems to be little desire or interest in the joy of food itself in the afterlife." A. Eastmond and L. James, "Eat, Drink . . . and Pay the Price," in *Eat, Drink, and Be Merry (Luke 12:19): Food and Wine in Byzantium: Papers of the 37th Annual Spring Symposium of Byzantine Studies, in Honour of Professor A. A. M. Bryer*, ed. L. Brubaker and K. Linardou (Aldershot, 2007), 183.

15 Shaw, *Burden of the Flesh*, 12–15.

Various textual sources describe the difficulty of living with a bodily sense of taste within a monastic environment. Some monks fasted often; others did not. Some could drink wine without becoming drunk; others could not even drink water for fear it would foster desire. Yet, there is more to the study of monastic taste than what appears in the *Lives* and other monastic literature. Egypt offers extensive evidence for early Byzantine monasticism, including monastic literature, monastic archives, architectural evidence, and now, archaeobotanical evidence from middens. Read together, the archaeology and textual sources become mutually informative for understanding how food was prepared in monastic kitchens and bakeries. Drawing upon a more diverse body of sources broadens our appreciation of who shaped monastic taste and how it was understood within the monastic community as a "structuring structure" that reinforced the community's identity.[16] The evidence associated with monastic cooks and bakers, in the form of archaeological evidence, illustrates that they were equally important in shaping monastic taste as were monastic authorities such as Pachomius, Shenoute, John Cassian, Barsanouphios, and Evagrios, who all addressed the dangers of taste and pleasure.

Methods for Approaching an Inquiry into the History of Monastic Taste in Early Byzantium

To write a history of Byzantine monastic perceptions of taste, I approach the topic from a few different directions by drawing upon literary sources, documentary evidence, and archaeology of monastic settlements. I draw upon recent archaeological, anthropological, historical, and philosophical studies of taste to frame the reading of the sources for early monastic taste. Research into the sense of taste, and more commonly food history, as an object of historical inquiry has generated several useful models for an inquiry into the history of the senses.[17]

16 P. Bourdieu, *The Logic of Practice* (Stanford, 1990), 53.

17 C. Korsmeyer, *Making Sense of Taste: Food and Philosophy* (Ithaca, NY, 1999); M. Serres, *The Five Senses: A Philosophy of Mingled Bodies*, trans. M. Sankey and P. Cowley (Cambridge, 2005).

The anthropology of the senses is a field of anthropological specialization of cultural anthropology, in which the senses are incorporated in fieldwork and analyses. When Paul Stoller wrote *The Taste of Ethnographic Things* in 1989 he argued for the importance of *sensorial* fieldwork in order to better ground one's anthropological understanding of culture.[18] He argued that taste, in particular, offered a variety of difficulties for anthropologists to document the "context specificity of taste" and the "semantic association with particular objects and events."[19] This anthropological study of food and taste has been augmented most recently by the study of synesthesia, or the union of the senses. Since consuming food is associated more with taste and smell, David Sutton argues that synesthetic studies "remind us that [the senses are] both socially cultivated and produced and that some of the distinct material properties of food go beyond the categorization of any five-sense model."[20] In considering Byzantine perceptions of taste within a monastic context, we can examine the social dynamics that constrain experiencing and expressing the sense of taste as it relates to food through a combination of documentary and hagiographical sources. The archaeological evidence related to food preparation and consumption takes us a step further to situate the sense of taste within the physical spaces of the kitchen, dining areas, and bakehouses.

Recent areas of study relating to food have exhibited an interest in dining, feasting, and banquets. These topics offer historians new directions in the cultural history of daily life from the view of the table in both secular and ecclesiastical settings.[21] Studies of Byzantine and medieval European dining illustrate the richness of our sources for reconstructing the social

18 P. Stoller, *The Taste of Ethnographic Things: The Senses in Anthropology* (Philadelphia, 1989).

19 J. C. Kupiers, "Matters of Taste in Weyéwa," in *The Varieties of Sensory Experience: A Sourcebook in the Anthropology of the Senses*, ed. D. Howes (Toronto, 1991), 125.

20 D. E. Sutton, "Food and the Senses," *Annual Review of Anthropology* 39 (2010): 209–23, at 219; idem, *Remembrance of Repasts: An Anthropology of Food and Memory* (Oxford, 2001); C. N. Seremetakis, ed., *The Senses Still: Perception and Memory as Material Culture in Modernity* (Boulder, 1994).

21 W. Mayer and S. Trzcionka, eds., *Feast, Fast or Famine: Food and Drink in Byzantium* (Brisbane, 2005).

variations surrounding food as a sign of status and wealth.[22] Food and drink has become a point of interest for several studies of Byzantium.[23] Scholars of monasticism had already undertaken discussions of the body, diet, and fasting as a way to better appreciate the cultivation of the self that monastic communities reinforced through daily restrictions on food and volume.[24] Michael Smith's *Sensing the Past* offered the first historical treatment of the senses and acknowledged that "senses are historical" and that they can be analyzed as "product[s] of place and, especially, time, so that how people perceived and understood smell, sound, touch, taste, and sight changed historically."[25] In 2003 Byzantinists considered the topic of food, drink, and eating in two diverse settings and the subsequent publications provided a valuable corpus for the foundation of our understanding of food in Byzantium. Papers presented at the *Feast, Fast or Famine: Food and Drink in Byzantium* conference approached the topic of foodways in Byzantium with an eye "toward understanding the role that food and drink, and its consumption, played within society."[26] At the thirty-seventh Spring Symposium of Byzantine Studies scholars examined food in a variety of mediums from preparation, consumption, presentation, and perceptions of real and imagined food.[27] The two publications introduced readers to the ubiquitous nature of food in a variety of arenas of Byzantine life, but ones that had not been previously examined.

One way to examine monastic taste is through the history of specific foods—those forbidden, those permitted, and those restricted.[28] Known more commonly as the archaeology of food, this approach places the food at the center of the study and the history of the foodways. Monastic typika, for example, are explicit in articulating what is good about food for a monastic diet and why. Yet, we learn little about how the meals are experienced. Therefore the archaeology of cooking, while related to food, is concerned with the type of human processes that transform ingredients into meals and in this case, how monastic cooks and bakers participated in the making of the sensorial meal. The importance of cataloguing and documenting what food was available, how ingredients transformed food, and what historical factors reshaped Byzantine cuisine is evident in *Flavours and Delights: Tastes and Pleasures of Ancient and Byzantine Cuisine* (2013), edited by Ilias Anagnostakes, and *Tastes of Byzantium: The Cuisine of a Legendary Empire* (2010), by Andrew Dalby. The two volumes illustrate the great variety of Byzantine tastes from high cuisine with visually rich delicacies to the more mundane food for the common table and the monastic refectory.

Delwan Samuel, an archaeologist and specialist in bread history, describes the complex limitations in studying premodern food as being compounded by "biological and cultural factors which affect food, the several phases involved in food provision, the profound transformations which food undergoes throughout these phases and the vulnerability of food, as organic material."[29] In Samuel's reading of the archaeological remains, the very food itself is hard to document as it has a history of its own that is difficult to reconstruct from its final depositional context. Additionally, textual descriptions of monastic taste are often overshadowed by an authoritarian voice that skews our ability to hear individual experiences with tasting food and drink.

For my contribution to a synesthetic treatment of food in Byzantine monasticism I employ methodologies from the archaeology of taste, a relatively new field of analysis, to explore how early monastic communities structured taste and consumption as a social habit. Like the developments in anthropology and history, archaeologists have found benefits by attuning their

22 G. Prinzing and D. Simon, eds., *Fest und Alltag in Byzanz* (Munich, 1990); E. Gowers, *The Loaded Table: Representations of Food in Roman Literature* (Oxford, 1993).

23 See the several works of A. Dalby, *Dangerous Tastes: The Story of Spices* (Berkeley, 2000); idem, *Flavours of Byzantium* (Totnes, 2003); idem, *Siren Feasts: History of Food and Gastronomy in Greece* (London, 1997).

24 L. Regnault, *La vie quotidienne des pères du hésert en Egypte au IVe siècle* (Paris, 1990).

25 M. Smith, *Sensing the Past: Seeing, Hearing, Smelling, Tasting, and Touching in History* (Berkeley, 2007), 3.

26 S. Trzcionka, "Introduction," in Mayer and Trzcionka, *Feast, Fast or Famine*, 3.

27 L. Brubaker, "Preface," in Brubaker and Linardou, *Eat, Drink, and Be Merry*, xxii.

28 V. Grimm, *From Feasting to Fasting, the Evolution of a Sin: Attitudes to Food in Late Antiquity* (London, 1996).

29 D. Samuel, "Approaches to the Archaeology of Food," *Petits propos culinaires* 54 (1996): 19.

analysis of material remains by considering the sensorial record of the past. The archaeology of taste, as Yannis Hamilakis explains, is a way to shift our understanding into one that "begins with the human body, or rather the *trans-corporeal, somatic landscape*" and is "culturally defined."[30] I have used the methodologies employed by monastic archaeologists working in Europe to inform my reading of taste and food production processes.[31] They have developed a two-pronged approach by first looking at the phases of food production, or showing "each stage the process involved, the location where activities take place, and the key influencing cultural factors" and then studying "the archaeological data associated with food production."[32] One of the significant challenges in investigating taste is the reliance upon written works to gain a sense of what we might call "ethnohistorical" evidence to articulate how monastics perceived the highly personalized sense of taste. Few sources offer specific monastic recipes, daily menus, or descriptions of the way food tasted in the numerous monastic communities of the Byzantine world. One can consider that much of the preparation of monastic food drew upon the apprenticeship of an experienced cook with a variety of assistants and thus recipes would change depending upon who was assigned to the monastic kitchen. Such mundane topics, including food preparation, were, as Johannes Koder states, "commonplace or self-evident" and therefore the evidence we wish to see "barely exists" for Byzantium.[33] By appropriating taste from a variety of related fields of anthropology, history, and archaeology it is possible to highlight what we can know about Byzantine monastic taste.

Monastic Foodways and Taste

The history of taste requires a consideration of foods, diet, and the methods of food preparation.[34] Eating and drinking fosters a complex sensory experience involving smell, touch, sight, and taste. Monastic diners could experience a range of pleasures at the smell of spiced food, at the touch of fresh baked bread, at the sight of delicacies on festival days, and at the taste of well-prepared food. Therefore, late antique and Byzantine monastic literature offers numerous examples of the danger of emotions associated with wanting and enjoying food. The *Longer Rules* and *Shorter Rules* of Basil of Caesarea (ca. 330–ca. 379) record his views toward several issues related to monastic eating. He warns "pleasurable tastes must not be followed as the goal of food—the need that serves life is sufficient, with indulgence being shunned. For if we serve pleasure, it is nothing other than to *make a god of our belly* (cf. Phil. 3:19)."[35] Basil equates pleasure and desire with indulgence and eventually with an overreliance upon food. Like rules, monastic handbooks and sermons present models of those who fast or monitor their food appropriately so as not to harm the asceticism of a community.[36] Shenoute (346–465) reminds monks not to try to sneak into other dining rooms for more food: "No person among us whether male or female shall finish eating and (then) go to the infirmary and eat there for a second time; or finish eating in the infirmary and (then) go the refectory and eat there a second time."[37] Fortunately, archaeological

30 Y. Hamilakis, "Archaeology of the Senses," in *The Oxford Handbook of the Archaeology of Ritual and Religion*, ed. T. Ingold (Oxford, 2011), 212; idem, "The Past as Oral History: Towards an Archaeology of the Senses," in *Thinking through the Body: Archaeologies of Corporeality*, ed. Y. Hamilakis, M. Pluciennik, and S. Tarlow (New York, 2002), 121–36.

31 D. Brooks Hedstrom, "Models of Seeing and Reading Monastic Archaeology," *Cistercian Studies Quarterly* 48, no. 3 (2013): 299–315.

32 Ibid. For evidence from Western monastic sites see J. Bond, "Production and Consumption of Food and Drink in the Medieval Monastery," in *Monastic Archaeology: Papers on the Study of Medieval Monasteries*, ed. G. Keevill, M. Aston, and T. Hall (Oxford, 2001), 54–87; P. Courtney, "Excavations in the Outer Precinct of Tintern Abbey," *Medieval Archaeology* 33 (1989): 99–143.

33 J. Koder, "Stew and Salted Meat—Opulent Normality in the Diet of Every Day?" in Brubaker and Linardou, *Eat, Drink, and Be Merry* (n. 14 above), 61.

34 S. Graff and E. Rodríguez-Alegría, eds., *The Menial Art of Cooking: Archaeological Studies of Cooking and Food Preparation* (Boulder, 2012).

35 *Rule of Basil* 9.9–10. *The Rule of St. Basil in Latin and English: A Revised Critical Edition*, trans. A. M. Silvas (Collegeville, MN, 2013), 101.

36 L. I. Larsen, "Monastic Meals: Resisting a Reclining Culture," in *Meals in the Early Christian World: Social Formation, Experimentation, and Conflict at the Table*, ed. D. E. Smith and H. Taussig (New York, 2012), 245–60.

37 *The Canons of Our Fathers: Monastic Rules of Shenoute*, ed. and trans. B. Layton (Oxford, 2014), no. 160; trans., 155.

and art historical studies of the spaces in which monks ate in private or in the communal refectory (*trapeza*) contextualize the spatial importance of where one ate.[38] The history of food and taste delineated by these sources offers a picture of Byzantine society as intellectually engaged with sensorial consumption and thus provides a broad framework for thinking about how monastic authors constructed the dangers and delights of tasting food.[39] As the lowest of the five Aristotelian senses, taste has received the least attention for the sense is embedded in the body and not the mind.[40]

Role models with a restrained passion for taste were found in scripture and frequently alluded to by authors to help teach monastic eaters how to control their sensorial experience with food. In *On Virginity*, Gregory of Nyssa (ca. 335–394) uses Elias and John as exemplars who controlled their taste to be "plain and simple" and shunned "the usual food and drink" of others. By doing so, they were "free from external disturbances."[41] For Gregory, a sense of taste was inseparable from the need for pleasure. He writes: "[A]nd be on guard, above all, against the pleasure of taste, because somehow this seems to be the most persistent, being practically the mother of all that is forbidden. Pleasures connected with eating and drinking abound in immoderate consumption, create in the body the necessity for a surfeit of undesirable evils, and this begets many similar sins among men." More succinctly Gregory states we must limit "every enjoyment connected with pleasure," including food.[42] Scriptural admonitions relating to food provided a clear framework for how monks should consider food and drink. When asked how one should follow Paul's directive to eat or drink "for the glory of God (1 Cor. 10:31)," Basil reminded monastics to "not eat carelessly" for otherwise one will become a slave to gluttony (γαστριμαργία).[43]

The baseness of taste was a clear path toward one of the greatest of sins—gluttony. Evagrios Pontikos (ca. 345–399), a resident at Kellia, offered his list of eight "generic thoughts" with gluttony (γαστριμαργία) as the first in the list.[44] His fellow monastic, John Cassian, also listed gluttony as the first vice in his *Conferences*.[45] In the *Institutes* Cassian outlines how Egyptian monastics guard against satisfying their palate, avoid eating tempting fruit, and keep from gratifying their appetite.[46] Self-control is essential, he argues, in resisting daily desires for food and avoiding gluttony. Cassian articulates that "it is not only the quality of food but also its quantity that dulls the heart's keenness" and thus both the quality (taste) and the quantity (volume) can cause equally damaging results for the monk.[47] In discussing gluttony, Cassian repeats the teaching of earlier monastic fathers who instruct that no one should "indulge to satiety of the belly, nor to be enticed by the pleasure of larynx."[48] Cassian admonishes monks to be aware of pleasure in taste and in fullness of the belly, for both can lead to intense sexual desires.[49]

How did monks navigate the warnings, but also not overly desire food? How did one monitor pleasure while tasting food so as not to undermine one's pursuit of *askesis*? In the late fourth-century text *History of the Monks in Egypt*, Abba Helle follows a strict fast in order

38 A.-M. Talbot, "Mealtime in Monasteries: The Culture of the Byzantine Refectory," in Brubaker and Linardou, *Eat, Drink, and Be Merry*, 109–26; S. Popović, "The Trapeza in Cenobitic Monasteries: Architectural and Spiritual Contexts," *DOP* 52 (1998): 281–303.

39 Philo of Alexandria (ca. 20 BCE–50 CE) explains how the "skill of pastry cooks and other experts at the art bewitches the taste, the most slavish of all the senses," and can attract the "lusts of the wretched belly."

40 Korsmeyer, *Making Sense of Taste*, 24–25.

41 Gregory of Nyssa, *On Virginity* 6 (*Traité de la virginité*, ed., trans., and comm. M. Aubineau, SC 119 [Paris, 1966], 504–10); St. Gregory of Nyssa, "On Virginity," in *St. Gregory Ascetical Works*, ed. and trans. V. W. Callahan, Fathers of the Church (Washington, DC, 1990), 29.

42 Gregory of Nyssa, *On Virginity* 21.2 (SC 199:506); trans. Callahan, 65.

43 *Rule of Basil* 57.1; Silvas, 155.

44 Evagrios of Pontos, *Ad Monachos* 6; trans. J. Driscoll, *The Ad Monachos of Evagrius Ponticus: Its Structure and a Select Commentary* (Rome, 1991), 13–15. G. Bunge, *Gastrimargia: Wissen und Lehre der Wüstenväter von Essen und Fasten dargestellt anhand der Schriften des Evagrios Pontikos* (Münster, 2012).

45 John Cassian, *Conferences* 5.14.

46 John Cassian, *Institutes* 18.

47 John Cassian, *Institutes* 5.5.

48 Cassian the Sabaite, *On the Eight Considerations of Evil*; trans., *A Newly Discovered Greek Father: Cassian the Sabaite Eclipsed by John Cassian of Marseilles*, ed. and trans. P. Tzamalikos (Leiden, 2012), 81.

49 Ibid.

to suppress his desire for honey (12.2). After a four-week fast, an angel provided him with spring water and "tender green plants." Helle followed the angel's invitation to partake in the divine provisions and "declared that he had never tasted anything more delicious (12.3)."[50] As a role model for acceptable conduct, Helle exemplified how one could achieve greater pleasure and taste through fasting.[51] If one could resist the temptation to eat, as Helle had, he would find even greater pleasures in the food provided by God, not by his fellow brothers. Pleasure in taste was permitted, therefore, if the food was granted by angelic beings. Similar stories of meals prepared by angels for the Virgin, saints, and other monastics illustrate that satisfaction in eating and drinking was permissible if one received the food from divine hands. Thus, in the *History of the Monks of Egypt* we read of several holy men, like Helle and Apollo, who did not rely upon the food provided by their communities or found in their own gardens, but rather they depended upon food prepared by angels. The food became a divine meal that highlighted the unique status of the monks as being pure, like Christ, the Virgin, John the Baptist, or Elijah. The fact that monastic authors spoke more about the dangers of eating than about the pleasure and benefits of eating suggests that tasting angelic food was not commonplace and only exceptional individuals could be singled out for divine feeding.

When we consider the different monastic settings in which monks encountered food and drink, we can begin to see how the social and spatial design of communities could shape monastic taste and attitudes toward experiencing food. Independent monks, living with either a few companions as at Mar Saba or in the loosely collected Egyptian monastic dwellings at Kellia, Wadi Natrun, and Manqabat, had apparently greater freedom in their meals than did monks in communal monasteries.[52] John Cassian recounts a story of visiting with Abba Serenus and how the monk offered food for them that departed, but did not exceed the cultural norm for dining in the more private dwellings.[53] Cassian goes to great lengths to explain a somewhat elaborate offering by Serenus to his guests who had returned to his cell after attending the liturgy. Rather than offer his guests just a few drops of oil, Serenus offered a "more liberal allowance of oil than usual" (8.1). Cassian explains to his community that this is not a sign of decadence nor for "any enjoyment from the taste of it," but rather it is for the practical purpose of "lin[ing] the passage of his throat and jaws" to allow the food to pass. For Cassian, he wants his readers to know that the Desert Fathers were not allowing the taste and pleasure of food to dictate their eating habits. Serenus provides a little extra oil for his guests because they are likely less accustomed to his more severe mode of eating, which required fewer drops of oil. Overall, the *Sayings of the Desert Fathers, The History of the Monks in Egypt,* and other early Egyptian sources point toward great diversity in monastic eating habits and taste in the independent settlements. An anonymous saying highlights the perceived freedom anchorites had in comparison with cenobites.[54] In one story some visiting monks from a communal settlement have a meal with a monk, who offers them food and fellowship. The guests comment to each other that the life of the ascetic seems more "restful" and thus the father decides to teach his guests a lesson about non-communal living. In the end, he sends them to a fellow monk who provides them with only a little bread and salt, and then pours a little vinegar on the salt. The meager food and lack of drink propelled the monks to sneak away as they feared the monk would keep them there and they wished to return to their own monastery, where they

50 *History of the Monks of Egypt* 12.2–4; trans., N. Russell, *The Lives of the Desert Father: The Historia Monachorum in Aegypto* (Kalamazoo, 1980), 90.

51 G. Frank, *The Memory of the Eyes: Pilgrims to Living Saints in Christian Late Antiquity* (Berkeley, 2000), 175. Frank discusses how Cyril of Jerusalem encouraged Eucharistic participants to taste and see God's goodness, but immediately Cyril discarded taste as being an unreliable sense.

52 For a survey of the archaeological evidence for independent monastic residences in Egypt see D. Brooks Hedstrom, "Divine Architects: Designing the Monastic Dwelling Place," in *Egypt in the Byzantine World, 450–700*, ed. R. Bagnall (Cambridge, 2007), 368–89; E. Wipszycka, *Moines et communautés monastiques en Égypte (IVe–VIIIe siècles)* (Varsovie, 2009), 206–17.

53 John Cassian, *Conferences* 8.1.

54 N229. English translation is *The Book of Elders: Sayings of the Desert Fathers: The Systematic Collection,* trans. J. Wortley (Trappist, KY, 2012), 180–81.

could eat better food. The story highlights the importance of not subjecting one's own ascetic taste for food and drink upon others, especially those coming from the communal monasteries. The stories illustrate how independent monks frequently found themselves offering hospitality to travelers, both monastic and lay, and unintentionally creating both anxiety and competition about what to eat or not for those not accustomed to personal choice.

In the communal monastic setting, the dangers in taste, pleasure, and emotional experiences with food appear throughout various rules and typika. In the establishment of a culture of communal living, there was a greater need to control food and drink to the point that monks were not allowed to eat in secret, were encouraged to eat what was given to them, and were admonished not to complain about the quality of the food. The early rules of Pachomius explicitly state that eating takes place in the monastic dining hall with little room for personal preferences or desires. Even the cook should not sample the food before the monks.[55] In his rules, Basil offers a fuller explanation about the interrelationship between the emotional, somatic, and sensorial associations with eating food: "Consequently, training in self-control is accomplished not only with regard to the pleasure of food, but also extends to abstinence from everything that harms us, by which we may be gratified but are also wounded in the soul."[56] In the thirteenth-century typikon for the convent of Lips in Constantinople, female monastics were warned that they should always be "satisfied" with the food set before them and not to use their rank, education, age, or virtue to extract different food to suit them.[57] By the fourteenth century, monastic typika describe in greater detail the dangers of devouring food and eating in secret. Makarios Choumnos's *Testament* for Nea Mone in Thesalonike offers a sophisticated understanding of taste as being individualized. He concedes that at times monks will observe variations within the community, especially when a brother is ill. He explains that standards differ and may require better wine to help cure a fellow monastic: "But everyone's constitution is not the same, nor are their bodies the same, but we know that just as there is a great difference in men's appearances, so too in their constitutions and bodies, and there is a great variety of knowledge and differentiation among them."[58] Nearly a millennium earlier than Choumnos, Shenoute warned that the men and women in his Egyptian communities should not touch or taste forbidden food. Even the mere thought could foster the emotional desire to attain coveted food items such as picked fish, garum, cheese, milk, and eggs.[59] In communal settings, the preparation of food for the monastic table was in the hands of a single cook and his attendants. They provided the food necessary for a community of healthy monks, along with additional foods for those who were in the infirmary or were nonmonastic visitors.[60] Grumbling led to envy and thus the lack of tasting what one wanted could foster disruptions within the community.[61]

In addition to offering daily admonitions about the monastic table, monastic authorities were equally concerned with the process of tasting and consuming the Eucharist.[62] If earthly food was dangerous, could the same be said of the Eucharist? Was the same restraint required when eating the bread and drinking the wine? Cyril of Jerusalem (ca. 315–386) invoked Psalm 34:8 (LXX 33:9), "O taste and see that the Lord is good!" saying that one must cultivate a spiritual palate. He writes, "It is not your bodily palate which is to be the judge of this, but unwavering faith. For tasting it is not bread and wine that

55 Precepts 74.

56 *Long Rules* 19–20. A. Silvas, *The Asketikon of St. Basil the Great* (Oxford, 2005), 207.

57 Lips 29, *BMFD* 3:1274.

58 Choumnos, *Testament* B21, *BMFD* 4:1451.

59 Layton, *Canons of Our Fathers*, nos. 74, 75.

60 B. Layton, "Social Structure and Food Consumption in an Early Christian Monastery: The Evidence of Shenoute's Canons and the White Monastery Federation A.D. 385–465," *Museon* 115 (2002): 25–56; A. Crislip, *From Monastery to Hospital: Christian Monasticism and the Transformation of Health Care in Late Antiquity* (Ann Arbor, 2005), 90.

61 Talbot summaries a satirical poem by Ptochoprodromos in which the monastic meal reflects the privileges afforded those of higher rank with delicacies for the senior monks and a diet of bare subsistence for the novices. "Mealtime in Monasteries" (n. 38 above), 118–19.

62 See A. McGowan, *Ascetic Eucharists: Food and Drink in Early Christian Ritual Meals* (Oxford, 1999).

you taste, but the body and blood of Chris which they signify."[63] Here, Cyril of Jerusalem presents a central concern that consuming the sacraments should not be based upon the sense of sight or taste. Instead he argues, "[Y]ou have learnt and are fully convinced that that which appears to be bread is not bread even though it seems so to the taste, but the body of Christ, and that which appears to be wine is not wine, even though taste suggests it, but the blood of Christ."[64] Eucharistic tasting is sacred tasting and therefore it negates the daily preferences of taste usually associated with food and drink. Like the sweet water that Abba Helle drank, the Eucharist provides heavenly food that cannot be tied to the base sense of bodily taste.

One of the clearest articulations of the role of taste as the enjoyment of the process of eating is from Dorotheos of Gaza (ca. 500–565). He describes two forms of gluttony in his discourse on the Lenten Fast. The first form of gluttony directly addresses taste as a sense by which one has a preference for good food. He recognizes that some individuals wish to eat because the food is appetizing. Taste, for Dorotheos, is inseparably linked to the pleasure of the act of eating. He describes how a monk "keeps the food in his mouth, rolling it round and round, and has not the heart to swallow it because he enjoys the taste."[65] The pleasure is literally a "madness of the palate" (λαιμαργία) in contrast to gluttony (γαστριμαργία), the second and better-known vice. Unlike the pleasure of the palate, or taste, gluttony is the pleasure of satiation and is not linked to the process of eating. More than the former pleasurable tasting, the consumption of food in large amounts is truly gluttonous. The monk who eats to please his stomach does not "ask for fancy food nor does he care especially about whether the taste is nice or not, he only wants to eat and fill his stomach."[66] Dorotheos's discussion of tasting and levels of consumption offers one of the more developed sensorial readings of taste. Often *laimargia* appears in lists of vices and can mean a love for delicacies, or special food. In a monastic context, reading *laimargia* as "madness for delicacies" reflects perhaps a very real temptation for some men and women who struggled with the mundane ascetic diet.[67]

Desire to have food could be engendered by one's work in the community as a farmer or gardener. Monastic gardens and fields provided a variety of grains, fruits, and vegetables for harvest and were supervised by monks.[68] The farmer and gardener then provided the needed food items to the cooks and their assistants. While the literary evidence outlines idealized habits for preparing foods and a limited course of food items, archaeological studies reveal that monks between the sixth and tenth centuries were eating a wide array of prepared foods from these kitchens.[69]

Archaeobotanical and Archaeozoological Clues to Monastic Taste

To assess the validity of the idealized relationship with monastic food, archaeobotantial remains recovered from monastic sites, such as in middens, latrines, monastic gardens, and samples from ceramic assemblages, contribute a diverse body of evidence for analysis.[70] Data recovered from archaeobotanical and archaeozoological samples demonstrate the limits of the literary narrative of monastic diet. The archaeological evidence

63 Cyril of Jerusalem, *On the Mysteries* 5.20; trans., *Documents in Early Christian Thought*, ed. M. Wiles and M. Santer (Cambridge, 1975), 193.

64 Cyril of Jerusalem, *On the Mysteries* 4.9; trans. Wiles and Santer, 190.

65 Dorotheos of Gaza, *On the Holy Lenten Fast*, trans. E. P. Wheeler, *Discourses and Sayings* (Kalamazoo 1970), 216–17.

66 Ibid.

67 In the eighth century, John of Damascus (ca. 660–750) wrote a short treatise *On Virtues and Vices* where he lists virtues and vices connected with food. Of the twenty-five virtues, four relate specifically to eating and drinking, including fasting, eating dry food, eating slowly, and drinking nothing but water. The positive habits of tasting, or the act of eating and drinking, counteract the passions of the body involving food. Gluttony (*gastrimargia*), eating delicacies (*laimargia*), drunkenness, and eating in secret are offered as the vices linking the sense of taste to passions of the body. John of Damascus, *On Virtues and Vices*; trans., G. E. H. Palmer et al., *The Philokalia*, vol. 2 (London, 1981), 334–35. PG 95:85–97.

68 Dalby, *Flavours of Byzantium*; idem, *Siren Feasts* (both n. 23 above).

69 Layton, "Social Structure."

70 D. Brooks Hedstrom, S. Davis, T. Herbich. S. Ikram, D. McCormack, M.-D. Nenna, and G. Pyke, "New Archaeology at Ancient Scetis: Surveys and Initial Excavations at the Monastery of St. John the Little in Wadi al-Natrun: Yale Monastic Archaeology Project," *DOP* 64 (2010): 217–28.

reflects a more complex story of what monks were growing, cooking, and possibly eating. As an essential part of the archaeology of food, archaeobotany can help us see what monks ate, what fuels they used, and if the food was locally available. Additionally, bioarchaeological studies of dental and skeletal remains offer clues to alterations in diet and overall health of monastic residents.[71]

A recent and comprehensive study of the bioarchaeological evidence from the Byzantine monastery at Kom el-Nana, in Middle Egypt, points to a diverse and nutritious monastic diet prepared by cooks.[72] Although monastic diets were primarily vegetarian in theory, the zooarchaeological assemblages at Kom el-Nana provide substantial evidence for the consumption of fish and mammals within an unquestioned monastic context. But what can we deduce from the presence of such bones? The discard areas for the bones appear in two separate middens, suggesting two areas for food preparation. One includes only bird and fish bones whereas the other includes bones of butchered mammals.[73] The location for these different categories of discarded bones reflects two workshops for food preparation. Does any evidence exist to demonstrate what animals monks were eating, if any? Based upon the recovered remains, we know dishes were prepared using beef, pork, sheep, goats, fish, chicken, pigeons, and doves.[74] However, the mere evidence of these meats in the remains is not enough to prove they were part of daily monastic cuisine. It is important to recognize that several animals were raised at monasteries to be used in meals for visitors and for ill monks. Cows could be used for milk, chickens for eggs, and sheep for parchment. In thinking about the multifaceted practical needs for such a wide range of animals, it may help us understand why monastics who subsisted on a more limited diet faced a constant temptation to want different food to taste.

In general, monastic textual accounts portray healthy monastics in late antiquity as embracing exclusively a plant-based diet. Yet, Sarah Clackson convincingly demonstrated that the monastic diet in Egypt included a healthy dose of fish, as she observed at the Monastery of Apollo at Bawit. Her analysis of both textual and archaeological evidence from the site illustrated the importance of interdisciplinary work on monastic material, but also showed how earlier scholars had overlooked the presence of fish due to an unwillingness to accept that monks were eating fish.[75] Bawit has yielded over 190 ostraca related to food items. Of those 45% related to wine, 25% address accounting of wheat, and 20% with the sale or collection of fish. The remaining 10% deal with all other organic material, such as onions, barley, and vegetables.[76] In reading the documentary evidence and reconsidering the earlier excavated remains, Clackson concluded that the inhabitants of the monastery regularly ate pickled and

71 Perhaps the most informative Byzantine Near East settlement to illustrate the importance of bioarchaeological analysis is the work at St. Stephen's in Jerusalem. See L. A. Gregoricka and S. G. Sheridan, "Ascetic or Affluent? Byzantine Diet at the Monastic Community of St. Stephen's Jerusalem from Stable Carbon and Nitrogen Isotopes," *Journal of Anthropological Archaeology* 32, no. 1 (2013): 63–73; eaedem, "Food for Thought: Isotopic Evidence for Dietary and Weaning Practices in a Byzantine Urban Monastery in Jerusalem," in *Bioarchaeology and Behavior*, ed., C. S. Larsen et al. (Gainesville, 2012). Few sites in Egypt have monastic burials available for analysis although the recent study at Naqlun, for example, offers an indication of promising results. See E. Jaskulska, "Skeletal Bilateral Asymmetry in a Medieval Population from Deir an-Nalqun (Nekloni), Egypt," *Bioarchaeology of the Near East* 3 (2009): 17–26; D. Dzierzbicka and M. Ozarek, "Two Burials from Cemetery A in Naqlun: Archaeological and Anthropological Remarks," *Polish Archaeology in the Mediterranean* 21 (2012): 233–43. For comparative illustrations in the monastic West see C. Polet and M. A. Katzenberg, "Reconstruction of the Diet in a Mediaeval Monastic Community from the Coast of Belgium," *Journal of Archaeological Science* 30, no. 5 (2003): 525–33.

72 W. Smith, *Archaeobotanical Investigations of Agriculture at Late Antique Kom el-Nana (Tell el-Amarna)* (London, 2003). Monastic burials were not available for comparative analysis.

73 R. M. Luff, "Monastic Diet in Late Antique Egypt: Zooarchaeological Finds from Kom el-Nana and Tell el-Amarna, Middle Egypt," *Environmental Archaeology* 12 (2007): 161–74. For a comparable study illustrating the richness of the monastic diet see Gregoricka and Sheridan, "Ascetic or Affluent?"

74 Polet and Katzenberg, "Reconstruction." The different types of middens at the monastery may suggest a wide variety of reuse activities associated with organic evidence in a secondary or tertiary process.

75 S. Clackson, "Fish and Chits: The Synodonts Schall," *Zeitschrift für ägyptische Sprache und Altertumskunde* 129, no. 1 (2002): 6–11, eadem, "Something Fishy in CPR XX," *Archiv für Papyrusforschung und verwandte Gebiete* 45 (1999): 94–95.

76 W. Van Neer et al., "Salted Fish Products from the Coptic Monastery at Bawit, Egypt: Evidence from the Bones and Texts," in *The Role of Fish in Ancient Time*, ed. H. H. Plogmann (Rahden, 2007), 154.

dried Nile catfish.[77] Fish provided the protein needed in a monk's diet, similar to that found in eggs, cheese, and milk.[78] Interestingly, the documents for the Monastery of Apollo, which is thirteen kilometers inland from the Nile, suggest that the salted fish products were produced on the monastic estates closer to the Nile and then delivered to the monastery. The study of the salted fish products at Bawit reconstructs an active monastic fishing industry at the monastery that included the use of monastic boats, the facilities for pickling fish, and the reuse of wine amphoras for storing pickled fish.[79]

The preparation of fish and the related fish sauce, *garum*, required both containers for long-term storage and physical space for the fish to rest in salt and ferment. Salt provided cooks with an essential ingredient not just for adding flavor to food, but also in preserving food such as fish and olives.[80] Salting was the most efficient way to preserve food. A cook would first clean the fish and then create two items: first, salted fish for meals and second, garum as a condiment. For salted fish, the ceramic vessel would need a lid and to be kept out of the sun, so as not to cook the contents. However, the production of garum needed intensive sun and for several months, likely requiring garum ceramic vessels to be kept in a courtyard rather than in the kitchen.[81]

77 R. M. Luff and Geoffrey N. Bailey, "Analysis of Size Changes and Incremental Growth Structures in African Catfish *Synodontis schall* (Schall) from Tell El-Amarna, Middle Egypt," *Journal of Archaeological Science* 27, no. 9 (2000): 821–35; eidem, "The Aquatic Basis of Ancient Civilizations: The Case of *Synodontis schall* an the Nile Valley," in *Human Ecodynamics*, ed. G. Bailey, R. Charles, and N. Winder (Oxford, 2000), 100–113.

78 C. Nash, *The History of Aquaculture* (Ames, IA, 2011), 6. A. Jotischky, *A Hermit's Cookbook: Monks, Food and Fasting in the Middle Ages* (London, 2011), 86–90.

79 W. Van Neer et al., "Salted Fish Products"; W. Van Neer and D. Depraetere, "Pickled Fish from the Egyptian Nile: Osteological Evidence from a Byzantine (Coptic) Context at Shanhûr," *Revue de Paléobiologie* 10 (2005): 159–70; W. Van Neer et al., "The Roman Trade in Salted Nilotic Fish Products: Some Examples from Egypt," *Documenta Archaeobiologiae* 4 (2006): 173–88.

80 Bo Pachomius 55. Veilleux, *Pachomian Koinonia*, 75.

81 Nash, *History of Aquaculture*, 4. "Salts in crystal form rubbed into the flesh before it is dried can preserve products for many weeks. If salts are applied instead in solutions of varying concentrations, they can pickle or ferment whole products that can be kept in pots for many months to years."

Archaeology of Byzantine Monastic Taste and Cooking

The archaeology of taste brings our attention to the spaces in which food was prepared by cooks and bakers. As ones who created meals for a variety of monastic communities, did cooks and bakers influence ascetic taste? A variety of facilities such as mills, olive presses, and wine presses helped cooks and bakers prepare and gather the ingredients for monastic meals.[82] A funerary relief from Rome of the baker Marcus Vergillius Eurysaces provides an excellent visual record of the production of bread. The tomb's first-century BCE frieze documents the arrival of grain, the milling process, the screening of the flour, kneading on boards, baking bread in a large beehive oven, and the eventual distribution of the bread.[83]

While the relief is several centuries removed from late antique monastic bakeries, many of the activities it records—of milling, kneading dough, and baking and distributing bread—appear also in monastic textual sources. In many cases the descriptions of Egyptian monastic kitchens and food production are embedded in stories where an author's food bias strongly overshadows stories of one's relationship to *prepared* food.[84] The cooks and the head bakers were given control over their spaces and other monks, even those who were housemasters of communal monasteries, were not allowed to enter the kitchen and demand special food.[85] Therefore the cooks monitored access to food in cenobitic communities such as the Pachomian and Shenoutean. The many Byzantine monastic kitchen facilities, storage areas, and cooking equipment assist us in thinking about how the act of cooking relates to taste. In shifting the focus away from the food consumed to the food produced, we can envision how the cooks and the bakers contributed to

82 K. Ahmet, "A Middle Byzantine Olive Press Room at Aphrodisias," *Anatolian Studies* 51 (2001): 159–67; P. Mayerson, "The Wine and Vineyards of Gaza in the Byzantine Period," *BASOR* 257 (1985): 75–80.

83 For frieze see P. Ciancio Rossetto, *Il sepolcro del fornaio marco Virgilio Eurisace a Porta Maggiore* (Rome, 1973); H. Lamer, *Römische Kulture im Bilde* (Leipzig, 1915), fig. 145.

84 D. Samuel, "Bread in Archaeology," *Civilizations* 49, nos. 1–2 (2002): 34.

85 Precepts 41.

perceptions of taste for their guests at the monastic table. By doing so, we are granting prominence to those monks who worked in the kitchens and bakeries, but are often not studied.

Difficulties in managing the preparation and distribution of food appear prominently in the writings associated with Shenoutean and Pachomian monastic communities. Bentley Layton's analysis of Shenoute's monastic rules reveals the complexity of concerns relating to how to live in a community and to monitor the eating of those who lived there.[86] Specifically related to food, Shenoute addresses serious concerns with monks stealing food from the storeroom; jealousies over the food eaten by the sick; and unhealthy power dynamics whereby a distributor of the food gave larger and tastier portions to her friends and not others.[87] Eating or drinking in secret is prohibited.[88] Cooking may have happened only once a week and those in charge of the food needed to monitor it for spoilage and not to be wasteful.[89] Knowing that even in the general refectory monks could envy the food of others, Shenoute and Pachomius both recognized the need to have separate eating areas for the sick, whose richer meals would certainly engender envy and grumbling by others. From these sources we learn about food anxiety and its importance for both physical and spiritual health. However, monastic authors do not address in-depth how food was prepared or produced.[90]

Cooks prepared food for four different populations: monks, young monks, ill monks, and visitors. These groups had different needs and expectations. But it was the monastic cooks who decided what was presented at the table. A famous story in the *Rules of Pachomius* illustrates how a cook made a decision to stop preparing cooked food and offer a completely raw diet of mustard greens and lettuce with garlic, vinegar, and oil. When Pachomius learned that the cook had refused to prepare cooked vegetables for the monks, he rebuked him, stating that it was not his place to interfere with monastic diet.[91] And yet, according to the story, the monks did not complain until a young boy brought the problem to Pachomius after two months. Shenoute also worried about the changes to the taste of food when he specified that "no omissions or additions shall be made, nor shall any extra ingredients be added to them so as to change their recipe, by adding oil to the brined anchovies (or garum) or salt or *charlock* or any thing else upon our tables in our refectories except only in the infirmaries."[92] Understanding that cooks were the gatekeepers of taste helps us appreciate the stories of monks pretending to be sick in order to get some variation in their diet.

Ethnoarchaeology and Experimental Archaeology

Ethnoarchaeology, both historical and contemporary, equips us to examine the kitchens and bakeries that were part of the early Byzantine world. We can see paths of continuity in cooking methods and the introduction of innovations in preparation methods. For ethnoarchaeologial examples of cooking, we can document the process of contemporary bread making and cooking in the villages that dot the Nile valley. The ovens (Ar. *furn*/pl. *afrān*) and stoves (Ar. *kānūn*/ pl. *kawānīn*) are made of the same materials used throughout Egypt's history (fig. 10.1). The modern examples provide informative parallels to assist us in understanding premodern food preparation activities (fig. 10.2). In employing the methodologies of experimental archaeology, whereby one recreates past materials and processes through replication, we can see what type of clay was needed to build an oven and then test similar materials found in excavations to study what fuels may have been needed to bake bread or cook vegetables.[93] Twigs, chaff, food

86 Layton, *Canons of Our Fathers*, 52.

87 R. Krawiec, *Shenoute and the Women of the White Monastery: Egyptian Monasticism in Late Antique Egypt* (Oxford, 2002), 35–36.

88 Shenoute, *Rules* 151; trans. Layton, 151.

89 Shenoute, *Rules* 179, 180; trans. Layton, 161.

90 Exception would be the long section in the *Regulations of Horsiesios*. It is Egypt's closest example of what will be known later in Byzantium as the monastic *typikon* (*BMFD* 1:34).

91 Rules 16. *Pachomian Chronicles and Rules*, 2, trans., 38.

92 Shenoute, *Rules* 316; trans. Layton, 223 (Canon 5. XS325 = L.IV:55).

93 See the results of one case study in N. Mulder-Heymans, "Archaeology, Experimental Archaeology and

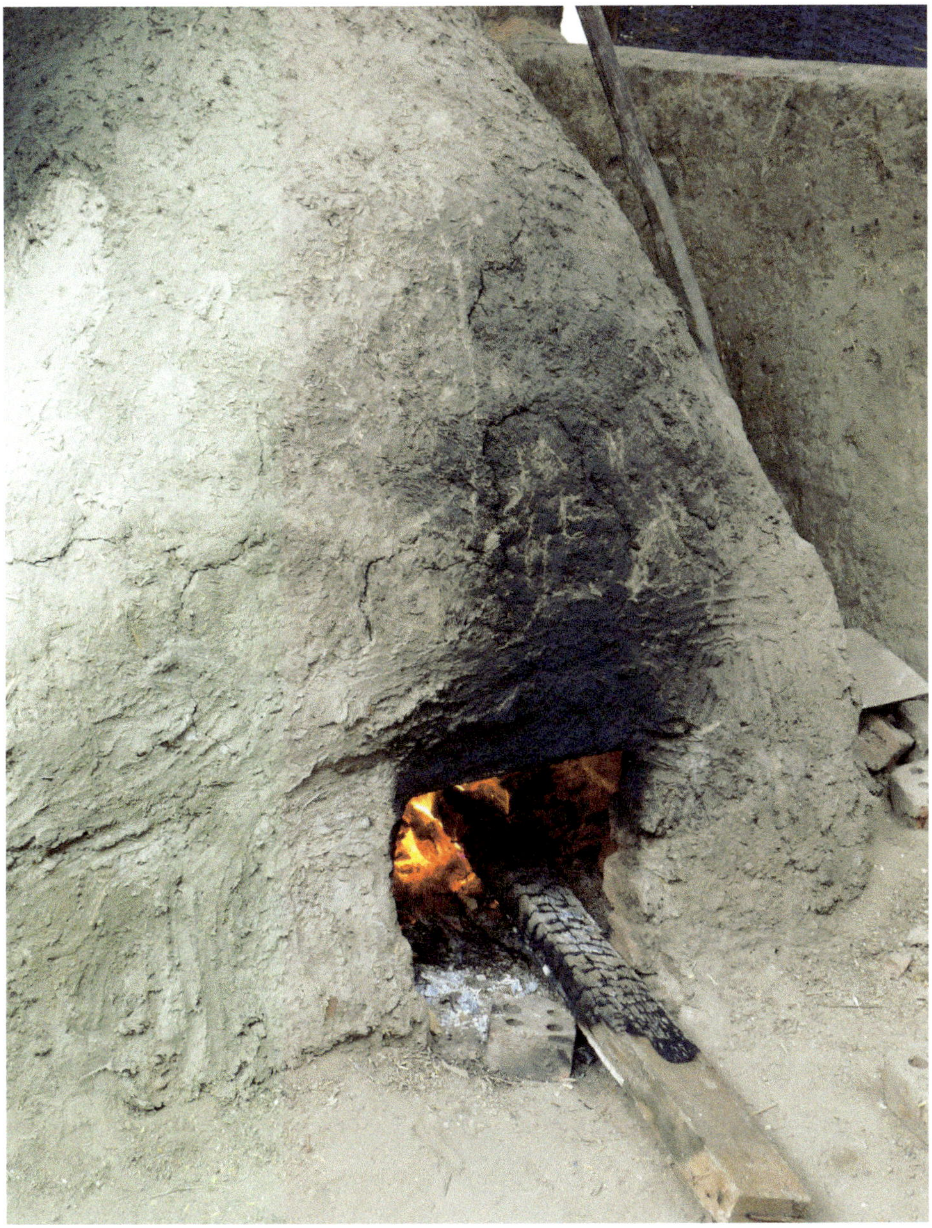

FIG. 10.1. Modern oven, Cairo, Egypt (photo: author)

by-products, and dung cakes provide different heating temperatures that help in the preparation of a variety of food items.[94] The documentary evidence from monastic sites recounts the delivery of firewood and the role of the dung carrier in distributing needed fuel to both the monasteries and the villages.[95] The variety of fuel sources reflects conscious choices by bakers and cooks in how to maintain low heat for cooking and high heat for the baking of bread.[96] The

Ethnoarchaeology on Bread Ovens in Syria," *Civilizations* 49 (2002): 197–221.

94 W. Smith, "Fuel for Thought: Archaeobotanical Evidence for the Use of Alternatives to Wood Fuel in Late Antique North Africa," *Journal of Mediterranean Archaeology* 11, no. 2 (1998): 191–205.

95 *P.Princ.* 3.154 is from Oxyrhynchos and is dated 7 Sept. 546. It is an account of an agreement between Christodorus, the dung carrier, and Aurelios Praous, the baker, regarding the receipt of 1 gold solidus, possibly for the delivery of dung brought on the baker's donkey.

96 We are fortunate to have at Dumbarton Oaks an additional source of ethnoarchaeological material to consult for the study of monastic kitchens in Egypt. Between 1929 and 1932, Thomas Whittemore traveled to Egypt, on behalf of the Byzantine Institute, to document the paintings at the Coptic Monasteries

FIG. 10.2.
Baking the Holy Bread, 1930–31. The Red Sea Monasteries, Egypt, Byzantine Institute Photographs, ICFA. BI_DO.REDSEA.0003 (photo: Dumbarton Oaks, Image Collections and Fieldwork Archives. Washington, DC, Trustees for Harvard University)

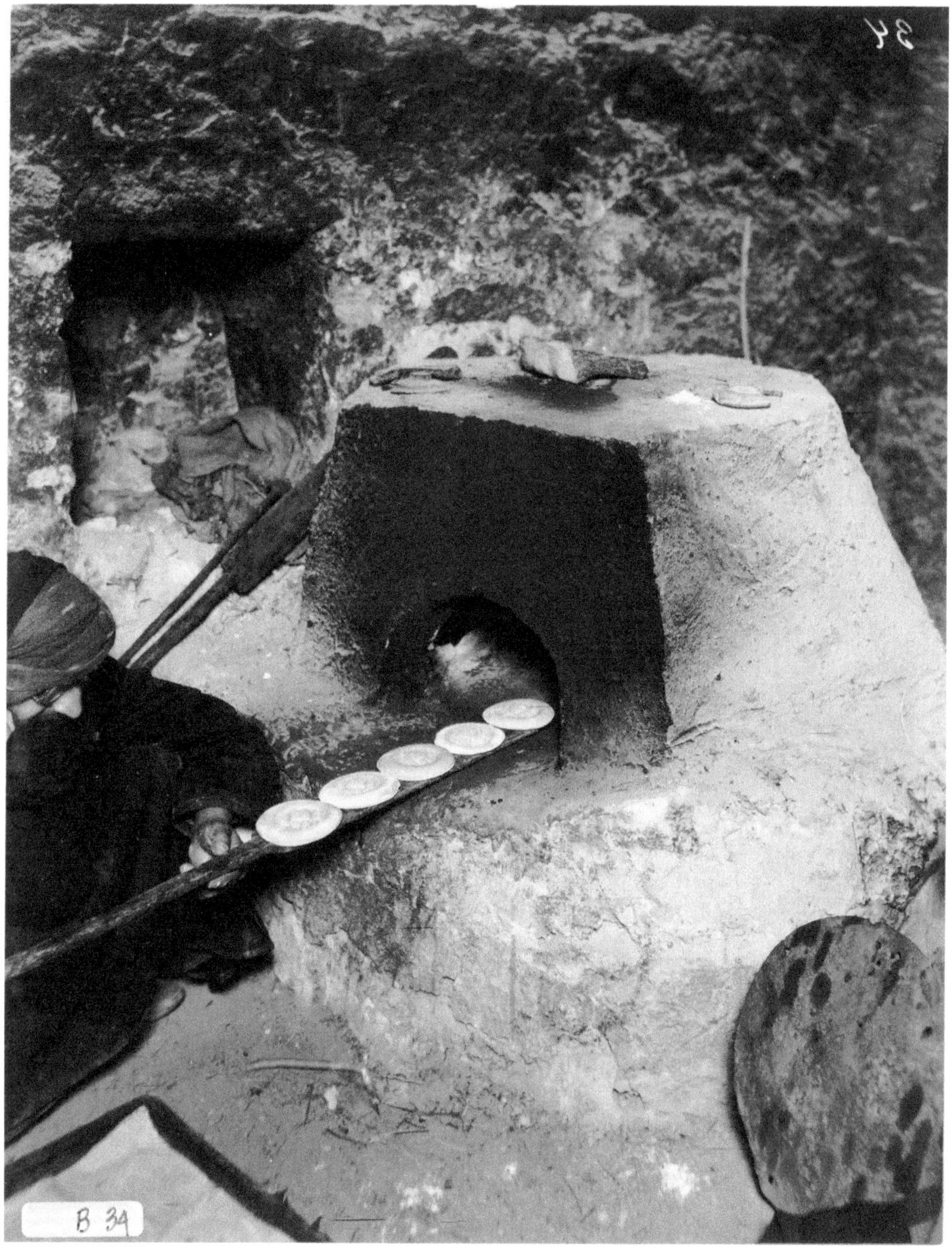

physical design of the ovens and the kitchens also provides clues for how to regard the ceramic vessels used in preparing food, and thus allow us to understand and more accurately interpret the use of cookers, lids, and large zirs for mixing or sorting food items.[97]

of St. Antony and St. Paul by the Red Sea. While his main objective was to document the Coptic art and not to produce an ethnographic account of early twentieth-century monasticism, his expedition produced a short, silent film of daily life at the monasteries and photographed several areas within. The film was recently digitized by Dumbarton Oaks. See Dumbarton Oaks, *Before Byzantium: The Early Activities of Thomas Whittemore (1871–1931); Red Sea Monasteries, Egypt.* http://www.doaks.org/resources/online-exhibits/a-truthful-record/history/red-sea-monastery (accessed 15 November 2016).

97 L. Joyner, "Cooking Pots as Indicators of Cultural Change: A Petrographic Study of Byzantine and Frankish

The Archaeology of Monastic Cooking and Taste

The majority of cooking areas in Byzantine and Islamic domestic housing were found in open courtyards of homes or shared between housing units in a communal areas. The closest parallel to these early Byzantine kitchens are those found in the Middle Byzantine Cappadocian elite estates.[98] The placement of monastic kitchens or cooking areas therefore provides important information about the spatial configuration of monastic settlements and how they compare with lay, domestic spaces. Excavated monastic kitchens from Egypt include two central components. The first feature is the bread oven, elevated on a platform for easy access. The second feature, located at the base of a pier, is the U-shaped fire pit that is not described in any detail in our written sources. Together the two heating features parallel those found in earlier pharaonic-, Roman-, and Byzantine-period sites.[99] The oven is essential for allowing a fire to burn within while a baker places bread along the walls of the oven. The oven is roughly 1.0–1.5 meters in height, to facilitate easy access to the fire and the bread.[100] The oven is ideally located in a corner of a room, especially in a courtyard, where it can generate heat without creating discomfort in other places in the house. Smoke from the fire then leaves the oven through the "eye" while the bread bakes. A flue, often made with the neck of a broken amphora, offers an easy access point for monitoring fuel.

The kānūn is a cooking feature that appears in later medieval Islamic cookbooks as a type of easily assembled stove or fireplace. The U-shaped firebox makes it easy for cooks to put in a variety of fuels and to allow food to simmer for several hours. In most cases the kānūn is a stove used for the cooking of vegetables, stews, soups, and any foods needing constant heat monitoring. In the monastic kitchens, multiple kawānīn were built directly onto a mud brick counter to create the Byzantine equivalent of a modern stove (fig. 10.3).[101] The feature is designed to allow the cook to stand and work efficiently without the need to crouch down and cook near the floor. The stove may include an opening for holding fuel or function as a warming chamber. While ash accumulated in kitchens, waste from the preparation of food rarely did so to the same degree within the buildings.[102]

The evidence available for studying the archaeology of monastic cooking in Egypt is remarkably rich. The Monastery of Jeremias at Saqqara offers a rare look into the spatial organization of a large communal monastery. Since we do not possess any physical remains of the monasteries that were part of Pachomius's *koinonia*, we can look at the sixth-century Monastery of Jeremias to see how a large community organized itself spatially. The site is also important as one of the first monasteries to be excavated in Egypt. The architectural layout reflects the communal cooking structure outlined in the communal monastic orders in Upper Egypt. One Pachomian rule clearly states, "No one may cook foods outside the monastery and the kitchen."[103] And Shenoute establishes similar parameters for those at the White Monastery in that all healthy monks followed the same diet and were not allowed to have food in greater quantity or quality than others.[104] Therefore, the Monastery

Cooking Wares from Corinth," *Hesperia* 76, no. 1 (2007): 183–227; Sarah R. Graff, "Culinary Preferences: Seal-Impressed Vessels from Western Syria as Specialized Cookware," in Graff and Rodríguez-Alegría, *Menial Art* (n. 34 above), 19–46; T. M. Brogan and K. A. Barnard, "Household Archaeology at Mochlos: Statistical Recipes from the Late Minoan I Kitchen," *Hesperia* Supplement 44 (2011): 185–98.

98 V. Kalas, "The Byzantine Kitchen in the Domestic Complexes of Cappadocia," in *Archaeology of the Countryside in Medieval Anatolia*, ed. T. Vorderstrasse and J. Roodenberg (Leiden, 2009).

99 D. D. E. Depraetere, "A Comparative Study on the Construction and the Use of the Domestic Bread Oven in Egypt during the Graeco-Roman and Late Antique/Early Byzantine Period," *MDAIK* 58 (2002): 119–56.

100 Mulder-Heymans, "Archaeology." More commonly in the archaeological record the oven is placed on the ground and the baker sits or stoops in order to access the opening for fuel and to place the bread inside the oven.

101 F. Bonnet, "Les cuisines des Kellia," in *Explorations aux Qouçoûr er-Roubâ'îyât: Rapport des campagnes 1982 et 1983*, ed. R. Kasser et al. (Louvain, 1994), 181–83.

102 Ibid., 264 (Room 9) in building QR 533.

103 Pachomius, *Rule* 80. *Pachomian Chronicles and Rules*, trans. A. Veilleux, vol. 2 (Kalamazoo, 1981), trans., 159.

104 Excavation work was generously supported in 2006 and 2007 by a Dumbarton Oaks Project Grant in Byzantine Studies. Unfortunately, we did not discover the location of the kitchens that Shenoute speaks of during those seasons.

FIG. 10.3. Modern kānūn from a village by Asyut (photo: author)

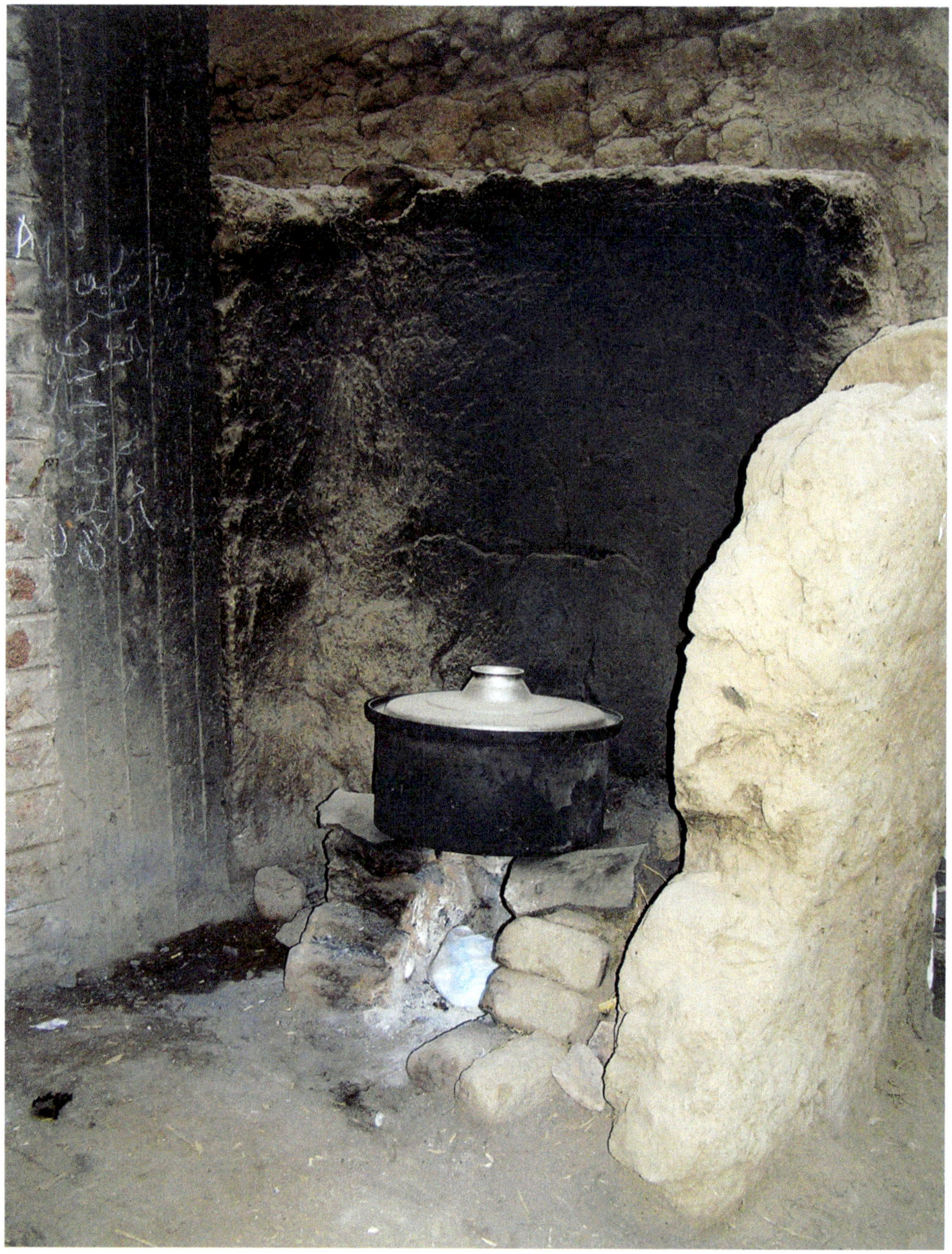

of Jeremias provides crucial information for us about site design.

The site plan for the monastery shows streets, footpaths, alleys, residential quarters, an infirmary, and churches (fig. 10.4). Overall, the entire site had nine formal cooking areas with freestanding ovens (fig., 10.5).[105] If the excavators observed any kawānīn, they did not record them or recognize them as such. It may also be the case that many residents used portable fireboxes in ceramic form to warm their dwelling. The ostraca from the site attest to the sale of dung, probably

105 J. Quibell, *Excavations at Saqqara*, vol. 4, *1908–9, 1909–10: The Monastery of Apa Jeremias* (Cairo, 1912). To the east and south of the church, Quibell excavated smaller residential areas, but did not always include details on his plans of the features of the rooms. His written description includes discussion of two rooms, 1943 and 2063, which both had ovens. Quibell included only seven of them on his comprehensive plan. Ibid., 10. Room 713 includes two mud brick ovens and a significant corpus of ceramics.

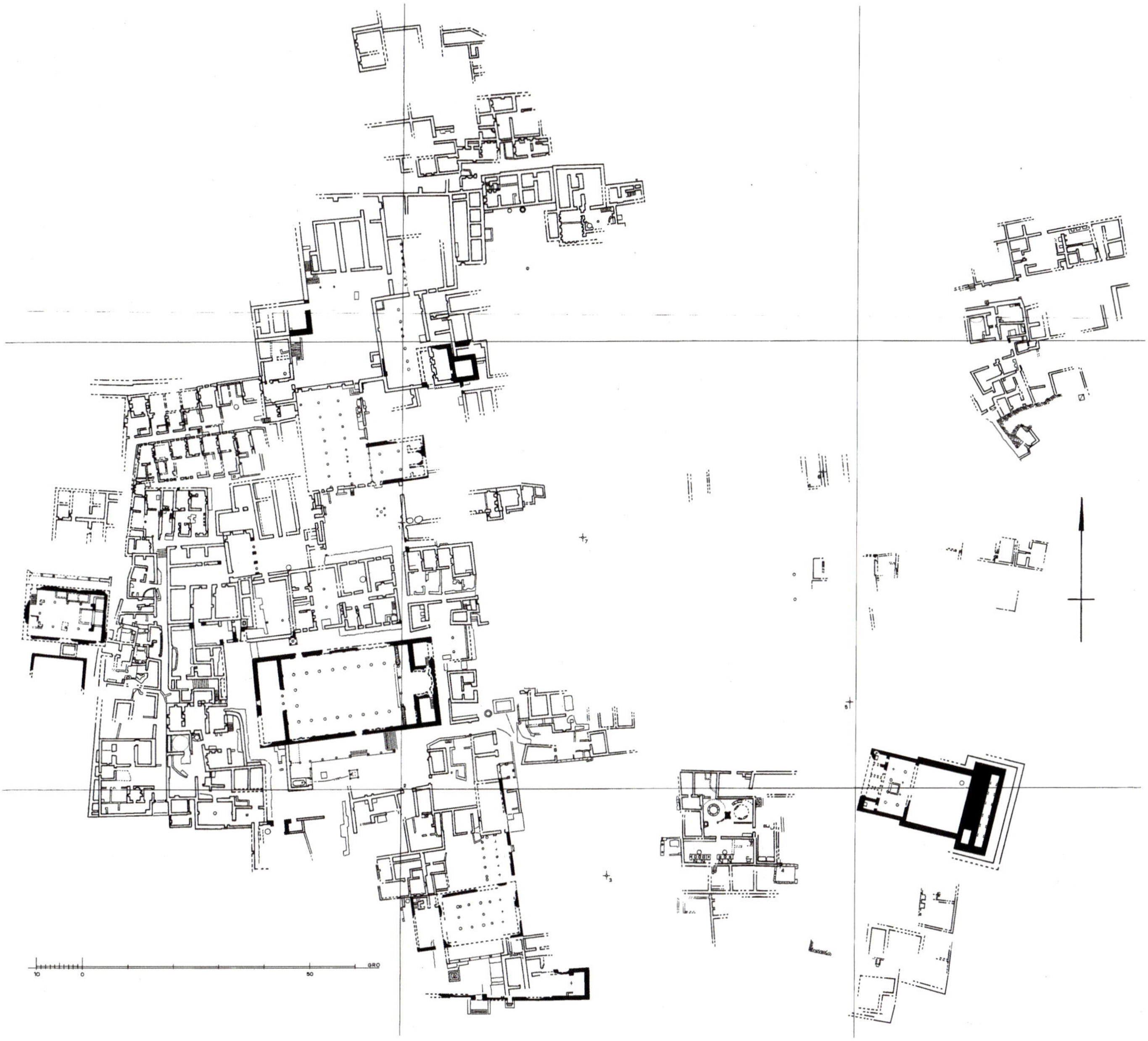

FIG. 10.4. Plan of the Monastery of Jeremias (plan: Peter Grossmann)

for fuel, the delivery of grain, and the use of wine and fish as payments.[106] All of these items would have moved through the monastic kitchens.

The ovens are spread across the site and reflect area bakeries within the monastery. The residential quarter on the west site of the settlement had three kitchens.[107] Other kitchens may have been used exclusively for the production of the Eucharistic bread, such as Rooms 704 and 713, adjacent to the main church.[108] In general, the bread ovens are made of bricks and built against the corner of rooms. The kitchen in Room 722 was accessible to both the refectory and the adjacent hospital.[109] The importance of cooking different foods for the ill is well attested in monastic sources.[110] Diets could

106 Ibid., #227; trans., 72.

107 Rooms 1835, 1843 and 1858. Ibid., 18 & 20.

108 Ibid., 9 and 101.

109 Ibid., 17.

110 See the work of Andrew Crislip and his examination of monastic health care. Crislip, *From Monastery* (n. 60 above); idem, *Thorns in the Flesh: Illness and Sanctity in Late Ancient Christianity* (Philadelphia, 2013).

FIG. 10.5. Two mud brick ovens in the food preparation area by the monastery's refectory. J. Quibell, *Excavations at Saqqara* 1905–1910 (Cairo, IFAO, 1907–12), plate II.

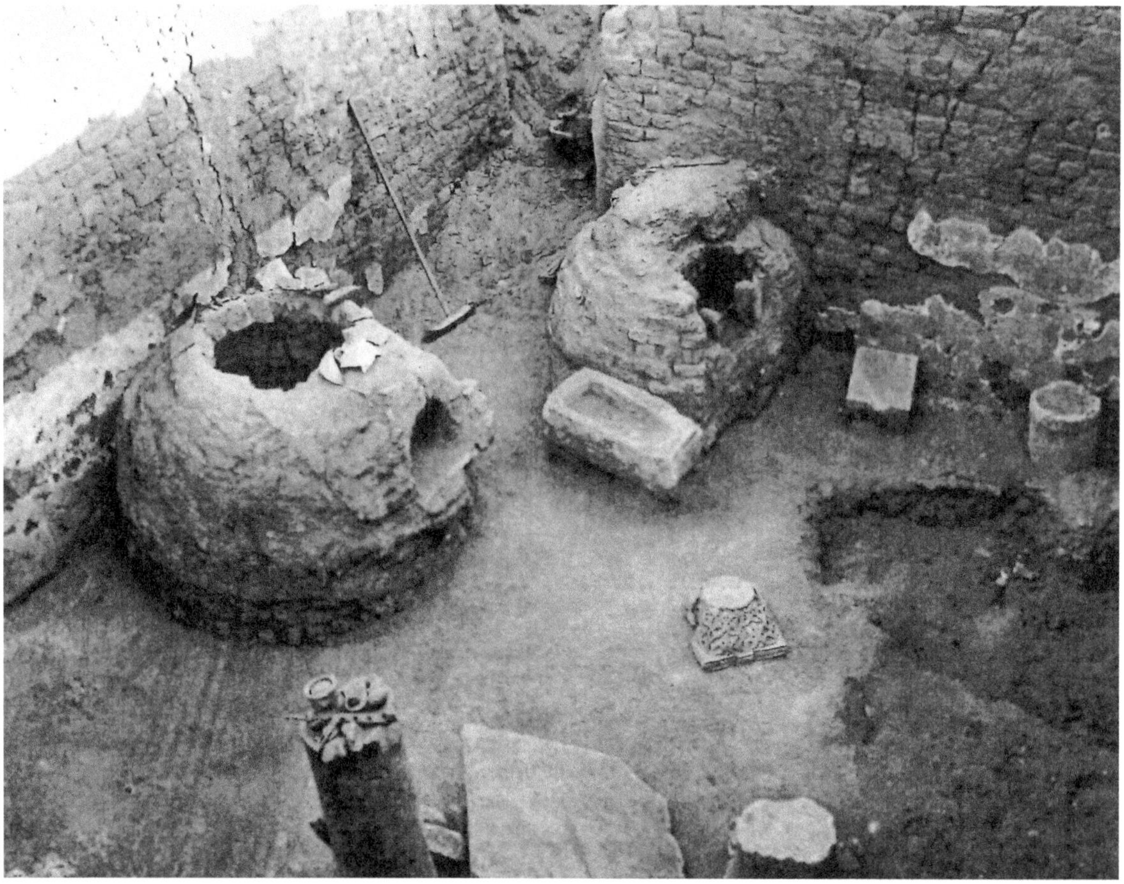

differ dramatically, and apparently temptingly so, between healthy and sick monks. Being sick certainly afforded one special privileges as many ailments were treated with variations in one's diet.[111] Healthy monks could not enter the communal kitchen, go to the storeroom, take food away from the infirmary, or even cook their own food; rather, they relied upon others for their specific dietary needs.[112]

The rules from Pachomius's and Shenoute's communities help contextualize the importance of refectories, kitchens, and bakeries as spaces linked to monitoring taste. For healthy monastics, the temptation to feign illness in order to gain access to tastier food was apparently a frequent occurrence.[113] Shenoute's *Rule* 427 explains that if ill monks want special food, they can have it prepared especially for them. Options included "boiled food, gruel, even *cauon*-drink, beer, or lentils."[114] Several other rules reveal monastics found opportunities to eat in private or to eat tastier food while working in the infirmary, traveling, or working at jobs associated with the bakery or the kitchen. At least three miracles occur in the *Life of Shenoute* that demonstrate Shenoute's ability to control milling; to increase bread in the storeroom; and to assist with the cleaning of the monastery's eleven ovens.[115] In the Pachomian rules, food production required complete quiet and spiritual diligence so that monastics would not imbue a product, such as dough, with unclean thoughts. In all these examples, the importance of regulating food production and consumption was a central concern for cenobitic members.

In contrast to the large communal monastery at Saqqara, the majority of Egyptian monasteries were smaller communities identified in Coptic

111 P. P. Bober, *Art, Culture, and Cuisine: Ancient and Medieval Gastronomy* (Chicago, 1999).

112 *Rules of Pachomius*, 41.

113 Layton, "Social Structure" (n. 60 above), 37–38.

114 Shenoute, *Rules* 427; trans. Layton, 273.

115 *Life of Shenoute* 20, 27–28, and 29.

dipinti and documentary evidence as "dwelling places" (*ma-n-shope*) or in Arabic, *manshubiyaat* (pl.). A *manshubiya* is a multiroomed residence that houses two to twenty monks; a collection of *manshubiyaat* may comprise a monastery. The southern settlements of Esna and 'Adaima are known for their unusual semi-subterranean dwellings, unique in Egyptian monastic architecture. Staircases lead from ground level to an open-air courtyard with clusters of rooms cut into the natural shale. Each of the sixth-century residences contains at least one kitchen.[116] The kitchen is usually a separate room located either to the east or west of the open-air courtyard.

Unlike the cenobitic sites that housed central kitchens, a *manshubiya* had its own, independent, kitchen as part of each residence. The monks in that house then had access to prepare their own food, to store it, and to create meals that would not be supervised by a chief baker or cook. In the example from Hermitage #5, the stove includes the kawānīn made with rims of broken ceramics to make an area for pots to rest over the fire. The kitchens had chimneys built directly into the wall to carry smoke up to the desert surface. The kitchens were not closed by doors, thereby allowing heat to move easily between the courtyard and the built-in chimney. All of the buildings had some built-in stove installation for a kitchen, but not all had bread ovens.[117] Unfortunately, we know little about the monks who lived here, but their kitchens reflect the spatial design of smaller, independent communities, in which the household was responsible for its own cooking.

Similar kitchen arrangements also exist north in the Fayuum at the site of Naqlun. The area consists of ninety *manshubiyaat* in the nearby hills with a church and cemetery for villagers at the base. The majority of the dwellings date to the late fifth and sixth centuries. The residences include a central courtyard, enclosed by a thin boundary wall, with radiating apartments cut into the cliffs on either side of a courtyard. In most cases, the excavators envisioned only one or two monks occupying each residence.[118] The largest *manshubiya* is a fifth-century residence with eighteen rooms around two courtyards for two monks.[119] The kitchen was located in the north corner of the courtyard in Room E and the smaller courtyard had two bread ovens.[120] The stove had two kawānīn. The monks who lived here could thereby make their own bread and be self-sufficient. Similarly, other dwellings at Naqlun have cooking facilities with at least one room dedicated specifically to cooking and built directly off of the courtyard. Hermitage 87 has a set of two kawānīn recessed in a niche and a bread oven in a separate room. The stove was made from a combination of mud daub (rough coating), stone, and mud mortar. The kawānīn sit side-by-side and allowed a cook to monitor two pots at the same time. Interestingly, most bread ovens were not built into the hill residences, but rather found on the desert plain below. Owing to the small nature of the rooms at Naqlun this building choice may reflect an environmental concern for the bakers and the heat generated in the smaller spaces.

Moving further north in Egypt, we have an abundance of archaeological evidence for the presence of independent monastic kitchens. The excavations at Kellia have recovered over 1500 monastic buildings and each includes at least one kitchen and as many as three. This would mean that in Kellia at any one time there could be over one thousand cooks preparing meals for the five to twenty monks living in each house. The archaeological evidence provides a very different picture of Kellia than what is found in the *Sayings of the Desert Fathers* and the writings of two of its most famous residents, John Cassian and Evagrios. In these sources we hear familiar

116 S. Sauneron and J. Jacquet, *Les ermitages chrétiens du désert d'Esna*, vol. 1 (Cairo, 1972), 18–24 and pl. VIII.

117 Ibid., 24–26 and pl. VII.

118 Hermitages 1, 2, 25, 44 and 89.

119 J. Leclant and A. Minault-Gout, "Fouilles et travaux en Égypte et au Soudan, 1997–1998," *Orientalia* 68, no. 4 (1999): 369. W. Godlewski, "Excavations 1997," *PAM* 9 (1998): 77–86; idem, "Naqlun: The Hermitage of Phibamon," in *Les civilisations du bassin méditerranéen: Hommages à Joachim Śliwa*, ed. K. M. Cialwicz and J. A. Ostrowski (Krakow, 2000), 93–98; idem, "Naqlun (Nekloni): The Hermitages, Cemetery and the Keep in the Early 6th Century," in *Graeco-Roman Fayum: Texts and Archaeology*, ed. S. L. Lippert and M. Schentulett (Wiesbaden, 2008), 101–12.

120 W. Godlewski and E. Parandowska, "Excavations 1996," *PAM* 8 (1997): 88–97.

themes about the concern with limiting consumption of food in general, avoiding pleasure in tasting, and the need to restrict one's attraction to tasty food. However, the individualization of the spaces at the *manshubiyaat* offer a physically close environment of monastic housing that is not immediately apparently in the *Sayings* nor in the accounts of Evagrios and Cassian. In one account, Makarios the Great observes Satan dressed as a pauper and heading toward Kellia.[121] Satan carries food for the brothers to "taste" and shares with Makarios that he has a variety of foods so that there will be something for everyone. In this account, it is clear that monastic authors recognized that taste was individualized. The story may reflect the reality of traveling monks such as Apollonios, who lived in nearby Nitria, and was known to take grapes, pomegranates, eggs, and cakes to the sick and elderly. It is interesting that in Palladios's accounting of Apollonios we do not read of any rebuke or judgment on such activity. Instead, the *Lausiac History* tells how a new monk assumed Apollonios's activities when he became too old to travel.[122]

While textual sources claim an early third-century date for the settlements in Nitria and Kellia, the earliest excavated material found at Kellia dates to the early fifth century.[123] Residence #39–40 was occupied during the sixth and seventh centuries and was remodeled as a pilgrimage center for visitors. The residence evolved from a dwelling for two to four monks to one that held over twenty monks and that offered a communal area for visitors. In particular the building has three different kitchens and each corresponds to a separate phase of building, thus documenting the changes in the archaeology of cooking for this community. The kitchen includes features typical of Kellian monastic kitchens: bread ovens and stoves with sets of three to four built-in kawānīn. The final phases had thirteen kawānīn and two bread ovens for a complex with over sixty rooms. In this configuration, in contrast to Naqlun, the ovens are built into the same room as the stove. The combination of bread ovens and stoves in the kitchen also indicates life in a *manshubiya* was different from communal monasteries, where bakeries were separate facilities linked to the kneading room.

The last example is the site that spawned my interest in the archaeology of cooking in the first place: the Monastery of St. John the Little in Wadi Natrun, which has over 80 *manshubiyaat,* with the largest over 90 meters in length (fig. 10.6). Recent excavations have recovered similar kitchen facilities to those found at other monastic sites in Egypt.[124] The site of John the Little continued from the sixth century and expanded until the tenth century.[125] The first *manshubiya* was excavated in the 1990s and is a twenty-roomed residence and its layout is akin to the more modest dwellings at Kellia.[126] The central kitchen is located off of a small courtyard that held a cistern and storage vessels. The kitchen includes both an oven and a three-burner stove (fig. 10.7). The

121 Makarios the Great 3.

122 Palladios, *Lausiac History* 13.2.; trans., Meyer, 49.

123 The settlement at Kellia and Pherme was inhabited until the eighth century. After the settlement was abandoned, it was left uninhabited.

124 Excavations by the Yale Monastic Archaeology Project under the direction and founder, Stephen J. Davis. From 2006 to 2010, Darlene Brooks Hedstrom served as the project's archaeological director; Gillian Pyke has served in this position from 2011 to the present. Excavation work was generously supported in 2006 and 2007 by a Dumbarton Oaks Project Grant in Byzantine Studies.

125 The date for the settlement is based upon ceramic material recovered during earlier Scriptorium excavations from 1992 to 1999 (see next note) and the current YMAP excavations of a monastic residence, Building B, which is dated on the basis of ceramics, glass, and epigraphic evidence to the ninth century. Material excavated from a midden by Building B points to parts of the site being occupied during the ninth century. S. J. Davis et al., "Life and Death in Lower and Upper Egypt: A Brief Survey of Recent Monastic Archaeology at Yale," *Journal of the Canadian Society for Coptic Studies* 3 (2012): 9–26. D. L. Brooks Hedstrom et al., "New Archaeology at Ancient Scetis: Surveys and Initial Excavations at the Monastery of St. John the Little in Wadi al-Natrun: Yale Monastic Archaeology Project," *DOP* 64 (2010): 217–228.

126 A joint American mission by Calvin Theological Seminary and Scriptorium Center for Christian Antiquites conducted sporadic work at the site from 1992 to 1999. The results of an excavation of a church and two domestic residences were not fully published aside from two brief communications. See S. el-Souriani, and P. Grossmann, "Researches in the Laura of John Kolobos (Wâdî Natrûn)," in *Ägypten und Nubien in spätantiker und christlicher Zeit: Akten des 6. Internationalen Koptologenkongresses Münster, 20.–26. Juli 1996,* vol. 1, ed. S. Emmel, M. Kruase, S. G. Richter, and S. Schaten (Wiesbaden, 1999), 360–64; S. el-Souriani, "Bâtiments monastiques anciens au Wadi Natroun," *Le monde copte* 21–22 (1993): 245–53. I served as field excavator in 1996 under the direction of Scott T. Carroll and later as field director (1997–1999) for the project under the direction of Bastiaan van Elderen.

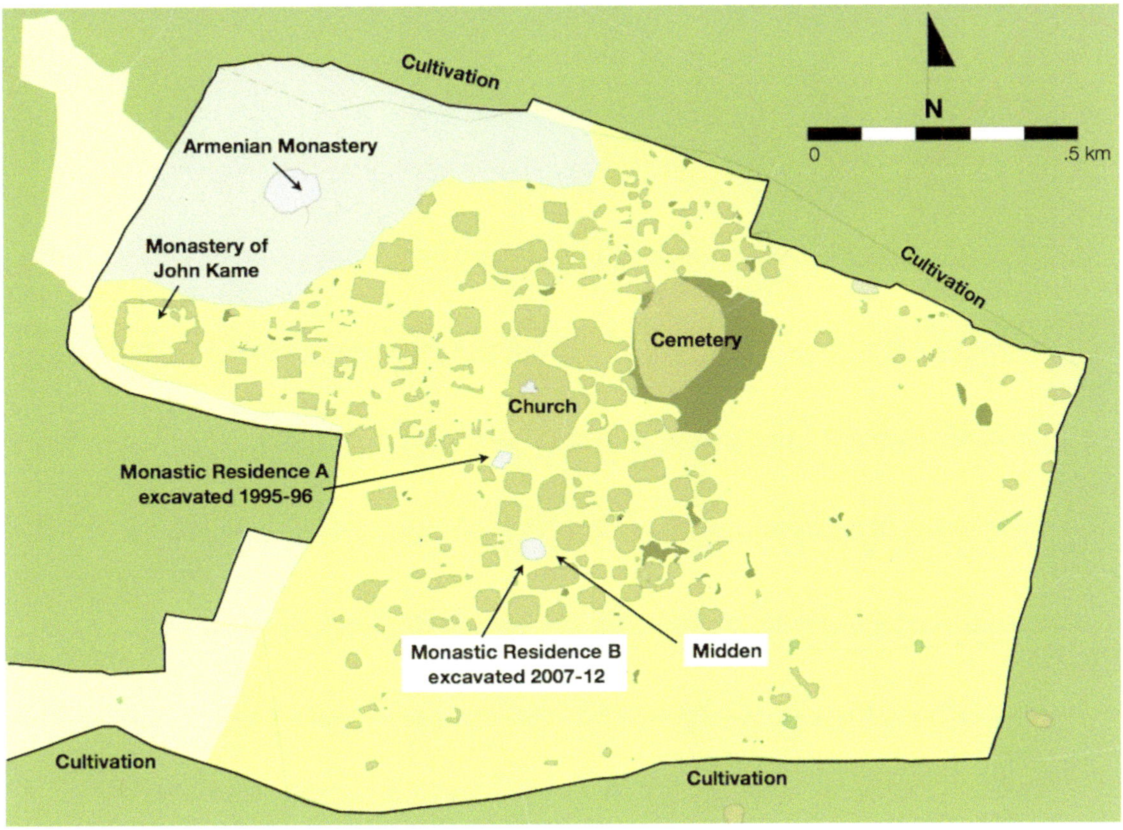

FIG. 10.6. General plan of the Monastery of St. John the Little, published in *DOP* 64 (2010): fig. 1 (survey and mapping: Dawn McCormack)

three kāwānīn hold the fuel in their base, while a niche, under the stove, was likely used to hold fuel for both the oven and the stove.

Residence B was excavated 2007–2012. Of the five kitchens excavated in the twenty-six roomed residence, three were in simultaneous use, whereas one oven and a fourth kitchen, being later additions, were built at a level higher than all other kitchen areas (fig. 10.8). Two ovens in Room 9 contain substantial archaeobotanical and archaeozoological material.[127] The earlier, west oven is made of mud and large ceramic body sherds, which is a departure in construction methods from ovens seen in earlier monastic contexts, in which the body of the oven is made of bricks or hand-packed mud, seen at sites such as Naqlun, Saqqara, and Thebes.[128] The later east oven is slightly different in its components, being made with a large collection of fired red bricks, which were placed on their ends to form a more conical oven. Narrow mud brick walls provide protection for the ovens from wind and may have helped contain the heat generated by these large features. The north kitchen facility is made of a small room, which was divided by an east–west arch and was likely unroofed.[129] Consisting of only two spaces, the kitchen was densely packed with three stoves comprising a total of ten kāwānīn and one, large bread oven in the east end of the south Room 19. On the east end of Room 20, a large oven fills the width of the small room. A set of four kawānīn flanks the south wall, with the westernmost kānūn actually crossing over into the entrance to the courtyard. Based upon the preliminary archaeobotanical and archaeozoological work at John the Little we now know that monks were baking bread in the building, but there is little evidence to suggest the inhabitants were using the building for

127 Davis, *Life and Death in Lower and Upper Egypt*, 11.

128 See G. Pyke and D. L. Brooks Hedstrom, "The Afterlife of Sherds: Architectural Reuse Strategies at the Monastery of John the Little, Wadi Natrun," in *Functional Aspects of Egyptian Ceramics within Their Archaeological Context*, ed. B. Bader and M. Ownby (Leuven, 2012), 307–26.

129 Similar designs for unroofed or light roofs made of reeds are found at Kellia. See E. Makowiecka, "L'ermitage QIZ 14 (55,42/20,14) Fouilles de 1981, 1982, 1986 et 1990. Hermitage QIZ 14. Description and Architectural Analysis," in *MSAC* (1999): 21–27.

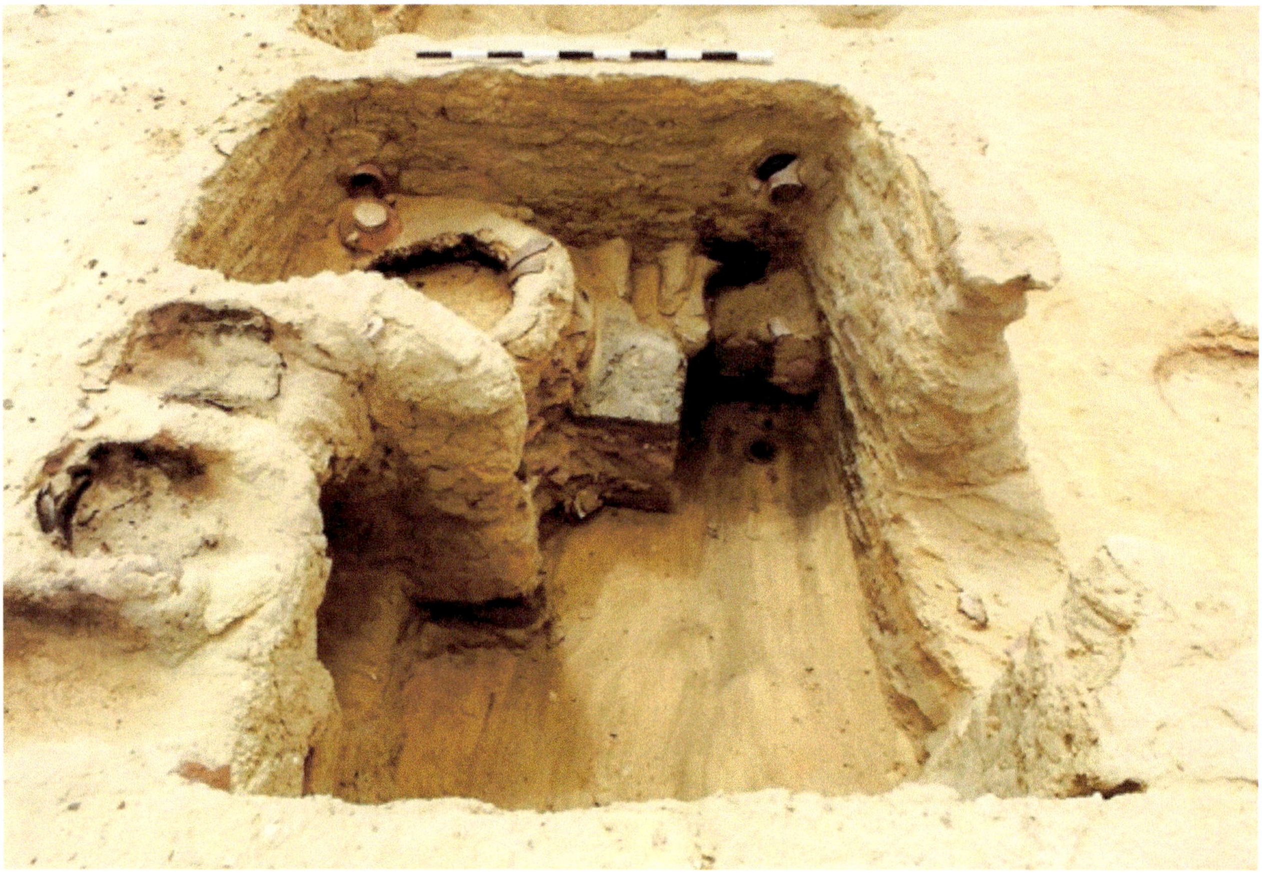

FIG. 10.7. Residence A at the Monastery of St. John the Little, 1996. Private kitchen with an oven and a stove with three kāwānīn (photo: author)

milling grain. They were also eating a diet of stews made of beans, lentils and possibly fish.[130] And based upon the living quarters, which could possibly house five or six monks, the presence of four operational kitchens suggests the ninth-century residents were engaged in food preparation for a community that extended beyond those living in the building.

Conclusion

What can the archaeology of food and cooking offer us in reconstructing how Byzantine monastics experienced taste? The monastic evidence from early Byzantine Egypt offers a unique data set to examine the relationship between religious practice, social structuring activities such as fasting and single meal times, and the spaces in which food was prepared, eaten, and eventually discarded. The numerous monastic kitchens and their spatial relationship to the larger monastic settlement allow us to see how those assigned to the kitchen could and did prepare bread and vegetables, the staples of a monastic diet, alongside salted fish, condiments, and other items.

Eating well in these communities could be at the mercy, or the delight, of the head cooks. The complaints about portions and the taste of the food illustrate the ways in which communities could and did regulate taste. At the White Monastery, there were evidently problems not just with the cooks but also with those who served the food. Complaints could be given to say that this was a "bad dish" or that "not all dishes are being made the same way or . . . being stirred."[131] Apparently it would take several complaints before anyone would address issues of bad taste in the food. In *Rule* 340 we learn that food

130 Mennet-Allah El Dorry public lecture at the International Conference of Life in Egypt during the Coptic Period, Alexandria, Egypt, September 2010; idem, public lecture, "Beyond Bread: A New Perspective on Monastic Diet and Food Procurement" at *Tenth International Congress of Coptic Studies*, Rome, September 17–22, 2012, Rome, Italy.

131 Shenoute, *Rules* 364; trans. Layton, 245.

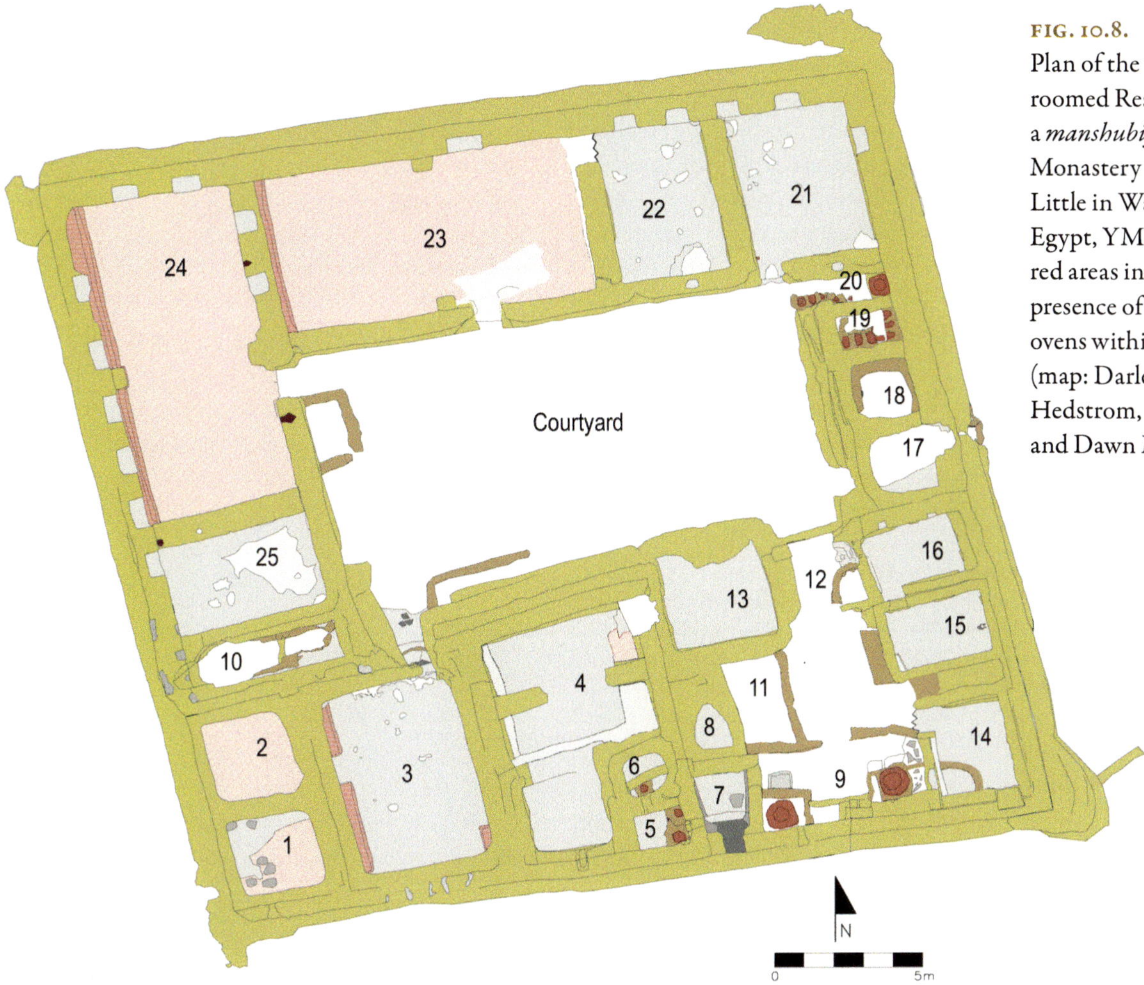

FIG. 10.8. Plan of the twenty-six–roomed Residence B, a *manshubiya* at the Monastery of St. John the Little in Wadi Natrun, Egypt, YMAP. The red areas indicate the presence of stoves and ovens within the building (map: Darlene L. Brooks Hedstrom, Elizabeth Davis, and Dawn McCormack).

could be salty, insipid, burned, stale, too pickled, or soppy.[132] Regardless of the quality, there certainly was oversight both in the dining area and in the kitchen or bakery. Together these sources help us see the complexity of reconstructing monastic taste and the need to integrate a variety of physical and textual sources. Thus, we may be able to discern particular concerns about monastic taste within a communal setting that would differ from those of the monastic settlements that were more independent and were not informed as obviously by a monastic order or by a particular rule.

In contrast to the large cenobitic monasteries, at the *manshubiya* or "dwelling place" sites, the story of cooking is significantly different and more elusive. We lack the monastic rules that might have governed daily life. In these settlements we see the pride of place of the private kitchen in every residence. The independent communities had greater autonomy in the preparation of food and in what was likely used for making meals. It is here that the archaeology of kitchens and the bioarchaeological remains become a crucial source for what was grown, imported, and cooked at the various residences. Only with greater archaeological study of middens, ash, and the cooking areas at such non-cenobitic sites can we test the possible diversity of diets *within* single communities. The recovery of fish bones, nuts, pomegranates, figs, bay leaves, onions, and other flavor enhancers point toward a varied diet enhanced by herbs and spices.[133] Although Shenoute, for example, expressly listed fish *garum*, cooked

132 Shenoute, *Rules* 340; trans. Layton, 235.

133 C. Ziegler et al., "La mission archéologique du Musée du Louvre à Saqqara: Résultats de quatre campagnes de fouilles

fish, and other fish as forbidden food, except for ill monastics, the recovery of evidence for salted and dried fish, mollusks, and oysters at several monasteries throughout Egypt suggests that monastic leaders were not able to fully monitor monastic taste.[134] While it is possible to understand the presence of the physical material as reflecting items for nonmonastic diets, the fact that the documentary evidence also speaks to fish consumption discloses a far richer story of monastic taste.

A multivariable approach that combines historical perceptions, daily practices, consumed food, and physical spaces is needed if we are to begin reconstructing a sensorial perspective of early Byzantine monastic taste. Studying monastic taste draws us onto several paths of inquiry to reconstruct the somatic landscape. Since taste is bounded in history by time and space, the archaeology of taste offers new methodological readings of physical evidence to assist us in reactivating the spaces where cooking and food preparation were performed. Further study is still needed to consider the intricate relationships between tasting and eating in the communal dining areas and in the private spaces of the *manshubiya*. Food also became a critical part of hospitality as monks welcomed guests and traveled to other monasteries or to the villages. By using the documentary and textual evidence in conjunction with the methodologies for the archaeology of taste we can now reconstruct with greater confidence how monastic cooks and bakers shaped ascetic taste and the food placed on the Egyptian monastic tables.

The kernel for this essay developed from a paper titled "Feeding Asceticism: Monastic Kitchens and Consumption Habits in Byzantine Egypt," which I presented in 2012 at the 38th Annual meeting for the Byzantine Studies Conference in Brookline, MA. I wish to thank Susan Ashbrook Harvey and Margaret Mullett for the invitation to further develop the project by engaging with the sense of taste as it relates to monastic cooking and baking for the symposium that led to this volume.

de 1993 à 1996," *Bulletin de la Institut Français d'archaeologie Oriental* 97 (1997): 272.

134 Clackson, "Fish and Chits," (n. 75 above) 11. T. Derda, ed., *Deir el-Naqlun: The Greek Papyri* (Warsaw, 1995), 141–46.

Touch

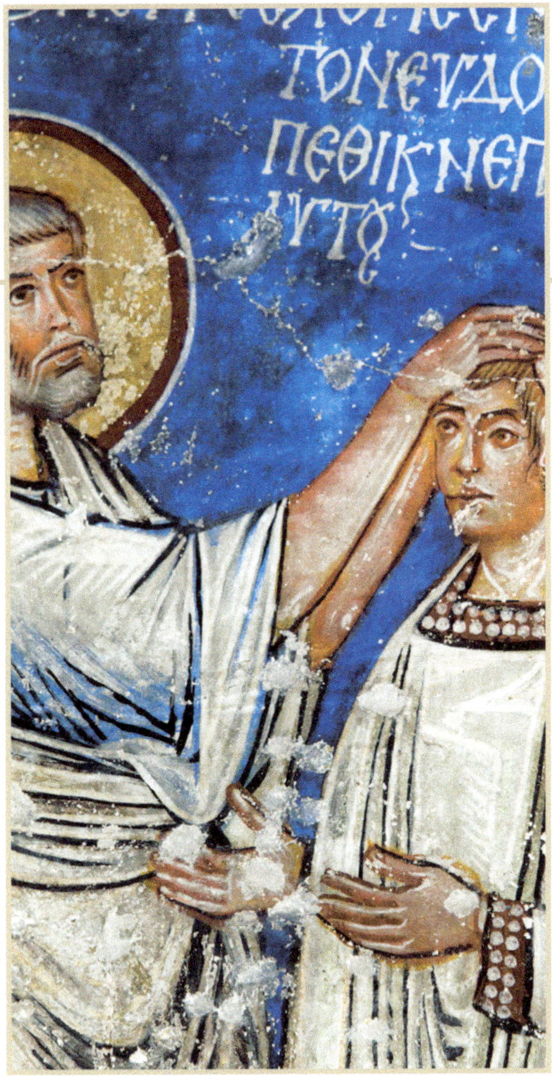

CHAPTER ELEVEN

Byzantine Christianity and Tactile Piety (Fourth–Fifteenth Centuries)

BÉATRICE CASEAU

The *Mandylion*, a piece of cloth that had reputedly touched the face of Jesus and on which his face was miraculously imprinted,[1] had been kept in Edessa for centuries until it was taken to Constantinople in August 944, to be cherished, from that point on, as an imperial relic, in the Great Palace church of the Pharos. On that August day, the relic was welcomed by Romanos Lekapenos and his two sons, as well as Constantine Porphyrogennetos, who, when he became sole emperor, commissioned a written narration of the translation of the relic.

The reception of the relic is illustrated in an illumination (fig. 11.1) in an ornate twelfth-century manuscript that preserves a copy of the *Chronicle* of John Skylitzes. In this illumination, the faces of Emperor Constantine Porphyrogennetos and of Christ meet in affectionate contact. Touching and kissing this precious piece of cloth was an imperial privilege, and its depiction highlights the legitimizing connection between God and the emperor.[2]

This image, perhaps more than any other, illustrates the importance of tactile piety. The organ of touch is the body itself and its medium is the flesh.[3] Whether an emperor or a poor fellow, touching a relic or an image was an active gesture, indicating an attachment to Christ and his saints, and the wish to pour out one's heart in a physical connection. Devotional gestures could be performed by all, clerics and lay people, men and women, young and old, rich and poor, and could help develop a nonliturgical and very personal relationship to Christ and his saints. Touch was the medium used to create and activate a link between this world and the next, between the frailty of human life and the healing strength of divine or holy beings. In their personal devotions, the Byzantines had relative freedom, and could choose their favorite saints and demonstrate their devotion through particular gestures, such as kissing icons. In Christian religious practices, tactile piety enabled both lay people and clerics to take an active role in ritual and devotional practices. Touching sacred objects was under clerical control and could be

1 *Histoire de Ya'yá ibn-Sa'íd al-An'ákí, Continuateur de Sa'íd ibn-Bi'ríq,* ed. and trans. I. Kratchovsky and A. Vasiliev, vol. 1, *PO* 18 (Paris, 1924), 730–31; E. Patlagean, "L'entrée de la Sainte Face d'Édesse à Constantinople en 944," in *La religion civique à l'époque médiévale et moderne (chrétienté et islam)*, ed. A. Vauchez (Rome, 1995), 21–35; A. M. Dubarle, "L'homélie de Grégoire le référendaire pour la réception de l'image d'Edesse," *REB* 55 (1997): 5–51; S. G. Engberg, "Romanos Lekapenos and the Mandilion of Edessa," *Byzance et les reliques du Christ*, ed. J. Durand and B. Flusin (Paris, 2004), 123–42.

2 E. Bozoky, *La politique des reliques de Constantin à Saint-Louis: Protection collective et légitimation du pouvoir* (Paris, 2007), 101–3.

3 T. K. Johansen, *Aristotle and the Sense-Organs* (Cambridge, 1998), 193–215.

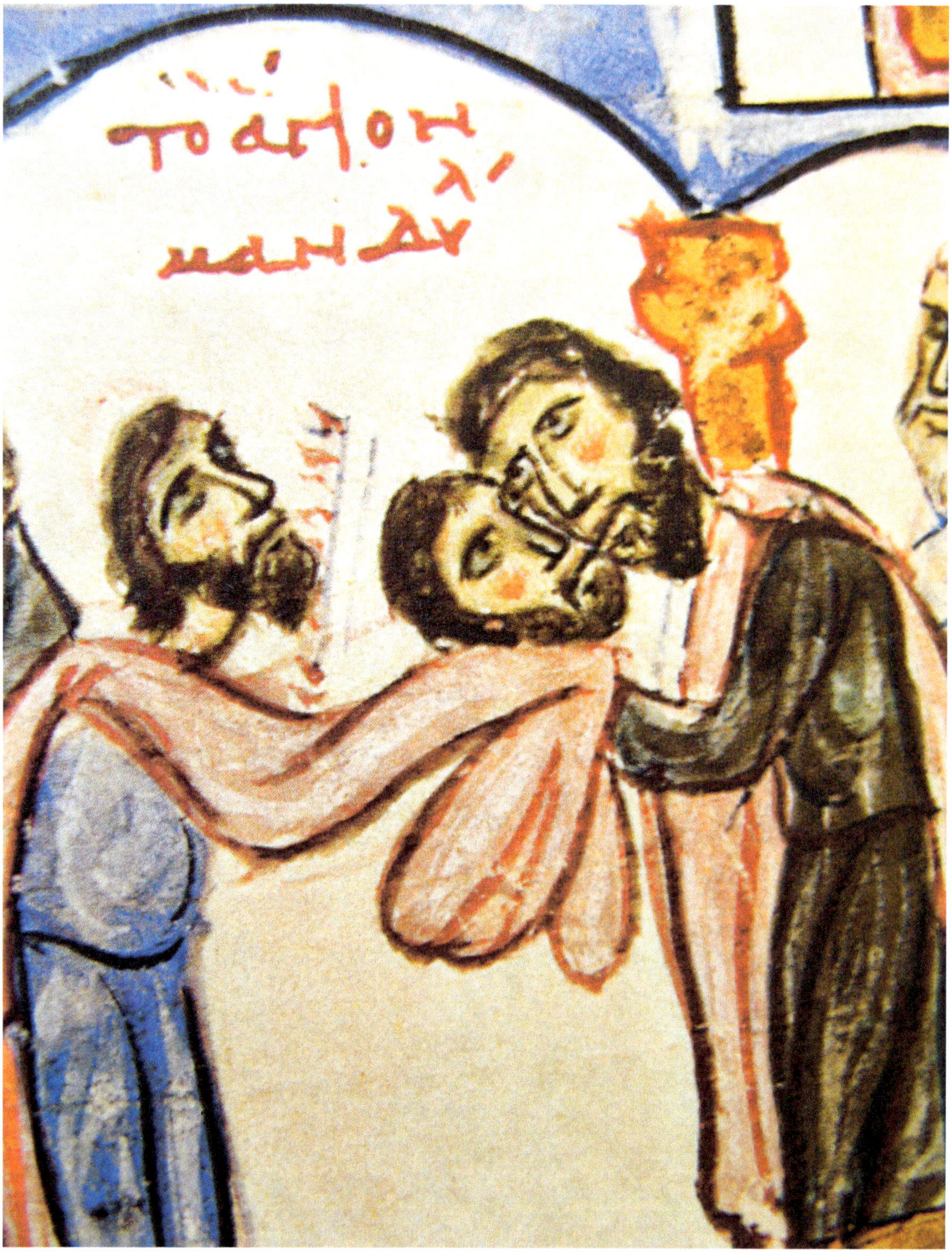

FIG. 11.1. Madrid, Bibl. Nac. Vitr. 26-2 (12th c.), fol. 131r: the emperor venerates the Mandylion (photo: Biblioteca Nacional de España)

both commendable and reprehensible, depending on what the object was, where it was located and who did the touching.

The sensory experience of a Christian entering a church is best described through the concept of *synesthesia*—the congruence of multiple sensory experiences.[4] Coming to church when a religious celebration took place involved different types of sensory experiences, mixing touch, sight, smell, and hearing, as well as taste, sometimes. Tactile piety often started with touching a church's doors, curtains, floor and icons. It was accompanied by sight, which was understood as a tactile sense establishing contact "between the eye and the thing seen."[5] Seeing the space and the interior decoration went together with smelling the faint or strong odor of incense and that of perfumed oils or burning wax, and hearing peoples' voices and chanting. While some of the senses, such as smell or even seeing, do not necessarily require an active, fully conscious, participation (odors strike the nostrils, one could see without focusing—the ears and the nose cannot avoid hearing and smelling), touch is different: it is both felt and produced. Touch involves intention and action. A hand clearing away a curtain door, or pushing a door open, tracing the cross on one's body, prostrating on the floor or kissing icons—all require intent and action. Action is required for the hands, the feet, the knees, the lips or the forehead to experience touch.

As Constance Classen reminds us, "touch is not just a private act. It is a fundamental medium for the expression, experience and contestation of social values and hierarchies."[6] Christians experienced the touch of a higher religious authority, when they were presented at church, during baptism and at different times, when the imposition of the hands accompanied blessings. The hand gesture, *manus impositio*, was understood as a sign of blessing, inherited from the Old Testament. It accompanied prayers asking God to bless and protect or heal the person. It also conveyed spiritual power. From top to bottom, touch was important in transmitting authority as well as blessing and healing. This kind of religious touch expressed hierarchical differences between lay people and clerics and inside the clergy, between the different ranks.

Touch was highly regulated inside the Byzantine religious culture. On the one hand, it was the privilege of spiritual authorities, clerics, or monastic holy men. By placing their hands on someone they could bless them or share their spiritual power. Among lay people, emperors had privileges, which included touching the censer inside the sanctuary, and also approaching and kissing relics, which were kept in the imperial palace's chapels. The touching of religious spaces, objects, and people, which can be subsumed under tactile piety and tactile piety, on the other hand, showed a range of emotions and feelings, such as respect and veneration. It was accessible to all, although the Byzantine church imposed limits on touching sacred objects or the Eucharist. Both tactile piety and clerical *manus impositio* are interelated. They both used physical contact as the proper gesture to signify spiritual realities.

Hand-laying was present in many Byzantine rituals, such as welcoming back penitents or churching heretics,[7] and it was especially fundamental to ordination rites.[8] Through touch, bishops transmitted their blessing and their sacerdotal power. Two gestures are recorded and often taken as interchangeable in Byzantine sources: χειροθεσία, actual hand-laying, and

4 *Synesthesis* is used in a different manner by neurologists, anthropologists, and art historians. A strict medical definition of the word concerns a rare neurological condition allowing certain persons to convert one sensory experience into that of another, e.g., seeing a word and feeling a taste, hearing a sound and seeing colors. It is also used to sum up multisensorial experiences in rituals. In this chapter, this second sense is implied.

5 L. James, "Senses and Sensibility in Byzantium," *Art History* 27, no. 4 (2004): 522–37, at 528; S. Biernoff, *Sight and Embodiment in the Middle Ages: Ocular Desires* (New York, 2002); B. V. Pentcheva, *The Sensual Icon: Space, Ritual and the Senses in Byzantium* (University Park, PA, 2010), 20.

6 C. Classen, "Fingerprints: Writing about Touch," in *The Book of Touch*, ed. C. Classen (Oxford and New York, 2005), 1.

7 M. Arranz, "Les sacrements de l'ancien Euchologe constantinopolitain (2): Ière partie: Admission dans l'Eglise des convertis des hérésies ou d'autres religions non chrétiennes," *OCP* 49 (1983): 42–90.

8 P. Bradshaw, *Ordination Rites of the Ancient Churches of East and West* (New York, 1990), 360–61; A. J. Chupungco ed., *Handbook for Liturgical Studies*, vol. 4, *Sacraments and Sacramentals* (Collegeville, MN, 2000).

χειροτονία, originally stretching out the hands, which can also mean contact with a person's head.[9] John Chrysostom explains that in this gesture it is the hand of a man, which is placed on someone's head, but that it is God who acts through him and ordains clerics.[10]

It was an episcopal privilege to perform hand-laying during the ordination ritual of members of the clergy. Who received the blessing of such a personal and powerful gesture? In book eight of the *Apostolic Constitutions* (fourth century), *cheirotonia* (χειροτονία), the hand-laying performed by the bishop on members of the clergy for their ordination, is mentioned for the priest, the deacon, the deaconess, the subdeacon and the reader.[11] For each clerical rank, specific prayers accompanied the cheirotonia, which was the visible gesture of the ordination. By touching the candidate's head, the bishop created a new identity as member of the clergy and formed a bond between himself and the new recruit. This bond was also a sign of authority of the bishop over members of the clergy.[12] It was not performed on virgins and widows, who dedicated their life to God but were not considered members of the clergy.

For the consecration of bishops, however, one notes some hesitation in the sources: the ceremony described in the *Apostolic Constitutions* did not include a cheirotonia. The Gospels were placed on the head of the new bishop during his consecration.[13] Although cheirotonia was applied to bishops as well as to priests and deacons in later sources, images of patriarchal consecration by other bishops sometimes show a gesture of stretching the hand rather than actual hand-laying, perhaps because in this second gesture, there is an element of submission on the part of the person who is touched. So if the word *cheirotonia* was indeed used for bishops as well as for other clerics, the actual gestures might have been different. Also the significance of hand-laying depended on other factors, such as the presence of other ministers and of the congregation. The location of the rite (e.g., inside or outside the sanctuary) was also important in order to distinguish between different types of ordinations that involved hand-laying. Touching someone's bowed head was the common gesture for transmitting spiritual power and asserting authority over somebody. Where and by whom it was performed changed its significance.

Touch was central to Byzantine Christianity because it inherited from ancient Judaism the idea that God's blessing was transmitted through sacerdotal touch. Christian bishops and priests shared the sacerdotal power to channel God's blessing by touching a person's head. Hand-laying was the mode to exert this power and demonstrate sacerdotal authority: it was performed on all Christians and created between them a physical bond, which was supposed to originate in Jesus's own practice of hand-laying and, further afield, to refer to Old Testament examples such as Moses imposing hands on Joshua (Num. 27:18). Byzantine Christians were touched on the top of their head during their baptism[14] and members of the clergy experienced this a second time during their ordination. If the prayers were different, the gestures were similar and revealed that all Christians were under clerical authority and that clerical mediation was important to reach God.

9 A. Papadakis, "Cheirothesia"; "Cheirotonia," *ODB* 1:417; J. Darrouzès, *Recherches sur les ΟΦΦΙΚΙΑ de l'Église byzantine* (Paris, 1970), 151.

10 Τοῦτο γὰρ ἡ χειροτονία ἐστιν· Ἡ χεὶρ ἐπίκειται τοῦ ἀνδρὸς, τὸ δὲ πᾶν ὁ Θεὸς ἐργάζεται. John Chrysostom, *Commentarii in Acta Apostolorum*, Hom. 14, PG 60:116.

11 *Apostolic Constitutions*, 8.16–22, in *Les constitutions apostoliques*, ed. M. Metzger, SC 320, 329, 336 (Paris, 1985–87), 3:216–24.

12 J. Coppens, *L'imposition des mains et les rites connexes dans le Nouveau Testament et dans l'Église ancienne: Étude de théologie positive* (Paris, 1925); C. Vogel, "Chirotonie et chirothésie: Importance et relativité du geste de l'imposition des mains dans la collation des ordres," *Irenikon* 45 (1972): 7–21, 207–38; idem, "L'imposition des mains dans les rites d'ordination en Orient et en Occident," *La Maison Dieu* 102 (1970): 57–72.

13 *Apostolic Constitutions*, 8.4.6 (Metzger ed., 3:142); P. F. Bradshaw, "Ordination: Theology and Rite, A.D. 200–400," *The Study of Liturgy*, ed. C. Jones, G. Wainwright, E. Yarnold, and P. Bradshaw (London, 1992).

14 V. Saxer, *Vie liturgique et quotidienne à Carthage vers le milieu du IIIe siècle*, 2nd ed. (Vatican City, 1969); idem, *Les rites de l'initiation chrétienne du IIe au VIe siècle: Esquisse historique et signification d'après leurs principaux témoins* (Spoleto, 1992); P. Cramer, *Baptism and Change in the Early Middle Ages, c. 200–c. 1150* (Cambridge, 1993); B. D. Spinks, *Early and Medieval Rituals and Theologies of Baptism: From the New Testament to the Council of Trent* (Aldershot and Burlington, VT, 2006).

Ordination cheirotonia distinguished lay people and clerics. Inside the clergy there was a clear distinction of ranks. The twelfth-century canonists Balsamon and Zonaras recall that the lower ranks of the clergy (e.g., readers, cantors . . .) now only received the *sphragis*, which refers to the sign of the cross traced on their body, while the higher ranks continued to receive the cheirotonia.[15] At that point, subdeacons still received the cheirotonia, but by the fifteenth century, this was no longer the case: Symeon of Thessalonike indicates that readers and subdeacons were offered a simple *cheirothesia* (χειροθεσία) outside of the sanctuary. Throughout its history, the Byzantine church felt the need to make distinctions to signify different functions and ranks inside the Church, but touching the head of a person, whether through *sphragis*, *cheirothesia*, or *cheirotonia*, remained the constant gesture common to all these ceremonies. The Byzantines were more or less aware that these gestures had a common root and could sometimes be equivalent. Zonaras for example equates *sphragis* and *cheirothesia* when it comes to describe the ordination of readers and cantors. He writes, "Some like bishops, priests, deacons, and subdeacons are ordained by laying on of hands, others like readers, chanters, and those with similar functions receive only the seal (and this is a form of imposition of hands)" (Οἱ μὲν γὰρ χειροτονοῦνται ὡς ἐπίσκοποι, καὶ πρεσβύτεροι, καὶ διάκονοι, καὶ ὑποδιάκονοι· οἱ δὲ σφραγίζονται μόνον (καὶ τοῦτο δὲ χειροθεσίας ἐστιν) ὡς ἀναγνῶσται καὶ ψάλται, καὶ οἱ τούτοις ὅμοιοι).[16]

Why did the Byzantine church feel the need to create these different categories of clerics? These distinctions between members of the clergy were connected to another issue relating to touch: only the higher ranks of the clergy were allowed to touch the sacred vessel used for the consecration of bread and wine. Only priests and bishops could consecrate these elements on the altar. Restriction on access and touch applied to the most sacred objects and spaces in a church.

The sacralization of space led to the differentiation of spaces inside the church building and gradients in sacrality: the narthex was less sacred, while the sanctuary was the most sacred area of the church building. Many Byzantine churches had a synthronon in the main apse of the church, for clerics to sit.[17] It was therefore quite clear that the first division of space was between lay people located in the nave, and most of the clergy sitting or standing in the sanctuary. Chancel barriers delineated visually the two areas. At the end of the seventh century, the council in Trullo forbade lay people to enter the holy sanctuary of a church.[18] This distinction between clerics and lay people was reinforced during the middle ages, when it seemed important to create boundaries around Christian sacred spaces and objects.[19]

This exclusion did not completely apply to the emperor, but it was enforced for empresses.[20] The exclusion from the area of the sanctuary was in fact particularly applied to women, with very few exceptions in convents.[21] Patriarch Luke Chrysoberges (1157–1170) was scandalized when he heard that little girls had been allowed in the sanctuary around the altar and he confirms that women, whatever their age, are not to enter inside the sanctuary.[22]

A second distinction was made between clerics who could touch the sacred vessel, especially the chalice and paten used in the Eucharistic celebration and those who were not allowed to do so.[23] Neither readers nor subdeacons were allowed

15 Darrouzès, *Recherches*, 87; Balsamon and Zonaras, PG 137:385.

16 Zonaras, *Canones XXX sanctae et oecumenicae quartae synodi Chalcedoniensis*, PG 137:385.

17 M. Altripp, "Beobachtungen zu Synthronoi und Kathedren in byzantinischen Kirchen Griechenlands," *BCH* 124 (2000): 377–412.

18 Council in Trullo, chap. 69, ed. and trans. G. Nedungatt and M. Featherstone, *The Council in Trullo Revisited* (Rome, 1995), 151.

19 S. Gerstel, ed., *Thresholds of the Sacred: Architectural, Art Historical, Liturgical, and Theological Perspectives on Religious Screens, East and West* (Washington, DC, 2006).

20 R. Taft, "Women at Church in Byzantium: Where, When—and Why?" *DOP* 52 (1998): 27–87, at 70–71.

21 V. A. Karras, "Female Deacons in the Byzantine Church," *Church History* 73 (2004): 272–316.

22 Luke Chrysoberges, *Canonical Answer to Euphemienos Hegoumenos of the Christ Savior Philanthropos Monastery*: V. Grumel, *Les Regestes des Actes du patriarcat de Constantinople*, vol. 1, Les Actes des patriarches, fasc. 2–3, *Les Regestes de 715 à 1206*, ed. J. Darrouzès, 2nd ed. (Paris, 1989), n. 1087.

23 B. Pitarakis, "La vaisselle eucharistique des églises d'Orient," in *Pratiques de l'eucharistie dans les Églises d'Orient et d'Occident (Antiquité et Moyen Âge)*, ed. N. Bériou, B. Caseau,

to touch the sacred vessel. When it came to the Eucharist, touch was highly regulated. Contact with the consecrated bread and wine sacralized objects. The result was a restricted access to sanctified objects. In the medieval Byzantine church, the use of a spoon to give communion meant that the hands of the faithful and lower clerics no longer touched either the consecrated bread that is the Body of Christ or the chalice containing the consecrated wine, transformed into the Blood of Christ. It is unclear when exactly the communion spoon started being used in Byzantium[24]—sometime after the seventh century and before the eleventh century, when it is clearly attested by Cardinal Humbert.[25] The hands of the faithful were no longer considered pure enough to touch the sacred vessel or the Eucharist.

This had not always been the case. In the early Byzantine period, catechetical homilies reveal that touching the Eucharist was expected and it was highly regarded as a moment of personal sanctification and spiritual benefit. Cyril of Jerusalem tells us that, for the communion ritual, the faithful were to approach with awe, and receive the Body of Christ in their hands before they could taste it.[26] This concrete touch provided them with a sense of intimacy with Christ. By taking the consecrated bread in their hands, the faithful came into contact with his Body. After drinking from the cup or chalice, they experienced the tincture of the Blood of Christ on their lips. Cyril of Jerusalem invited the communicant to take this opportunity to sanctify the other senses.[27] A simple contact was enough to sanctify the senses and open the mind.

Expressions of gratitude and affection are also recorded in connection with the Body of Christ in the Eucharistic bread. Theodore of Mopsuestia (d. 428) recommends kissing the Eucharistic bread before eating it.[28] The different Eastern churches shared a common culture of touch as a means to connect with divine beings. One can also find references to kissing the consecrated parcels of bread, called the pearls, in different authors belonging to Syriac churches, such as Narsai or Cyrus of Edessa.[29] In the early seventh century Gabriel bar Lipeh of Qatar explains: "Whenever we take them in our hands we ought thus to think that we are embracing and kissing our Saviour himself, as if we mingle his Body in our body, and mix his Blood in our blood."[30] Touching the sacred was beneficial for these Christians and touching the Eucharist was the next best thing after touching Christ himself, which they could no longer do. A whole culture of tactile piety developed because of this belief in the spiritual and physical benefit of contact with Christ's Body. Depictions of the communion of the apostles such as on the Riha paten (fig 11.2) show Jesus himself giving the bread and the wine to his disciples, as if the apostles were waiting to receive communion as the faithful did at church. This scene reveals that communion is about personal contact between Jesus and the communicant.

This shared tactile culture was nevertheless challenged at the end of the late antique period. Attitudes toward the body evolved. This change concerned the perception of nudity, the care of the self, as well as notions of ritual purity. These

and D. Rigaux, Collection des études augustiniennes (Paris, 2009), 309–29.

24 R. F. Taft, *A History of the Liturgy of St. John Chrysostom*, vol. 6, *The Communion, Thanksgiving, and Concluding Rites* (Rome, 2008), 288–300; B. Caseau, "L'abandon de la communion dans la main (IVe–XIIe s.)," in *Mélanges Gilbert Dagron*, Travaux et Mémoires 14 (Paris, 2002), 79–94; R. Taft, "Byzantine Communion Spoons: A Review of the Evidence," *DOP* 50 (1996): 209–38.

25 Cardinal Humbert: "accipite et cum cochleari comedite; hoc est enim corpus meum," PL 143:951.

26 Cyril of Jerusalem, *Mystagogical Homily* 5.21, in *Catéchèses Mystagogiques*, ed. A. Piédagnel, *Cyrille de Jérusalem*, SC 126 (Paris, 1966), 170–73; trans. Leo P. McCauley and A. Stephenson, *The Works of Saint Cyril of Jerusalem*, vol. 2 (Washington, DC, 1970), 203.

27 Cyril of Jerusalem, *Mystagogical Homily* 5.22 (Piédagnel ed., 172–73; McCauley and Stephenson trans., 203).

28 Theodore of Mospuestia, *Second Homily on the Mass*, 27–28, *Les Homélies catéchétiques de Théodore de Mopsueste. Reproduction phototypique du Ms. Mingana Syr. 561*, trans. R. Tonneau, with R. Devreesse (Vatican City, 1949), 577–79; see also D. L. Schwartz, *Paideia and Cult: Christian Initiation in Theodore of Mopsuestia* (Washington, DC, 2013).

29 Narsai, *Homily* 17, *The Liturgical Homilies of Narsai*, trans. J. A. Robinson (Cambridge, 1909), 29. Cyrus of Edessa, *Six Explanations of the Liturgical Feasts by Cyrus of Edessa, An East Syrian Theologian of the Mid Sixth Century*, trans. W. F. Macomber, CSCO 356, Scr. Syr. 156 (Louvain, 1974), 18.

30 S. Brock, "Gabriel of Qatar's Commentary on the Liturgy," *Hugoye* 6, no. 2 (2003), http://www.bethmardutho.org (accessed 9 June 2016); S. H. Jammo, "Gabriel Qatraya et son commentaire sur la liturgie chaldéenne," *OCP* 32 (1966): 39–52.

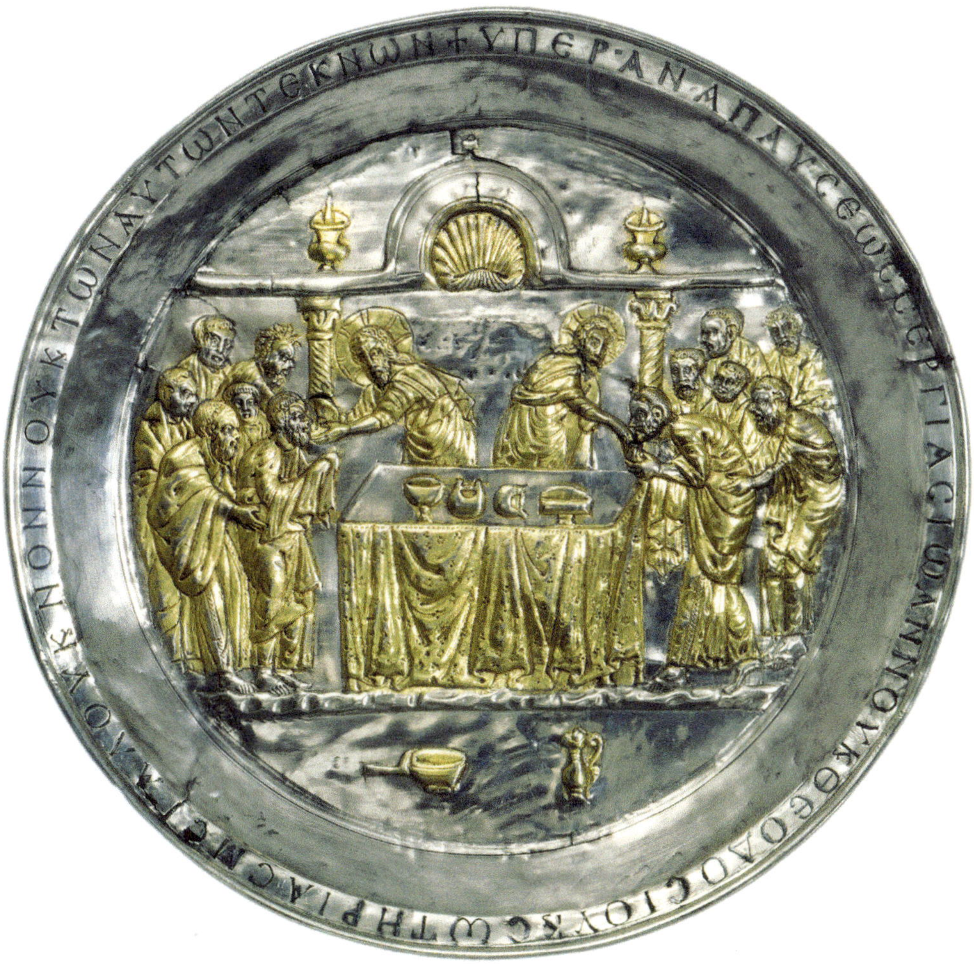

FIG. 11.2.
Riha paten with Communion of the Apostles, Dumbarton Oaks, BZ.1924.5 (photo: Dumbarton Oaks Research Library and Collection)

anthropological changes had consequences not only in bathhouses but also inside churches. The faithful did not consider that they could approach the altar and take communion easily. They also started to avoid hand contact with the Eucharistic bread. We hear about this evolution by the protest launched in 691–692 during the council in Trullo. Canon 101 condemns those who bring vessels for receiving consecrated bread rather than extend their hand. Ordinary worshippers were told to be in awe before the Eucharist and most felt too sinful or too impure to touch the Body of Christ with their own hands. Council members attempted to maintain the tradition of personal contact of the communicant's hand with the Body of Christ: "if anyone desires to partake of the immaculate body during the service and to become one with it through participation, he shall hold his hands in the form of the cross and in this wise approach and receive the communion of grace."[31] They explain that Christians are the temple of God and that they are "sanctified in soul and body."

This sanctification of the body was somehow lost from view by some ecclesiastical authorities when it concerned women's bodies. As early as the third century, discussions took place to forbid women from touching the Eucharist during periods of menstrual or postpartum blood flow. A letter of Dionysios of Alexandria (d. 264), later incorporated in Byzantine canon law compilations, explained that women should not even enter the church building when they are impure.[32] In his opinion, pious women would not touch the body and blood of Christ during

31 *The Canons of the Council in Trullo*, 101, ed. Nedungatt and Featherstone (n. 18 above), 182.

32 Dionysios of Alexandria, *Letter to Basilides*, in *Discipline générale antique*, vol. 2, *Les canons des Pères grecs*, ed P. Joannou (Rome, 1963), 12.

menstrual periods. This amounted to introducing Jewish laws of purity in Christian practice.[33]

During the third and fourth centuries, the role of Jewish practices in Christian worship was hotly debated. Arguments against incorporating Jewish ritual purity laws inside the Church appear in the *Didascalia of the Apostles* and the *Apostolic Constitutions*, which rejected such laws. To make their point, both sides in the debate used the same episode in which Jesus is touched by the woman suffering from a constant flow of blood (Mt. 9:20–22; Mk. 5:25–34; Lk. 8:43–48). Those in favor of excluding women explained that the woman touched only his clothes not his body;[34] those in favor of admitting women to communion insisted on the fact that she was allowed to touch Jesus, although she experienced a flow of blood, and that she was not rebuked but healed.[35] Eventually, however, Byzantine practice came to exclude women from touching the Eucharist during menstrual and post-partum periods.[36] Patriarch Nicholas III Grammatikos (1084–1111), for example, confirmed this exclusion. He wrote that women who gave birth during Lent would not be permitted to take communion at Easter: they needed to be purified before they could set foot in a church again and touch the Body of Christ.[37] Only dying women would receive communion, after a prayer (of purification). Women would not be baptized (unless they were dying)[38] or married during their menstrual periods. This exclusion from churches and touching the Eucharist also applied to midwives, who were in contact with blood and were considered impure for the same reason.[39]

Although some discussion arose concerning the impurity of sperm emissions, men were not excluded from entering churches or taking communion on that account.[40] While Dionysios of Alexandria had called on men to refrain from approaching the altar after nocturnal emissions, Athanasios of Alexandria rejected the idea that it made men impure.[41] Finally, Timothy of Alexandria established a distinction between monks for whom nocturnal emissions called for penance, and married men who should not be excluded from communion for involuntary nocturnal emissions.[42] The tendency was to recommend sexual abstinence before taking communion: it was mandatory for a priest before celebrating the Eucharist. All in all, numerous rules of ritual purity prevented Christians from approaching the altar and receiving communion. Touching the Eucharist had become highly regulated, which made taking communion an event that required a lot of preparation for lay people.[43]

As a result, the laity replaced taking communion with other forms of devotions. When too many sins tarnished their baptismal robe, the Byzantines preferred taking blessed bread instead of consecrated bread.[44] Following Saint Paul's advice and warning (1 Cor. 11:27), they considered taking communion too lightly risky for one's

33 S. J. D. Cohen, "Menstruants and the Sacred in Judaism and Christianity," in *Women's History and Ancient History*, ed. S. B. Pomeroy (Chapel Hill, 1991), 273–99; J. Beaucamp, "Exclues et aliénées: Les femmes dans la tradition canonique byzantine," in *Strangers to Themselves: The Byzantine Outsider*, ed. D. Smythe (Aldershot, 2000), 87–103.

34 Dionysios of Alexandria, *Letter to Basilides*, Joannou ed., 12.

35 *Apostolic Constitutions*, 6.28.7, Metzger ed., 386–87.

36 Hesychios of Jerusalem, PG 93:978; S. Tampellini, "L'esegesi del Levitico di Esichio di Gerusalemme," in *La purità e il culto nel Levitico*, ed. M. Pesce and M. Simonetti, *Annali di storia dell' esegesi* 13, no. 1 (1996): 201–9.

37 Nicholas III Grammatikos, *Answers to the Bishop of Zetounion* 5, ed. J. Darrouzès, "Les réponses de Nicolas III à l'évêque de Zétounion," *Καθηγήτρια: Essays Presented to Joan Hussey for Her 80th Birthday*, ed. J. Chrysostomides (Camberley, 1988), 327–43.

38 Leo VI, *Novella* 17, in *Les novelles de Léon VI*, ed. P. Noailles and A. Dain (Paris, 1944), 62–65.

39 *Canons of Hippolytus*, canon 18, in *Canons d'Hippolyte, édition critique de la version arabe*, ed. R. G. Coquin (Paris, 1966) (PO 31.2), 375; B. Caseau, "Sancta sanctis: Normes et gestes de la communion entre Antiquité et haut Moyen Âge," in Bériou, Caseau, and Rigaux, *Pratiques* (n. 23 above), 1:371–420.

40 D. Brakke, "The Problematization of Nocturnal Emissions in Early Christian Syria, Egypt and Gaul," *JEChrSt* 3 (1995): 419–60; for a late Byzantine discussion of the same question, see P. D. Viscuso, *Sexuality, Marriage, and Celibacy in Byzantine Law: Selections from a Fourteenth-Century Encyclopedia of Canon Law and Theology; The Alphabetical Collection of Matthew Blastares* (Brookline, MA, 2008), 19–20; idem, "Purity and Sexual Defilement in Late Byzantine Theology," *OCP* 57 (1991): 399–408.

41 Athanasios of Alexandria, *Letter to Amoun the Monk*, ed. Joannou (n. 32 above), 66; T. Vivian, "Everything Made by God Is Good: A Letter concerning Sexuality from Saint Athanasius to the Monk Amoun," *Église et théologie* 24 (1993): 75–108.

42 Timothy of Alexandria, canon 20, ed. Joannou, 253.

43 Taft, *History* (n. 24 above), 378–89.

44 B. Caseau, *Nourritures terrestres, nourritures célestes: La culture alimentaire à Byzance* (Paris, 2015), 89.

salvation. Eating a piece of blessed bread rather than consecrated bread was an easy solution. Patriarch Nicholas III Grammatikos encouraged the faithful to take blessed bread, because, in his opinion, it chased away bad thoughts and restored the body's health.[45] It could be divided into small bites or offered for festivals as whole breads, on which a marker had imprinted either an image of the saint, or a drawing of the sanctuary, or some text calling for God's blessing, such as ЄVΛΟΓΙΑ KVΡΙΟV ЄΦ ΗΜΑC.[46]

Another solution, often adopted by Christians who did not share the faith of the clergy of a particular church but wanted to worship a local saint, was to ask for oil burning in the lamps on top of saints' tombs or reliquaries. In the early seventh century, the Egyptian healing shrine of Cyrus and John welcomed both Monophysites and Chalcedonians. As the priests were Chalcedonians, those who did not share their faith would not receive communion from their hands. Instead they asked for some oil, which they drank or rubbed on themselves.[47]

Even for the pilgrims who shared the faith of the clergy in charge of a church, obtaining some holy oil was a favorite activity, which helped develop the manufacture and trade of *ampullae* and other small flasks to carry the precious oil.[48]

Sanctioned by clerical approval, different gestures of devotions allowed Christians, men and women, to be active participants in religious rituals. Most of these gestures were spontaneous, even if promoted by society and perhaps performed under peer pressure. These gestures could take place at home as well as in churches, or anywhere else as a matter of fact. They represented an area of personal involvement for each person with religious objects at home or with the church building and its content.

For example, when entering a church, bowing, kneeling or touching the floor was a way to show respect to the holiness of the church and the presence of God and his angels. Veneration within the church could take diverse forms, such as kissing columns or doors and mostly bowing and kissing icons. What took place behind the iconostasis was no longer visible and accessible to lay people, but the icons were. Personal devotion to particular saints could be expressed by paying a visit to their image.[49] The council of Nicaea II approved kissing icons and offering the saints represented in the image gestures of affection, lights, and incense. After the members of the council gathered in 787, they decided that these were proper gestures of veneration.[50] Kissing became an official part of the Byzantine religious culture after 843. Not that the Byzantines had ignored kissing religious objects before that date or were alone in expressing devotion through kissing. Western Christians, Jews, and Muslims also venerated tombs and used reliquaries and other sacred objects, incorporating kissing into their gestures.[51] Yet in the Byzantine religious culture, more than in any other contemporary one, kissing icons became a trademark. Physical and affectionate relations with the saints depicted in

45 Nicholas III Grammatikos, *Canonical Answers to an Athonite Monk*, ed. J. Oudot, *Patriarchatus Constantinopolitani Acta selecta* (Rome, 1941), 19.

46 G. Galavaris, *Bread and the Liturgy: The Symbolism of Early Christian and Byzantine Bread Stamps* (Madison, 1970); examples of bread stamps bearing the image of saints and sanctuaries: N. Ševčenko, "Bread Stamp with St. Philip," in *Age of Spirituality: Late Antique and Early Christian Art, Third to Seventh Century*, ed. K. Weitzmann (New York, 1979), 590–91. On donations of bread and its marking, see B. Caseau, "Autour de l'autel: Le contrôle des donateurs et des donations alimentaires," in *Donations et Donateurs dans le monde byzantin, Actes du colloque international de l'Université de Fribourg (13–15 mars 2008)*, ed. J.-M. Spieser and E. Yota (Paris, 2012), 47–73.

47 Sophronios, *Miracles of Cyrus and John* 38.1–3, in *Los* thaumata *de Sofronio*, ed. N. F. Marcos (Madrid, 1975), 333.

48 A. Grabar, *Ampoules de Terre Sainte: Monza*, Bobbio (Paris, 1958); C. Metzger, *Les ampoules à eulogie du musée du Louvre* (Paris, 1981); G. Vikan, "Byzantine Pilgrims' Art," in *Heaven on Earth: Art and the Church in Byzantium*, ed. L. Safran (University Park, PA, 1998), 229–66; J. Witt, *Werke der Alltagskultur*, pt. 1, *Menasampullen* (Wiesbaden, 2000); M. Gilli, *Le ampolle di San Mena: Religiosità, cultura materiale e sistema produttivo* (Rome, 2002); L. Lavan, E. Swift, and T. Putzeys, eds., *Objects in Context, Objects in Use: Material Spatiality in Late Antiquity* (Leiden, 2007); G. Vikan, *Early Byzantine Pilgrimage Art*, 2nd ed. (Washington, DC, 2010).

49 H. Belting, *Likeness and Presence: A History of the Image before the Era of Art*, trans. E. Jephcott (Chicago, 1994), 172.

50 Pentcheva, *Sensual Icon* (n. 5 above), 71–72; context for iconoclasm in L. Brubaker and J. Haldon, *Byzantium in the Iconoclast Era, c. 680–850: A History* (Cambridge, 2011).

51 J. W. Meri, "Relics of Piety and Power in Medieval Islam," *Past and Present* 206, suppl. 5 (2010): 97–120, at 101–2; idem, *The Cult of Saints among Muslims and Jews in Medieval Syria* (Oxford, 2002); D. M. Gitlitz and L. K. Davidson, *Pilgrimage and the Jews* (Westport, CT, 2006); J.-C. Schmitt, *La raison des gestes dans l'Occident médiéval* (Paris, 1990).

ritual objects became a tradition, later adopted by other Orthodox sister or daughter churches.

Kissing was not the only possible devotional gesture in front of religious images. Lighting a lamp and putting one's forehead in contact with the icon were accompanied by prayers sent to God through the saints. Lighting a censer and bringing offerings were also frequent ways of attracting the saints' attention. The cult of saints developed in Byzantine Christianity on different levels: through the Church calendar, with festive days; through art, with paintings, mosaics and icons. The cult of one's favorite saints could thrive on a personal level when one chose to carry portable objects such as *enkolpia* or small icons close to the body, sewn into the hems of a coat, kept in a pocket, or worn around the neck.[52] The choice of a specific saint for one's seal also revealed either a group or a personal attachment to a particular saint.[53] Thus Byzantine Christians could relate to the saints liturgically, by attending the liturgy or by joining the prayers of the hours on a saint's feast day as well as, in a private devotional manner, by choosing patron saints, by carrying their image, by naming children after them, by visiting churches devoted to them, by praying in front of their icon, and by embracing their images. Many of these devotional gestures included touching. Tactile piety developed because the Byzantines believed that objects such as relics could be filled with the power to bless, protect, and heal. They expected that the saints transmitted some of their holiness to objects on which they were depicted or which had come into contact with remains of their bodies.

Relics' efficacy was judged by their ability to cure. Stories of miracles spread the news that such and such a saint was indeed attentive and powerful at healing.[54] Some saints specialized in curing specific illnesses. It was important for sanctuaries to properly identify God as the source of healing, through the intercession of his saints. This is why, although clerics often had some medical or pharmaceutical knowledge, the means to cure the sick were very different from actual medicines provided by doctors. In healing shrines, ailments were cured with lamp oil, *myron*, perfumed oil, or *kerote*, a mixture of wax and oil.[55] Other less conventional curative means were also imagined by storytellers who had a sense of humor.[56] In the Kosmidion, the sanctuary of Saints Kosmas and Damian, a patient had experienced a strange cure in a vision: he was to be cured by taking a pubic hair from "Kosmas." Puzzled, he asked other patients if such a strange cure had been offered in the past. It appeared that "Kosmas" was in fact the nickname of a lamb offered to the healing shrine.[57] In comparison, being offered a cure with some perfumed oil to rub on one's body must have been much more pleasant.

Myroblite saints were very popular and pilgrims came from far away to visit their shrine, in order to be healed and protected or to bring back home some of the miraculous oil that came from their reliquary, or icons.[58] Some pilgrims drank the perfumed oil offered by the saints, others preferred to anoint themselves with it. The oil was an efficient medium to capture a saint's *virtus*. Pilgrims hoped it would heal and protect their families or themselves. The phenomenon had probably started in Cyprus with John the Almsgiver and had spread to other cults after the Arabic invasion: it is also recorded at Aegina for

52 B. Pitarakis, *Les croix-reliquaires pectorales byzantines en bronze* (Paris, 2006); eadem, "Objects of Devotion and Protection," in *A People's History of Christianity*, vol. 3, *Byzantine Christianity*, ed. D. Krueger (Minneapolis, 2006), 164–81.

53 J. Cotsonis, "The Contribution of Byzantine Lead Seals to the Study of the Cult of the Saints (Sixth–Twelfth Century)," *Byzantion* 75 (2005): 383–497; J.-C. Cheynet, *La société byzantine: L'apport des sceaux*, vol. 1 (Paris, 2008); B. Caseau, "Saint Mark, a Family Saint? The Iconography of the Xeroi's Seals," *Ἠπειρόνδε: Proceedings of the 10th International Symposium of Byzantine Sigillography* (Ioannina, 1–3 October 2009), ed. C. Stavrakos and B. Papadopoulou (Leiden, 2011), 81–110.

54 V. Déroche, "Pourquoi écrivait-on des recueils de miracles? L'exemple des miracles de saint Artémios," in *Les saints et leurs sanctuaires: Textes, images et monuments*, ed. C. Jolivet-Lévy, M. Kaplan, and J.-P. Sodini (Paris, 1993), 95–116.

55 B. Caseau, "Parfum et guérison dans le christianisme ancien et byzantin: Des huiles parfumées au myron des saints byzantins," in *Les Pères de l'Eglise face à la science médicale de leur temps*, ed. V. Boudon-Millot, B. Pouderon, and Y. M. Blanchard (Paris, 2005), 141–91.

56 B. Caseau, "Ordinary Objects in Christian Healing Sanctuaries," in Lavan, Swift, and Putzeys, *Objects in Context*, 625–54.

57 L. Deubner, *Kosmas und Damian*, Texte und Einleitung (Leipzig, 1907), 105*.

58 J. O. Rosenqvist, *The Hagiographic Dossier of St. Eugenios of Trebizond in Codex Athous Dionysiou 154* (Uppsala, 1996), 45.

Saint Athanasia,[59] at Myra for Saint Nicholas,[60] at Thessalonike for Saint Demetrios[61] and later Saint Theodora,[62] at Trebizond for Saint Eugenios,[63] to cite just a few examples.[64] Oil was the main ingredient in many medicines. It is not so suprising to find it in many cults. Oil burning in front of a reliquary was a longtime favorite for pilgrims, yet oil miraculously offered by the saints contained the promise of a powerful efficiency to heal and protect. This list of cults reveals the need for an easy to carry "holy matter," charged with the blessings of the saints.

Water was even more affordable than *myron* and the *hagiasma*[65] attached to a sanctuary often remained popular even after the fall of the Byzantine Empire and its capital, Constantinople. Holy fountains had the reputation of holding water with healing powers. The monastery of the Theotokos of Pege had such a miraculous fountain, with water deemed blessed by the Theotokos herself. Miracles stories were compiled from the tenth through the fourteenth centuries to spread the reputation of this healing shrine.[66] Sick people rubbed water and mud on their diseased bodies, while other pilgrims simply drank the water. The shrine received visits from all sorts of people, including members of the imperial family. At the end of the eighth century, Empress Irene drank from the holy water and recovered from a hemorrhage. In return, she and her son offered vessels and curtains to the church.[67] In the tenth century, Empress Zoe Karbonopsina thought she owed her pregnancy to a skein of silk that she wrapped around her loins after it had been in contact with an icon of the Theotokos in that shrine. Also, she recovered from a fever thanks to the mud and the holy water of the Pege.[68] In 1330, Emperor Andronikos III felt better after some of the water was rubbed on his forehead.[69]

One can be surprised to see the imperial family simply drinking water from Pege, when emperors and empresses had access to very important relics, not to mention doctors. It is a testimony to the reputation of some healing shrines and to the imperial family's devotion to the Theotokos.[70] It reveals the importance of matter in capturing holiness and its healing powers and the infusion of divine and saints' presence at hot spots.

Still, members of the imperial family had privileged access to relics and could ask to come into personal contact with objects having belonged to saints, or even better to the Theotokos or to Christ. These relics were sought out in the hope that through their agency suffering could be alleviated. For example, the belt of the Theotokos was a very precious relic, probably brought to Constantinople during the fifth century.[71] It was once lent to Zoe Zaoutsaina,

59 F. Halkin, "Vie de sainte Athanasie d'Egine," 15, *Six inédits d'hagiologie byzantine* (Brussels, 1987), 179–95; *Life of Saint Athanasia of Aegina*, trans. L. F. Sherry, *Holy Women of Byzantium*, ed. A.-M. Talbot (Washington, DC, 1996), 142–58.

60 G. Anrich, *Hagios Nikolaos: Der Heilige Nikolaos in der griechischen Kirche* (Leipzig, 1913–17).

61 Iohannis Caminiatae, *De expugnatione Thessalonicae*, ed. G. Böhlig (Berlin, 1973), 3 line 66; D. G. Frendo, "The Miracles of St. Demetrius and the Capture of Thessaloniki: An Examination of the Purpose, Significance and Authenticity of John Kaminiates' *De expugnatione Thessalonicae*," *Byzantinoslavica* 58 (1999): 216; Rosenqvist, *Hagiographic Dossier*, 302 (cites the healing cult of Demetrios).

62 *Life of Saint Theodora of Thessalonike*, trans. A.-M. Talbot, in eadem, *Holy Women of Byzantium*, 164–237; eadem, "Family Cults in Byzantium: The Case of St. Theodora of Thessalonike," *ΛΕΙΜΩΝ: Studies Presented to Lennart Ryden on His Sixty-Fifth Birthday*, ed. J. O. Rosenqvist (Uppsala, 1996), 55–69.

63 Rosenqvist, *Hagiographic Dossier*.

64 Caseau, "Parfum."

65 R. G. Ousterhout, "Water and Healing in Constantinople," in *Life Is Short, Art Long: The Art of Healing in Byzantium*, ed. B. Pitarakis (Istanbul, 2015), 65–77.

66 S. Efthymiadis, "Le monastère de la Source à Constantinople et ses deux recueils de miracles: Entre hagiographie et patriographie," *REB* 64–65 (2006–7): 283–309; A.-M. Talbot, "The Anonymous *Miracula* of the Pege Shrine in Constantinople," *Palaeoslavica* 10 (2002): 222–28; eadem, "Two Accounts of Miracles at the Pege Shrine in Constantinople," *TM* 14 (*Mélanges Gilbert Dagron*) (Paris, 2002), 605–15; trans. A.-M. Talbot and S. F. Johnson, *Miracle Tales from Byzantium* (Cambridge, MA, 2012).

67 *Anonymous Miracles of the Pege* 8, ed. and trans. Talbot and Johnson, 222–23.

68 *Anonymous Miracles of the Pege* 26, ed. and trans. Talbot and Johnson, 266–67; B. Pitarakis, "Female Piety in Context: Understanding Developments in Private Devotional Practices," *Images of the Mother of God: Perceptions of the Theotokos in Byzantium*, ed. M. Vassilaki (Aldershot 2005): 153–66.

69 *Nicephori Gregorae Byzantina historia, graece et latine*, ed. L. Schopen, vol. 2 (Bonn, 1830), 442.

70 C. Angelidi and T. Papamastorakis, "Picturing the Spiritual Protector: From Blachernitissa to Hodegetria," in Vassilaki, *Images*, 209–23.

71 J. Wortley, "The Marian Relics at Constantinople," *GRBS* 45 (2005): 171–87.

who had become the mistress of Leo VI while his first wife Theophano still lived. She eventually became his second wife, but she did not live long and her reputation was tainted. The *synaxarion* and Basil's *menologion* record a story about her stating that she was possessed by a demon but was cured by touching the belt of the Theotokos.[72] A political rehabilitation of the lady might be read in this story. If the Theotokos cured her from her evil ways, it might mean that she was forgiven.

Marian relics and objects that Christ himself had been in contact with were at the top of a hierarchy of holy relics to be touched and kissed.[73] The Byzantines expected a lot from touching the Holy Cross, whose pieces began to be dispersed in the late fourth century. Macrina, the sister of Basil of Caesarea and Gregory of Nyssa, had managed to obtain a piece of the Cross that she wore close to her heart.[74] The Byzantine emperors offered small pieces of the Cross as diplomatic gifts. Justin II offered a piece of the precious relic to Queen Radegund, for her convent in Poitiers.[75] Eventually, after the defeat of the Sassanians, who had confiscated the relic, Emperor Heraklios took control of the rest of the relic and most of it was kept in the Great Palace, in Constantinople. Each year, the emperor shared the precious relic, and the *staurotheke* containing the Cross was brought to Hagia Sophia cathedral for three days of veneration, during Holy Week. A Western pilgrim, who had travelled to Constantinople in the 680s, described the ceremony. Men and women, lay people and clerics took turns to touch and kiss the relic. The emperor led the men, the women followed the empress, and members of the clergy approached it after the patriarch of Constantinople. Each group had a day set aside for this ceremony. On the Thursday, the emperor and his soldiers came to kiss the relic; on Good Friday, it was the turn of the empress, the ladies of the aristocracy, and the women of Constantinople to come and kiss the relic with "great veneration." Finally, on the Saturday before Easter, the bishop and the clergy approached the relic with "awe and trembling" and kissed it with great reverence.[76]

The same signs of veneration were offered on different, less formal, occasions. Whether they came to visit a distant shrine, after a long pilgrimage, or entered a neighborhood chapel, worshippers performed similar gestures. They came, they bowed, they touched, and they kissed. They often liked to mark the holy shrines they had visited with a sign of their presence, many times by incising graffiti on the walls or leaving ex-votos. Tactile piety was the natural manner for the Byzantines to relate to their saints and capture some of their holiness. When Russian pilgrims write about their visit to the churches, they mention what they kissed. Ignatius of Smolensk, for example, visited Hagia Sophia in 1389 and he recalls all the wonderful relics he came into contact with. "We kissed the table on which the Relics of the Passion of Christ are placed, and [the body of] St. Arsenius the Patriarch and the table at which Abraham welcomed Christ manifest in Trinity, as well as the iron pallet on which Christ's martyrs were burned."[77]

Christians naturally wished they could still touch Jesus, and because the Eucharist was highly revered and somehow kept at a distance, the Byzantines developed substitute devotions based on touch. Instead of touching Christ directly, they approached his divine being though objects, or through the cult of saints. The wish to touch Christ and benefit from his divine contact through the objects he himself had touched created the frame for developing tactile piety. These devotional gestures could be performed by all,

72 H. Delehaye, *Synaxarium Ecclesiae Constantinopolitanae e codice Sirmondiano nunc Berolinensi adiectis synaxariis selectis opera et studio* (Brussels, 1902), 936; *Menologion of Basil*, PG 117:613.

73 Durand and Flusin, *Byzance* (n. 1 above); C. Hahn and H. A. Klein, eds., *Saints and Sacred Matter: The Cult of Relics in Byzantium and Beyond* (Washington, DC, 2015).

74 Gregory of Nyssa, *Life of Macrina*, 30, ed. P. Maraval, *Vie de sainte Macrine*, SC 178 (Paris, 1971), 238–40; on the discovery attributed to Helena, the mother of Constantine, J. W. Drijvers, *Helena Augusta: The Mother of Constantine the Great and the Legend of Her Finding of the True Cross* (Leiden, 1992); idem, "Helena Augusta, the Cross and the Myth: Some New Reflections," *Millenium* 8 (2011): 125–74.

75 A. Frolow, *La relique de la Vraie Croix: Recherches sur le développement d'un culte* (Paris, 1961).

76 Adomnan, *The Holy Places*, 3.3.5–12, trans. J. Wilkinson, *Jerusalem Pilgrims before the Crusades* (Warminster, 1977), 202; text in *Adamnani, De locis sanctis libri tres*, ed. L. Bieler, CCSL 175–76 (Turnhout, 1965).

77 G. Majeska, *Russian Travelers to Constantinople in the Fourteenth and Fifteenth Centuries*, DOS 19 (Washington, DC, 1984), 92.

clerics and lay people, men and women, young and old, rich and poor, and they helped develop a non-liturgical and very personal relationship to religious matters. Tactile piety played a key role in Byzantine Christianity, first because it was an embodied religion and second because, besides sacramental life, lay people expressed their religious agency through devotion.

There is a theological reason for this approach to the divine. The development of tactile piety is linked to the incarnation of Christ, which made the Son of God reachable through the senses. He could be touched, kissed, or embraced while living on this earth. He also touched the sick in order to heal them (e.g., Mt. 8:3, 8:15; Mk. 7:31–37, etc.), let his favorite disciple recline on him (Jn. 13:23–26), and allowed a woman to rub perfumed oil on his feet (Jn. 12:3; Lk. 7:37–38). Even after the Resurrection, Jesus encouraged doubting Thomas to place his hand in his wounds and testify that he was no ghost (Jn. 20:25–28). The development of tactile piety is steeped in Christian incarnation theology.

After his ascension, Jesus Christ having left this earth, it was no longer possible to touch him directly.[78] But the Church offered another means of contact, through the Eucharistic bread and wine, transformed into his Body and Blood. Starting in the fourth century, newly discovered objects he had been in contact with during his lifetime created other ways for devout Christians to establish a personal connection with Christ or his saints.[79] The constant need to reach God through gestures and touch was answered by an also constant wish on the part of Church authorities to control devotion and keep the sacred at a distance from unholy or impure hands. Touching the Eucharist and its containers with the hand became a clerical privilege, and precious relics were approached only under clerical supervision. This is perhaps why touching icons and kissing them became such a popular devotion for all Byzantine Christians of the middle ages.[80]

78 On the anguish of this separation see G. Frank, "Sensing Ascension in Early Byzantium," in *Experiencing Byzantium*, ed. C. Nesbitt and M. Jackson (Farnham, 2013), 293–309, at 306–7.

79 P. Maraval, *Lieux saints et pèlerinage d'Orient*, 2nd ed. (Paris, 2004); Durand and Flusin, *Byzance*; J. Wortley, *Studies on the Cult of Relics in Byzantium up to 1204* (Farnham, 2009); *Treasures of Heaven: Saints, Relics, and Devotion in Medieval Europe*, ed. M. Bagnoll, E. A. Klein, and G. Griffith Mann (Cleveland, 2010); C. Freeman, *Holy Bones, Holy Dust: How Relics Shaped the History of Medieval Europe* (New Haven, 2011).

80 A. Cutler, *The Hand of the Master: Craftsmanship, Ivory and Society in Byzantium* (Princeton, 1994), 22–29.

CHAPTER TWELVE

A Touch of Violence

Feeling Pain, Perceiving Pain in Byzantium

GALINA TIRNANIĆ

Modern science distinguishes between active and passive aspects of the sense of touch—the active haptic perception, or touching, and the passive tactile perception, or feeling. While Béatrice Caseau in the previous chapter explores the active aspect of holy touch in Byzantium and in the next Ingela Nilsson examines a specific instance of touch that affects body and soul—erotic touch by women—I address here the passive aspect of the sense of touch, that is, the feeling of being touched.[1] The focus of the essay is the perception of pain, a particular category of sensation caused by touch, and the specific nature of pain considered is that caused by the violent touch of a public executioner.[2] Needless to say, this essay will scratch the surface of the phenomenon of touching and feeling in Byzantium.

The most obvious organ of touch, skin, is the largest body organ, but it is only a membrane, a container, albeit a container that feels. The pain is sometimes felt on the surface at the location of touch, but often also beyond the surface, underneath, internally. Writing about the sense of touch in the eighth century, John of Damascus recognized that its "organs are nerves which come from the brain and ramify all through the body. Hence the body as a whole, including even the other organs of sense, possesses the sense of touch."[3] Our brain maps the body and we understand where the pain is located.[4]

1 For an exploration of what it meant for objects to perceive and feel in Byzantium, see the chapter by Glenn Peers in this volume.

2 Receptors for pain, known as *nocireceptors*, are different from those for nonviolent tactile sensation, such as those caused by temperature or fine touch. For introduction to sensory perceptions of pain see for example D. Purves et al., *Neuroscience*, 5th ed. (Sunderland, 2011), 209–28.

3 John of Damascus, *De fide orthodoxa*, ed. B. Kotter, *Die Schriften des Johannes von Damaskos* (Berlin, 1972), 2: ch. 18. See also *Esposizione della fede = De fide orthodoxa*, with Ital. trans. by M. Andolfo (Bologna, 2013). Engl. trans. S. D. F. Salmond in "Exposition of the Orthodox Faith," *Nicene and Post Nicene Fathers*, vol. 9, *Hilary of Poitiers, John of Damascus*, ed. P. Schaff and H. Wace (1899; repr. Peabody, MA, 1994), 625–26. John of Damascus also notes that all other organs come in pairs, but "touch is spread over the whole body with the exception of bones, nerves, nails, horns, hairs, ligaments, and other such structures." John relies heavily on Aristotle, directly or indirectly. M. Frede, "John of Damascus on the Human Action, the Will and Human Freedom," *Byzantine Philosophy and Its Ancient Sources*, ed. K. Ierodiakonou (Oxford, 2002), 63–95. In the East, "the tradition of commenting on Aristotle continues uninterrupted until the 15th century or even beyond the fall of Constantinople in 1453," K. Ierodiakonou, "Psellos's Paraphrasis on Aristotle's *De interpretatione*," *Byzantine Philosophy*, 157–82, at 157. Aristotle's *De anima* was widely read in Byzantium, especially through the lens of Alexander of Aphrodisias and other commentators. See A. Towey, *Alexander of Aphrodisias on Aristotle's "On Sense Perception"* (Ithaca, NY, 2000). For Aristotle touch is the most "imperfect" of senses, but also most "essential" and taste is also a function of/kind of touch. Touch and taste are assigned the element of earth: they are associated with the heart because of their hot quality. Sight is associated with water, hearing and smell with air; these are related to the brain because they are cold.

4 In contemporary terms, the cortical homunculus maps the body onto the brain.

By considering a selection of visual and textual references to corporal punishment from a variety of sources aimed at different audiences, from manuscript illuminations and frescoes to histories and saints' lives, I hope to open the discussion about what it meant to be physically touched by the law in Byzantium. Far from a systematic survey, instances of lashing, burning, and blinding discussed here will provide an initial exploration of the connection between these events and the Byzantine understanding of the sense of touch and the perception of pain.

During actual punishment spectacles in medieval Constantinople, spectators were implicitly asked to understand the message of what they saw, and the contemplation of the physical pain experienced by the condemned was a component of that message.[5] Eyewitnesses of these events could all see the same thing, hear the same thing, even smell the same thing, and attest to the visual, audio, and olfactory experiences of others with a great deal of certainty, but they could not feel the pain of the condemned. So how was this sensation transmitted to the observers?

In her groundbreaking book, *The Body in Pain*, Elaine Scarry argues that language fails to describe and express pain and that this inexpressibility of pain through language has political consequences.[6] Not only patients and other sufferers of pain struggle to express what they feel, even medical professionals have difficulty assessing and describing pain verbally. Scarry notes that there are essentially two categories of metaphors that people use to express pain through language: the "external agent of pain, a weapon that is pictured as producing the pain" and the "specific bodily damage that is pictured as accompanying the pain."[7] One *pictures* a weapon and a wound in order to understand the quality of pain.

In Constantinople, the sense of vision was called upon to perceive pain in the imagination of the onlookers of punishment spectacles. Relationship between vision and touch was addressed by Byzantine thinkers, such as John of Damascus, who notes that certain qualities perceived by touch are also perceived by vision.[8] The instruments of causing pain and the wounds on the flesh of the condemned were not only metaphors, but actual means of comprehending the sensation. Similarly, readers of saints' lives and viewers of martyrdom images had to imagine punitive events and assess the pain of martyrs by visualizing instruments and wounds. While the suffering of martyrs was meant to elicit empathy and the suffering of criminals, a satisfaction, the distinction between the two was not always clear—for example both early Christian and iconophile martyrs were criminals with regard to the imperial laws. The following cases of public punishments as well as the textual and visual accounts of actual and legendary events provide a variety of examples through which to investigate how instruments and wounds, the two visible indicators of the severity and quality of the otherwise inexpressible and incomprehensible pain, helped the onlookers, readers, and viewers in perceiving the pain of both martyrs and criminals in Byzantium. While the primary focus will be on translating tactile into visual, I will also take into consideration instances when other senses were

5 Punishment spectacles were an extension of the imperial ceremony. See for example M. McCormick, "Analyzing Imperial Ceremonies," *JOB* (1985): 1–20. For explorations in punishment of emperors and usurpers, see for example B.-P. Maleon, "Le rôle de la mutilation dans la lutte politique à Byzance: Genèse et évolution jusqu'au XIe siècle," in *Le corps et ses hypostases en Europe et dans la société roumaine du Moyen Âge à l'époque contemporaine*, ed. C. Vintilă-Ghitulescu and A.-F. Platon (Bucharest, 2010), 125–46; and his "The Impossible Return: About the Status of Deposed and Mutilated Emperors," *Medieval and Early Modern Studies for Central and Eastern Europe* 3 (2011): 31–49.

6 E. Scarry, *The Body in Pain: The Making and Unmaking of the World* (Oxford and New York, 1985).

7 Ibid., 15.

8 He continues: "Further it is to be observed that sight is possible only in straight lines, whereas smell and hearing are not limited to straight lines only but act in all directions. Touch again, and taste act neither in straight lines, nor in every direction, but only when each comes near to the sensible objects that are proper to it." When John of Damascus actually discusses pain he does not mention physical pain, but four kinds of psychological pain: anguish (pain without utterance), grief (pain that is heavy to bear like a burden), envy (pain over the good fortune of others), and pity (pain over the evil fortune of others). He touches on wounds and disease but not much on other aspects of physical pain. He does address pain when he discusses passion: "For pain succeeds passion, but it is not the same thing as passion. For passion is an affection of things without sense, but not so pain. Pain then is not passion, but the sensation of passion: and it must be considerable, that is to say, it must be great enough to come within the scope of sense." *De fide orthodoxa* 2.14 ("Concerning Pain") and 2.22 ("Concerning Passion and Energy").

called upon as additional aids in perceiving the pain of others.[9]

Beaten by Wood and Hide: Lashing/Flogging

It makes sense to begin with the most common kind of corporal punishment sanctioned by the Byzantine law, lashing, which features prominently in a variety of sources.[10] While such punishment is often mentioned in chronicles and histories, the authors of these sources tend not to dwell on the details and the physiological effects. By contrast, textual accounts of martyrdom provide more cues as to the experience of the lashed persons. Numerous images of lashing in illuminated manuscripts, frescoes and icons, while iconographically repetitive, offer some insight into the nature of the pain undergone by martyrs. Rare visual references to historical instances of lashing are iconographically similar to these martyrdom scenes. In both categories, we encounter a variety of punitive beating: the lashed individuals are standing up, lying down, or hanging upside down, they are beaten by clubs or whips, they are nude or clothed.[11]

For instance, in a rare illustrated history, that of John Skylitzes (Madrid, Bibl. Nac. Vitr. 26-2), we see an example of lashing in the agora (Forum of Constantine), observed by Emperor Theophilos (r. 829–842) on a horse (fig. 12.1).[12] As is common to a variety of corporal punishment in Byzantium, the body as a whole was activated in the punishment process, stripped to its nude state to emphasize its vulnerability to the elements, as well as to the hand of the law. The vertical positioning of the lashed man, his wide open arms forming a cross shape, as well as his tilted head, all invite the viewer to compare this body to the body of Christ in Crucifixion images. Two executioners support an arm each, holding and restraining the wrists of the condemned upon their shoulders. Two others perform the lashing upon the back of his nude torso. The instruments seem to consist of only one wide strap. Would it produce sharp or dull pain? Would it be felt on the surface or deep inside the body, or both? As I struggle to find correct words for the pain experienced by the lashed person, something that can arguably be correctly understood only by those who had experienced such, or a similar, pain, it becomes even more poignant how difficult it is to verbally convey the precise nature of someone else's pain, or even describe our own.

To the right of the lashed culprit, Emperor Theophilos on the horse extends a hand toward the punishment scene. With this gesture, he reveals himself as the ultimate source of this lashing: he both points out the functioning of a healthy legal system to the group of mounted figures behind him, and also implies that he is the one who ordered it. He is the one who touches the bodies through the agency of the executioners and the instruments they hold.

Yet the visual paralleling of the lashed person to the crucified Christ subverts the message of the text that presents Theophilos as a just emperor observing the practice of law in his ordered city. Because of the Christ-like figure

9 On synesthetic experience in Byzantium, see L. James, "Senses and Sensibility in Byzantium," *Art History* 27, no. 4 (2004): 522–37.

10 For its legal uses, see for example L. Burgmann, ed., *Ecloga, das Gesetzbuch Leons III und Konstantinos V* (1983). The Greek text was originally edited by P. and I. Zepos, *Jus Graeco-Romanum* 2 (Athens, 1931), 3–62. See also L. Burgmann, ed., "Appendix *Eclogae*," *Fontes Minores* 3 (1979): 24–125; *The Ecloga: A Manual of Roman Law*, trans. E. H. Freshfield (Cambridge, 1927); and *Revised Manual of Roman Law*, trans. E. H. Freshfield (Cambridge, 1927).

11 While other examples are discussed in this essay, for upside-down bodies see Psellos, who describes the lashing of a man who plotted to assassinate Constantine IX: "He was stripped, hoisted up to a wooden beam, and suspended from it by his feet, then flogged till he was half-dead. This punishment had a crushing effect on him." Engl. trans. by E. R. A. Sewter, *Fourteen Byzantine Rulers: The Chronographia of Michael Psellus* (London, 1966), 227. Greek text in recent edition by D. R. Reinsch: *Michaelis Pselii Chronographia*, 2 vols. (Paris, 2014), 6.137. See also Niketas Choniates on deposed emperor Andronikos, who was beaten while hanging upside-down at the Hippodrome. *Historia*, ed. J. L. van Dieten (Berlin and New York, 1975), 350. Eng. trans. by H. Magoulias, *O City of Byzantium, Annals of Niketas Choniates* (Detroit, 1984), 193 [350]. For a visual example, see Vat. gr. 1613, fol. 138.

12 Madrid, Bibl. Nac. Vitr. 26-2, fol. 43v. Interestingly the image is not backed up by Skylitzes's text, but the premise is supplied by Zonaras: a woman complained about the empress's brother Petronas. When Theophilos spotted the accused at the Forum of Constantine, he ordered that he be whipped on the back and chest. V. Tsamakda, *The Illustrated Chronicle of Ioannes Skylitzes in Madrid* (Leiden, 2002), 85. *Ioannes Zonaras: Epitome historiarum*, ed. M. Pinder and M. Büttner-Wobst (Bonn, 1841–97), 3:356–357.

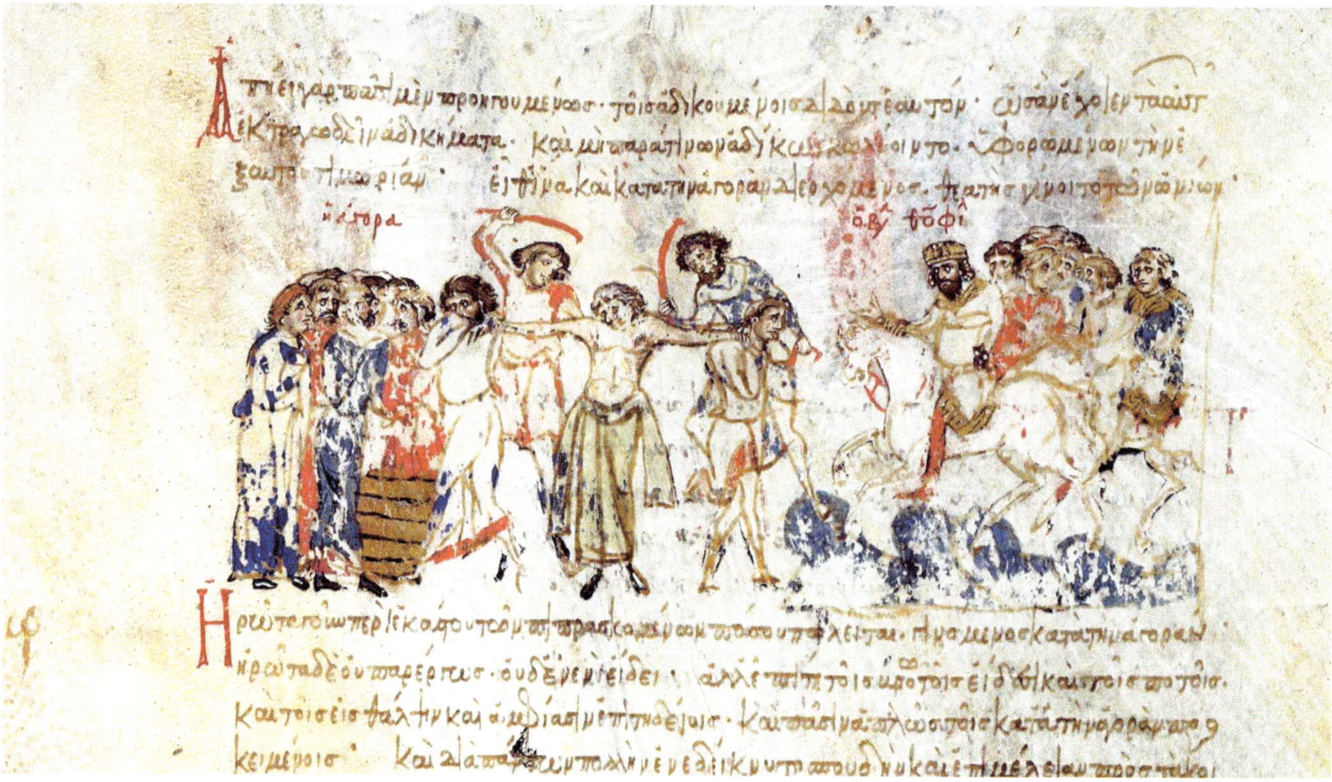

FIG. 12.1. Madrid, Bibl. Nac. Vitr. 26-2 (12th c.), fol. 43v, detail: Theophilos observes lashing in the agora (photo: Biblioteca Nacional de España)

of the punished, the judgment of the emperor who punishes him is called into question. The emperor easily slips into the role of a wrongdoer, perhaps as a reference to his iconoclastic policies.

As we read in Zonaras's description of the man lashed by Theophilos, not only the back but sometimes also the front of the torso was exposed to the punitive blows, which is also described in the life of St. Stephen the Younger.[13] In an episode from this account Emperor Constantine VI (r. 780–797) allegedly threatens to beat a nun, Anna, on the back *and* front if she does not admit fornicating with the monk Stephen, a false accusation. The emperor gathers a crowd and exposes the nun's nude body before the observers. He shows her the ox-hide whip (βούνευρον) to instill in her fear of the imminent pain. He hopes that by looking at the instrument of torture she will imagine the blows on her naked skin and foresee the pain that is coming. As she awaits the actual beating, her body, accustomed to being covered, is introduced to new sensations in its stripped state: she can feel the air upon the naked skin, and also the gaze of the crowd, for the rays of vision often touch and "grab" in Byzantium.[14] The emperor expects that the imagination of the future pain itself will be enough to scare her into admitting her alleged crime. Elaborating on the nature of fear, John of Damascus distinguishes between the fear of imminent pain and the pain itself: "when a bad thing is expected it gives rise to fear, but when it is present it causes pain."[15] The fear that that the nun is expected to feel could be characterized as "terror," which John defines as "fear arising from a strong mental impression."[16] The emperor seeks to activate

13 *La Vie d' Étienne le Jeune par Étienne le Diacre*, ed. M.-F. Auzépy (Birmingham, 1997), 230–31. It must have been common to witness lashing in the city.

14 See R. S. Nelson, "Descartes's Cow and Other Domestications of the Visual," and "To Say and to See: *Ekphrasis* and Vision in Byzantium," in *Visuality Before and Beyond the Renaissance: Seeing as Others Saw*, ed. R. S. Nelson (New York and Cambridge, 2000), 1–21 and 143–68. By contrast, Aristotle does not see vision as haptic, grabbing.

15 *De fide orthodoxa*, 2.12 (Concerning Man). Alternate translation by Salmond: "an evil thing in anticipation begets fear, and in realisation it begets pain."

16 *De fide orthodoxa*, 2.14 (Concerning Fear). Alternate translation by Salmond: "Consternation is fear originating in some huge product of the imagination." Also, "Shrinking is fear of some act about to take place."

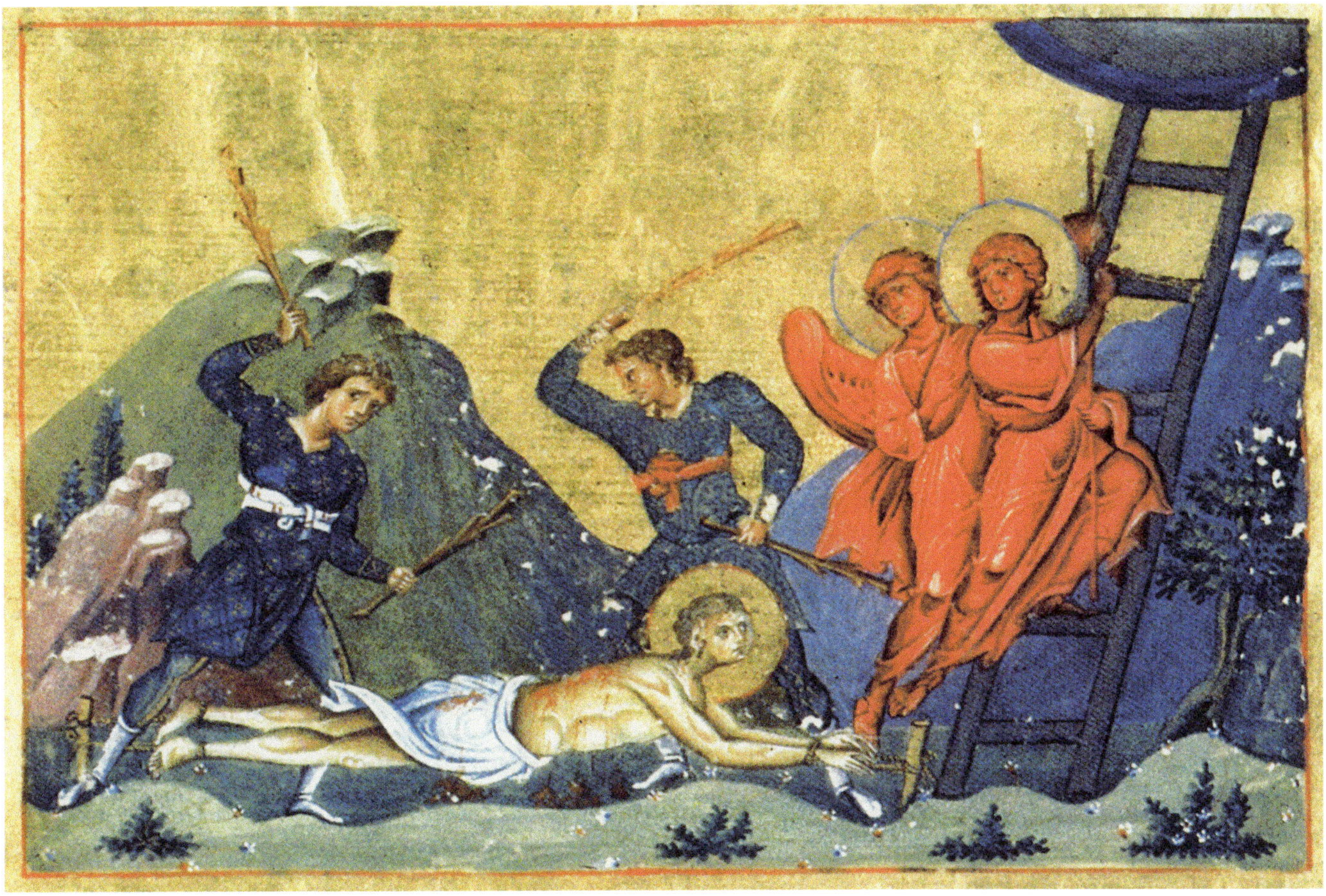

FIG. 12.2. Biblioteca Apostolica Vaticana, Vat. gr. 1613 (11th c.), p. 217: Martyrdom of Ananias the Persian (photo: Biblioteca Apostolica Vaticana with all rights reserved)

Anna's imagination, but she does not succumb to the fear and is eventually faced with actual pain. She is subdued by eight "robust men" who take her arms and make a cross of her body (similar to what we see in the Skylitzes image) and then one beats her "mercilessly" on the back, and another on the front. Readers are implicitly expected to imagine the blows on their own naked bodies in a show of empathy for the martyr.[17] The cross her body forms serves to connect the suffering of the nun with that of the ultimate suffering of Christ on the cross. In this way, her righteous imitation of Christ is juxtaposed to the error in judgment of Constantine VI, whose action in effect parallels that of Pontius Pilate. In addition, her servant is ordered to slap her on the face, adding another conduit for the nun to experience pain, this one produced by someone's bare palms. The reader is invited to hear the sounds of the lashes on the body as well as the slaps on the face. After a while, the nun loses her voice and her body collapses.[18]

Another, more commonly represented version (to the point of being a topos) of punitive beating is exemplified by a number of images in the so-called Menologion of Basil, an early eleventh-century illuminated manuscript produced in Constantinople containing brief notices of saints' lives (Ms. Vat. gr. 1613).[19] One such image illustrates the martyrdom of the early Christian martyr Ananias the Persian (fig. 12.2).[20] Ananias

17 Auzépy wonders if this is a reference to an actual kind of punishment or a symbolic implication that Constantine is flagellating the cross, *La Vie d'Étienne*, 231, n. 246.

18 This story has all the elements of torture that also appear in many accounts of the lives of the early Christian martyrs.

19 *Il menologio di Basilio II (cod. Vaticano Greco 1613)* (Turin, 1907). H. C. Evans and W. D. Wixom, *The Glory of Byzantium: Art and Culture of the Middle Byzantine Era, A.D. 843–1261* (New York, 1997), cat. no. 55. "Menologion of Basil II," *ODB* 2:1341–42. I. Ševčenko, "The Illuminators of the Menologium of Basil II," *DOP* (1962): 248–76. F. D'Aiuto, *El "Menologio de Basilio II," Città del Vaticano, Biblioteca Apostolica Vaticana, Vat. Gr. 1613; Libro de estudios con ocasión de la edición facsimile* (Madrid, 2008).

20 Ms. Vat. gr. 1613, p. 217. As much as the stories of martyrs suffering are repetitive, so do the images resemble one another.

is stripped to a loincloth, his body stretched between two short poles. His hands and feet are bound by rope and attached to the poles. Each executioner has a club in each hand, and is about to deliver another forceful blow with the club in the outstretched arm. Ananias's back is covered with blood, a visual indication that the two executioners are breaking the skin on his back as they beat him with clubs. The only indications of pain experienced by the martyr are the red blood of the wound and the implied force of the blows to come, expressed through the dynamic poses of the executioners' bodies, the force of their stance extending into the instruments they wield. While the source of this punishment is not visible in the scene, Ananias's gaze leads the viewer to the two red-colored angels busy holding a ladder and pointing to the heavenly ascent that awaits the suffering martyr. The implication is that the terrestrial pain has already earned Ananias a place in heaven. While his body succumbs to the two executioners, who are extensions of the emperor and his laws, the angels, who represent the will of God, the ultimate Judge, remind him and the viewers that his soul will be rewarded.[21]

The visual topos of the extended hand is repeated in a damaged thirteenth-century fresco from the church of St. Euphemia at the Hippodrome in Constantinople, where we find another early Christian martyr, St. Euphemia, stripped to a loincloth and being beaten in the arena by two executioners wielding their instruments in both hands (fig. 12.3).[22] As is common in Byzantine art, her nude female body is represented with masculine characteristics, not much different than that of St. Ananias discussed above. Although this and other frescoes in the cycle are about the life of an early Christian saint, the proximity of the building to the Hippodrome, where many public punishments took place over the centuries, is important for understanding the nature of public punishment in Constantinople.[23] The outstretched arm of the proconsul Priskos, who orders the punishment from an open window of a building, reminiscent of the emperor observing events in the Hippodrome from the *kathisma* (the imperial box), is a reference to the imperial power. This image is labeled, "πάλιν ὁ τύραννος, ῥάβδοις τὴν μάρτυρα βαρυτάταις κελεύει τύπτεσθαι" ("again the tyrant orders that the martyr be beaten with heavy rods").[24] The proconsul stands in for his emperor Diocletian, but also visually references the living emperor in Constantinople. The positioning of the bodies, both of the martyr and of the two executioners, is similar to that of the numerous scenes of lashing in the Menologion. But in the case of the fresco, instruments of torture seem to be double-tongued whips, as opposed to the clubs in the Ananias image, and as opposed to the rods mentioned in the label. It must be different to feel the wooden clubs on one's body as opposed to supple strands of raw hide, and it is here again that the instruments cause the viewer to imagine the nature of the pain they inflict by coming into violent contact with the body of the naked saint. Furthermore, a blunt object hitting the relatively soft surface of the skin would produce a thumping sound, as opposed to a swishing sound produced by a thinner, suppler instrument. The envisioned instruments and the imagined sounds imply the dullness or the sharpness of the sensation felt by the body.

This instrument, βούνευρον, or "strap of raw ox-hide," is attested as an instrument of punishment in a variety of sources, including the *Oneirokritikon of Achmet*, a tenth-century book of dream interpretation popular at the Byzantine court.[25] "If someone dreams that he was beaten

See, for example, very similar scenarios on pages 36, 79, and 313, as well as 71 and 325.

21 Because the Menologion was made for or at least commissioned by Emperor Basil, could it be possible that bad emperors are not represented here lest they be confused with the current emperor?

22 For images and a thorough description of the program, see R. Naumann and H. Belting, *Die Euphemia Kirche am Hippodrom zu Istanbul und ihre Fresken* (Berlin, 1966).

23 I discuss this fresco cycle in relation to public punishments in Constantinople in "Politics of Martyrdom and Punishment in Byzantine Visual Culture: St. Euphemia at the Hippodrome," in *Autopsia: Blut- und Augenzeugen: Extreme Repräsentationsformen des christlichen Martyriums*, ed. C. Behrmann and E. Priedl (Munich, 2014), 23–41.

24 Naumann and Belting, *Die Euphemia Kirche*, 132. The labels closely follow the text of Symeon Metaphrastes.

25 M. Mavroudi, ed., *A Byzantine Book on Dream Interpretation: The Oneirocriticon of Achmet and Its Arabic Sources* (Leiden, 2002), 318. E. Patlagean first connected *Ecloga*'s mutilations to the symbolic importance given to different parts of

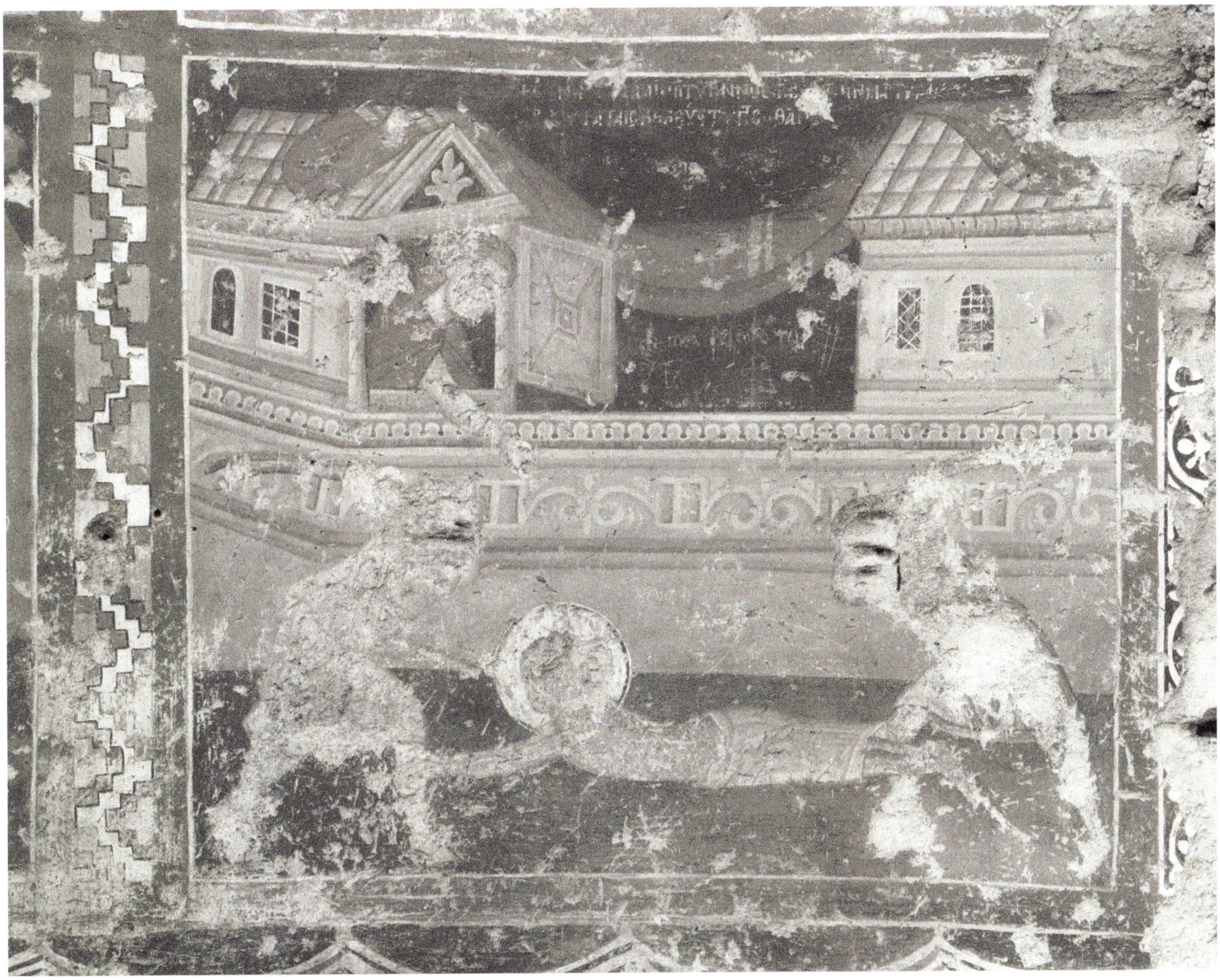

with a strap of ox-hide (βούνευρον) by someone he knew, he will find gold in coins commensurate with the number of blows. If the one who beat him is a person of authority he will give some authority to the dreamer."[26] Other related punitive instruments include strap (μαγκλάβιον), whip (χαρζάνιον) and staff (ῥάβδος). For example, "If the king dreams that he ordered somebody to be beaten with a strap (μαγκλάβιον) the person who was beaten will receive from the king great joy and wealth commensurate with the number of blows."[27]

If dreams are indicators of the dreamer's psyche, these quotes confirm the role that lashing played in the psychological landscape of people in Constantinopolitan imperial circles. It must have been a common enough dream to warrant interpretation. Instruments of punishment may have been used by the executioner in real life, but were clearly understood as an extension of the emperor's hand in the Byzantine subconscious. In the *Oneirokritikon*, the king sometimes beats with a rod (ῥαβδος), which could be interpreted as his imperial staff; in dreams the staff is paralleled to the executioner's βούνευρον or μαγκλάβιον.[28] It is ultimately the emperor's hand

FIG. 12.3. Church of St. Euphemia at the Hippodrome, Istanbul, fresco, 13th century: Lashing of St. Euphemia (photo: Deutsches Archäologisches Institut, Istanbul)

the body in Byzantine and Arabic books of dream interpretation: "Byzance et le blason pénal du corps," in *Du chatîment dans la cité: Supplices corporels et peine du mort dans le monde antique* (Rome, 1984), 405–26.

26 Mavroudi, *Byzantine Book*, 318.

27 Ibid.

28 In Heb. 1:8 ῥαβδος refers to a king's staff: "thy righteous scepter is the scepter of your kingdom." In 1 Cor. it is used as a rod for punishment. In Acts 16:22 "to beat with a rod." Nestle-Aland, *Greek–English New Testament* (Stuttgart, 1998).

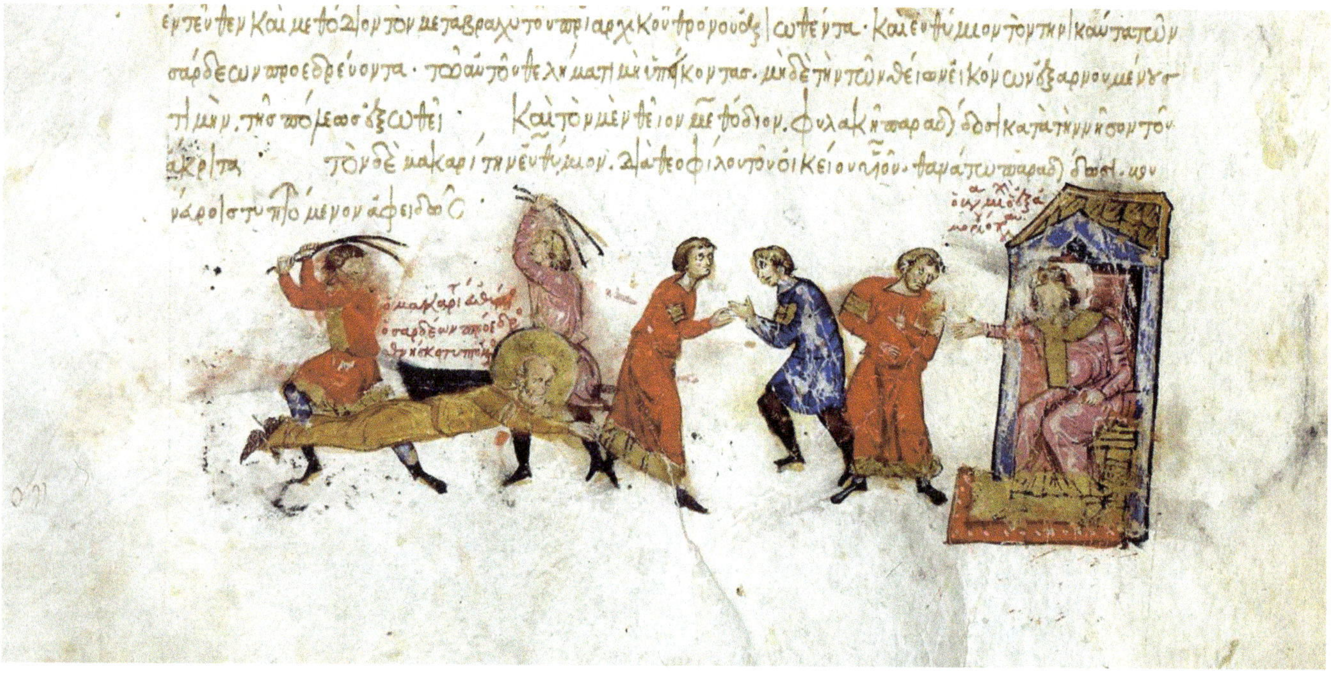

FIG. 12.4. Madrid, Bibl. Nac. Vitr. 26-2, fol. 28v, detail: Lashing of Bishop Euthymios (photo: Biblioteca nacional de España)

that leaves marks of the imperial rule on the bodies of the condemned.

In some visual examples the condemned are not stripped but beaten through their garments and we see this in the Skylitzes manuscript on fol. 28v, where on the bottom of the page the iconophile Bishop Euthymios of Sardis is shown lashed by the order of the iconoclast Emperor Michael II (r. 813–820) (fig. 12.4). According to the text, Michael "put the blessed Euthymios to death by a merciless flogging with bull's sinews [βούνευρον] at the hand of Theophilos, his [Michael's] own son," which sounds like Theophilos, the future emperor beat him himself.[29] The bishop is fully dressed, yet stretched out on the floor in a manner similar to Ananias and Euphemia, while two animated executioners each hold a double ox-hide strap with both hands (the whip on the right has two prongs on both the top and the bottom; it is in fact unclear whether these are double-pronged instruments or just two thin straps held together).[30] On the throne, the emperor orders the punishment with an outstretched arm gesture. The order is taken up by the figure in red, supposedly his son Theodosius, and travels left along a line formed by the arms and bodies of two more figures, each one in physical contact with the next, ending with the body of the bishop lashed by the executioners. The viewer understands that the executioners are the extensions of the emperor's hands. The colors of their short tunics match the pink and red of the longer robes worn by Michael and Theodosius respectively, solidifying this connection. Through them and their instruments the emperor touches the punished bishop. His word becomes violence; law becomes punishment.

Touched by the Elements: Punishment by Fire

Another punishment designed to cause pain to the whole body was execution by burning. While flogging was very common, punishment by burning was rare, yet undoubtedly memorable.

29 J. Wortley, trans., *John Skylitzes: A Synopsis of Byzantine History, 811–1057* (Cambridge, 2011), 31 and n. 19. See also J. Gouillard, "La vie d' Euthyme de Sardes (*ob* 831), une œuvre du patriarche Méthode," *TM* 10 (1987): 1–101.

30 E. N. Boeck explains why Skylitzes' images are not representations of real experiences but visualizations of events by remote interpreters in "Engaging the Byzantine Past: Strategies of Visualizing History in Sicily and Bulgaria," in *History as Literature in Byzantium, Papers from the 40th Spring Symposium in Byzantine Studies*, ed. R. Macrides (Farnham, 2010), 215–35; and more recently in *Imagining the Byzantine Past: The Perception of History in the Illustrated Manuscripts of Skylitzes and Manasses* (Cambridge, 2015).

It does appear often as one in a slew of punishments of early Christian martyrs—it was meant to elicit extreme compassion on the part of the reader, listener, or viewer. In the twelfth century, Constantinopolitans got to witness two spectacular burnings at the Hippodrome: the Bogomil Basil was burned in the vicinity of the *spina* by Alexios Komnenos (r. 1081–1118) and Mamalos was burned at the *Sphendone* by Andronikos I Komnenos (r. 1183–1185), the former accused of heresy and the latter of treason.[31] Princess Anna Komnena, Alexios's daughter, describes in great detail the punishment of Basil in 1118:

> The Emperor . . . had an immense pyre built in the Hippodrome. A very large trench was dug and a quantity of wood, all tall trees piled up together, made the structure look like a mountain. When the pile was lighted, a great crowd slowly collected on the floor and steps of the circus in eager expectation of what was to happen. On the opposite side a cross was fixed and the impious man was given a choice, for if he dreaded the fire and changed his mind, and walked to the cross, then he should be delivered from burning. . . . He shewed himself contemptuous of all punishment and threats, and while he was still at a distance from the fire he began to laugh and talk marvels, saying that angels would snatch him from the middle of the fire. . . . But when the crowd stood aside and allowed him to have a free view of that terrifying sight, the burning pyre (for even at a good distance he could feel the fire, and saw the flames rising high and as it were thundering and shooting out sparks of fire which rose to the top of the stone obelisk which stands in the centre of the Hippodrome), then the bold fellow seemed to flinch from the fire and be disturbed. For as if wholly desperate, he constantly turned away his eyes and clapped his hands and beat his thigh. . . .
>
> So there stood that abominable Basil, unmoved by any threat or fear, and gaped now at the fire and now at the bystanders. And all thought him quite mad for he did not rush to the pyre nor did he draw back, but stood fixed and immovable on the spot he had first taken up. . . . Then they . . . took him and pushed him, clothes, shoes and all, into the middle of the pyre. And the flames, as if deeply enraged against him, ate the impious man up, without any odour arising or even a fresh appearance of smoke, only one thin smoky line could be seen in the midst of the flames. For even the elements are excited against the impious; whereas, to speak truthfully, they spare those beloved of God, just as once upon a time in Babylon the fire retreated from those young men who were dear to God, and enclosed them like a golden chamber. In this case the men who lifted up the accursed Basil had scarcely placed him on the pyre before the flames seemed to dart forward to snatch hold of him.[32]

The instrument of this punishment was fire, one of the four elements that the Byzantines believed their world consisted of, air, water, and earth being the other three. In Plato's *Timaeus*, particles that constitute fire have the shape of tetrahedrons, geometric forms with many pointy edges. Plato explains this choice with the description of the heat of fire as "sharp and stabbing," befitting the sharpness of tetrahedron's edges.[33] By

31 For Basil, see Anna Komnena, *The Alexiad of the Princess Anna Comnena, Being the History of the Reign of Her Father, Alexius I Emperor of the Romans, 1081–1118*, trans. E. A. S. Dawes (New York, 1967), 417–18. For Mamalos, see Magoulias, *O City* (n. 11 above), 172 [311]. Other examples include the praepositus Nikephoros (grand chamberlain of the palace), who was burned alive at the Hippodrome under Theophilos (829–842). T. Preger, ed., *Scriptores originum Constantinopolitanarum* (Leipzig, 1901–), 2:224. R. Guilland, "The Hippodrome at Byzantium," *Speculum* 23, no. 4 (1948): 681–82.

32 Trans. from Dawes, *Alexiad*, 417–18. See also G. Buckler, *Anna Komnena: A Study* (Oxford, 1968), 520–21. Zigabenos also gives an account of this event: Euthymios Zigabenos, *De heresi Bogomilorum narratio, in Die Phundagiagiten: Ein Beitrag zur Ketzergeschichte des byzantinischen Mittelalters*, ed. G. Ficker (Leipzig, 1908), 110–11. Michael Angold, *Church and Society in Byzantium under the Comneni, 1081–1261* (Cambridge, 1995), 485–87.

33 "First, let us enquire what we mean by saying that fire is hot; and about this we may reason from the dividing or cutting power which it exercises on our bodies. We all of us feel that fire is sharp; and we may further consider the fineness of the sides, and the sharpness of the angles, and the smallness of the particles, and the swiftness of the motion; all this makes the action of fire violent and sharp, so that it cuts whatever it meets. And we must not forget that the original figure of fire [i.e., the

contrast, Aristotle does not see elements in terms of geometry, but assigns them a combination of qualities of hotness, coldness, dryness, and wetness. For him, fire is hot and dry and also fast acting and therefore produces acute sensation.[34] It is this "sharp and stabbing" (in Platonic terms) or excessively hot and quick (in Aristotelian terms) instrument that gets in touch with the exposed body of the condemned.[35]

Anna begins with the statement that "The Emperor . . . had an immense pyre built in the Hippodrome." It is again the emperor who provides the instrument of punishment. In the beginning, Basil is brave and vociferous but as he gets a "free view of that terrifying sight, the burning pyre," he begins to flinch, turn away in fear, beat his hands and slap his thighs. In other words, as he visually takes in the instrument in the form of "flames rising high and as it were thundering and shooting out sparks of fire which rose to the top of the stone obelisk," language escapes him and the terror caused by envisioning what will happen to his body sets in. The executioners obey the emperor's wishes by pushing him into the fire, applying physical pressure to his body. The flames of the fire seem to obey the emperor as they "snatch hold" of the terrified Basil. "For even the elements are excited against the impious," Anna adds, not least to absolve her father from staging such a gruesome punishment and wielding such a destructive instrument of justice.

While Anna did everything to excuse her father's decision, over half a century later, historian Niketas Choniates disapproved of Emperor Andronikos I's choice to burn Mamalos at the Hippodrome. Mamalos had been found guilty of treason for predicting that Alexios Komnenos would ascend the throne. Choniates recounts:

> The fire was ignited, and the flame shot up high into the air along the turn of the racecourse, equal to that of the Chaldean furnace; kindled by naphtha and brushwood, it burned seven times hotter than usual. Mamalos was brought forward bound by ropes and as naked as when he first saw the light of day as he emerged from his mother's womb. The furnace workers who stood beside the youth garlanded, with the first down upon his lip and cheeks, prodded him with long poles, as though he were a sacrificial victim and threw him into the midst of the flames. As he neared the furnace and felt great pain, he became fainthearted as would any man, and hoping to escape what was already an inescapable death, he now threw himself against the thrusting poles, deeming the pain inflicted by them to be less than that of the licking flames spreading out from the charcoals; but pushed again into the midst of the fire . . . and engulfed by the flames, he would then jump out of the furnace like the quick-darting serpents. . . . This drama continued for some time, moving the spectators to tears. Finally exhausted, he fell, and the raging flames engulfed his flesh and quickly snuffed out his life. The savor of burnt flesh ascending upwards to the heavens polluted the air, while the stench of the acrid smoke and soot was unbearable for the bystanders.[36]

There are some differences in the description of the two burning events. For example, while Basil is fully clothed ("shoes and all"), Mamalos

pyramid], more than any other form, has a dividing power which cuts our bodies into small pieces, and thus naturally produces that affection which we call heat; and hence the origin of the name." Plato, *Timaeus* 22–23, trans. B. Jowett, in *The Dialogues of Plato* (London, 1892), 3:483. See also G. Vlastos, *Plato's Universe* (Seattle, 1975), 66–82 and J. N. Findlay, "Notes on Plato's Universe," *The Philosophical Forum* 38, no. 2 (2007): 159–71. Neoplatonist Proclus in his commentary on Plato's *Timaeus* describes fire as sharp, subtle, and moveable, while earth is blunt, dense, and immobile.

34 Air is hot and wet, water is cold and wet, and earth is cold and dry. When discussing perception of sound, Aristotle uses tactile perception to explain it: "Acute and grave are here metaphors, transferred from their proper sphere, viz. that of touch, where they mean respectively (a) what moves the sense much in a short time, (b) what moves the sense little in a long time. Not that what is sharp really moves fast, and what is grave slowly, but that the difference in the qualities of the one and the other movement is due to their respective speeds. There seems to be a sort of parallelism between what is acute or grave to hearing and what is sharp or blunt to touch; what is sharp as it were stabs, while what is blunt pushes, the one producing its effect in a short, the other in a long time, so that the one is quick, the other slow." *De anima* 8. In part 11 he discusses the property of touch in some detail, emphasizing how difficult it is to pinpoint its qualities.

35 Both traditions are attested to and expanded upon in Byzantium.

36 Magoulias, *O City*, 172 [311].

is "nude as when he first saw the light of day." Choniates invites us to imagine his naked skin in direct contact with the fire, and by noting the "first down" on Mamalos's face, he emphasizes his gentle age and perhaps the suppleness of the skin that burns. While Basil's burning allegedly resulted in no smell, Mamalos's burned body produced intense stench and "acrid smoke." The pain his body experienced and that the viewers could contemplate by observing his reactions is here reinforced by the odor and smoke that they could smell and arguably taste. Anna deprives the reader of the smell of Basil's burning body, diminishing the sensory reality of the event, and therefore taking away a means of accessing his suffering.

The terror however is common to both men and they both resist getting close to the flames. When confronted with the two instruments, that is to say the executioners' poles on the one hand and the flames of fire on the other, Mamalos prefers the violent stabs of the poles to the heat of the fire and throws his nude body against them. While poles are long and arguably sharp objects, relative to the tactile response to the fire, they produce a blunt sensation. Choniates observes that as Mamalos neared the furnace "he felt great pain," which the historian deduces from the jerking of the youth's body back and forth. Rather than express their pain and fears through words, the condemned writhe, jump, scream, and shriek. Their nonverbal expressions, the movements of the bodies and the sounds they produce, aid the observer in understanding their physical and psychological pain. The touch of the law is intended to make the recipients passive, yet their bodies respond in a very active fashion. These involuntary reactions last long enough to produce an emotive reaction in the observer.[37] Unlike the jeering crowd observing the punishment of Basil, the spectators here are moved to tears—they show empathy for the condemned young man.

A contrast to the experiences of Basil and Mamalos is provided by another episode from the life of Saint Euphemia. Two different representations of St. Euphemia tortured in a pyre at the arena in Chalcedon show her fully clothed

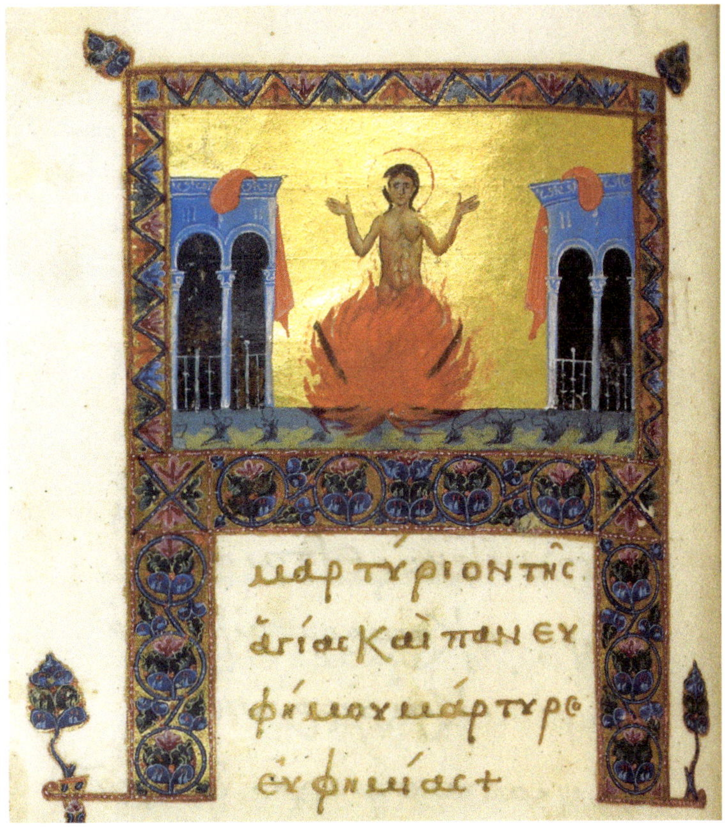

FIG. 12.5. London, BL, MS. Add. 11870, fol. 121v, detail: St. Euphemia burned alive (photo: British Library)

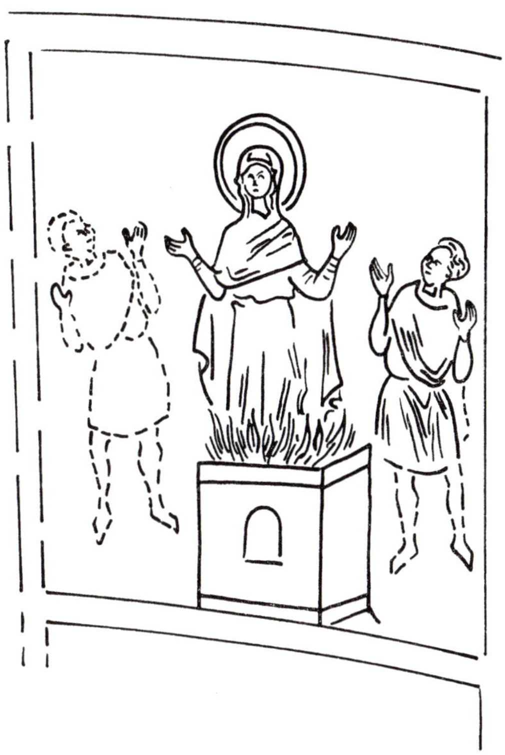

FIG. 12.6. Church of St. Euphemia at the Hippodrome, Istanbul (drawing: after R. Naumann and H. Belting, *Die Euphemia Kirche am Hippodrom zu Istanbul und ihre Fresken* [Berlin, 1966], fig. 38)

37 I thank Susan Harvey for pointing out that my original premise of passive response belies the dynamic responses of the bodies in pain.

and nude respectively—she appears clothed in the fresco cycle at the church of St. Euphemia of Chalcedon and nude in the same scene in the manuscript known as the London Additional 11870 (figs. 12.5, 12.6). Because the London Additional illustrates stories of other martyrs with the images of their final martyrdom, one would imagine the text of Euphemia's vita here is based on that recorded by Asterios in the fourth century, in which she succumbs to the fire as the last in a series of punishments she undergoes.[38] However, the text follows the later version by Symeon Metaphrastes, a version also followed by the fresco cycle at St. Euphemia at the Hippodrome, in which fire is just one of the instruments used in a series of unsuccessful attempts to execute the saint. In this later version, like the three youths in the fiery furnace in the Old Testament story, and like the Burning Bush seen by Moses at Sinai, she was enveloped in fire, but protected from burning by God, in a miraculous confirmation of her holiness. Unlike Basil and Mamalos, in both versions Euphemia stands in the midst of the flames, unaffected, her arms in the gesture of prayer. Fire is in contact with her body but it does not seem to affect her; it does not obey the orders of the emperor but takes its cue from the higher authority—that of God. She is not touched, her skin is not singed, no mark is left on her body, no pain is experienced by the saint.[39] Her sanctity lies somewhere between experiencing pain and being relieved from that pain. Both versions of the vita could be read into both images. The viewer could imagine the possible pain experienced by the martyr amid the flames, and interpret that pain as a testament to her steadfastness and her proximity to the ultimate sacrificial figure: Christ on the Cross. On the other hand, the viewer can contemplate the fact that Euphemia's willingness to suffer physical pain for her faith ultimately relieved her from the reality of that pain.

38 Asterios of Amasea, *Description of a Painting of the Martyrdom of Saint Euphemia*, in C. Mango ed., *The Art of the Byzantine Empire 312–1453: Sources and Documents* (Toronto, 1986), 37–39. F. Halkin, ed., *Euphémie de Chalcédoine* (Brussels, 1965), 4–8.

39 The tension between extreme pain experienced by martyrs and moments of complete deliverance from painful sensations is common in the lives of martyr saints.

Deprived of Other Senses: Punishment by Blinding

In some instances of corporal punishment, particular body parts were affected by the targeted violence of the punitive touch, and in the process the bodies of the condemned were deprived of other senses. As John of Damascus observes, the sense of touch is contained in organs of other senses.[40] By extension, through violent touch these organs can be damaged and other senses compromised. Some punishments targeted specific body parts associated with other senses, such as blinding, hand, nose, and tongue mutilation.[41] The most common punishment that involved intense legal violence and at the same time deprived the touched and mutilated person of another sense was blinding. The instrument sometimes mentioned in cases of blinding is a *kauter*, actually a medical instrument, also used for branding.[42] The primary target was the eye itself, which was touched by a hot iron and burned until it melted. By applying solid pressure and temperature, a combination of pressing and burning, qualities perceived by the sense of touch, the executioners left the condemned deprived of the highest in the hierarchy of the senses—vision.[43] In some instances, the iron, specified as *siderion,* was not heated, and the procedure was more of a gouging.[44]

40 John of Damascus, *De fide orthoxa,* ch. 18.

41 These are attested in Byzantine legal tradition. See for example Freshfield, *Ecloga* (n. 10 above) and idem, *A Manual of Eastern Roman Law, The Procheiros Nomos* (Cambridge, 1928).

42 On blinding see O. Lampsides, "Ἡ ποινή της τυφλώσεως παρά Βυζαντινοίς" (PhD diss., Athens, 1949); J. Herrin, "Blinding in Byzantium," in *Polyplerous Nous: Miscellanea für Peter Schreiner zu seinem 60. Geburstag*, ed. C. Scholz and G. Makris (Munich and Leipzig, 2000), 56–68; J. Laskaratos and S. Marketos, "The Penalty of Blinding during Byzantine Times: Medical Remarks," *Documenta Ophthalmologica* 81 (1992): 133–44 and "Blinding," *ODB* 1:297–98.

43 When Alousianos "arrested Dolianus, he cut off his nose and blinded his eyes, using a cook's knife for both operations." Psellos, *Chronographia*, 4.49 (Sewter, *Fourteen* [n. 11 above], 115). Crudity of this punishment implies a nonmedical nature of the procedure and by extension that it was not backed up by a just legal system.

44 For the distinction between instruments in the medical profession, see L. J. Bliquez, "Two Lists of Greek Surgical Instruments and the State of Surgery in Byzantine Times," *DOP* 38 (1984): 187–204.

Michael Psellos witnessed the double blinding of the overthrown emperor Michael V and his uncle Constantine on 21 April 1042 and provides us with a written recollection of these events. When Michael and Constantine sought asylum at the Stoudios monastery, supporters of Theodora sent "bold, resolute men" to blind the fugitives as soon as they saw them outside the sacred building.[45] Another group brought them out, "intending to drive them through the center of the city, but they had not gone far on the journey when they were encountered by the man who had been commanded to blind the two miscreants."[46]

Psellos notes that the executioners prepared for the procedure by sharpening the iron for the branding, perhaps calling the reader's attention to the "sharp" nature of the pain caused by the sharpened instrument.[47] He describes the reactions of the blinded men: while Constantine was calm and collected, Michael "moaned and wailed aloud," raised hands in supplication, and had to be tied down. When his turn came, he did not acquiesce to the handing out of the punishment; he reacted violently to being violently touched. Michael first observed the blinding of his uncle: "Meanwhile the emperor, seeing in the other's torment the fate that was about to overtake him too, lived through Constantine's anguish in himself, beating his hands together, smiting his face and bellowing in agony."[48]

45 Psellos, *Chronographia* 5.38–51 (Sewter, 144–51).

46 Apparently this took place at the Sigma: Sewter, 151, n. 79. This scene is illustrated in the Skylitzes manuscript (Madrid, Bibl. Nac. Vitr. 26-2, fol. 221r): on the left of the scene Constantine and Michael are dragged out of the church, and then in the middle of the scene they are being blinded. They had voluntarily removed their courtly dress and donned supplicant robes before seeking asylum in the monastery. As they were dragged outside their heads and other body parts must have felt the bumps on the ground. Their skin must have been chafed, their wrists and ankles bruised. While they had touched/grasped the altar in the hopes of reaching Christ, the new imperial power established itself by grasping their bodies and touching their eyes and leaving a visual proof of their punishment.

47 Psellos, *Chronographia* 5.47 (Sewter, 149). There is no indication that the σιδήριον was heated.

48 Psellos, *Chronographia* 5.49 (Sewter, 150). Psellos also describes equally opposed reactions to blinding by two other men who were accused of plotting against the emperor Constantine IX: while Tornicius "emitted a cry of anguish and basely lamented his fate," Vatatzes "straight away lay down on the ground, face upwards, and nobly submitted to his punishment." Psellos, *Chronographia* 6.123 (Sewter, 219–20).

While he did not get to hear the sounds of his stoic and silent uncle screaming to aid his imagination of the imminent pain, Michael still "lived through Constantine's anguish in himself." He bellowed out the agony of Constantine; he gave voice to someone else's pain. His terror was a combination of what he was seeing and what he was imagining on his own body. By witnessing his uncle's punishment, he imagined it on his own skin, on his own eyes. While other observers could empathize through bodily imagination, Michael had the added certainty that he would go through the same process momentarily, giving rise to his terror.

An instance of a feigned blinding described by Anna Komnena gives us an insight into how both sound and vision played a part in witnessing someone's blinding.

> Ursel was laid flat on the ground, the executioner applied the iron, while the victim howled and groaned like a lion roaring; but all this was only a feint of depriving him of his sight, for he who apparently was being blinded had been ordered to shout and shriek, and he who seemingly was gouging out the eyes, to stare harshly at his prisoner on the ground, and do everything savagely, and yet only to act the blinding. And so Ursel was blinded, yet not blinded, and the rabble clapped their hands, and the blinding of Ursel was buzzed about everywhere.... Thus the admirable commander, having got Ursel into his power, kept him like a lion in a cage, with bandages still over his eyes as symbol of his supposed blinding.[49]

Ursel was ordered to shout and shriek, as audible proofs of him actually undergoing the pain and terror of being blinded. Then his eyes were bandaged, covering the fact that they were left intact by the violent surgery, but also serving as proofs that there were wounds underneath. Senses of hearing and vision were called upon to attest to the tactility of the experienced pain. Those who heard the sounds of anguish "buzzed" about the event. When a certain Dokeianos saw Ursel "bearing the marks of blinding, and led

49 Dawes, *Alexiad* (n. 31 above), 9.

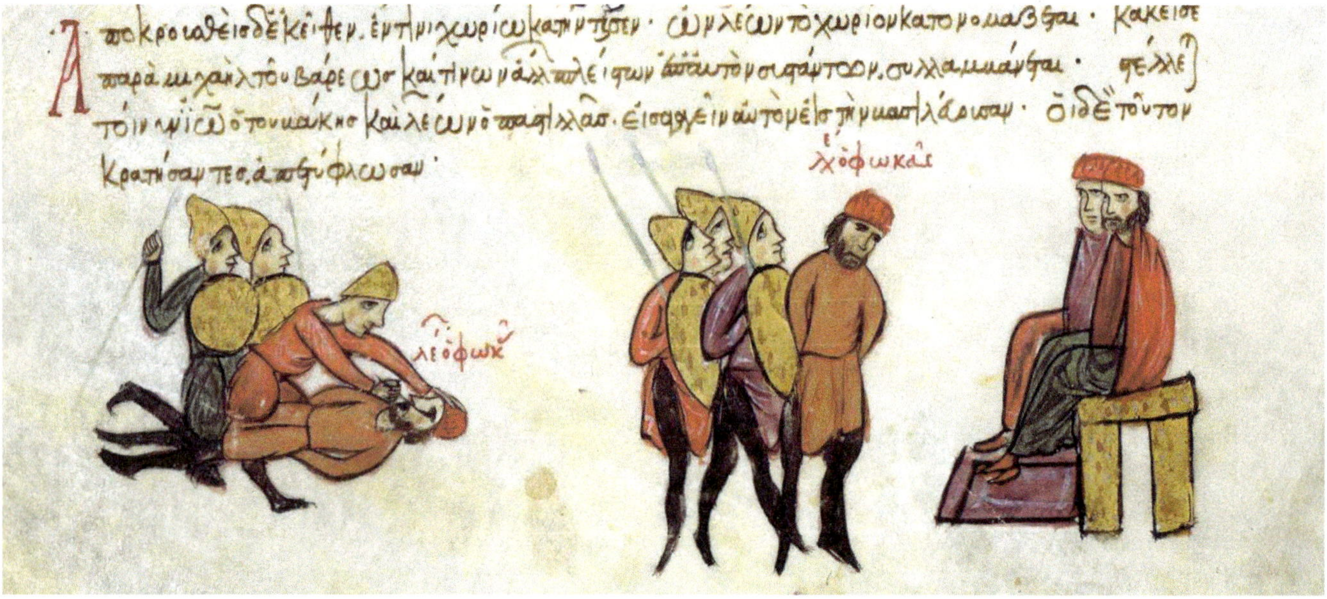

FIG. 12.7. Madrid, Bibl. Nac. Vitr. 26-2, fol. 126r, detail: Blinding of Leo Phokas (photo: Biblioteca nacional de España)

by the hand," he "heaved a deep sigh, burst into tears over him, and denounced the General's cruelty."[50] To Dokeianos, the bandages were a mark of the pain undergone by Ursel and the sight of this mark elicited his empathy. However, he did not associate the cruelty of this act with the executioner but with the general himself, the future emperor Alexios, who in the end is revealed as compassionate.

An image of another blinding procedure provides us with a close detail of the instrument and wounds of blinding. On the bottom of fol. 126r of the Madrid Skylitzes, we see an executioner straddling the usurper Leo Phokas and vigorously attacking his eye with a sharp slender tool, while two other executioners constrict the movements of Leo's legs by sitting on his knees (fig. 12.7). This is the moment of inscribing the punishment onto the body of the condemned usurper. The direct contact of the instrument of branding with the eye of the condemned makes the viewer contemplate the pain by imagining what kind of sensation a tool like that would produce on the viewer's own eyes. On the right, the branded face is displayed to the two seated emperors (Constantine VII and Romanos Lekapenos), to whom the wounded eyes of Leo are the indication of the meted justice. To the viewer of the image, the blackness of the marks indicates not only the physical pain experienced by the condemned but also the psychological pain of no longer being able to see. Leo acquiesces to the hand of the law during the act of punishment and afterward he can no longer see those who look at him. He has become a passive object of other people's gaze.

Conclusion

One of the goals of public punishment was to make the pain of the condemned visible to the observers. That perception was augmented by the audible input of screams and jeers and in some instances smell and taste. Instruments of punishment left visible marks on the bodies of the condemned, and these punitive wounds served as permanent marks of the violent touch. The law made its touch visible to onlookers who were supposed to understand both the haptic power of the lawgiver and the tactile sensation of the pain experienced by the condemned. The feeling of the pain was a one-time event, while the visual perception was something that was meant to endure and to be recalled in the imagination of those contemplating the events at a later date.[51] Specific instruments of inflicting pain and the particular wounds they produced

50 Ibid.

51 This image "imprints itself on the *phantasia* like a seal." G. Mathew, *Byzantine Aesthetics* (London, 1965), 118–19.

during punishment procedures served as visual indicators of the pain to be perceived by the spectators. Similarly, they aided the imagination of those who contemplated images and stories of punishment. People's approaches to suffering of others were shaped by both reality and myth, by experience and imagination.

To be touched by the law in Byzantium meant to actually be touched by the Byzantine emperor. We saw visual examples of this with Theophilos ordering the lashing at the agora, with Priskos (representing imperial power) ordering the beating of Euphemia, and with Constantine and Romanos inspecting the wounds of Leo. Furthermore, in texts of dream interpretation, and therefore in the anticipated Byzantine subconscious, the king was clearly seen or understood to be the one who not only authorizes punishment but actually metes out the blows.

The touch of the law effected by the emperor was meant to be corrective and therefore healing. Michael Psellos uses the metaphor of a surgeon to describe the actions of Emperor Isaac Komnenos:

> Isaac... abhorred anything that was physically diseased or corrupt. But his hopes were disappointed, for he found nothing but disease and festering sores.... In the one case he ought to have waited for the appropriate moment before he applied surgical remedies and cautery; it was wrong to operate on the internal organs with the surgeon's heated iron without reasonable premeditation.... He wanted to see the sick body restored to health immediately. What with his burning and cutting here, and his mighty pulling and tugging with the reins on his runaway horses there, he somehow or other failed to notice that he himself had caught the disease before he got control over these troubles and restored them to order.[52]

Healers, or doctors, did not always have a good reputation in Byzantium and were on occasion compared to executioners, a comparison that was intended to debase the profession of a surgeon.[53] The inversion of the metaphor, however, elevates the executioner, who assumes the role of a healer. As the doctor-surgeon disrupts the integrity of the body in order to make the system better, so the executioner disrupts the body of the condemned to repair the body of the community. Yet, as the executioner is just an extension of the emperor's hand, the real doctor is the emperor himself. An interesting parallel is provided in the life of Saint Loukas the Younger: the healing saint appears in a dream of a monk Gregory holding a *kauter*, a branding iron, ready to perform surgery on Gregory's stomach.[54] The saint claims that he is not the doctor and that the real healer, "the doctor of soul and body," is God himself, while the saint is but an instrument of God's will.[55] In a similar fashion, the real executioner/doctor is the Byzantine emperor, who causes corporal pain in the condemned in order to heal the suffering body and soul of the empire.

52 *Chronographia* 7.58 (Sewter, 236).

53 A. Kazhdan, "The Image of the Medical Doctor of the 10th to 12th Centuries," *DOP* 38 (1984): 43–51. See also B. Baldwin, "Beyond the House Call: Doctors in Early Byzantine History and Politics," *DOP* 38 (1984): 15–19.

54 Kazhdan, "Image," 47, Greek in PG 111:441–80 and E. Martini, "Supplementa ad acta S. Lucae iunioris," *AB* 13 (1894): 106:17–18.

55 Kazhdan, "Image," 47; Martini, "Supplementa," 101:15–17.

I would like to thank Margaret Mullett for inviting me to participate in this exciting project, Susan Harvey for her constant encouragement and extraordinary kindness, Michael Maas for his generosity and patience, and my anonymous readers for their constructive comments and attention to details.

CHAPTER THIRTEEN

To Touch or Not to Touch

Erotic Tactility in Byzantine Literature

INGELA NILSSON

Among the five senses, touch is the most diffuse—it involves the entire body and not just one part of it, like seeing or hearing. Owing to its relation to the body, most notably the skin and flesh, it is closely associated with corporeality. Touch seems to reproduce the outside world most indisputably and yet the sense of touch can be surprisingly difficult to locate and define.[1] While Aristotle praised touch as both an indispensable sense and a primary form of sense, uniting all living beings,[2] touch is also known as the basest sense. This is related to the classical attitude that theoretical activity is distinct from and superior to the practical, and it agrees with the Platonic metaphysic, which relegates the physical to an inferior status.[3] This belief was reinforced in Neoplatonic and Christian thought, and touch thus became closely associated with the lower, bodily senses.[4] This idea still strongly influences our general attitude toward aesthetic experience: the fine arts—pictorial representation and music—are experienced by means of sight and hearing, while touch is rarely expected to be part of the aesthetic experience. This division between sight and hearing on the one hand (so-called distance receptors), and contact senses on the other (that is, taste, smell and touch), corresponds to the distinction between the sensuous and the sensual. In the words of Arnold Berleant, "The sensuous is admissible only when made safe by being perceived through the senses of sight and hearing, while the senses of taste, smell, and especially touch, are ineradicably suggestive of the sensual."[5] This may seem obvious; touch is indeed sensual in that it is closely related to the erotic experience, which is what I will focus on here. But while the major sensory channel through which love (or desire) is experienced is indeed the tactile, we cannot completely ignore the other senses: sight, hearing, smell, and taste are probably as important for the erotic experience as is touch. This is true also for the way in which love and desire are described in numerous literary texts from antiquity onward.

Before discussing the Byzantine material, let us note that touch should not be seen as completely confined to physical experience. Instead, physical touch can, and often does, induce a mental or

1 For lucid introductions to and contextualization of touch in early modern culture and onward, see E. D. Harvey, ed., *Sensible Flesh: On Touch in Early Modern Culture* (Philadelphia, 2003), 1–21, and C. Classen, *The Deepest Sense: A Cultural History of Touch* (Urbana, 2012), xi–xvii.

2 Aristotle, *De anima* 413b and *De sensu* 436b.

3 See M.-L. Veyron, *Le toucher dans les Évangiles* (Paris, 2013), 20–29, for a useful survey of touch as both a secondary and suspect sense and as a primary sense throughout the premodern and modern tradition.

4 A. Berleant, "The Sensuous and the Sensual in Aesthetics," *Journal of Aesthetics and Art Criticism* 23, no. 2 (winter 1964): 185–92, at 186–87. See also Harvey, *Sensible Flesh*, 1, and G. M. Spiegel, "Paradoxes of the Senses," in *Rethinking the Medieval Senses: Heritage, Fascinations, Frames*, ed. S. G. Nichols et al. (Baltimore, 2008), 186–93, on Christian thought versus the Aristotelian heritage in the middle ages.

5 Berleant, "Sensuous and the Sensual," 186.

emotional process. Two aspects are useful to consider in the following analysis. First, the sense of touch allows our bodies to experience both pleasure and pain. Regardless, however, of whether we feel pleasure or pain (or in some cases both at the same time), the tactile experience affects more than just the body; touch can cause physical reactions that also affect our minds. Second, sensations—whether sensuous or sensual—are often seen as a way of getting in touch with the inner self, a sacred part of the human being that cannot be reached without proper ritual.[6] We may consider here the crucial role of the tactile in both pre-Christian and Christian religion, spanning from healing rituals and erotically charged mystery religions to mortification of the flesh and, indeed, the marriage ritual.[7] The sexual experience that comes with marriage, since it involves mixing of hitherto unmixed, virginal entities, changes not only the bodies of the persons involved, but also their minds.[8] Even if this is less pronounced in Christian ideology than in pre-Christian thought, we can see erotic imagery being transferred to the relation between man and God, the good Christian desiring to be united with a higher being.

In this chapter I shall examine discourses of erotic touch that appear in Byzantine literature, that is, descriptions of tactile experiences that are erotically charged, negatively or positively.[9] Such discourses are often imbued with a tension between touching and not touching: the desire to be touched mixed with the reluctance to give in to that desire, but also the desire *not* to be touched and how to avoid unwanted tactile experiences. Averil Cameron has put it very aptly: "In Byzantium, I would argue, there was a constant dialectic between the language of denial and the language of desire."[10] This tense dialectic is at the core of the present investigation, with a focus on eroticized touch. Erotic dreams and visions will not be included in my survey, and I shall look only at passages that include explicit touch and women touching men.[11] I have chosen this narrow focus on female touch because I want to follow the trace of seductive provocation that starts with Eve and that is so prevalent in the Byzantine patriarchal view of women: women are guilty of deceit and yet gullible, easily led into weakness and sin.[12] Certainly, not only women seduce in Byzantine literature, but touch, as a central aspect of seduction and sin, seems to be gendered. The implication is that a female touch, which is equivalent to sexual provocation, differs from a male touch, which is most often identical with sexual violence.[13] In search of suitable passages, I have turned primarily to hagiographical and novelistic texts, simply because questions of denial and desire are at the core of these genres. Accordingly, this brief survey is not to be seen as a complete study of erotic touch in Byzantine literature, but rather as a point of departure for future analysis.

The Forbidden Fruit

Let us begin by looking at the overarching haptic event of Christian literature: the picking of the

6 Cf. the discussion of physical pain and holiness in S. Constantinou, "The Saint's Two Bodies: Sensibility under Self-Torture in Byzantine Hagiography," *Classica et Mediaevalia* 66 (2017): forthcoming.

7 See also B. Caseau, "Christian Bodies," in *Desire and Denial in Byzantium*, ed. L. James (Aldershot, 1999), 101–9, on the use of the body in sacred space in Byzantium, esp. 103–4 on touch.

8 On this mixture as a conflict and a taboo, see H.-G. Beck, *Byzantinisches Erotikon* (Munich, 1986), 17–19; cf. S. Lalanne, *Une éducation grecque: Rites de passage et construction des genres dans le roman grec ancien* (Paris, 2006), on the ancient novels as depicting the transition to adulthood and marriage.

9 Touch that is not erotically charged will not be included in this survey; the cultural history of touch in Byzantium remains to be written, but for touch in a primarily religious context see the contribution by Béatrice Caseau in the present volume.

10 Av. Cameron: "Desire in Byzantium—the Ought and the Is," in James, *Desire and Denial*, 205–13, at 211; cf. also M. Cunningham, "Spiritual Treatises on Resisting the Passions," in the same volume, 21–32, at 31, on Christian texts expressing thoughts rather than sexual acts themselves.

11 Dreams and visions are indeed crucial since a fairly large part of the tactile experience takes place in dreams in Byzantine literature, but they have been treated in an excellent manner in a recent article by C. Messis, "Fluid Dreams, Solid Consciences: Erotic Dreams in Byzantium," in *Dreaming in Byzantium and Beyond*, ed. C. Angelidi and G. T. Calofonos (Surrey, 2014), 187–205. See also A. Kazhdan, "Byzantine Hagiography and Sex in the Fifth to Twelfth Centuries," *DOP* (1990): 131–43, at 142. For some tactile experience during dreams and visions, see also P. C. Miller, *The Corporeal Imagination: Signifying the Holy in Late Ancient Christianity* (Philadelphia, 2009).

12 I adhere to Catia Galatariotou's definition of a patriarchal society as "a system of social order in which power and the means of acquiring and perpetuating it... have been assumed by the male sex": "Holy Women and Witches: Aspects of Byzantine Conceptions of Gender," *BMGS* 9 (1984–85): 55–94, at 56.

13 See Messis, "Fluid Dreams," 204–5.

forbidden fruit. This major narrative implicitly permeated the discourse of touch in Byzantium and thus provides an important background for the texts that shall be discussed below. The *noli me tangere* imperative is most often associated with Mary Magdalene's encounter with the risen Christ in John 20:17. She first mistakes Jesus for a gardener, but then she recognizes him and he speaks the famous words: Μή μου ἅπτου, traditionally rendered as "Touch me not," but linguistically closer perhaps to "Stop clinging to me" or "Don't hold on to me."[14] A number of explanations of why the resurrected Christ does not want to be touched or kept by Mary Magdalene have been presented,[15] but what is more interesting to us here is the tactile prohibition as such, which may be seen as an echo of another encounter between a man and a woman in a garden: God's command to Adam and Eve in Genesis 2:16–17, telling them not to eat from the tree of knowledge.[16] Eve's disobedience to the command, under the influence of the snake, leads to the expulsion from Paradise; Eve is accordingly to be blamed not only for all women's sins but also for Adam's—that is, man's—fall from grace.[17] As Gregory of Nazianzos put it in the fourth century, Adam lost his glory in Paradise "because of the envy of the devil and the influence of a woman, an influence which she herself suffered as she was softer [than Adam], and which she brought [unto Adam] as she was more persuasive [than he]" (φθόνῳ διαβόλου καὶ γυναικὸς ἐπηρείᾳ, ἥν τε ἔπαθεν ὡς ἀπαλωτέρα καὶ ἣν προσήγαγεν ὡς πιθανωτέρα).[18]

Touch—and especially erotic touch—is thus often imbued with forbidden temptation, as is also the garden. Eden as *the* garden of Byzantine literature is accordingly a place of ambiguous feelings toward pleasure. It is the most beautiful and pure place on earth, and at the same time it has connotations of impure temptation. In the Byzantine novels, both of these aspects are integrated as innocent as well as erotic action is played out in the setting of beautiful and fragrant gardens, enticing the protagonists and yet reminding them of paradises both Christian and pagan.[19] This inherent ambivalence of the garden is brought out by the twelfth-century author (and novelist) Theodore Prodromos in a series of poems under the title *On a Garden*. Of particular interest for us is the third strophe:

> Ὁρῶν σε, κῆπε, καὶ τὰ δένδρα σου βλέπων,
> ἀγάλλομαι μὲν τῇ θέᾳ τὴν καρδίαν,
> φαντάζομαι δὲ τῆς Ἐδὲμ τὸ χωρίον,
> καὶ βούλομαι μὲν τοῖς φυτοῖς προσεγγίσαι.
> Πλὴν τοῦ φυτοῦ τὴν γεῦσιν εἰς νοῦν λαμβάνω,
> ἐξ οὗ φαγὼν ὤλισθον εἰς ἁμαρτίαν·
> θέλω τρυγῆσαι καὶ φαγεῖν, ἀλλὰ τρέμω,
> μὴ γνώσεως τὸ ξύλον ἐκφαγὼν θάνω.

> Seeing you, o garden, and looking at your trees,
> I exult in my heart over the sight,
> I imagine you to be the place of Eden,
> and I want to approach the plants.
> But the tasting of the fruit comes to my mind,
> the fruit from which I ate and fell into sin;
> I wish to reap and eat, but I tremble and fear
> that I will die eating from the Tree of Knowledge.[20]

14 See also Mk. 5:24–34 and Lk. 8:42–48.

15 See e.g. J.-L. Nancy, *Noli me tangere: On the Raising of the Body*, trans. S. Clift, P.-A. Brault, and M. Naas (New York, 2008), 1–54, at 52–53; cf. Veyron, *Le toucher*, 125.

16 For a brief discussion of this echo, see E. Sauer and L. M. Smith, "Noli me tangere: Colonialist Imperatives and Enclosure Acts in Early Modern England," in Harvey, *Sensible Flesh* (n. 1 above), 141–58: esp. 141. While God's command is expressed simply as "Do not eat" (οὐ φάγεσθε ἀπ᾽ αὐτοῦ) in Genesis 2:17, Eve's recapitualation of the command to the snake in 3:3 includes a command also against touch (οὐ φάγεσθε ἀπ᾽ αὐτοῦ, οὐ δὲ μὴ ἅψησθε αὐτοῦ). On the use of the verb ἅπτομαι in the Gospels, see Veyron, *Le toucher*, 40–51.

17 See Beck, *Byzantinisches Erotikon*, 32, and (in greater detail) Galatariotou, "Holy Women and Witches," 59–62.

18 Greg. Naz., *Or.* 38.12, ed. C. Moreschini and P. Gallay, *Grégoire de Nazianze, Discours 38–41*, SC 358 (Paris, 1990), 128–30; English trans. (here revised) in S. Papaioannou, "Michael Psellos on Friendship and Love: Erotic Discourse in Eleventh-Century Constantinople," *EME* 19 (2010): 43–61, at 50.

19 See A. R. Littlewood, "Romantic Paradises: The Rôle of the Garden in the Byzantine Romance," *BMGS* 5 (1979): 95–114; C. Barber, "Reading the Garden in Byzantium: Nature and Sexuality," *BMGS* 16 (1992): 1–19; I. Nilsson, "Nature Controlled by Artistry—The Poetics of the Literary Garden in Byzantium," in *Byzantine Gardens and Beyond*, ed. H. Bodin and R. Hedlund (Uppsala, 2013), 15–29, at 24–26.

20 Theodore Prodromos, *On a Garden* (Hörandner no. 158), strophe 3. I cite the new edition by N. Zagklas, "Theodore Prodromos: The Neglected Poems and Epigrams (Edition, Translation, and Commentary)" (PhD diss., University of

From this perspective, the garden may also represent or reflect the female body: the most beautiful, and yet the most dangerous. Pleasure can be pure and chaste, but it can also be dangerous and sinful. At the same time, the garden, just like a pure relationship, can be enjoyed if approached with caution and moderation. Prodromos goes on, in the fourth strophe:

> Ἄνθρωπε, δεῦρο καὶ τρύγησον καὶ φάγε·
> ἀκινδύνως γὰρ καὶ τρυγήσεις καὶ φάγῃς,
> μόνον τὸ λίχνον ἐκδιώξας μακρόθεν
> τὸν ὑάκινθον κεῖρε, τοῦ κρίνου δρέπου,
> τρύγα τὸ μύρτον, λαμβάνου τοῦ βαλσάμου,
> οὐχ' ὡς δι' αὐτῶν θηλυνεῖς τὴν καρδίαν,
> ἀλλ' ὡς τρυγήσῃς μυστικὴν εὐωδίαν,
> τοῖς κτίσμασι γνοὺς τὸν κτίσαντα δεσπότην.

> Come here, o mortal, reap the fruits and eat!
> For without danger you may reap and eat,
> once you have driven gluttony far away.
> Cut off the hyacinth, pluck the lily,
> reap the myrtle, partake of the balsamum,
> not because of them to become soft in your heart,
> but to reap their mystical fragrance,
> knowing by his creations the Lord Creator.

We are reminded here not only of the ambiguous garden, representing both chaste heaven and erotic sin, but also of the paradoxical character of touch. Touch is physical, corporeal, but as already noted above it also entails something beyond the body, something potentially spiritual. In a Christian literary context we may refer to this as "chaste tactility."

Chaste Tactility

By chaste tactility I refer to metaphorical touch, frequently employed in Christian texts and then most often as a means of describing man's relation to God. We might compare it to Cameron's discussion of the language of passionate love in the context of Christian literature: "It presents a grammar of desire, a pattern on which the soul aspires to heavenly truth."[21] This "grammar of desire" is used, for example, as a way of representing the indescribable touch that the Virgin somehow experienced in order to become the Theotokos.[22] There are numerous examples in Byzantine literature, but it suffices here to consider one case of this contrast between touch and virginity, a rather crucial aspect of many tactile discourses in Byzantium. We can stay in the fourth century and again turn to Gregory of Nazianzos. One of Gregory's less known texts is an autobiographical poem in which he described a dream that convinced him to remain chaste and devote himself to God.[23] In the dream, he was visited by two beautiful women. This sight caused him great pleasure and he accepted their kisses on his mouth. They presented themselves as Purity (Ἁγνεία) and Moderation/Chastity (Σωφροσύνη), and thus appeared to be Christian virtues rather than dangerous seductresses. As Charis Messis has recently argued, the dream of Gregory thus turned out to be a "revisionist game," since it resulted not in sex or marriage, but in celibacy—a sort of inverted erotic dream.[24]

If we move forward in time and turn to another author we have already met, namely Theodore Prodromos, he picked up this pseudo-erotic dream in a set of tetrastichs devoted to Gregory of Nazianzos. Prodromos took over the motif, elaborated the scene, and created a dialogue between Gregory and Chastity.

> – Γρηγόριε, προτιόσσευ ἐμὸν πολυήρατον εἶδος·
> ἥν με λάβησθα βίοιο συνέμπορον, αἰθέρα δ' ἔλθῃς.
> – Τίς δὲ σύ, παρθενίη; περὶ χείλεσι χείλεα βάψα,

Vienna, 2014), 395–402. For an earlier text, see C. Welz, *Analecta Byzantina: Carmina inedita Theodori Prodromi et Stephani Physopalamitae* (Leipzig, 1910), 62–63. English trans. and discussion in Nilsson, "Nature Controlled by Artistry," 20–24.

21 Cameron, "Desire in Byzantium," 210. See also further below.

22 For a recent study of erotic language employed for describing the experiences of the Virgin, see T. Arentzen, "Virginity Recast: Romanos and the Mother of God" (PhD diss., University of Lund, 2014), esp. 59–118.

23 Gregory of Nazianzos, *Θρῆνος περὶ τῶν τῆς αὐτοῦ ψυχῆς παθῶν*, PG 37:1369–75.

24 C. Messis, "Fluid Dreams," 202. We may also note that Gregory's dream echoes the ancient dream of Hercules, where the two women personify vice and virtue, one preferable to the other. The motif is thus well established in the Greek tradition.

σὸν λέχος ἀμφιέποιμι, γάμος δ' ἀποτῆλε μολείτω.

– O Gregory, look at my much-loved appearance! / If you take me as companion for life, you will enter heaven!
– Who are you, Virginity? I dip my lips to your lips, / I want to tend your couch, and the wedding may last a long time.[25]

Prodromos thus imitated the inverted dream, written by Gregory himself, and staged it as a suggestive dialogue between Gregory and Virginity (that is, Gregory's life in celibacy). The erotic tension lies primarily in the choice of words; we may note, for instance, the πολυήρατον εἶδος of the girl, reminiscent of Eros, and the entering of heaven as a hint of sexual climax. The forbidden touch has in this manner been turned into accepted touch: you may not touch a virgin, but you may kiss and go to bed with virginity, just like you may have intercourse with God. Erotic language can accordingly express, in the words of Mary Cunningham, "the legitimate longing of the soul for union with God, as well as the snares which the Devil sets for the soul by means of the appetitive passions."[26] This particular characteristic of eroticized discourse in Byzantium provides us with yet another important background for the understanding of eroticized discourse in Byzantine literature, so let us keep it in mind as we move on to the discourse of forbidden touch.

The Forbidden Touch

Hagiographical writing and sexual expression are most often seen as incompatible. As pointed out by Alexander Kazhdan in his well-known article on this topic, hagiography presents its audience with the system of Christian values, "among which chastity naturally holds a place of honor."[27] The body along with its impure desires—the demon of fornication—should be suppressed and ultimately eliminated. And yet, a number of hagiographical texts include episodes that appear to be highly erotic, sometimes even slightly pornographic. Kazhdan understood this as part of the entertainment value of hagiography, which he described as "the mass media [*Triviallitteratur*] of the time,"[28] an idea that has been further discussed and developed by Stavroula Constantinou.[29] I shall return to the question of hagiography as sexy entertainment below, while my primary focus in the following readings is the narrative and ideological meaning of erotically charged episodes.

With chastity being crucial for the life of unmarried men and monks, staying chaste and untouched was of course a primary concern.[30] The shameful body had to be kept under strict control, appropriately covered, and the ambivalence of human beauty had to be carefully considered. While outer beauty could be a reflection of a beautiful soul, it could also cover spiritual ugliness and thus, by using a fake appearance, pose a threat to a chaste man.[31] The demon of fornication could appear in both male and female

25 Theodore Prodromos, *Εἰς Γρηγόριον ὄναρ τῇ παρθενίᾳ ὡς γυναικὶ ὁμιλοῦντα*; M. D'Ambrosi, *I tetrastici giambici ed esametrici sugli episodi principali della vita di Gregorio Nazianzeno: Introduzione, edizione critica, traduzione e commento*, Testi e Studi Bizantino-Neoellenici 17 (Rome, 2008), 146–47, with commentary at 176–77. English trans. in Zagklas, "Neglected Poems," 191, who discusses the hexametric tetrastich in relation to Prodromos's *Similar [Verses] on Gregory the Theologian* (Ὅμοιοι εἰς τὸν Θεολόγον Γρηγόριον) (Hörandner 120.2).

26 M. Cunningham, "Spiritual Treatises" (n. 10 above), 30–31. See also I. Nilsson, "Desire and God Have Always Been Around, in Life and Romance Alike," in *Plotting with Eros: Essays on the Poetics of Love and the Erotics of Reading*, ed. I. Nilsson (Copenhagen, 2009), 235–60.

27 Kazhdan, "Byzantine Hagiography and Sex" (n. 11 above), 131.

28 Ibid. Cf. Beck, *Byzantinisches Erotikon*, esp. 201–13, and C. Cupane, "Byzantinisches Erotikon: Ansichten und Einsichten," *JÖB* 37 (1987): 213–33, esp. 217.

29 S. Constantinou, *Female Corporeal Performances: Reading the Body in Byzantine Passions and Lives of Holy Women* (Uppsala, 2005), esp. chapters 1–2 on the female martyr and the repentant prostitute respectively.

30 See Cunningham, "Spiritual Treatises," 28–29, on what causes desire and how to resist it. Chastity was an issue also for lay saints who were married; see D. Krausmüller, "Chastity or Procreation? Models of Sanctity for Byzantine Laymen during the Iconoclastic and Post-Iconoclastic Period," *Journal for Late Antique Religion and Culture* 7 (2013): 51–71. On male chastity, see also S. Tougher, "Holy Eunuchs! Masculinity and Eunuch Saints in Byzantium," in *Holiness and Masculinity in the Middle Ages*, ed. P. H. Cullum and K. J. Lewis (Cardiff, 2004), 93–108.

31 Cunningham, "Spiritual Treatises," and Kazhdan, "Byzantine Hagiography and Sex," 135. On beauty and its challenges in Byzantium, see M. Hatzaki, *Beauty and the Male Body in Byzantium: Perceptions and Representation in Art and Text* (New York, 2009), and eadem, "The Good, the Bad and the Ugly," in *A Companion to Byzantium*, ed. L. James (Malden, MA, 2010), 93–107.

disguise, sometimes as a pretty young man, but often as a beautiful woman coming on very strongly and almost forcing the monk or holy person to touch her in an indecent manner.[32] As we shall see in the examples below, the man has to find various ways of escaping this unwanted attention and, above all, the dangerous touch, so that it does not affect his body and upset his self-control.

Women were by definition a threat to the chaste man, just as Eve had been to Adam and indeed all humanity. Female behavior was accordingly of interest for the early Church Fathers, as can be seen for instance in the writings of John Chrysostom. John took a special interest in women's negative conduct,[33] arguing that women *want* to seduce men—an idea that of course went against all accepted rules for female behavior in both late antique and Byzantine society.[34] Women therefore had to be particularly careful in order to keep their desires under control, behaving and dressing modestly so as not to lead men into temptation. Meetings with men in public should at all costs be avoided, and touching a man in public, even unintentionally, could lead to a severe punishment.[35] The worst-case scenario seems to have been a situation in which a woman deliberately touched or came on to a man, strictly censured by the Church.[36] This is the kind of event that is repeatedly envisioned in hagiography, probably as an edifying example of how to deal with female temptation.

There are numerous examples of such edifying tales, but we shall look at the version told in *Barlaam and Ioasaph*, the Christian version of the life story of Buddha, probably reaching Greek via a Georgian adaptation in the eleventh century.[37] Here, the temptation is not caused directly by a woman, but is the result of male intervention. After having met the monk Barlaam, who introduces him to Christianity, the Indian prince Ioasaph does not care for worldly things but only for philosophy. This greatly worries his father the king. Nothing seems to help, but a certain magician by the name Theudas comes up with the plan to remove all male servants and surround the young man with only beautiful women; after he has "once only had intercourse with but one of these women" (ἅμα τῷ συγγενέσθαι αὐτὸν μιᾷ καὶ μόνῃ τῶν τοιούτων γυναικῶν), says Theudas, Ioasaph will not bother with philosophy anymore: "For there is nothing like the sight of women to allure and enchant the reasoning of men" (Οὐδὲν γὰρ ἕτερον ὡς ὄψις γυναικῶν ἐπαγαγέσθαι καὶ θέλγειν τοὺς τῶν ἀρρένων λογισμοὺς πέφυκε).[38]

The king is then presented with an example of how well this had worked in the past (chapter 30), and to him it sounds like a splendid idea. He has beautiful women replacing men in the palace: "These then flocked around him, embraced him, and provoked him to filthy intercourse, by all words and gestures inviting him to

32 See D. Brakke, *Demons and the Making of the Monk: Spiritual Combat in Early Christianity* (Cambridge, 2006). For a recent study of the demon of fornication and transgression in hagiography, see Z. Ainalis, "De l'Éros et d'autres démons: Les représentations littéraires du tabou et de la transgression dans la société tardo-antique de l'Orient chrétien (IVe–VIIe siècles)" (PhD diss., University of Paris, 2014).

33 See A. Hartney, "Manly Women and Womanly Men: The *Subintroductae* and John Chrystostom," in James, *Desire and Denial in Byzantium* (n. 7 above), 41–48, on the negative attitudes to the female as an expectation placed on the male. On misogyny in Byzantium (including a discussion of Chrysostom), see Galatariotou, "Holy Women and Witches" (n. 12 above), 66–69.

34 Hartney, "Manly Women and Womanly Men," 44–45, and Beck, *Byzantinisches Erotikon* (n. 8 above), 49–55. See also K. Zamfir, "Men and Women in the Household of God: Chrysostom's Homilies on 1 Tim 2,8–15," *Sacra Scripta* 6, no. 2 (2008): 144–64.

35 Beck, *Byzantinisches Erotikon*, 59–60; on the social and legal context for appropriate female behavior, see A. E. Laiou, "Sex, Consent, and Coercion in Byzantium," in *Consent and Coercion to Sex and Marriage in Ancient and Medieval Societies*, ed. A. E. Laiou (Washington, DC, 1993), 109–221, esp. on legal categories, 113–32.

36 Cf. Plutarch, *Moralia* 12 (Γαμικὰ παραγγέλματα, "Advice to Bride and Groom"), stating that a woman should never take the initiative. There is clearly a late antique tradition preceding and influencing Christian thinkers in these matters.

37 For a thorough discussion and presentation of all evidence in this complicated question, see R. Volk, *Die Schriften des Johannes von Damaskos,* vol. 6, pt. 1, *Historia animae utilis de Barlaam et Joasaph,* PTS 61 (Berlin and New York, 2009), 1–157.

38 *Barlaam and Ioasaph,* 29.98–103, ed. R. Volk, *Die Schriften des Johannes von Damaskos,* vol. 6, pt. 2, *Historia animae utilis de Barlaam et Joasaph,* PTS 60 (Berlin and New York, 2006), 300. English trans. G. R. Woodward and H. Mattingly, Loeb (Cambridge, MA, 1937), revised. We may note that this episode reflects an episode in later versions of the life of Buddha; see D. S. Lopez Jr. and P. McCracken, *In Search of the Christian Buddha: How an Asian Sage Became a Medieval Saint* (New York and London, 2014), 26–27.

pleasure" (Αὗται λοιπὸν περιεφύοντο αὐτῷ, συνεπλέκοντο, πρὸς τὴν μυσαρὰν συνουσίαν ἠρέθιζον, διὰ πάντων ῥημάτων τε καὶ σχημάτων πρὸς ἡδονὴν ἐκκαλούμεναι).[39] Ioasaph does not let himself be provoked, seeing through the ruse and focusing on the beauty of Christ rather than the women, who are "fair of face, but uncomely of soul" (αἱ δὲ τὴν ὄψιν εὐπρεπεῖς, τὴν δὲ ψυχὴν καὶ λίαν δυσειδεῖς).[40] Satan becomes annoyed and enters the soul of the most beautiful girl, convincing her to work even harder:

> πολλὰ δὲ τοιαῦτα εἰπόντος αὐτοῦ εὐθὺς τὸ πονηρὸν πνεῦμα ὑπαγορεύει τῇ γυναικὶ τὰ τῆς ἀπάτης ὑφαπλῶσαι θήρατρα καὶ πρὸς τὸν ἐμπαθείας βόθρον κατασῦραι τὴν θεοφιλῆ ἐκείνην ψυχήν, καθά ποτε τῷ γενάρχῃ πεποίηκε διὰ τῆς Εὔας, τοῦ παραδείσου καὶ τοῦ θεοῦ ταλαιπώρως, φεῦ, ἐξορίσας καὶ θανάτῳ ὑπόδικον αὐτὸν γενέσθαι παρασκευάσας ἀντὶ τῆς μακαρίας καὶ ἀθανάτου ζωῆς.
>
> Having said many such things, immediately the evil spirit suggests to the girl to spread under his [Iosaphat's] feet the nets of deceit and drag his blessed soul into the pit of lust, as he once did to our first ancestor by means of Eve, thus miserably banishing him, alas! from Paradise and God, and making him subject to death instead of bliss and everlasting life.[41]

The audience is thus reminded of Eve, the garden, and the apple, but also of Satan's ultimate responsibility for that event. Just as within the story, Theudas the deceitful magician rather than the girls themselves are responsible for the seduction, Satan rather than Eve is responsible for the original sin.[42]

Whereas the story of Ioasaph seems rather innocent and at times almost naïve, erotically charged episodes in Byzantine hagiography are often described in an aggressive and brutal manner, so as to describe the severe affliction suffered by the protagonist. Even imagined or proposed touch may lead to painful consequences, as in the *Life of James*, where a woman is employed in order to tempt the hero-saint. The woman comes on to James and wants him to touch her breasts, but instead he puts his hands in the fire and burns them.[43] As a result the woman is so impressed by his strong faith that she converts. A number of similar stories of temptation appear in the *Apophthegmata patrum*. One adheres rather closely not only to the theme, but also to the motif, and is thus of particular interest here. A woman sets out to seduce a hermit, inspired by the devil (κατ' ἐνέργειαν τοῦ Σατανᾶ). She pretends to be lost and cries in order to be let into his dwelling, and the devil causes the monk to feel desire for her.

> Ὁ δὲ νοήσας τὸν πόλεμον τοῦ ἐχθροῦ ἔλεγε καθ' ἑαυτόν· Αἱ μεθοδεῖαι τοῦ ἐχθροῦ σκότος εἰσίν, ὁ δὲ Υἱὸς τοῦ Θεοῦ φῶς ἐστιν. Στὰς οὖν ἀνῆψεν τὸν λύχνον. Ἐκκαιόμενος δὲ τῇ ἐπιθυμίᾳ ἔλεγεν ὅτι· Οἱ τὰ τοιαῦτα πράσσοντες εἰς κόλασιν ἀπέρχονται· δοκίμασον οὖν σεαυτὸν ἐντεῦθεν, εἰ δύνασαι ὑπενέγκαι τὸ πῦρ τὸ αἰώνιον. Καὶ βαλὼν τὸν δάκτυλον αὐτοῦ ἐπὶ τὸν λύχνον, ἔκαυσεν αὐτὸν καὶ οὐκ ᾐσθάνετο διὰ τὴν ὑπερβολὴν τῆς πυρώσεως τῆς σαρκός. Καὶ οὕτως ποιῶν ἕως πρωΐ, ἔκαυσεν ὅλους τοὺς δακτύλους αὐτοῦ.
>
> As he realized the war of his enemy he said to himself: "The crafts of the enemy are darkness, but the Son of God is light." So he stood up and lit the lamp. And burning with desire he said: "Those who do such things go to Hell; put yourself to the test, then, and see if you can stand the eternal fire." And he put his hand to the lamp and due to the excessive fire he did not feel his flesh. Doing that until the morning, he burned all his fingers.[44]

The monk thus saves himself, while the poor girl—"daughter of the devil" (θυγάτηρ τοῦ

39 *Barlaam and Ioasaph* 30.33–35 (Volk 303).

40 *Barlaam and Ioasaph* 30.47 (Volk 304).

41 *Barlaam and Ioasaph* 30.107–12 (Volk 308).

42 Cf. Galatariotou, "Holy Women and Witches," 61 on the guilt shared by the devil and Eve, the latter being an easily persuaded organ.

43 BHG 770, 279–81. For a brief discussion, see Kazhdan, "Byzantine Hagiography and Sex," 138.

44 *Apophthegmata patrum (collectio systematica)*, 5.42, ed. J.-C. Guy, *Les apophtegmes des pères: Collection systématique, chapitres I–IX*, SC 387 (Paris, 1993), 284. My translation.

διαβόλου)—rather than being converted in fact dies from fear. From a tactile perspective it is interesting to note that the fire of desire—an internal pain, burning from within—in both these cases is quenched by actual fire, the external pain of the burned skin. We shall have reason to return to that imagery below.

Let us now consider two motifs in which women act shamelessly toward men, apparently not convinced by someone else and at least not explicitly by the devil (although he is implicitly involved in any shameful behavior). First, an episode from the *Life of Elias Spileotes*, in which the hero saint had to go to Patras and was invited for dinner by a local man. The wife of the host was so taken by the sight of the young monk's face, that she stared at him openly across the table, but also stretched out her foot under the table and rubbed his leg.[45] Her desperate attempts to seduce him had no effect; Elias—"the new Joseph"—was not affected in his heart and wanted none of her affection; in fact he did not even feel her touch, as he told his companions afterward. The "new Joseph" refers, of course, to the biblical story of Potiphar's wife, who began to desire the young and beautiful Joseph—the servant of her husband—and wanted to have an affair with him. When he ran away, leaving her with only his garment, she accused him of rape and he was put into jail. This narrative is central to the kind of motif that we are considering here: the lust of an impure woman for a pure male body; all such women are accordingly "Egyptian women," and men who find themselves in this situation are "new Josephs."[46] The motif appears not only in Genesis and in hagiography, but also in hymnography, in iconographical representations, in various folkloristic tales, and—as we shall see below—in the novel.[47]

Now to our second motif: the washing of male feet as an opportunity for indecent female behavior. In the *Life of St. Meletios*, in the version written by Theodore Prodromos in the twelfth century,[48] a young monk is sent to a village nearby to buy wine, and he and his fellow monks are received by a local. As we have already seen, an invitation into the home of a worldly person is a situation in which indecent behavior may occur. In this case, the host himself is "a genuine lover of God and a friend of monks" (ὡς ἀκριβῶς φιλόθεός τε καὶ φιλομόναχος), but his wife is a "wicked trollop of a woman" (ἑταιριστικῷ γυναίῳ). The passage in question is intriguing, being one of the most vivid representations of this kind.

> ὃ τὸν λίχνον τινὶ τῶν μοναχῶν ἐπιβαλὸν ὀφθαλμὸν καὶ οὐ βιώσιμα οἱ τοῦ λοιποῦ ἡγούμενον ἔσεσθαι, εἰ μὴ ῥυπαρῶς τῷ τοῦ καθαροῦ συγγένοιτο μαθητῇ, ὑπήρχετο παντοίως τὸν ἄνδρα, τί μὲν οὐ λέγον ἐκ τῶν τῆς ἐμμανοῦς ἐκείνης καρδίας περισσευμάτων, τί δὲ οὐ πράττον τῶν ὅσα καὶ μαχλάδες πράττειν εἰώθασιν. ὑπήντα προσερχομένῳ τὰς βλαύτας ὡς μὲν ὑπέλυε τῶν ποδῶν, ὡς δὲ ἀπεμόργνυ καὶ διεκάθαιρε, προσέβλεπεν ὑγρὸν, θερμὸν προσεδάκρυεν, ὅλους ὡς εἰπεῖν διένευεν ἔρωτας καί· ὢ τῆς βίας, πολλάκις λαθὸν ὑπεφώνει, τί σοι καὶ τῇ ἐρήμῳ; τί σοι καὶ τῷ αὐχμῷ; οὐκ ἐπιπρέπει σου τῷ ποδὶ τὸ ἀγροικικὸν τοῦτο σανδάλιον, οὐ προσαρμόττει σου τὸ τρίχνιον τῇ σαρκί. τίς σου τῇ κεφαλῇ τῆς καλῆς ἐφθόνησε κόνης; εἴθε τὸ ἄστυ παρὼν ἐκόσμεις, καὶ τὰ πρῶτα παρὰ τοῖς ὑπατεύουσιν ἔφερες. ὡς δ' ἀδάμαντα παίειν ἐῴκει, καὶ ἄντικρυς τοξεύειν πρὸς οὐρανὸν, τέλος ἐνεδρεῦσαι τούτῳ λάθρα διαγινώσκει καὶ ὀμόσε χωρῆσαι κατὰ τῆς ἀηττήτου ἐκείνης ψυχῆς.

45 BHG 581, 857AB. For a brief discussion, see Kazhdan, "Byzantine Hagiography and Sex," 139; see also C. Jouanno, "Sur un topos romanesque oublié: Les scènes de banquets," *REG* 109 (1996): 157–84, at 180, n. 42.

46 It might be worth noting that Joseph is known in the Orthodox tradition as *pankalos*—beautiful both internally and externally—and represented iconographically as a pretty young man.

47 See S. Goldman, *The Wiles of Women / The Wiles of Men: Joseph and Potiphar's Wife in Ancient Near Eastern, Jewish, and Islamic Folklore* (New York, 1995); on Romanos the Melodist see also R. J. Schork, *Sacred Song from the Byzantine Pulpit: Romanos the Melodist* (Gainesville, 1995), 31–33, and S. Gador-White, "Changing Conceptions of Mary in Sixth-Century Byzantium: The Kontakia of Romanos the Melodist," in *Questions of Gender in Byzantine Society*, ed. L. Garland and B. Neil (Surrey, 2013), 77–92, at 80.

48 For a comparison of the two extant versions of this life, see C. Messis, "Deux versions de la même 'vérité': Les deux vies d'Hosios Mélétios au XIIe siècle," in *Les Vies des saints à Byzance: Genre littéraire ou biographie historique?* ed. P. Odorico and P. A. Agapitos (Paris, 2004), 303–45.

> Casting a lecherous glance at one of the monks and thinking that life was no longer worth living unless she could have the disciple of the chaste one in her dirty bed, there were no words from the crazed fullness of her heart and no acts that sluts normally perform that she did not try in her efforts to seduce the man. She would meet him when he came and first would untie the slippers from his feet, and then would wipe and clean them; she would give melting looks and shed warm tears at him and would beckon all the passions, so to speak. "O the violence," she often whispered to him secretly, "What is there for you in the wilderness? What is there for you in the drought? This rustic sandal does not suit your foot, the hair shirt does not fit your body. And who was envious of the lovely hair on your head? If only you came to the city and dressed up, you would win the foremost place among the ruling class." When it seemed that she was striking a man of steel and shooting straight at the sky, she eventually determined to ensnare him by cunning and join battle against his indomitable soul.[49]

We recognize here the beauty of the man—to be understood as the beauty of his soul reflected in his outer appearance—and the vain efforts of the woman, since the beautiful man is indifferent to any female temptation. She makes one more attempt, following him into the vineyards.

> ὡς δὲ κατὰ ταυτὸ τῆς ὁδοῦ ἐγενέσθην, καὶ ἀνανθρωπία τοῦ λοιποῦ κατεῖχε τὸν χῶρον, εὐθὺς τὴν ἀλωπεκῆν ἀπεκδὺν, γυμνῷ τῷ πόθῳ κατὰ τοῦ μεγάλου νεανιεύεται καὶ τοῦ ῥυτῆρος ἀμφοτέραις ἐπιλαβόμενον, ἕλκειν ἐπιχείρει πρὸς ἑαυτό· καὶ ὢ τῆς τοῦ μοναχοῦ γενναιότητος, μᾶλλονδὲ τῆς ἀοράτου τῶν προσευχῶν τοῦ Μελετίου ἐπικουρίας. ἐπικαλεῖται τὰς τοῦ διδασκάλου εὐχὰς συμμάχους ὁ μαθητὴς πρὸς τὸν πόλεμον, καὶ πρὸς τὴν ἐκεῖθεν διαθαρσήσας βοήθειαν, ὕβρεσι μὲν ὡς εἶχε τὸ μεμηνὸς ἐκεῖνο ἀποκρούεται γύναιον, τῆς δὲ προκειμὲνης ἔχεται ἀμεταστρεπτί. εἴδετε τὸν Ἰωσὴφ ἐντεῦθεν καὶ τὴν Αἰγυπτίαν αὐτοῦ κυρίαν ἐνθυμήθητε, καὶ τὸν ἔρον ἐκείνης καὶ τὴν ἐπὶ τούτῳ βίαν, καὶ τὴν ὁλκὴν καὶ τὴν ἀνθολκὴν, καὶ τὴν σωφροσύνην τοῦ μειρακίου, καὶ τὴν ῥῆξιν τοῦ χιτωνιοῦ, καὶ τὴν ἐκ τοῦ κακοῦ ἀποπήδησιν, καὶ ὡς ἁρμοδιώτητά γε καὶ οὐ παρά μοῖραν ἐνθυμήθητε.
>
> When they had reached a point on the road where the area was for the time being deserted, she stripped off her slyness and with naked lust molested the great man, and seizing hold of the reins in both hands she tried to haul him towards her.[50] O the noble courage of the monk, even more, the unseen succor of the prayers of Meletios! The disciple summoned his teacher's prayers as allies for the battle, and heartened by the help received from that quarter, as best he could he beat off with blows that demented female, and continued unswervingly with the job in hand. So think of Joseph and call to mind his Egyptian mistress and her passion and violence against him, her onslaught and his resistance, the self-control of the youth, the tearing of his tunic, and his escape from evil, and consider how very fitting and proper was his conduct.

Here we are reminded again of the narrative archetype, Joseph and Potiphar's wife. The episode has a somewhat unexpected end, as the monk is reprimanded by his teacher Meletios when he recounts this event: the young monk should not have met the woman's attack with blows, says Meletios, but instead he should have corrected her behavior by speaking to her "in a gentle and fatherly voice" (πραείᾳ καὶ πατρικῇ τῇ φωνῇ).[51] So presumably the young monk lacked self-control, while he should have remained completely indifferent to the naked body and the touch.

In this context it is worthwhile returning to the question of entertainment: are episodes of this kind meant to be erotic or sexy? As already mentioned, Kazhdan assumed that this was the case, arguing that "the average listener of

49 Theodore Prodromos, *Life of Meletios* 28, ed. V. Vasilievskii, *Pravoslavnyj palestinskij sbornik* 17 (1886): 40–69, at 57–58. English trans. by P. Armstrong, *Sanctity and Monasticism in Middle Byzantine Greece: The "Lives" of Meletios of Myoupolis* (Leiden, forthcoming).

50 The "reins" probably refer to the rope tied around the monk's waist.

51 Theodore Prodromos, *Life of Meletios* 28 (Vasilievskii, 59).

hagiographical works wanted sexy stories."[52] It indeed seems reasonable to assume that everyday life in Byzantium was very different from the official message of the church—to stay chaste or get married, and never to talk or think about sex. The textual tradition that has come down to us is prescriptive, and not necessarily a reflection of historical reality.[53] As pointed out by Hans-Georg Beck in his pioneering *Byzantinisches Erotikon*, the majority of Byzantines lived a secular life, often far from the capital and sometimes perhaps even unaware of the regulations laid down by the Church,[54] and the "grammar of desire" employed in Christian texts, as pointed out by Cameron, had "little to do with the everyday pragmatics of sexual or emotional experience."[55] However, this does not necessarily mean that hagiography partly replaced the presumed need for erotic imagery in people's life. In fact, in the context of the hagiographical narrative, the erotically charged episodes do not seem to appear as "sexy" in our modern positive sense. The erotic advances of the women may indeed be a temptation, but they are also aggressive and threatening for someone who has promised to stay chaste. The sexual attacks are rather a trial that has to be endured, so that the monk can return to being subject to Christ rather than to the demon of fornication.[56] Now, what any given reader felt, we cannot know. But the sensations experienced by the literary characters at the erotically charged touch depend on the narrative and ideological context: it can be pleasurable or painful, it may sincerely "touch" you emotionally or spiritually, or not. That noted, we shall move on to the discourse of erotic tactility in the physical and positive sense.

Erotic Tactility

In order to find examples of the discourse of erotic tactility, we need to turn to secular literature and romance.[57] Here I will focus only on the Komnenian novels, written in the twelfth century, even if erotic touch certainly appears also in the later Palaiologan romance.[58] However, we should note that touch is not a crucial part of the novelistic genre as a whole. The novels of Theodore Prodromos and Niketas Eugenianos contain rather few and brief tactile moments. Prodromos's *Rhodanthe and Dosikles* is very focused on chastity: the couple share "a solemn relationship and desire without passion / and the pure bond of bodies that are not linked" (σχέσις δὲ σεμνὴ καὶ πόθος πάθους δίχα / καὶ δεσμὸς ἁγνὸς σωμάτων ἀσυνδέτων),[59] and erotic touch is thus more or less absent.[60] The modest Rhodanthe

52 Kazhdan, "Byzantine Hagiography and Sex," 131; cf. also p. 143 on monasticism as an escape from sexual activities, but not from sexual desire. Note also the work of S. Constantinou, cited above, n. 29.

53 Note Cameron, "Desire in Byzantium" (n. 10 above), 205.

54 Beck, *Byzantinisches Erotikon* (n. 8 above), 76–78, underlining the presence of a secular Byzantium, not always to be clearly distinguished from the Orthodox part; note also p. 202: "Die Sünde ist auch in Byzanz intergraler Bestandteil des christlichen Alltags." Cf. the useful comments in Cupane, "Byzantinisches Erotikon" (n. 28 above).

55 Cameron, "Desire in Byzantium," 210.

56 See Messis, "Fluid Dreams" (n. 11 above), 194–95, arguing that the subject in hagiography experiences "an intense and undefined threat which is interpreted as a kind of erotic aggressiveness that must be endured so that he and she may be reconstituted as a Christian subject." Cf. also Ainalis, "De l'Éros" (n. 32 above), 242, arguing that erotic episodes could function as a sort of ascetic exercise, as suggested by D. Krueger, *Writing and Holiness: The Practice of Authorship in the Early Christian East* (Philadelphia, 2004), 94–109.

57 There is indeed erotic discourse beyond the novels (e.g., erotic epigrams, some of the progymnasmata of Nikephoros Basilakes, certain passages of historiography), but I have not come across any that include the specific motif that I investigate here (a positive representation of women coming on to men and physically touching them).

58 See, e.g., P. A. Agapitos, "The Erotic Bath in the Byzantine Vernacular Romance *Kallimachos and Chrysorrhoe*," *Classica et Mediaevalia* 43 (1990): 231–60. For a general introduction to the Komnenian novels and the Palaiologan romances, see R. Beaton, *The Medieval Greek Romance* (London, 1996). See now also the useful introductions to the respective novels in the translation by E. Jeffreys, *Four Byzantine Novels: Theodore Prodromos, Rhodanthe and Dosikles; Eumathios Makrembolites, Hysmine and Hysminias; Constantine Manasses, Aristandros and Kallithea; Niketas Eugenianos, Drosilla and Charikles* (Liverpool, 2012), with an updated bibliography.

59 Theodore Prodromos, *Rhodanthe and Dosikles* 2.66–67. Cf. *Rhodanthe and Dosikles* 6.195–206 on the impossibility of separating the couple, possibly with philosophical connotations, and also Niketas Eugenianos, *Drosilla and Charikles* 1.324–29 and 7.229–34. All Komnenian novels are cited with Greek text from F. Conca, ed., *Il romanzo bizantino del XII secolo: Teodoro Prodromo—Niketa Eugeniano—Eustazio Macrembolita—Constantino Manasse* (Turin, 1994) and English trans. in Jeffreys, *Four Byzantine Novels*.

60 Note, however, Theodore Prodromos, *Rhodanthe and Dosikles* 8.200–209, on the effect of Dosikles on young women, one of whom even dares to touch his tunic. Cf. Niketas Eugenianos, *Drosilla and Charikles* 2.334–35.

may at some point wish to touch Dosikles, "urged by passion / to cling to him and to kiss his mouth" (καὶ προσφύναι μὲν καὶ φιλῆσαι τὸ στόμα / ἠλίκον οἷον ἠρέθιστο τῷ πόθῳ), but she is held back by modesty and fear.[61] Eugenianos's *Drosilla and Charikles* is more daring and the lovers do at times engage in some heated kissing and embracing, both in reality and in reveries. They are also surrounded by suggestive imagery and playful love songs, creating an erotic atmosphere that inspires both of them to think and behave rather immodestly.[62]

We should note, though, that erotic sensations in the novels often are provoked not as much by touch as by sight: in accordance with the ancient topos, love and desire enter the soul via the eye, as a small reflection of the beloved travels from the pupil down to the heart.[63] This is how love at first sight appears, and it is also how this first love transforms into love proper, by finding a place to rest in the other.[64] Here we have, I think, an interesting tactile aspect of sight, since seeing is turned into a very physical process. Even the chaste Rhodanthe is affected by the tactile memories associated with the visual memory of her beloved Dosikles, as she describes him to a certain Myrilla:

> ... τί χρή μοι λέγειν
> κόρης, παρειᾶς, ὀφρύος, χείλους πέρι,
> τῆς τετραγώνου, τῆς κεκανονισμένης,
> τῆς κυπαρίττῳ ξυγγενοῦς ἠλικίας,
> ὤμων ἐκείνων καὶ σφυρῶν, χειρῶν, ποδῶν;
> καλὴ μὲν ἡ χείρ, ἀλλὰ πολλῷ καλλίων
> ὅταν ἐνήργει φυσικῶς κινουμένη
> (ἐρυθριῶ μὲν τὴν ἐνέργειαν λέγειν,
> ἐρῶ δ' ὅμως, Μύριλλα, καὶ τί γὰρ πάθω;),
> ἐμοῦ τραχήλου γνησίως ἠρτημένη.

> What should I say / of his eyes, his cheeks, his eyebrows, his lips, / his sturdy, well-proportioned figure / close kin to a cypress, / his shoulders, his ankles, his hands, his feet; / his hand is beautiful, but much more beautiful / when it has made advances, moved by forces of nature / (I blush to speak of advances, / but yet I am in love, Myrilla, and what have I to lose?), / and it is clinging enthusiastically to my neck.[65]

No enthusiastic clinging has actually appeared in the novel, but this is still what the girl remembers when she visualizes the hands of her beloved at the end of the story.[66] Sight and imagination thus often replaces touch in the Komnenian novels, creating an erotic tension that depends to a large degree on the lack of actual touch.[67]

There is, however, one significant exception, because in one of the novels, *Hysmine and Hysminias* by Eumathios Makrembolites, touch plays a significant role. In comparison to the other ancient and Byzantine novels, where tragedy and misfortune are most often starting-points for the story, touching is here the trigger of the love story. Moreover, it is the girl—Hysmine—whose touch awakens the desire and eventual love of the hero, Hysminias.[68] Hysminias, the narrator of the story, is a young man, a virgin, who travels as the holy ambassador of Zeus to another town, where he is received by a local, Sosthenes. Sosthenes has a beautiful garden, in which he throws a dinner

61 Theodore Prodromos, *Rhodanthe and Dosikles* 8.294–96.

62 See, e.g., Niketas Eugenianos, *Drosilla and Charikles* 2.334–35 and the erotic songs in book 3. Note also the description of the heroine in 4.122–23 and the following erotic imagery in Charikles' dream, 4.276–90.

63 In the novelistic tradition, see, e.g., Achilles Tatius, *Leukippe and Kleitophon* 1.4.4 and 1.19.3 and Eumathios Makrembolites, *Hysmine and Hysminias* 3.6.2, 3.7.3, 4.4.3, 4.17.2, and 5.11.6.

64 On the mechanics of vision and the ancient background to such ideas, see H. Morales, *Vision and Narrative in Achilles Tatius' Leucippe and Clitophon* (Cambridge, 2004), 130–40.

65 Theodore Prodromos, *Rhodanthe and Dosikles* 7.213–32.

66 Cf. J. Burton, "Abduction and Elopement in the Byzantine Novel," *GRBS* 41 (2000): 377–409, at 404, who sees a development in Rhodanthe's character: "Rhodanthe becomes more outspoken and erotically assertive as the novel progresses."

67 Cf. Nancy, *Noli me tangere* (n. 15 above), 21 and 49: "What is seeing if not a deferred touch?".

68 On female behavior in the novels, see L. Garland, "Be Amorous, but Be Chaste: Sexual Morality in Byzantine Learned and Vernacular Romance," *BMGS* 14 (1990): 62–120; C. Jouanno, "Les jeunes filles dans le roman byzantin du XIIème siècle," in *Les personnages du roman grec*, ed. B. Pouderon, C. Hunzinger, and D. Kasprzyk (Lyon, 2001), 329–46; eadem, "Women in Byzantine Novels of the Twelfth Century: An Interplay between Norm and Fantasy," in *Byzantine Women: Varieties of Experience A.D. 800–1200*, ed. L. Garland (Aldershot, 2006), 141–62; E. Jeffreys, "The Depiction of Female Sensibilities in the Twelfth Century," in *Το βυζάντιο ώριμο για αλλαγές: Επιλογές, ευαισθησίες και τρόποι έκφρασης από τον ενδέκατο στον δέκατο αιώνα*, ed. Ch. G. Angelidi (Athens, 2004), 73–85 (a comparative study of female behavior in novels and occasional poetry).

party on the evening of Hysminias's arrival. His daughter, Hysmine, is in charge of serving the wine, and this is the first encounter of the protagonists. Hysminias, who is the narrator of the story, watches the girl baring her arms, drawing water from the garden fountain, and mixing the wine. When she comes to serve him the first cup, she whispers "Welcome," to which Hysminias does not respond; he is thirsty, so he drinks with pleasure. Then she comes for the second round of drinks, and this is when it happens.

> Ἧκεν οὖν ἡ παρθένος καὶ ἐπ' ἐμὲ καὶ μάλα βραχείᾳ φωνῇ "ἔχεις" φησὶν "ἐξ ὁμωνύμου παρθένου τὴν κύλικα" καὶ τὸν πόδα ταύτης ἐπὶ τὸν ἐμὸν ἐπιτέθεικε καὶ προσεπέθλιβεν ἐφ' ὅσον ἐγὼ τοῦ πόματος ἔπινον· ἐγὼ δ' ἠρυθρίων, νὴ τοὺς θεούς, καὶ τάχ' ἂν καὶ ἀπέσκωψα πρὸς αὐτήν, εἰ μὴ τύχῃ γενέσθαι τὸ πρᾶγμα νενόμικα.
>
> Πάλιν οὖν ἐτρεφόμεθα καὶ πάλιν ἐπίνομεν. Ἧκεν ἡ κόρη κιρνῶσά μοι καὶ προὐτείνετο τὸ ποτήριον, ἐγὼ δ' ἐξέτεινα τὴν χεῖρα λαβεῖν· καὶ τῆς μὲν κύλικος ἐλαβόμην, ἡ δ' οὐκ ἀπεσπᾶτο τῶν τῆς παρθένου χειρῶν· ἡ γάρ μοι παρθένος καὶ παρετίθετο τὸ ποτήριον καὶ παρακατεῖχεν αὐτό· καὶ τῷ μὲν σχήματι παρετίθετο, τῇ δ' ἀληθείᾳ κατεῖχεν.
>
> Ἔρις οὖν ἐν χερσί, καὶ χεὶρ παρθένου κόρης νικᾷ χεῖρα κήρυκος ἀνδρὸς παρθένου. Ἐγὼ δ' αἰσχυνθεὶς τὴν ἧτταν εἶπον πρὸς τὴν παρθένον γλώσσῃ κήρυκος, ἐλευθέρᾳ φωνῇ, παρθένῳ ψυχῇ "οὐ βούλει μοι δοῦναι; Τί δ' ἄρα βούλει;" Ἡ δὲ συναρπάζει τῷ λόγῳ τὴν χεῖρα τῆς κύλικος, ὅλη δ' ἔντρομος ἐγεγόνει καὶ τὴν παρειὰν ὑπὲρ τὴν φύσιν ἠρύθρωτο, τοὺς ὀφθαλμοὺς ὅλους ἀφῆκε τῇ γῇ καὶ ἦν ὡς ἐκ κεραυνοῦ βληθεῖσα τινὸς καὶ ὅλην ἐπὶ τοῦ προσώπου φέρουσα τὴν αἰδῶ.

> So the maiden came and said to me, in a very quiet voice, "You are receiving the cup from a maiden with the same name." And she placed her foot against mine, and kept it there for as long as I drank from the cup. I blushed, by the gods, and I might have made a joke of it, except I thought that this had happened accidentally.
>
> Then we ate once again and then we drank again. The girl came up, she mixed the wine for me and held out the cup. I held out my hands to take it and grasped the cup, but she did not let it out of her maidenly hands. For the maiden both offered me the cup and kept hold of it and though she was apparently offering it, in reality she was holding on to it.
>
> So there was a contest between our hands, and the hand of the virgin girl is victorious over the hand of the virgin herald. I was shamed by the defeat and addressed the girl in my herald's mien, with my full voice, with a virgin soul, "Do you not want to give it to me? What do you want to do?" At this she snatched her hand away from the cup and was quite abashed and her cheek grew more red than was natural; she kept her eyes completely on the ground and looked as if she had been struck by a thunderbolt, with her shame visible all over her face.[69]

There are a number of interesting things to note in this passage. First, from a literary perspective, we recognize the motif that we have already seen in the *Life of Elias Spileotes*: the female foot pressing against the male foot under the table.[70] But Hysmine is not a mature woman, trying to seduce an inexperienced man: she is a virgin, just like Hysminias. And yet, she breaks all the rules of female behavior, to which the young man apparently reacts; then first comes the virginal shame, at the realization of what she has done, or rather at having been caught in the act of doing it. Second, from a transtextual perspective, Hysminias's reaction to the touch of Hysmine may be seen as a reflection of the behavior of Jesus at the touch of Mary Magdalene: "Touch me not" or, perhaps more fitting here, "Stop clinging to me." There is thus at least one potential Christian subtext at work here. Third, from the tactile perspective, we may note the combination of sensorial impressions in this passage. To begin with, Hysminias simply watches the girl as she

69 Eumathios Makrembolites, *Hysmine and Hysminias* 1.9.1–4.

70 For the Byzantine habit of sitting at the table rather than reclining (a prerequisite for the erotic play under the table), see J. Grosdidier de Maton, "Note sur le sens médiéval du mot κλίνη," *TM* 7 (1979): 363–73. On dinners as an occasion for flirting and erotic play in the Greek novel, see Jouanno, "Sur un topos" (n. 45 above).

prepares herself and the wine;[71] so we have the visual impression, pregnant with erotic tension as she bares her arms and shows her skin.[72] Then we have the whispering, which we also recognize from the hagiographical scenes; whispering is a sign of improper behavior and virgins, in particular, are not supposed to whisper things to strangers. Hysminias drinks and describes the refreshing moment: "the cup was very delightful and the wine very sweet and the water clear and very cold: nothing can be more agreeable than this for a man who is thirsty and very hot and sweaty" (τὸ ἔκπωμα μάλα τερπνὸν καὶ τὸ πόμα γλυκὺ καὶ τὸ ὕδωρ διειδὲς καὶ μάλα ψυχρόν, ὧν οὔτι γένοιτ' ἂν ἥδύτερον ἀνδρὶ διψῶντι καὶ καυματουμένῳ καὶ ζέοντι).[73] Then the girl comes up, touching him. So basically Hysminias moves from sight and hearing—the higher senses—to taste and touch, the more bodily experience.[74]

Moreover, one should also note how the paradoxical behavior of the girl is reflected in the linguistic and rhetorical character of the passage: "For the maiden both offered me the cup and kept hold of it and though she was apparently offering it, in reality she was holding on to it" (*Hysmine and Hysminias* 1.9.3, cited above). This "touching but not touching" becomes programmatic for the way in which the erotic experience is described throughout the novel, first repeated in a series of dinner scenes, and then reflected in a series of erotic dreams in which Hysminias does all the things he did not dare to do in reality:

> Τὴν ἡμέραν ἐπεθύμουν ἰδεῖν· ὠνειροπόλουν τὴν τράπεζαν καὶ τὴν Ὑσμίνην κιρνῶσαν, "Ἂν θλίψῃ" λέγων "τὸν δάκτυλον, ἀντιθλιβήσεται γενναιότερον. Ἀλλ' ἔθλιψε χθές. Ναὶ θλιβέτω καὶ πάλιν. Ἂν θλίψῃ, θλιβήσεται· εἰ δ' οὐ θλίψει, θλιβήσεται. Ἂν τὸν πόδα ταύτης ἐπιθήσῃ μου τῷ ποδί, τοῖν ποδοῖν ἐγὼ προσεπιθήσω τὸν ἕτερον."
>
> I longed to see the day; I went into a dream about the banquet and Hysmine mixing the wine, saying, "If she squeezes my finger, she will be squeezed more firmly in return. But she did squeeze it yesterday! Very well, let her squeeze it yet again; if she does, she will be squeezed; but if she doesn't, she will still be squeezed. If she puts her foot on mine, I'll add my other foot to the two already there."[75]

The touch is thus repeated in the imagination or subconscious of the hero, emphasizing the importance of the tactile events in the experience of the young man.[76]

If we return to the main narrative of *Hysmine and Hysminias*, we find another familiar motif strategically placed right after the first touch at dinner. Hysminias is brought to his bedroom and his feet are being washed by Hysmine. She greedily grasps this second opportunity to touch him:

> ἡ δὲ παρθένος Ὑσμίνη ὀκλάσασα τὼ πόδε καὶ λαβομένη μου τῶν ποδῶν ἐκπλύνει τῷ ὕδατι (καὶ τοῦτο γὰρ τοῖς κήρυξιν ἀφωσίωται)· συνέχει τούτους, κατέχει, περιπλέκεται, θλίβει, ἀψοφητὶ φιλεῖ καὶ ὑποκλέπτει τὸ φίλημα· καὶ τέλος ἀμύττουσα τοῖς ὄνυξι γαργαλίζει με.
>
> The maiden Hysmine, crouching down by my feet and taking hold of them, washes

71 Eumathios Makrembolites, *Hysmine and Hysminias* 1.8.1: "She girt up her tunic, she bared both her arms to the elbow, she tied with a fine cord about her neck the light fabric that was round them and, sitting by the dove, washed her hands (ἡ δ' ἀνεζώσατο τὸν χιτῶνα, ἐγύμνωσε τὼ χεῖρε μέχρις ἀγκῶνος, τὴν περὶ ταύτας ὀθόνην μηρίνθῳ λεπτῇ περὶ τὸν τράχηλον ἀναδήσασα, καὶ παρακαθίσασα τῇ περιστερᾷ τὰς χεῖρας ἐνίπτετο).

72 See Garland, "Be Amorous, But Be Chaste," 72, n. 40, on girls showing their elbows in public.

73 Eumathios Makrembolites, *Hysmine and Hysminias* 1.8.3.

74 The close relation between sight, hearing, and touch is also indicated a little later, as the girl comes up with the third drink: "The girl stands beside me, putting the cup with her hand into mine and entwining her eyes intently with mine, I hold out my hand to take the cup and she presses my finger, and as she does so she moans and breathes a gentle sigh as if from her heart" (*Hysmine and Hysminias* 1.11.2–3: Ἡ δὲ κόρη παρίστατο, τῇ μὲν χειρὶ τῇ χειρί μου παρατιθεμένη τὸ ἔκπωμα, τοὺς δ' ὀφθαλμοὺς ὅλους τοῖς ὀφθαλμοῖς μου συμπλέκουσα. Προτείνω τὴν χεῖρα λαβεῖν, ἡ δὲ τὸν δάκτυλον ἐπιθλίβει μου καὶ θλίβουσα στένει καὶ φύσημα λεπτὸν ὡς ἐκ καρδίας φυσᾷ). Cf. C. Angelidi, "Αισθήσεις, σεξουαλικότητα και οπτασίες," in *Ανοχή και καταστολή στους μέσους χρόνους*, ed. K. Nikolaou (Athens, 2002), 221–29, at 226, on the many sensory impressions of the sexual encounter in the novels.

75 Eumathios Makrembolites, *Hysmine and Hysminias* 3.4.2–3.

76 Note Messis, "Fluid Dreams" (n. 11 above), 194, on the unclear distinction in hagiography between the dream experience and the waking event: temptation-filled dreams are often described as true experience. This device is probably at play also in *Hysmine and Hysminias*.

> them in the water (this is an honor accorded to heralds); she holds them, she clasps them, she embraces them, she presses them, she kisses them silently and sneaks a kiss; eventually she scratches me with her fingernails and tickles me.[77]

It has been suggested that the tickling, which causes Hysminias to laugh, is a sign of the presence of Eros, a plausible interpretation in view of the tense situation in the bedroom of the hero.[78] This tickling, too, is reexperienced in the dream we just looked at, and then expanded with some medical "treatment" on part of the hero:

> ἂν γαργαλίσῃ μου τὸν πόδα, καταγαργαλίσω τὴν κόρην αὐτός, καὶ πείσω ταύτην ἐξ ἡδονῆς ἀνακαγχάσαι καὶ ἔρωτος· ἂν μετὰ τὸ δεῖπνον ἀλγήσῃ τὸν πόδα, ἂν δευτέρα τοῦ πατρὸς ἐρχομένη μονωθῇ τῆς μητρός, ἐπιλάβωμαι τοῦ πληγέντος ποδός, καταφιλήσω τὸ τραῦμα, τὴν πληγὴν πολυπραγμονήσω, ζητήσω τὰ πρόσφορα φάρμακα, κατεπιθήσω ταῦτα, τὴν οὐλὴν καταμαλάξω πᾶσαν ἰατρικῶς, ἐπιστημονικῶς ἐρευνήσω καὶ ὅλην ἰάσομαι.

> If she tickles my foot, I too will tickle the girl, and I will make her burst out laughing from pleasure and passion. If after dinner her foot hurts, if as she goes out following her father she is separated from her mother, I will take hold of the sore foot, I will kiss the hurt, I will make a fuss of the wound, I will ask for the right ointments, I will put them on, I will massage the scar like a doctor, I will make a professional examination and I will make it all better.[79]

The pseudo-medical aspect of touching is probably drawn from the ancient novels, where similar treatments are employed as means of seduction or simply erotic games. It can be understood in light of the idea of desire as an illness, a pain impossible to cure. The treatment of a wound thus meets and merges with the treatment of love, so that a lover in practice functions like a doctor, "curing" someone struck by desire.[80] As Longus has one of his characters express it in his *Daphnis and Chloe*, "There is no medicine for Love, no potion, no drug, no spell to mutter, except a kiss and an embrace and lying down together with naked bodies" (Ἔρωτος γὰρ οὐδὲν φάρμακον, οὐ πινόμενον, οὐκ ἐσθιόμενον, οὐκ ἐν ᾠδαῖς λαλούμενον, ὅτι μὴ φίλημα καὶ περιβολὴ καὶ συγκατακλιθῆναι γυμνοῖς σώμασι).[81] While this idea is only implicitly present in *Hysmine and Hysminias*, it is echoed in one of the fragments of the novel by Constantine Manasses: "Bed and night and kisses, embraces and a couch / are balm to the souls of those tormented by love" (Εὐνὴ καὶ νὺξ καὶ φίλημα, περιπλοκὴ καὶ κοίτη / ψυχῶν θεραπευτήρια τοῖς ἐρωτοκεντήτοις).[82]

It is clear that the repetition of tactile experiences in dreams is used by the author of *Hysmine and Hysminias* as a means of multiplying the erotic action and thus creating even more tension.[83] At the actual event, as Hysmine is washing Hysminias's feet, we may again note that Hysmine behaves like an older woman making advances at a younger chaste man, echoing narrative situations known from hagiography. Hysminias, however, is clueless and does not really understand what is going on. He initially has the characteristics of a young monk: he is a virgin, he is on a mission and he is received in a

77 Eumathios Makrembolites, *Hysmine and Hysminias* 1.12.3.

78 Conca, *Il romanzo bizantino* (n. 59 above), 510, n. 14, with reference to *Anacreontea* 6.5–7 West. Jeffreys, *Four Byzantine Novels*, 183, n. 23, notes that this is used also at Longus, *Daphnis and Chloe* 3.142–43.

79 Eumathios Makrembolites, *Hysmine and Hysminias* 3.4.5–6. On this kind of repetition of episodes as a central narrative device of the novel, see I. Nilsson, *Erotic Pathos, Rhetorical Pleasure: Narrative Technique and Mimesis in Eumathios Makrembolites' Hysmine & Hysminias* (Uppsala, 2001), 64–74.

80 For instance as Kleitophon "cures" Melite in Achilles Tatius, *Leukippe and Kleitophon* 5.26–27 and 6.1, cf. 5.13 on which J. König, "Body and Text," in *The Cambridge Companion to the Greek and Roman Novel*, ed. T. Whitmarsh (Cambridge 2008), 127–44, at 133. Note also Theodore Prodromos, *Rhodanthe and Dosikles* 8.501–6, where the hero rubs the heroine with a herb all over, a surprisingly physical procedure in view of their overall chaste relationship.

81 Longus, *Daphnis and Chloe* 2.7.7. English trans. by C. Gill in *Collected Ancient Greek Novels*, ed. B. P. Reardon (Berkeley, 1989), 306. The pain of Eros is thematized not only in the novels, but also in in the epigram tradition; for a discussion of John Geometres in the 11th century, see Beck, *Byzantinisches Erotikon* (n. 8 above), 120–21.

82 Constantine Manasses, *Aristandros and Kallithea*, fr. 111.

83 See Nilsson, "Erotic Pathos, Rhetorical Pleasure," 107 and 110.

home where a woman makes advances, while he wishes to remain chaste.[84] He finds himself in a conflict between Zeus and Eros, tearing him apart, and he eventually realizes what an experienced reader of novels already knows, namely that desire can be very painful. He spends sleepless nights in anguish:

> ἐμοῦ δὲ τοὺς ὀφθαλμοὺς ὁ ὕπνος ἐξέφυγε καὶ ἐδόκουν νὴ τοὺς θεοὺς ὅλας ὀρύττεσθαι τὰς πλευράς, καὶ νὴ τὸν Ἔρωτα τὴν στρωμνὴν ἀκάνθινον εἶχον, καὶ ὡς ἐπὶ πυρᾶς ὀπτούμενος πυκνὰ στρεφόμενος ἦν, ὥσπερ τι θῦμα καινὸν ἐξωπτημένον τῷ Ἔρωτι.

> sleep had fled from my eyes and I seemed, by the gods, to have my ribs gouged out and, by Eros, I was lying on a bed of thorns and I tossed and turned as though I was being roasted on coals, like some strange sacrifice being cooked up for Eros.[85]

We may compare this pain of being roasted on a spit to the episodes drawn from hagiographical texts that I referred to above (*Life of James* and *Apophthegmata*), where the hero put his hands in the fire in order not to be tempted, or rather to withstand the female temptation. Hysminias's pain—the fire of Eros—is internal, so that the potential pleasure of Eros is turned into torture, strongly reminiscent of some physical experiences of Christian martyrs.[86] When Hysminias eventually falls asleep he experiences a series of dreams in which he finally manages to touch the breasts of Hysmine, and then seems to experience an orgasm.[87]

> Ἤλγουν, ἠθύμουν, καινόν τινα τρόμον ἔτρεμον, ἠμβλυνόμην τὴν ὄψιν, ἐμαλθακιζόμην τὴν ψυχήν, τὴν ἰσχὺν ἐχαυνούμην, ἐνωθρευόμην τὸ σῶμα, ἐπείχετό μοι τὸ ἄσθμα, πυκνὸν κατεπάλλετό μοι τὸ περικάρδιον, καί τις ὀδύνη γλυκάζουσα κατεπέδραμέ μου τὰ μέλη καὶ οἷον ὑπεγαργάλισε, καὶ ὅλον με κατέσχεν ἄρρητος ἔρως ἀνεκλάλητος, ἄφραστος· καί τι πέπονθα, νὴ τὸν Ἔρωτα, οἷον οὐδέποτε πέπονθα.

> I was in pain, I was in anguish, a strange trembling came over me, my sight was dimmed, my soul softened, my strength weakened, my body grew sluggish, my breath choked, my heart beat faster and a sweet pain poured over my limbs with a kind of tickling sensation and an ineffable, unspeakable, inexpressible passion took possession of me. And I experienced, by Eros, what I had never experienced before.[88]

This sexual climax—indeed an accumulation of sensory impressions—is, in a way, also the climax of the tactile relation of the couple. Rather soon after this episode—paired with more or less daring events in real life—the girl starts behaving like a chaste virgin should, protecting her virginity. As convincingly argued by Messis, once Hysminias has found his masculine identity, Hysmine "is reduced to modesty (αἰδώς), the social rhetoric of femininity"; Hysminias, on the other hand, "progresses from painless pleasure to guilty reality."[89] She willingly elopes with the hero, but they both stay virgins until the very end.

In the second half of the novel, Hysminias is instead the subject of unwanted attention from other women, now much more in coherence

84 Cf. J. Burton, who proposes a Christian reading of this scene, based on Luke 7:36–50 and John 13:3–20, "Reviving the Pagan Greek Novel in a Christian World," *GRBS* 39 (1998): 179–216, at 208–11. Cf. also the "mystical" interpretation of the novel by K. Plepelits, *Eustathios Makrembolites, Hysmine und Hysminias* (Stuttgart, 1989), esp. 29–69.

85 Eumathios Makrembolites, *Hysmine and Hysminias* 3.4.1–3.

86 See Burton, "Pagan Greek Novel," 211–12, on this passage and Hysminias as a martyr. Cf. Eumathios Makrembolites, *Hysmine and Hysminias* 3.10.4: "The table is bedecked with various dishes; my hand is concerned with these, my eyes with Hysmine, my mind with passion while my limbs were wracked and my fibers torn apart" (Ἡ τράπεζα ποικίλλεται ταῖς τροφαῖς· ἡ χείρ μοι περὶ ταύτας, ὀφθαλμοὶ πρὸς Ὑσμίνην, καὶ νοῦς μοι πρὸς ἔρωτα· οὕτω μοι τὰ μέλη διέσπασται καὶ τὰ μέρη διέσπαρται·), and Niketas Eugenianos, *Drosilla and Charikles* 2.354: "a woman is an unquenchable fire in the heart" (γυνὴ δὲ πῦρ ἄσβεστον ἐν τῇ καρδίᾳ). On the tortures of female martyrs, see Constantinou, *Female Corporeal Performances* (n. 29 above), 19–58.

87 On this passage, see M. Alexiou, "A Critical Reappraisal of Eustathios Makrembolites' *Hysmine and Hysminias*," *BMGS* 3 (1977): 23–43, at 41; I. Nilsson, "In Response to Charming Passions: Erotic Readings of a Byzantine Novel," in *Pangs of Love and Longing: Configurations of Desire in Premodern Literature* (Cambridge, 2013), 176–202; Messis, "Fluid Dreams," 198–200.

88 Eumathios Makrembolites, *Hysmine and Hysminias* 3.7.6–7.

89 Messis, "Fluid Dreams," 199–200.

with the motif we know from Potiphar's wife. When the loving couple have been separated, Hysminias is taken prisoner and sold as a slave. The mistress of his new household comes on to him, much like the women in hagiographical tales: "How much my mistress sported with me passionately and sat beside me incessantly, and how much she slandered me to my master, and how much she threatened me with her hand and tongue and head, it would not be for me to say in words" (Ὅσα μὲν οὖν μοι συνέπαιζεν ἡ δεσπότις ἐρωτικῶς καὶ κατεπετίθετο συνεχῶς καὶ ὅσα παρὰ τῷ δεσπότῃ κατελοιδόρει μου καὶ ὅσα μοι κατηπειλεῖτο καὶ χειρὶ καὶ κεφαλῇ, οὐ τῆς ἐμῆς ἂν εἴη ταῦτα γλώσσης λαλεῖν).[90] He just barely escapes her advances as he travels with his master, ambassador of Apollo, to another town and there finds Hysmine, who also has become a slave. Now her mistress, the young Rhodope, falls in love with Hysminias, and Hysmine, pretending to be Hysminias's sister, is used as her mediatrix—carrying kisses from the one to the other. "Whatever you think should be said to please Rhodope," says Hysminias, "say it as if from me":

> "Ὅσα σοι δοκεῖ πρὸς χάριν Ῥοδόπης εἰπεῖν, ὡς ἐξ ἐμῆς ταῦτα φάθι φωνῆς. Εἰ δὲ καὶ φιλεῖσθαι ζητεῖ, καταφίλησον, καὶ μετάθου φιλήματα, ὅσα τῶν ἐμῶν τούτων χειλέων ἔχεις πολλὰ στόματι παρατεθειμένα τῷ σῷ. Εἰ δ' οὐ μόνοις ἀρκεῖται φιλήμασιν οὐδ' ἐν χείλεσι παραμυθεῖται τὸν ἔρωτα, κατὰ δὲ τὰς τῶν φοινίκων θηλείας πτόρθον ἐξ ἄρρενος φοίνικος περὶ μέσην αὐτῆς ζητεῖ τὴν ψυχήν, καταπράξομαί σοι καὶ τοῦτο τῇ Ῥοδόπῃ διαπεμπόμενος."

> If she asks to be kissed, kiss her, and give her all the many kisses that my lips have stored on your mouth. And if she is not satisfied with kisses alone and her passion is not assuaged with lips but, like female palm trees,[91] she seeks a shoot from the male palm to penetrate her innermost soul, I shall demonstrate first with you, conveying this to Rhodope."[92]

However gallant this offer is, Hysminias never has to penetrate Rhodope, since the end is close and the young couple is soon rescued by their parents and brought back to their home and, finally, a proper marriage.[93]

This kind of highly suggestive language, representing sexual intercourse which in fact does not take place in reality, appears also in the novel by Eugenianos. The hero Charikles once draws the heroine Drosilla's attention to the lovemaking of birds in order to seduce her:

> Καὶ συγκεκυφὼς εἰς τὸν αὐτῆς αὐχένα
> καὶ τρὶς φιλήσας, θεὶς ὑπ' αὐτὴν ἀγκάλην
> τὰ τῶν γυναικῶν ἀντιπάσχειν ἠξίου
> "ὁρᾷς" λέγων "τὰ δένδρα"—δείξας δακτύλῳ—
> "ὅσας νεοττῶν καλιὰς ὑπερφέρει·
> ἐκεῖ τελεῖται στρουθίων πάντως γάμος·
> παστὰς τὸ δένδρον ἐστί, νυμφὼν ὁ κλάδος,
> κλίνην ἔχει δὲ τὰς ἑαυτοῦ φυλλάδας·
> ναὶ καὶ τὸν ὑμέναιον ἐξᾴδει μέγα
> τὰ πτηνὰ συρρέοντα τοῦ κήπου πέριξ.
> Δός μοι, Δροσίλλα, καὶ σὺ τὸν σαυτῆς γάμον. . . ."

> And bending over her neck / and kissing her three times, he grasped her by the elbow / and asked her to give a womanly recompense, / saying, as he pointed with his finger, "You see the

90 Eumathios Makrembolites, *Hysmine and Hysminias* 8.17.1. Cf. also 8.16.4: "In the middle of all this my mistress suddenly appeared and said, 'Why are you so drenched with tears? Look, who is beside you; you have me as your Hysmine, your mistress and your slave in passion.' I made no reply but immediately jumped up and respected my love for Hysmine alone, and imagined only her" ("Τί τοσοῦτον καταβαπτίζῃ τοῖς δάκρυσιν; Ἰδού σοι παρίσταται· ἔχεις Ὑσμίνην ἐμέ, δέσποιναν σὴν καὶ δούλην ἐξ ἔρωτος." Ἐγὼ δ' οὐδὲν εἰπὼν εὐθὺς ἀνεπήδησα, καὶ μόνης Ὑσμίνης ἐτίμων τὸν ἔρωτα, καὶ ὅλην ἐνωπτριζόμην αὐτήν).

91 Cf. *Leukippe and Kleitophon* 1.17.3–5 (a male palm tree is "cured" by a shoot from the female palm), and also the same story in Constantine Manasses, *Aristandros and Kallithea*, fr. 21a (Plan §4).

92 Eumathios Makrembolites, *Hysmine and Hysminias* 10.3.1–2.

93 The motif appears also in the ancient novels, most notably in *Leukippe and Kleitophon*, the main model of Makrembolites, where the beautiful widow Melite indeed succeeds in seducing the hero Kleitophon (cf. above, n. 80). Similar episodes appear in the other Komnenian novels, though never harming the chastity of the protagonists: Myrilla falls in love with Dosikles and tries to poison Rhodanthe (Theodore Prodromos, *Rhodanthe and Dosikles*, esp. 8.415–43) and the queen of barbarians Chrysilla is taken by Charikles while her son falls in love with Drosilla (Niketas and Eugenianos, *Drosilla and Charikles*, esp. 4.77–79, 5.65–106 and 5.197–327). The fragmentary state of Manasses' novel allows us only occasional glimpses of the plot, but fr. 164–66 are indicative of a similar subplot; see also Jeffreys, *Four Byzantine Novels*, 280.

trees, / how many bird's nests with heir nestlings there are in them; / there regularly the sparrows celebrate their marriages: / the tree is a bridal bower, the branch the bridal chamber, / which has its leaves as the bridal couch; / yes the great bridal hymn is sung / by the winged creatures fluttering around the garden. Grant me, Drosilla, marriage with you."[94]

He reminds her of the sufferings they have endured together, bringing in mythological exempla in order to convince her, ending with a final plea: "All this is your bridal ode; grant me marriage. / The sparrow can make love, it can have a marriage; / but we who are in the throes of passion, can we not be united?" (Σὸς Ὑμέναιος ταῦτα· δός μοι τὸν γάμον. / Ὁ στρουθὸς οἶδε μίξιν, οἶδε τὸν γάμον· / ἡμεῖς δὲ καὶ ποθοῦντες οὐ μιγνύμεθα;).[95] Drosilla does not let herself be talked into anything unseemly, but rather accuses him of using force, although he is only touching her elbow: "Do not struggle, do not force me, do not make pointless efforts" (Μὴ κάμνε, μὴ βίαζε, μὴ μάτην πόνει).[96] Since there is no physical force per se, the discourse of erotic touch that Charikles presents to Drosilla may be considered safe—according to the definition by Berleant, cited at the beginning of this essay—since it is perceived primarily through the senses of sight and hearing. The same could be argued for the erotic songs and much of the erotic imagery in *Rhodanthe and Dosikles* and *Drosilla and Charikles*, but hardly for the more explicitly tactile action in *Hysmine and Hysminias*.

Numerous attempts have accordingly been made to explain Hysmine's indecent behavior, in light of the overall novelistic focus on marital bonds and chastity, coherent with Byzantine moral rules and social codes. Their underlying message of the novels is indeed, as stated by Elizabeth Jeffreys, "that marriage is an excellent and essential institution."[97] Is Hysmine then to be seen as a negative example of indecent female behavior? Little in the novel seems to suggest that, in spite of her breaking a number of social and legal rules,[98] often in a manner that is reminiscent of "bad" women in hagiography. Is the author then playing with convention,[99] or is he staging a moral debate on the question of virtue?[100] Should we perhaps read the novel against the metaphorical discourse of desire discussed above, the "grammar of desire," and see Hysminias as a young Christian, struggling toward being united with Hysmine, the Church?[101] While all these interpretations seem plausible, the tactile experiences in *Hysmine and Hysminias* are here read against the Byzantine dialectic, perhaps to be seen even as a negotiation, between the language of denial and the language of desire.

The Ambiguity of Tactile Rhetoric

This brief survey of Byzantine discourses of erotic touch has presented us with a number of partly overlapping, partly contradicting motifs, which together may be seen as layers of narrative and ideological underpinnings of erotic literature. We have seen how the negative or positive charge of the very same motifs is controlled by the narrative and ideological context, so that the tentative female touch—always potentially threatening in an androcentric society—can be experienced as aggressive or pleasurable, sometimes within the same narrative. In *Hysmine and Hysminias*, the touch of Hysmine is threatening to begin with, since Hysminias is chaste, but once he has gained his ground and, under the influence of Eros,

94 Niketas Eugenianos, *Drosilla and Charikles* 8.81–91.

95 Niketas Eugenianos, *Drosilla and Charikles* 8.128–30.

96 Niketas Eugenianos, *Drosilla and Charikles* 8.141. On this passage, see Jouanno, "Women in Byzantine Novels" (n. 68 above), 154. The passage seems to partly mirror the fictional story made up by Charikles in book 4, staging a meeting with a girl described in highly suggestive garden imagery (4.276–88; cf. also 6.572).

97 Jeffreys, "Depiction of Female Sensibilities" (n. 68 above), 83.

98 See Jouanno, "Sur un topos" (n. 45 above), 181–84, on Hysmine and her indecent behavior (cf. Rhodanthe, who refuses even to take part in a banquet until invited by a woman; Theodore Prodromos, *Rhodanthe and Dosikles* 2.74–75); cf. Jouanno, "Women in Byzantine Novels" (n. 68 above), 159–60, on a possible influence from the western *chanson de geste*. See also Beck, *Byzantinisches Erotikon*, 146–50.

99 Jouanno, "Sur un topos," 182.

100 Ibid., 184; cf. Beck, *Byzantinisches Erotikon*, 211, on what he describes as the Byzantine *Doppel-leben*.

101 Plepelits, *Eustathios Makrembolites* (n. 84 above), esp. 29–69; cf. Beck, *Byzantinisches Erotikon*, 154–55 on the absence of critique and the possible readership of novels (including men of the church).

becomes a man (rather than being a boy), he finds the idea of her touch very exciting. Thereby he also adopts the male touch—he goes from wishing to reciprocate her touch (caress her hand if she caresses his) to trying to convince her to have sex with him; "to do something more erotic," as it is put in the novel.[102] The dream leading up to his first orgasm is a description of such a physical battle between the two, in which she tries to protect her body and he "wins" by managing to touch her breasts. Hysminias is certainly a fairly gentle seducer, but we are still reminded of the violent male touch that we find in, for instance, *Digenis Akritas*.[103]

These two categories of gendered touch do not seem to depend on generic or moral context. They appear in hagiography and romance alike, and they are likely to reflect—within the frame of fiction—an ideological approach to gender. In the novels, both categories appear in a subdued form: the touch of Hysmine is indeed a seductive touch, but it is less indecent than what we have seen examples of in hagiography; the reaction of Hysminias is an expression of subdued violence, but much more controlled than in *Digenis Akritas*. In the passage from Eugenianos just mentioned above, Drosilla assumes force even though Charikles is barely touching her. If we look at the novel by Prodromos, the heroine Rhodanthe is once the victim of a tentative rape, but she easily escapes, leaving part of her tunic in the hands of the violent brute.[104] This is, in fact, a gender reversal of the story of Joseph and Potiphar's wife, and here much more in conformity with traditional gender roles.[105] So both female temptation and male violence appear in the novel, but they are never allowed to defeat chastity.

While erotic touch was officially seen as problematic in Byzantium, in literature we find a number of ways of describing the tactile experience, both physical and metaphorical touch. In view of this inherent ambiguity of erotic touch, we may run the risk of offering interpretations that are based on very modern concepts of categorization, such as the clear boundary between spiritual and secular, sexual and chaste. Perhaps we should not see the erotically charged episodes of hagiography merely as sexual repression, or Hysmine's behavior in the novel as a way of sexing up a rhetorical text, but try to reach beyond our ever Freudian perspective and look at the tactile experience rather from a literary and rhetorical angle. The linguistic and rhetorical construction of such experience may then be seen to reflect the paradoxical sensorial impression itself. Contrary to Michel Serres' idea that rhetoric is cold and distancing, opposed to the immediacy of "lived" experience, rhetoric could also be seen as a way to express or indeed embody sensory and sensual experience.[106] Let me add one last quotation from *Hysmine and Hysminias* in order to illustrate what I mean, drawn from a passage in which the two lovers kiss by drinking from the same cup:

> Οὕτως ἐκοινούμεθα τὸ ποτήριον, καὶ ἦμεν ὅλοι συμπίνοντες καὶ λίαν ἐρωτικῶς καταπίνοντες· οὕτω τὰ χείλη παραδόξως ἀνακεκράμεθα, ὅλον ἐρώτων ἐρατὸν ὀπὸν ἀμελγόμενοι καὶ ὅλους ἀλλήλους τοῖς ὀφθαλμοῖς μεθέλκοντες ἐπὶ τὰς ψυχάς.
>
> So we shared the cup, and imbibed together and drank very passionately; thus we mingled our lips in no ordinary manner, sucking the passionate juices of our love and each drawing the other into our souls with our eyes.[107]

We should note the mingling of senses—sight, taste, and implicit touch—and the paradox of the situation: kissing, but not kissing, touching, but

102 Cf. Messis, "Fluid Dreams," 198–202. Cf. also Jouanno, "Women in Byzantine Novels," 148, on the concept of "sexual symmetry" (homonymity as a dream of symmetry) in the Komnenian novels.

103 On *Digenis Akritas*, see Garland, "Be Amorous" (n. 68 above), 82–95, esp. 86 on rape.

104 Theodore Prodromos, *Rhodanthe and Dosikles* 3.265–88, on which see Garland, "Be Amorous," 73.

105 Noted by Jeffreys, *Four Byzantine Novels* (n. 58 above), 59, n. 104.

106 M. Serres, *The Five Senses: A Philosophy of Mingled Bodies*, trans. M. Sankey and P. Cowley (London and New York, 2008), first published as *Les cinq sens* (Paris, 1985). See also S. Connor, "Michel Serres' Five Senses," in *Empire of the Senses: The Sensual Culture Reader*, ed. D. Howes (Oxford and New York, 2005), 318–34.

107 Eumathios Makrembolites, *Hysmine and Hysminias* 5.10.5.

not touching, all expressed and reflected in the rhetorical and linguistic structure of the passage. The senses are thus entwined with each other, as is the sensory experience with the text. Rhetoric is not lived, as Serres would argue, nor is it necessarily a complete alienation from lived experience.[108]

The author of *Hysmine and Hysminias*, just like his contemporary Nikephoros Basilakes, indeed seems to test foundational cultural values as regards the relation between man and woman,[109] but he also draws on an arsenal of sensory imagery that had been developed throughout the centuries in both secular and spiritual literature, from Sappho to the New Testament. In my view, the various scholarly explanations for Hysmine's indecent behavior need not exclude one another; Makrembolites might well have been playing with convention while discussing virtue and opening up for spiritual or Neoplatonic interpretation.[110] What he certainly did was to explore the tactile experience by turning it into rhetoric, and to combine touch with other sensory impressions, in order to express the ambiguity of erotic sensations.

108 In fact, Serres' own text seems to witness of a similar eroticized relationship between the experienced and the written, as he describes the relational character of tactility, the fact that you cannot touch without at the same time being touched (even by yourself): "I touch my lips, which are already conscious of themselves, with my finger. I can then kiss my finger and, what amounts to almost the same thing, touch my lips with it" (Serres, *Five Senses*, 22); "Je touche mes lèvres de mon doigt, mes lèvres conscientes d'elles-mêmes, déjà. Je puis, alors, baiser mon doigt et, presque indifféremment, toucher mès lèvres de mon doigt" (*Les cinq sens*, 19). Cf. Veyron, *Le toucher* (n. 3 above), 9 and 30–33 on touch as a reciprocal/relational sense.

109 Cf. S. Papaioannou, "On the Stage of Eros: Two Rhetorical Exercises by Nikephoros Basilakes," in *Theatron: Rhetorische Kultur in Spätantike und Mittelalter*, ed. M. Grünbart (Berlin and New York, 2007), 357–76, at 373: "Basilakes is ready to use erotic fiction in a manner that tests—even if it does not transgress—foundational cultural values of contemporary Byzantium," among which is androcentric authority (*andreia*).

110 Cf. Garland, "Be Amorous," on the Byzantine obsession with virginity which in the novels merges with the taste for the erotic, for us a rather disconcerting mixture.

My warmest thanks to Charis Messis, Stavroula Constantinou, and Dimitrios Iordanoglou for critical comments and inspiring discussions; to Pamela Armstrong for allowing me to cite her unpublished translation of Theodore Prodromos's *Life of Meletios*; to Saskia Dirkse for pointing me to the interesting passage in the *Apophthegmata patrum*; and to David Konstan for reading my final version and offering useful advice.

The Sensorium

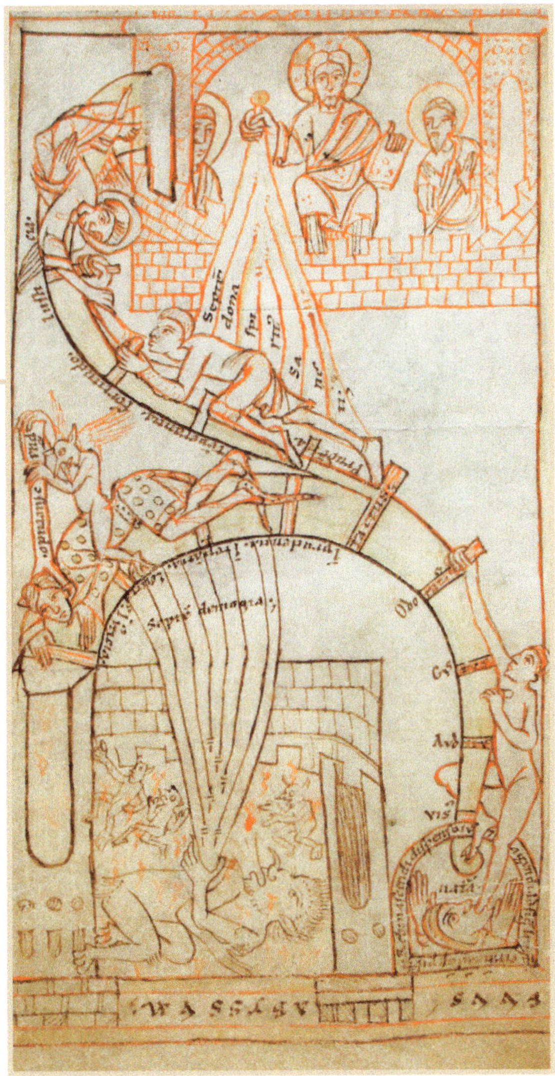

CHAPTER FOURTEEN

Virtual Sensations and Inner Visions

Words and the Senses in Late Antiquity and Byzantium

RUTH WEBB

The word, whether spoken or written, has a particular relationship to the senses and to the sensations that we feel. The spoken word appeals most obviously to the sense of hearing while the written word is perceived through sight, sometimes aided by touch in the case of inscriptions, for example. But the reception of both individual words and verbal messages (whether in the form of speeches, poems, or simple conversations) sets in motion processes that are both intellectual and sensual. Beyond its immediate sensory appeal, the word can convey information both about perceptible entities (people, objects, architecture) and about the experience of perceiving them, both for members of the same community and, later, for historians such as ourselves in search of information about perceptions and the senses. However, talk about perceptions is not merely informative for, in addition to telling the reader or listener about the impact made on both body and mind through the senses, words can themselves evoke responses. They can create the impression in readers or listeners that they are perceiving the entity that is described or, what is more, feeling as they would if they were in the physical presence of that entity or if they were performing the actions described.

This dimension of language, although often overlooked in modern critical studies which, understandably, prefer to focus on more objectively observable features of texts, was widely acknowledged in ancient and Byzantine rhetoric and discussed under the headings of *enargeia*, *ekphrasis*, and *hypotyposis*. It has also been brought to light by several recent studies of the ways in which the brain reacts to language, suggesting that hearing about objects and actions stimulates parts of the brain involved in the physical interaction with those objects or in accomplishing the actions.[1] I will approach the twin topics of how words create an illusion of sensation and of the nature and quality of the resulting experiences through a selection of different texts from the fourth to the ninth century, not in order to construct a history of linear development, though I think that there are important changes that take place in the use and conception of appeals to the senses, but primarily in order to explore some different uses of such appeals and the differing relationships between the word, the virtual sensation that it creates, and reality, whether that reality is understood as sensible, intelligible, or both.

1 Action words especially have this effect. See O. Hauk et al., "Somatotopic Representation of Action Words in Human Motor and Premotor Cortex," *Neuron* 41, no. 2 (2004): 301–7, M. Jeannerod, *Motor Cognition: What Actions Tell the Self* (Oxford, 2006), 161; V. Gallese, "Mirror Neurons and Art," in *Art and the Senses,* ed. F. Bacchi and D. Melcher (Oxford, 2013), 457. For an exploration of the implications of such findings in Western medieval and modern literature see G. Bolens, *The Style of Gestures: Embodiment and Cognition in Literary Narrative* (Baltimore, 2012).

Making Visible and Bodily Involvement

First of all, it is clear that when a scene is evoked in words we are not dealing with the mere communication of factual details about an entity and its appearance. Rather, the authors or speakers are often attempting to produce an effect that is analogous to that of sense perception. In one way, such effects bypass the body, in that the impression of seeing, hearing, or touching does not result from stimulating the physical sense organs, aside from the ear or the eye perceiving the oral or written word. It would be wrong, however, to assume that the body of the listener is left unaffected by the impact of the word. Here, the explicit discussions of *enargeia* and related terms in rhetorical treatises are less than helpful as their authors so often use an abbreviated form of words to evoke complex phenomena that were familiar from experience. Instead, we can turn to some of the uses made of words to appeal to the senses to see what they can tell us.

One of the most startling examples of the use of the word to arouse a sensory impact is John Chrysostom's demonstration of the impact of merely hearing the name of a famous pantomime dancer or of an actress (two of his favorite bêtes noires). He is complaining about idle gossip about worldly matters that distracts people from discussions of theology. The topics of conversation that harm the soul include the private business of neighbors and, worst of all, discussions of favorite entertainers from the stage. Here, Chrysostom changes his strategy in order to evoke in greater detail the tenor of such conversations:

> Ἅμα γὰρ ἐφθέγξατο ἡ γλῶττα τοῦ ὀρχουμένου τὸ ὄνομα, καὶ εὐθέως ἀνετύπωσεν ἡ ψυχὴ τὴν ὄψιν, τὴν κόμην, τὴν ἐσθῆτα τὴν ἁπαλὴν, αὐτὸν ἐκεῖνον τούτων μαλακώτερον ὄντα. Ἕτερος πάλιν ἑτέρωθεν ἀνεῤῥίπισε τὴν φλόγα, γυναῖκα πόρνην εἰς τὴν διάλεξιν εἰσαγαγὼν, κἀκείνης τὰ ῥήματα, τὰ σχήματα, τῶν ὀμμάτων τὰς διαστροφὰς, τῆς ὄψεως τὸ ὑγρὸν, τῶν τριχῶν τὰς στρεβλώσεις, τῶν παρειῶν τὰ ἐπιτρίμματα, τὰς ὑπογραφάς.
>
> The moment the tongue has pronounced the name of the dancer, your soul has represented his appearance, his hair, his soft garments, the man himself who is softer than all of these. Another stirs up the fire in a different way, introducing a harlot into the conversation along with her words, her gestures, her sidelong glances, her languid expression, the curls of her hair, the rouge on her cheeks, her made up eyes.[2]

These details are part of a deliberate strategy that relies on the ability of words (spoken in this case, at least in their first performance) to provoke a response in the listener and the passage is particularly clever in that it appears at first to be about something else. Ostensibly, Chrysostom is bringing before the eyes of his audience the misbehavior of the anonymous individuals who waste their time in gossip. In the very act of speaking about these third parties, however, he goes on to reproduce the very behavior he is condemning, along with its consequences. The observation is interesting in its own right: Chrysostom claims that a single word suffices to summon a mental image of the person named.[3] If this is the case it is because speaker and audience both have a mental image of what that particular word refers to. Chrysostom's evocation of the details of the appearance of the dancer and the mime actress seems at first to be included as a kind of scientific commentary on this behavior, revealing for the edification of his audience precisely what is happening inside the minds of the chatterers, minds that are separate from those of the listeners. But he immediately reveals that his own audience within the Church are concerned too. After the passage quoted above, he asks them directly: Ἆρα οὐκ ἐπάθετέ τι καὶ ἐμοῦ ταῦτα διηγουμένου; ("Didn't you feel something [or rather 'You felt something, didn't you'] even while I was saying that?").

With this dramatic switch from the third person to the second he challenges—even teases—his audience. If he is able to predict that

2 John Chrysostom, *Homily on John* 18, PG 59:119–20. Unless otherwise indicated, all translations are my own.

3 Compare Augustine's *De Trinitate* 8.6.9, in which the enunciation of the name "Carthage" is said to be preceded by the activation of the corresponding image (*phantasia*) in the speaker's mind. On this passage see R. Webb, "Sight and Insight: Theorising Vision, Emotion and Imagination in Ancient Rhetoric," in *Sight and the Ancient Senses,* ed. M. Squire (London, 2015).

the evocation of the dancer's eyes, hair, and soft clothing would have an impact on them it was surely because he knew what was in their mental gallery, sensations that had been imprinted there by culture and experience. The effect, he claims, is natural: Ἀλλὰ μὴ αἰσχυνθῆτε, μηδὲ ἐρυθριάσητε· ἡ γὰρ τῆς φύσεως ἀνάγκη τοῦτο ἀπαιτεῖ, καὶ οὕτω διατίθησι τὴν ψυχὴν, ὡς ἂν ἡ τῶν ἀπαγγελλομένων δύναμις ἔχῃ ("Don't be ashamed, don't blush, the necessity of nature demands this and disposes the soul in accordance with the power of the subject matter of the speech.")

In a strikingly similar passage in his homily on Ephesians, Chrysostom uses the more standard techniques of verbal evocation of a scene in order to illustrate the evils of dissent. He describes an imaginary attack on a ruler whose purple robe is shredded before he himself is torn limb from limb. This leads to a (mock) invitation addressed specifically to the women in the church to beat the preacher himself: "Beat me, spit on me when you meet me in public and aim blows at me" (ῥάπισον, ἔμπτυσον ἐντυχοῦσα δημοσίᾳ, καὶ πληγὰς ἔντεινον). He then asks: "Do you shudder when you hear these words?" (Φρίττεις ταῦτα ἀκούουσα;) before pointing out that divisions in the Church are even worse.[4]

Here, the evocation of a strikingly transgressive crime (the attack on the imaginary ruler) leads to an invitation to certain members of the congregation to perform similarly violent acts on the body of the speaker, acts whose transgressive nature becomes clear when we recall that the imperatives are addressed to women and that the very fact of being publicly beaten would assimilate the victim to the lowest of the low. Most importantly, this sequence of ideas is assumed by Chrysostom the speaker to provoke a physiological response in his listeners (the shudder expressed by the verb φρίττω) that is parallel to the physical response felt, or rather "undergone" (πάσχω), by the male members of his audience when they hear talk about actresses and dancers. In both cases it is legitimate to assume, I would argue, that Chrysostom is talking about an effect that was real for at least some of his listeners and that they did therefore feel an impact from his words that went far beyond the perception of articulated sounds. In both cases we can assume that the words evoked an image in the mind. In the first case, the visual nature of the impact is made clear through the presence of terms denoting details of the appearance and movements of the characters, but other senses are also engaged as Chrysostom refers to the sound of the unspoken name (the nonspecific nature of these descriptions would have made it even easier for each listener to supply their own details), the actress's words, and the tactile qualities of the dancer's clothing and the hair of both. It is reasonable to assume that the pathos that Chrysostom is so sure of having provoked involved different senses. In the case of the imaginary act of violence, the visual element is less prominent as Chrysostom invites his listeners to imagine that they are accomplishing actions, beating and spitting on him, before calling on them to reflect on the horror of those actions by attributing to them the shudder of disgust and fear. I am aware that it might seem naïve to take Chrysostom at his word regarding the physical, mental, and emotional impact of his words but the findings regarding the reception of action words suggest that these effects could be real and the examples discussed above suggest in turn that orators like John were well aware of their potential.

These two examples from the homilies of John Chrysostom are as valuable (perhaps even more so) than many pages of rhetorical theory in that they represent speeches given in front of an audience. We can see how the word does far more than convey *information about* an entity; in addition—above all perhaps—it creates an *experience of* perceiving that entity and, what is more, the listener, like a member of a theater audience, participates in the production of the effect. More than this, in the case of objects and actions, the listener is made to experience the act or the physical interaction with the object (feeling the softness of the dancer's clothes, all but participating in the imaginary attack on the preacher).

I would like now to examine some further examples that bring out another aspect of verbal evocation: although sight is the sense most often spoken of, often the only sense mentioned by rhetorical theorists, other senses are engaged by these texts. As suggested above, the whole range

4 John Chrysostom, *Homily on Ephesians* 11 (PG 62:87). Translation in W. Mayer and P. Allen, *John Chrysostom* (London, 2000).

of senses is potentially engaged by speech, as are the judgments that can accompany these feelings, such as the feeling of horror at the thought (or rather, at the virtual act) of physically attacking the preacher.

Spatiality and the Senses

One of the most striking examples of the engagement of senses other than sight is to be found in Chorikios's ekphrasis of the church of St. Sergios at Gaza. The ekphrasis is at first organized as a tour around the building, a common structuring device in the genre. As he leads his listeners in their imagination through the courtyards, Chorikios evokes the particularly pleasant breeze to be felt there:

> ἡ πρὸς ἑσπέραν εὐμήκης στοὰ μεστὸν εὐθυμίας εἰσάγει παγκάλης αὔρας ἐκ τοῦ πρὸς ζέφυρον πνεούσης προτεμενίσματος, πνεῖ γὰρ ἡδύς τε καὶ ἄλυπος καὶ τῶν ἱματίων ἐντὸς ὑποδὺς ἠρέμα διαψύχει τὰ σώματα τῶν ἐσθήτων αἰωρουμένων τῷ πνεύματι.
>
> The long stoa to the West leads one in full of contentment as a delightful breeze blows from the western atrium, for it blows pleasantly and gently and, penetrating inside your clothing, it gently cools your body as the fabric is lifted up by its breath.[5]

The evocation of the wind and its cooling effect on the body as it gently lifts the clothing is startlingly sensual. The describer and his listeners go from being controllers and interpreters of the space to being acted upon by it as it draws us in, and caresses us.[6] The evocation of the breeze is a highly effective way of making us aware of the *space* of the church, the empty volume that surrounds one. The passage therefore combines the sense of sight with touch and a spatial awareness that places the listener in imagination within the building, surrounded by it and "in touch" with it, no longer occupying the position of the detached observer.

5 Chorikios, *Laudes Marciani*, 1.22.

6 See the chapter by Glen Peers, 11–30.

Thus, we see that a perfectly standard ekphrasis, like that of Chorikios, may make an overt appeal to senses other than sight. Even if it does not do so, these other senses may still be involved. As James Porter has pointed out concerning ancient aesthetics in general, sight brings along with it other sensations: to see a pool of water can evoke the associated tactile sensations; a verbal evocation of appearance can do the same even when sounds and smells are not explicitly evoked.[7]

So the feeling of "being there" produced by the word does not concern the sense of sight alone but involves other senses too. Describing a place as if one was moving through it, as many ekphraseis of buildings do, is much more than a convenient way of organizing one's material; it reproduces the experience of being in the space, of being a sentient body within a three-dimensional space. When I say "reproduce," the resulting "reproduction" is to be understood not as a technical reconstruction (though that may be possible) but as the production of an effect of presence. What is offered is not a static, two-dimensional picture but a space to be moved through, a space that involves the whole body and this spatiality is, as we will see, a recurrent element in the passages despite their differences. Here, neuroscience again offers a valuable perspective. Antonio Damasio argues that memory images are never purely visual but are corporeal, involving the whole body and its relation to the thing remembered.[8] It is remarkable how ekphraseis of buildings correspond in their attempts to position the listener in imagination. There is a suggestion then of a sixth sense that is spatial—the feeling of the body's placement in space in relation to the tangible objects around it. Chorikios's words thus have a twofold function: they remind us of this sense and evoke it in us.

7 J. Porter, *The Origins of Aesthetic Thought in Ancient Greece* (Cambridge, 2010), 65 quoting John Dewey. On synesthesia in antiquity see the remarks of J. Toner, "Introduction: Sensing the Ancient Past," in *A Cultural History of the Senses in Antiquity, 500 BCE–500 CE*, ed. idem (London, 2014), 2–4.

8 His work is particularly relevant to us here because of the importance he attributes to mental images. See in particular A. Damasio, *Self Comes to Mind* (London, 2012), esp. 132: "The organism interacts with objects, and the brain reacts to the interaction. Rather than making a record of an entity's structure, the brain actually records the multiple consequences of the organism's interaction with the entity."

Having set out these principles, I would like to move on to a different aspect of the evocation of sensation: the relation of rhetorically induced visions to reality. In traditional rhetorical theory, the connection to tangible reality can be loose. In order to be effective, rhetorical *enargeia* needs to fulfill two criteria: it must succeed in making the audience imagine the scene in question and that scene must be plausible, that is to say, it must correspond to the audience's expectations of what usually happens. The rhetorical image is, therefore, its own justification; what counts is that it achieves its desired effect. Other conceptions of the relationship between word-induced imaginings and reality did exist in classical sources. These relate them to a type of transcendent reality of different types. One configuration is to be found in pseudo-Longinus (fl. 3rd century CE?).[9] Speaking of particularly intense evocations in tragedy, the author claims that it is as if the poet had himself witnessed the scene. This claim is a topos of course, but it is also highly significant. It implies that the image conveyed through words may give us access to the mind of another individual and, in this case, through them to realities that are not normally available to the senses.

With these questions in mind, let us look at some other examples of the presentation of events of various types in the writings of John Chrysostom, once again, and from the particularly vivid homilies of Andrew of Crete. In both authors we find phenomena that recall Chorikios and his church: a concern to create an illusion not just of a visible scene but of bodily presence that engages all the senses. This bodily presence is closely linked to the sense of space and of the position of the viewer/listener—or of his intratextual representative—within that space. This illusion of presence will also lead to an understanding of realities that are not available to the senses.

John Chrysostom *On the Priesthood:* Conveying Emotions through the Senses

The first example takes us back to John Chrysostom and to his dialogue *On the Priesthood,* which is in itself an exercise in making absent people present as he justifies to his friend, Basil, his refusal to accept ordination. The text—we are very much in the domain of written communication—ends on a remarkable series of comparisons (6.12) that call upon the reader to imagine a variety of scenarios in order to understand the writer's state of mind at the moment when he decided against becoming ordained. These similes are interesting because they both engage the senses in their detailed exposition of the imaginary scene and play a cognitive role, altering the listener's perception of the thing compared.[10] As I will show, this effect is not a purely intellectual matter but relies in large part on the appeal to the senses, including the spatial sense that we saw so strikingly in Chorikios's ekphrasis.

Chrysostom begins with some brief similes (marked by the paired adverbs ὥσπερ... οὕτω...) that express moral and emotional states through comparisons with perceptible phenomena. If he returns to the world he will be like a man who, swept away by a rapid current, can see the danger that awaits him but finds himself entirely unable to escape (6.12.26–33). Just as wild beasts become impossible to control if they are fed and are full of vigor, so Chrysostom's own passions would be fed by vainglory, desire for money, and fame and become uncontrollable if he were to return to the world (6.12.38–57). He was paralyzed by the idea that the Church as the bride of Christ would be dishonored by being entrusted to such an unworthy individual as himself (76–87): ὥσπερ οἱ παραπλῆγες ἐκείμην ἀχανής, οὔτε ὁρᾶν οὔτε ἀκούειν τι δυνάμενος, "I lay dumbstruck like paralyzed men do, unable to see or hear anything."

Up until this point, the images have been relatively brief and general: although they can certainly be said to appeal to the senses, in particular through the use of a wide range of verbs to convey actions, there is no attempt to "place before the eyes" of the reader the particular details, for example, of an individual beast. In what follows, however, the technique changes and Chrysostom has recourse to far more developed images. The

9 On the arguments for the later date see M. Heath, "Longinus *On Sublimity,*" *Proceedings of the Cambridge Philological Society* 45 (1999): 43–74.

10 C. Perelman and L. Olbrechts Tyteca, *Traité de l'Argumentation* (Brussels, 1988), 512–17 discuss the argumentative functions of various kinds of analogy.

first is a miniature romance in which the suitor of the beautiful and supremely virtuous daughter of a powerful king hears that she is engaged to be married to a man of lesser birth, with a mutilated body. The story—parable even—serves to illustrate his sense of despondency (ἀθυμία).[11] The other, which is the example I will focus on, is a developed image of a battle, or rather, of a young country boy being shown around a battlefield, and serves to convey the feelings of terror that led to his decision not to enter the priesthood and to let Basil be ordained alone. It is here that the most direct and intense appeals to the senses are made. Before analyzing the battle image, however, it is worth quoting in detail the transitional passage in which Chrysostom sets out his aims and his methods:

> Τοσαύτη ζάλη τὸν παρελθόντα συνέζων χρόνον· σὺ δὲ ἠγνόεις καὶ ἐν γαλήνῃ με διάγειν ἐνόμιζες. Ἀλλὰ νῦν σοι ἀποκαλύψαι πειράσομαι τὸν χειμῶνα τῆς ἐμῆς ψυχῆς· τάχα γάρ μοι καὶ ἀπὸ τούτου συγγνώσῃ, τὰ ἐγκλήματα ἀφείς. Πῶς οὖν σοι, πῶς αὐτὸν ἐκκαλύψωμεν; Εἰ μὲν σαφῶς ἐθέλοις ἰδεῖν, ἑτέρως οὐκ ἐνῆν ἀλλ' ἢ τὴν καρδίαν γυμνώσαντα τὴν ἐμήν. Ἐπειδὴ δὲ τοῦτο ἀδύνατον, δι' ἀμυδρᾶς τινος εἰκόνος, ὡς ἂν οἷός τε ὦ, πειράσομαί σοι τὸν τῆς ἀθυμίας τέως ὑποδεῖξαι καπνόν· σὺ δὲ ἐκ τῆς εἰκόνος τὴν ἀθυμίαν σύλλεγε μόνην.[12]
>
> This was the type of storm with which I lived in the past. You, however, had no idea and thought that I was spending my time peacefully. Now I shall try to reveal to you the storm in my soul and perhaps this will lead you to pardon me and stop your complaints. How, then, how shall I reveal this to you? If you wished to see clearly, there would be no other way than by stripping bare my heart. Since this is impossible, it is through a dim image [*eikon*] that I will try, to the best of my ability, to indicate to you the smoky shadow of my despondency and you must extract my despondency alone from the image.

11 As Chrysostom himself was the one to refuse the priesthood, rather than being refused, as in the case of the rejected suitor, the comparison is not a neat fit.

12 John Chrysostom, *On the Priesthood*, 6.12 (91–101).

Here, the language of perception is clear in the use of the verb of sight (ἰδεῖν) and the metaphors of revealing (ἀποκαλύψαι, ἐκκαλύψωμεν, γυμνώσαντα) and showing (ὑποδεῖξαι). Chrysostom announces that he is not only going to appeal to the senses but that his images will have an effect that is both cognitive and transformative, leading his reader to understand his state of mind and to change accordingly his evaluation of Chrysostom's actions.

The *eikon* of the battle (121–76) is particularly interesting as it is so clearly a very standard ekphrasis. The image created by Chrysostom is full of visual detail: armor gleaming in the sun, for example (127–29), but also aural sensations such as the sound of clashing weapons, the neighing of horses (129–30). Like them, too, it has a temporal and a spatial dimension: first the encampment is described, then a battle is evoked, and the consequences of the battle (with an emphasis on the experiences of the losing side) is related, as in the standard school ekphraseis of battles.[13] The presentation is important: Chrysostom creates his image by means of a series of third-person imperatives: "let there be an encampment [ἔστω στρατόπεδον] . . . let the sheer number of ships cover the sea [καλυπτέτω μὲν τὴν θάλατταν ὁ τῶν τριήρων ἀριθμός] . . . let the bronze of the weapons shine equally to the sun [ἀντιλαμπέτω μὲν ἡλίῳ τῶν ὅπλων ὁ χαλκός]. . . . Let the enemy be drawn up against them [Ἀντιπαρατάττέσθωσαν δὲ αὐτοῖς καὶ πολέμιοι]."

Chrysostom does not, as we might expect, issue commands to his interlocutor to picture or imagine the scene but speaks as if it were already happening, co-created by the two of them as part of the dynamic interaction of the dialogue.[14] The picture is developed further by the introduction, attributed to an unspecified person (τις), of an internal viewer in the shape of an imaginary

13 See, for example, Aphthonios, *Progymnasmata*, 12.1, pseudo-Hermogenes, *Progymnasmata*, 10.4.

14 The use of the third-person imperative in the context of a description recalls both technical treatises and the narrative of the Creation. On the former see E. Cancellu, "Mathematical Constructive Demonstrations," in *La trame et le tableau: Poétiques et rhétoriques de récit et de la description dans l'Antiquité grecque et latine,* ed. M. Briand (Rennes, 2012), 203–16 and C. Roby, *Technical Ekphrasis in Greek and Roman Science and Literature: The Written Machine between Alexandria and Rome* (Cambridge, 2016), esp. 166–91.

country boy, a picture of innocence and ignorance, who knows nothing beyond "pipes and shepherds' crooks." The imaginary boy is to be pictured in the process of being armed and of being shown around the camp and seeing its commanders, each element being introduced with the imperative δεικνύτω "let him (i.e., the anonymous person) show." Then the boy is to be told in detail (καταλέγω) of the events of battle: the dust, the darkness and confusion, the rivers of blood, the cries of the fallen, the victors' shouts, and the piles of corpses, complete with graphic details of brains smeared on swords and broken lances still transpiercing eyeballs. The reader is then asked to imagine that the boy is told that he has to take charge of all this. What, asks Chrysostom, would he do? The point of the image is clear. The boy's reaction, which the reader is left to supply, is analogous to Chrysostom's refusal to accept ordination. This *eikon* is remarkable for its developed, hyperbolic character and for the way in which it takes longstanding topoi to a new cognitive level. It is possible to detect here echoes of Thucydides, echoes perhaps of Homeric battle narratives, echoes certainly of school rhetoric in the form of ekphraseis of battles and declamation themes. Moreover, the effect of the sights of battle on a coward was also the subject of an *ethopoiia* (speech in character) by Libanios, who may have taught John and who, even if he was not John's teacher, was representative of the same milieu.[15]

What is different about John's battle evocation is the use of the battle description not to evoke its referent but to illustrate and convey an internal state that we would call psychological, his *athumia*. As Chrysostom explains, the perceptible (the boy being shown around the camp) is being used as a way of expressing the invisible: Chrysostom's inner turmoil and despondency. More precisely, the reader, through the ekphrastic elements, is invited to place himself in the position of the imaginary boy and then to transfer his imagined response to Chrysostom. It is true that the *eikon* or image was a common rhetorical exercise, even if it has not survived among the *Progymnasmata* that were selected for use in Byzantine schools.[16] But its use to convey an inner state is, I think, new in the late fourth century and is paralleled in other patristic writers.[17] It involves a movement back and forth between the emotional and the perceptible (John perceives his emotions, he uses an analogy in the world to explain those emotions, and he translates that analogy via rhetorical composition into a text that encourages the reader to move from the realm of the sensual to that of ideas).[18] At the end of this journey, the reader has achieved a new understanding.

Why does Chrysostom go to all this trouble to convey a thought that could be conveyed by a simple statement or a far simpler simile ("I was as scared as a country boy would be on seeing an army")? One answer I think is that his developed narrative is a way of placing his interlocutor into the situation which he is presenting as analogous to his own, getting him not just to understand it intellectually but to feel it, to share it, to be in it. An important aspect of that feeling with ("empathy" at one remove if you like) is the spatiality that marks the account of the battle. The boy is brought in from the country; he is shown around the encampment. We follow him in imagination through this journey, or rather Basil, the supposed addressee, follows him through an extended simile that is part of a dynamic dialogue meant to persuade.

Andrew of Crete: Bodily Knowledge in the Mind

I would like finally to turn to some Byzantine examples of vivid evocation which attempt to make present episodes from the New Testament. These are the extraordinarily dramatic sermons of Andrew of Crete (fl. 8th c.),[19] rich in evocations

15 Libanios, *Ethopoiia* 19 in *Opera*, ed. Foerster, 8:460–64. Text and translation in C. A. Gibson, *Libanius' Progymnasmata: Model Exercises in Greek Prose Composition and Rhetoric* (Atlanta, 2008), 404–7.

16 L. Pernot, "Aspects méconnus de l'enseignement de la rhétorique dans le monde gréco-romain à l'époque impériale," in *L'enseignement supérieur dans les mondes antiques et médiévaux*, ed. H. Hugonnard-Roche (Paris, 2008), 283–306.

17 See, for example, Gregory of Nazianzos's (similarly autobiographical) *Poem on His Life*, PG 37:1039–40.

18 We may also compare with Plotinus's frequent use of metaphors drawn from the perceptible to convey abstract ideas.

19 See M. Cunningham, "Andrew of Crete: A High-Style Preacher in the Eighth Century," in *Preacher and Audience:*

of sensual detail and, particularly, in appeals to the sense of hearing through speeches attributed to the characters, notably the angel Gabriel, who, in front of Mary's door, wonders how exactly to deliver his message to her (showing a very precise concern for rhetorical niceties, like *captatio benevolentiae*).[20] In two homilies in particular, the homily on the Transfiguration and that on Palm Sunday, as Mary Cunningham has pointed out, Andrew seeks to move from the sensual to what he calls mystical perception. In the former homily, the anagogical language is explicit as Andrew invites his listeners—using the jussive subjunctive—to go with him onto the mountain and then, later in the homily, into the cloud itself in order to see or to contemplate its meaning (*logos*).[21] This speech takes us into a different realm and yet the vocabulary of spatiality is still active, expressing an entirely intellectual perception.

In the *Homily on Palm Sunday*, Andrew speaks as if he and his congregation were present at the events themselves. "What is this great throng?" he asks, "Crowds everywhere, children everywhere."[22] In a vivid narrative—an ekphrasis—using the historic present, he describes the crowds massing, setting out where they stood in a clear effort to establish the relative positions of the participants. Then he involves his listeners directly: ἀλλά μοι δεῦρο, συναναβάντες ἐπὶ τὸ ὄρος τῶν Ἐλαιῶν, Χριστῷ συναντήσωμεν ἐκ Βηθανίας ἐπανιόντι σήμερον, καὶ πρὸς τὸ σεπτὸν ἐκεῖνο καὶ μακάριον ἐθελουσίως χωροῦντι πάθος, ἵνα πέρας ἐπιθῇ τῷ μυστηρίῳ τῆς ἡμῶν σωτηρίας ("Come here, going up together onto the Mount of Olives, let us meet Christ as he comes from Bethania today and as he travels toward the sacred and blessed Passion, in order to accomplish the mystery of our salvation").

Note how Andrew does not simply describe the scene but evokes it through his own reactions, particularly the rhetorical questions. Rather than stating "there was a mass of people," he responds verbally as if he were a witness, thereby drawing his listeners to share his reaction through a mimetic identification. There could hardly be a clearer illustration of the way in which the word provokes a sense of perception and of interaction with an entity rather than reproducing the external appearance of that entity. Second, this passage illustrates the importance of imagined space to the creation of a feeling of presence. As we have seen, Andrew makes clear the spatial disposition of the various elements of his scene and, what is more, invites his listeners to travel in imagination through that space. It is particularly interesting to note that the imagined movement upward onto the Mount of Olives brings knowledge and is thus integral to the achievement of understanding aimed at by Andrew. A little further on, we come to the explicit expression by Andrew of what his listeners are to do: Λαβὲ σεαυτῷ νοητὴν εἰκόνα, τὴν ἐν καρδίᾳ τυπουμένην μυστικῶς θεωρίαν, καὶ ἀναζωγράφει μοι τῶν τότε πραγμάτων ἀνατύπωσιν ("Conceive an intelligible image/icon the contemplation [*theoria*] impressed/represented [*tupoumenon*] mystically in your heart and picture, I pray, an image/impression [*anatuposin*] of what was done at that time").[23]

There is picturing in this sermon, there is descriptive language in abundance, and above all, there are calls to "be with." The image to be conceived is not purely visual but involves different senses. Above all, the audience are asked to immerse themselves in the scene, to imagine that they are fully present as Andrew invites them to be one of those leading Christ or to hold the palm. Most strikingly of all, he calls on the listener to become the ass (πῶλος) carrying Christ. In answer to the listener's imagined objection that he is a creature of the word and of intellect (λογικός) and cannot therefore be a creature devoid of these capacities (ἄλογος, playing on the term for "horse"), Andrew urges him or her to imitate the beast in its ἀλογία.[24] This extraordinary passage invites the listener first to imagine the sensation of weight, to become a

Studies in Early Christian and Byzantine Homiletics, ed. M. Cunningham and P. Allen (Leiden, 1998), 267–93.

20 Andrew of Crete, *Homily on the Annunciation*, PG 97:892B–893C.

21 Andrew of Crete, *Homily on the Transfiguration*, PG 97:936B: ἀλλ' ἐπὶ τὸ προκείμενον ἔωμεν, μᾶλλον δὲ προθύμως ἐπὶ τὸ ὄρος ἀνίωμεν; ibid., 952D: ἀλλὰ καὶ τῆς νεφέλης εἴσω χωρήσωμεν.

22 Andrew of Crete, *Homily on Palm Sunday*, PG 97:988A: τίς ἡ τοσαύτη συνάθροισις; . . . πανταχοῦ πλήθη, πανταχοῦ παῖδες.

23 PG 97:1008A–B.

24 Ibid., 1008C: γενοῦ πῶλος, εἰ βούλει . . . βάστασον Χριστὸν ἐπὶ τὴν Ἰερουσαλὴμ ἀφικόμενον.

pure body bearing Christ and then to abandon all human intellectual endeavor, to move beyond understanding.

Conclusion

The capacity of the word to evoke sensations was powerful and there are reasons to take seriously the claims of the rhetoricians that words alone could provoke feelings analogous to those produced by the perceptions of real actions or events. The rhetoricians strongly emphasized sight as the principal sense involved in verbal evocations but, as we have seen, in practice orators often found it more effective to induce their audiences to follow them through space, reenacting in imagination a bodily engagement with the entity evoked, whether a building, as in the case of the Church in Gaza, a typical scene, like Chrysostom's battle, or an event from the life of Christ.

The ability of the word to stimulate the brain to mimic physical sensations is confirmed by neuroscience, but this observation goes only so far. The question remains of the ontological and epistemological status of these word-induced sensations. In his evocation of the impact of merely speaking about the dancer, Chrysostom plays on the unsettling nature of these verbal phenomena, that is to say, he exploits the ability of the word to provoke a response in the listener, even to stoke the fires of physical desire. In *On the Priesthood* Chrysostom's extended ekphrastic metaphor shows his ability and his willingness to "place before the eyes," in this case to move beyond the evocation of perception (of the imaginary army) in order to achieve a shared understanding of his own state of mind. He goes further still in what follows to compare (in a *synkrisis*) the armies of the Devil which, being invisible, are more formidable still, thus initiating a movement from the imaginary perceptible entity to two different types of invisible phenomena: his mental state and the works of the Devil. Similarly, Andrew starts from the evocation of the concrete, in this case the details of an event authenticated as true, to move through the impression of participation that he creates in the listener to a "feeling like" the beast of burden that is purely physical. And yet, it is not purely physical, precisely because it is an imagined mental state that brings with it a form of cognition that is simultaneously bodily and spiritual.

CHAPTER FIFTEEN

Bitter Waters and Dew of Rest

Corruption and Creation in Two Late Ancient Jewish Hymns

LAURA SUZANNE LIEBER

In the sixth century CE, on a Sabbath morning in a Galilean synagogue, the liturgical poet Yannai[1] presented his congregation with a dramatic juridical scene: a wife, accused of infidelity, finds her crime revealed by divine ordeal. The ritual culminates in a moment of graphic horror:

> And just as she betrayed the nature of (her) Creator
> He will make her drink curses from a created vessel
> The mere mention of the Holy Name, written with holiness
> Will be blotted out with holy water to put to proof the (un)holy woman
> The curves of her thighs will abruptly rot
> And the depths of her belly will there empty out
> Her lovely face will yellow and her eyes bulge
> Her fingernails fall off and her sinews give way
> They will see her and say, "Take her out! That alien woman,
> Before she renders the Temple Court impure!"[2]

The suspected adulteress, having consumed the bitter waters which will reveal the truth of the accusation, has her guilt exposed with violent, visual immediacy. The vivid manifestation of justice elicits collective revulsion from the spectators in response to the spectacle. At the same time, the shared experience also conjures individualized, interior sensations: the literal bitterness of the cursed water and the metaphorical sourness of intimate betrayal; the stench of decay and rot. The poet transforms the biblical scene into exegetical theater: through words that were heard and gestures that were seen, Yannai conjures the experience of a long-defunct rite that enters the ears, eyes, and even mouth of his audience. The faithless woman ingests the bitter waters; the witnesses—conceptual and congregational—participate alongside her until they can endure it no longer and cry for her removal.

The literary category of hymnography—poetry that by definition exists at the intersection of aesthetics, exegesis, and performance—offers a unique point of access into the lived and constructed

1 Yannai ranks among the most important early Jewish liturgical poets; for a detailed exploration of his history and significance within the context of Piyyut studies more broadly, as well as a translation of thirty-two of his poems, see L. S. Lieber, *Yannai on Genesis: An Invitation to Piyyut* (Cincinnati, 2010).

2 From Yannai's poem for Numbers 5 (*Poem* 5, lines 6–10); for the full text, see appendix A.

reality of late antiquity. The rich works that fall under this category function as lyric, homily, and prayer simultaneously, and as a consequence they appeal to the listener from an array of perspectives. As textual works experienced in the context of both religious ritual and Torah teaching, the poems engage their listeners intellectually, elicit emotional and intellectual responses, and create immersive and even transformative experiences which had the power to shape and alter the worldviews of their listeners through liturgical experience. The poets deploy strong and vivid sensory language as part of constructing the alternative reality of the liturgical world.[3]

Background on the Texts

In order to explore the sensorially evocative richness of this hymnography, the present essay focuses on two Hebrew-language synagogue poems from the late sixth century in Palestine. The two texts, read with and against each other, articulate deep elements of the experience of life in Jewish late antiquity as expressed, experienced, and shaped through sensory-engaging and evocative language.

The first, by Yannai, quoted above, was composed for a routine Sabbath when the Torah portion began with Numbers 5:11. Composed of nine distinct units, it imaginatively amplifies the ordeal of the accused adulteress (*sotah*)—the ritual of the bitter waters—depicted in the scriptural reading and recasts private marital discord as public trial and demonic apocalypse.[4] The liturgical poem does not merely poetically retell the biblical text, however; in keeping with rabbinic traditions, Yannai—who occasionally quotes Mishnah Sotah[5] in this work—recasts the isolated biblical ritual involving husband, wife, and priest, as a public test of her virtue. He amplifies the drama that the rabbinic authors of the Mishnah imagined.[6] In the hand of a hymnographer, biblical law and rabbinic ritual become liturgical theater: a multisensory, immersive, even transformative experience connecting author, performer, and audience.

The second poem, by Eleazar berabbi Qallir (late 6th–early 7th century, Galilee), was performed on the specific festival occasion when the first day of Passover coincided with the Sabbath. This work is a special kind of poem, called a *tefillat tal* (prayer for dew), as it celebrates the special blessing inserted into the liturgy that marks the turn from the rainy winter season to the drier summer, when dew becomes, quite literally, a source of life.[7] This second work displays an even more elaborate structure and a radically positive set of themes: it transforms the minutiae of daily life into augurs of immanent paradise.[8] In Yannai's poem, bitter waters exorcise a fatal corruption blamed on Eve and extended to all womankind; in Qallir's composition, heavenly "dew of rest" restores land and people, here envisioned as a faithful woman, to an Edenic fecundity that triumphs over death. These two works stake out extremes: Eden and exile, promise and failure, attraction and disgust, life and death.

Both texts are *piyyutim*. The Hebrew term *piyyut* (a borrowing from the Greek *poesis* and thus related to English *poetry* and *poet*) can refer to any postbiblical synagogue hymn but applies generally to Hebrew hymnography from late antiquity and the middle ages. Piyyutim, as suggested by their Greek name,[9] were recognized as something new in the Jewish world, different

3 See L. S. Lieber, "The Rhetoric of Participation: The Experiential Elements of Early Hebrew Liturgical Poetry," *Journal of Religion* 90, no. 2 (2010): 119–47.

4 For a translation of this text, see appendix A. This particular piyyut makes a striking companion to Mishnah Sotah, the tractate of the Mishnah anthologizing early (pre-220 CE) rabbinic legal tradition devoted to the topic of the accused adulteress. In many instances, Yannai seems to draw on mishnaic traditions and even employs mishnaic language; but to an equally strong degree, Yannai marks out a distinctive interpretation of the biblical passage. A full comparison of the two texts falls beyond the scope of the present essay, but those who are interested in the mishnaic treatment should consult I. Rosen-Zvi, *The Mishnaic* Sotah *Ritual: Temple, Gender, and Ritual*, trans. O. Scharf (Leiden, 2012).

5 On the Mishnah Sotah see previous note.

6 On the ritual trial of the accused adulteress in rabbinic writings, see Rosen-Zvi, *Mishnaic* Sotah *Ritual*.

7 On the liturgical significance of this benediction, see R. Ulmer, "Consistency and Change in Rabbinic Literature as Reflected in the Terms 'Rain' and 'Dew,'" *Journal for the Study of Judaism* 26, no. 1 (1995): 55–75.

8 For a translation of this text, see appendix B.

9 That is, rabbinic sources do not call these works by biblical terms for poetry such as *mizmor*, *shir*, or *tehillah*, nor do they use terms such as *hodayah*, as we see in Qumran.

from the biblicizing hymns of earlier periods. These works were tremendously popular and offered an important Jewish complement to Christian hymnography from the same period, works such as those of Ephrem, Narsai, and Romanos, as well as Samaritan liturgical poetry (also called *piyyutim*). Piyyutim came in various genres, including *qedushta'ot* (sg. *qedushta*), popular in the sixth through seventh centuries. In a fashion akin to a cantata, qedushta'ot synthesized the themes of statutory blessings of the central prayer of the Jewish liturgy—the *Amidah*[10]—with the language and content of the lectionary, thereby making the rituals of the synagogue new every week. That is, the poem weaves verses from the Sabbath or Festival Torah portion and its prophetic complement (*haftarah*) into the scaffolding of the fixed liturgical benedictions. These works were most likely sung by the cantor (*hazzan*) alone, or accompanied by a choir, or with congregational participation. Qedushta'ot were organically linked to the ritual practices of the synagogues in Byzantine Palestine, as they were composed for the Palestinian triennial Torah-reading cycle, in which the entire Pentateuch was read over the course of three to three-and-a-half years. As the Babylonian annual cycle supplanted the Palestinian triennial cycle, the vast body of weekly qedushta'ot became, abruptly, outdated.

Yannai, the author of the poem on the *Sotah*, was the first master of the qedushta. When his body of writing became liturgically obsolete, Yannai was lost to history for over a millennium, until his complete works were recovered amid the treasures of the Cairo Genizah.[11] By contrast, Qallir, author of the second text examined here, ranks among the most prolific and best-known poets of Jewish late antiquity; his works survived in many medieval and modern rites, in part because he composed only for festivals and special occasions and thus his works remained viable.[12] By the middle ages, Qallir remained famous but Yannai was just a name on Saadia Gaon's tenth-century list of fathers of Hebrew poetry.

As much as the two poems examined here differ from each other, they emerged from the same milieu. Both poems were performed by cantors in the synagogues of late ancient Galilee and were embedded among statutory prayers and rituals that included psalms, prose prayer texts, and the centerpiece of synagogue ritual, the Torah service. While piyyutim were in many ways performance pieces, they afforded ample opportunities for the congregation—composed of women as well as men[13]—to participate actively, in the form of joining in refrains; and "intellectually," as sympathetic participants in, subjects and objects of, the experience these poems created. The popularity of these poems in antiquity suggests that they were performed in diverse synagogue settings, which would have influenced the experience. A wealthy urban congregation (such as the gorgeously decorated structure at Sepphoris, the kind of community that could have supported a professional poet and perhaps even a choir) could have enabled far more elaborate modes of performance than might have been the custom in a smaller, rural synagogue.[14] The differences between these two poems dramatize the power of payyetanic rhetoric, performance,

10 The *Amidah* ("standing prayer") is also known as the *Shemoneh Esre* ("Eighteen Benedictions") or simply the *Tefillah* ("the prayer"). It is the central prayer of the synagogue liturgy, recited communally every day as part of the morning and afternoon services and silently in the evening service. The Sabbath and festival version of the Amidah contains only seven benedictions: the three initial and three final blessings are unchanged but the intermediate benedictions are replaced by a single prayer on the theme of the day. The qedushta'ot typically embellish the first three blessings of the Amidah, on the themes of God's relationship with the ancestors ("Blessed are You ... shield of Abraham"), his power ("Blessed are You ... who resurrects the dead"), and his holiness ("Blessed are You ... the holy God") and culminate in the recitation of the *Qedushah* (Isa. 6:3 and Ezek. 3:12).

11 On the Cairo Genizah generally, see A. Hoffman and P. Cole, *Sacred Trash: The Lost and Found World of the Cairo Genizah* (New York, 2011). The Ben Ezra synagogue in Fustat (Old Cairo) provides much of our knowledge of the Palestinian prayer rites. See U. Ehrlich, "The Contribution of Genizah Texts to the Study of the *Siddur of Rabbi Solomon ben Nathan*," in *From a Sacred Source: Genizah Studies in Honor of Stefan C. Reif*, ed. B. M. Outhwaite and S. Bhayro (Leiden, 2011), 127–37. On Yannai, see Lieber, *Yannai on Genesis*.

12 Tradition rendered history more melodramatically. A medieval source tells that Yannai's works were intentionally suppressed as punishment for Yannai's jealousy-fueled attempt to murder his pupil, Qallir, by putting a scorpion in his shoe. For text and an analysis, see E. Hollender, *Piyyut Commentary in Medieval Ashkenaz* (Berlin, 2008), 152.

13 See L. I. Levine, *The Ancient Synagogue: The First Thousand Years*, 2nd ed. (New Haven, 2005), 499–518.

14 On the populations of the Galilean synagogues, see C. S. Spigel, *Ancient Synagogue Seating Capacities: Methodology, Analysis and Limits* (Tübingen, 2012).

and oratory to create sensory, and sensual, experiences embedded within the liturgical drama.[15] The formal and contextual differences that make these two poems seem quite unrelated to each other at first glance can, in fact, cast their common elements of audience engagement and performance in that much sharper relief.

Analytical Approaches

My analysis of these intricate works, which integrate prayer and scripture in the context of liturgy, psalms, and Torah readings, highlights three performative-rhetorical registers and their embedded and implicit appeals to the senses (particularly, but not exclusively, to sight and sound). Both move along a continuum from empathy to active participation, their transformative power enacted through sensory evocation. In the first step of the continuum, here labeled "the performance of seduction," the poet appeals to his listeners to imagine themselves in scenes and situations far from ordinary reality—with the poet's appeal to and upon his listeners itself echoing the act of seduction. Through the second, "the performance of fantasy," the poet crafts experiential tours of hell and paradise with the purpose of making remote and abstract past and future not only tangible but urgent, so that the listeners begin to see the world through new eyes. And by means of the third, "the performance of magic," the poet deploys the power of poetic rhetoric to make and break spells—to alter reality—in concert with his audience. The sounds of the words, the sight of the performer, and the perception of the multisensory images and sensations he conjures in the listeners' imaginations possess a transformative potency.

In both poems, these three rhetorical modes overlap and intersect, with the cumulative effect reinforcing the overall vividness and experiential immediacy of the poems. Yannai and Qallir carve out an imaginative space within the liturgical drama and craft within it a dynamic, community-engaging experience, one simultaneously of and not-of the present day world. The liturgical setting amplifies and transforms the rhetorical concept of *enargeia*—forceful vividness—through the implicit potency of the ritual (rather than theatrical) setting. The poems' appeals to the senses and verbal clarity augment a sense of imaginative immediacy and thus imbue the performance with additional constructive power.[16] After participating in the praying of these poems, the community returns to the world beyond the synagogue walls, finding it subtly transformed.

Performance of Seduction

I use the term "performance of seduction" here to describe a rhetoric of enticement rooted in empathy: the ways in which the adulteress is accused of entrapping her lover with her promises, stated and unstated, of sensual pleasure, with Yannai effectively transforming the synagogue and its rituals into a court of law; and, conversely, the ways in which Qallir entices his listeners, already attuned to the heavenly realm through their participation in the liturgical rites, to imagine, in concrete detail, a reality more lovely and in some ways more intensely real than the present one. At issue here is the transformative power of imagination, particularly as shaped by the liturgical setting which works to suspend one's sense of the present before the poet visualizes an alternative world: the prayer service, with its participatory and highly visual elements and its dramatic

15 My approach to the power and effectiveness of liturgy is shaped strongly by ritual theory, both in the modern sense (as in C. Bell, *Ritual Theory, Ritual Practice* [Oxford, 1992]) and the understanding of the power of words and actions in antiquity. On ritual theory in the realm of late antiquity see especially N. Janowitz, *Icons of Power: Ritual Practices in Late Antiquity* (University Park, PA, 2002) and the chapters in *Jewish Studies at the Crossroads of Anthropology and History: Authority, Diaspora, Tradition*, ed. R. Boustan, O. Kosansky, and M. Rustow (Philadelphia, 2011), particularly chapter 13, M. Swartz, "Judaism and the Idea of Ancient Ritual Theory," 294–317. My earlier article, "The Rhetoric of Participation," delineates many of the key hypotheses understood to be in operation here.

16 As Nicholas the Sophist of Myra (5th century, Constantinople) explains: "We say that ecphrasis [ἔκφρασις] is descriptive speech, bringing what is described clearly [ἐναργῶς] before the eyes. 'Clearly' is added because in this way it most differs from narration; the latter [narration] gives a plain exposition of actions, the former [ἔκφρασις] tries to make the hearers into spectators." From G. A. Kennedy, *Progymnasmata: Greek Textbooks of Prose Composition and Rhetoric* (Atlanta, 2003), 166; see also R. Webb, *Ekphrasis, Imagination and Persuasion in Ancient Rhetorical Theory and Practice* (Farnham and Burlington, VT, 2009).

conceptual underpinnings (such as the belief that Israel joins the angels in heavenly prayer) provides a highly attuned and rich-with-potential canvas which amplifies the poet's ability to paint a picture of how the adulteress seduced her lover, even as it provides the poet with an audience primed to be persuaded. Religious ritual creates an openness to imagined worlds.[17] The seductress's manipulation of her lover finds a potent echo in the poet's seduction of his listeners.

Yannai's piyyut recreates in lurid detail the ways in which the accused adulteress enticed her lover. Vituperative descriptions of the woman texture the entire poem. She is "brazen" (poem 4, line 3) and bestial (poem 5, line 3); she is conspicuous (poem 5, line 4) even as she is secretive (poem 5, line 5). Her every action is Other, foreign and animalistic. The poet ascribes guilt not merely to a single woman but to womankind, with vehemence: "From among a thousand, one can find at least one man; but a single woman? Not among any of these" (poem 6, line 13). Yannai's language conjures within the framework of synagogue service the atmosphere of a court, and places the performer in the role of the prosecuting attorney. He appeals to the deity as "the Judge" (poem 6, line 12); the congregation (women as well as men) constitutes both the witness and jury. The ritual of the adulteress's test constitutes a trial: she is "put to proof" (poem 5, line 7). But by deploying the language of accusation (by "sounding like" an official charge) and segueing immediately to a highly visual yet entirely imaginary depiction of instantaneous punishment through the woman's physical decomposition, the poet presents her guilt not as hypothesis but as fact.[18] The poet-performer-prosecutor describes her guilt with vividness and verve, certain the community will answer "amen" to his accusation.[19] The more fully the listeners can be engaged, through a multiplicity of senses, the more persuasively the poet's argument will be realized.

While these motifs recur throughout the poem, in poem 7A, the poet's performance reaches a heated climax. So visually vivid is his catalogue of the woman's misdeeds that one can almost envision even now the performer of this poem pantomiming her salacious actions: she *binds* jewels upon her head, *fastens* the braids of her hair, *paints on* her makeup, and—setting her face brazenly to conceal her perversity—she *opens* her thighs to the stranger who *embraces* her belly. Her lascivious ways are catalogued from head to loins, drawing the mind's eye down her body with scandalous directness. While the mishnaic treatment of this passage (a text that would have been studied rather than prayed) pays fair attention to the woman's male counterpart in the crime, amplifying his presence beyond what it is in the biblical text, here he barely merits mention. Who could help but succumb to such blandishments? Even in poem 7B, which considers, hypothetically, the woman's innocence, her virtue is described in terms of what she did not do: she did not revel in her sensuality, she did not flaunt herself, she did not spread her knees for the stranger or summon him to her belly. In short, not sinning sends the poet's imagination, and his trailing listeners, down the same road as sinning does. The woman's actions, alive in the mind's eye through the power of heard word and seen gesture, becomes in some sense real even when they are *not* done.

Within the Hebrew Bible we find similarly forceful rhetoric, such as in the depictions of Israel as a harlot in Hosea and Ezekiel.[20] But there, the figurative significance of the reading is never far from view; here such a reading can be discerned but does not lie at the surface. In the

17 For a study of how piyyutim, in particular, engaged listeners through a variety of techniques, see Lieber, "Rhetoric of Participation."

18 Forensic rhetoric would have relied just as heavily on imagination, as a way of persuading listeners that events transpired just as the lawyers had argued; the persuasiveness of the argument relies in the vividness and sense of "realness" of the oratory. Orators and actors learned a great deal from each other. See W. Batstone, "The Drama of Rhetoric at Rome," in *The Cambridge Companion to Ancient Rhetoric*, ed. E. Gunderson (Cambridge, 2009), 212–27.

19 It is worth exploring whether the woman described here should be understood figuratively as representing Israel. Such a reading is certainly feasible and draws the male listeners into the drama in a different way if they are to identify with the woman rather than the betrayed husband or duped lover.

20 My trans. For example, Ezek. 16 verges upon the pornographic in its depiction of Israel's wanton behavior; see T. Frymer-Kensky, *In the Wake of the Goddess: Women, Culture, and the Biblical Transformation of Pagan Myth* (New York, 1992), 144–52.

concrete vividness of this poem, the poet brings to mind some of the most effective techniques from the world of ancient declamation and oratory.[21] For example, in his *Progymnasmata* (rhetorical exercise book), Nicholas the Sophist of Myra (5th cent. CE, Constantinople) distinguishes the *koinos topos* (commonplace) from invective using the example of adultery: "[*Koinos topos*] is 'common' because it is directed not against a specified person, for example, against Timarchus for prostitution of Lycophron for adultery, but simply against a prostitute or adulterer."[22] Yannai's treatment of adultery—the sexual transgression of one woman and all women—reflects this same generalizing sensibility. This poem attacks a presumed evil with the intent of convicting, shaming, and condemning a whole category of wrongdoer.[23]

Perhaps the most powerful rhetorical element in the trial of the accused adulteress, however, is that, even in the biblical text, it requires and presumes an audience; the humiliation of the woman (even should she be found innocent) cannot take place in private.[24] Despite the fact that the *Sotah* ritual, if it ever were practiced at all, was defunct by Yannai's time, the presence of the living community (as witnesses, accusers, and—for the women—the accused) was vital to its effective, if imaginary, re-creation. The poet had to make the scene real for the ritual to work. The poet thus appeals, like a good lawyer, to his listeners' imaginations. He does so through both graphic imagery and language itself. In long stretches, his vocabulary relies on a baseline of sibilant and guttural sounds—whispering, rushing, and scurrying—causing the performer to embody and make real the very behaviors the poem condemns.[25] Hearing these words would have reinforced their content as the sounds creeped into the ears and across the skin of the listeners. The poem induces emotional and even physiological responses in its performer and audience, primed by setting and sound to participate in the shared vision.

The spectacle of the trial of the accused adulteress culminates, plotwise if not structurally, in the conclusion of poem 5, where the audience—merging the present community into the imagined audience—points to the woman and exclaims (perhaps in actual participation with the performer): "Take her out! That alien woman / Before she renders the Temple Court impure!" As Ishai Rosen-Zvi notes, the cry of "Take her out! Take her out!" (also quoted in Mishnah Sotah 1:4) derives from the ritual of capital punishment in the Roman arena. The woman's presence, her existence, has become

21 The poem also should be understood in relationship to Mishnah Sotah, not just because of the similarities (e.g., the measure-for-measure punishment of the adulteress) but also because of its differences. Most significantly, the Mishnah addresses and actually amplifies the guilt of the male party in the sin, a subject that seems willfully neglected here, by contrast.

22 Kennedy, *Progymnasmata,* 148. Nicholas defines a commonplace as "an amplification and attack on an acknowledged evil . . . a running attack on an acknowledged and ascertained human evil. . . . The main difference between common-place and invective is that in the case of common-place the judges are being urged to punish the wrongdoer, while in invective hearers are being incited to hatred of the individual against whom the attack is being made. They differ further in that in the common-place the person attacked is not specified but in invective he is named, since we are making an attack on a person rather than on a deed" (ibid., 148, 149).

If the *Progymnasmata* suggests a rhetorical theory beneath such presentations, then centuries earlier, the great Roman orator Cicero provided memorable examples, such as when he accuses Clodia (who was not even the defendant) of adultery, prostitution, drunkenness, and incest, and speaks to her in the voice and with the mannerisms of her illustrious ancestor, Appius Claudius Caecus (§34 of *Pro Caelio*). Likewise, in his *Pro Cluentio,* Cicero depicts Sassia as a seductress and murderer. Immorality, especially sexual transgression, depicted as graphically as possible, is how one convicts a woman—or defeats one who has not been accused. In practice, the boundary between commonplace and invective can be thin, and in the Yannai piyyut, the fact that the poem begins, early on, with a condemnation of Eve (the paradigmatic female) suggests that in the case of women, the difference between attacking an individual person and a generic category has collapsed.

23 Yannai's attack on adultery is particularly striking since Hebrew poetry in late antiquity lacks the sort of moralizing topical poems (e.g., "On Drunkenness") that we find in Christian hymnography.

24 This treatment echoes God's language in Ezek. 16:37, where Israel's collective shame is described: "Indeed, I will gather all your lovers, to whom you were pleasing, all those whom you loved and all those whom you loathed; and I will gather them against you from all around, and I will expose your nakedness to them, that they may see all your nakedness" (my translation).

25 On the important relationships among action, sound, and objective reality, see A. Corbeill, "Gesture in Early Roman Law: Empty Forms or Essential Formalities?" in *Body Language in the Greek and Roman Worlds*, ed. D. Cairns (Swansea, 2005), 157–74.

toxic and polluting, and having been judged via spectacle, she is condemned in one, too.[26]

If this poem conjures an emotionally fraught, sexually charged, luridly vindictive spectacle of toxicity, then Qallir's piyyut for dew offers its listeners a sensory antidote. Whereas Yannai's poem displays a horrified, highly visual fascination with female destructiveness as manifest through the ritual of bitter waters, Qallir's poem offers a paean to the gentle, nurturing power of life-giving dew. He offers balm to the ears and eyes, the cool of dew after the heat of transgressive passion. Yannai sears with his vision of violence while Qallir's words drip with healing salve. This second poem, approached from the perspective of the "performance of seduction," inserts the listeners into the drama as participants rather than positioning them as witnesses to an ancient rite. That is, the listeners, embracing a kind of willing vulnerability as soon as they enter the heightened world of the liturgy, become the seduced: Qallir entices them to imagine a world just beyond the current horizon, a vision of an Eden layered over the dim disappointment of exilic reality. Rather than being spectators witnessing a spectacle, the assembled community stands as imminent beneficiaries. The stakes, then, are that much higher; attentiveness, the physical sensation of leaning in for a better listen, increases.

The seductive-forensic rhetoric of the poem appears most forcefully in poems 4 and 5, which celebrate the abundant plant life of the Land of Israel. The two poems share a common structure and function in tandem as a single unit: the first consists of an alphabetical acrostic from *alef* to *tav*, while the second mirrors that structure with a *tav*-to-*alef* (*tashraq*) acrostic, yielding a visual but also audible sense of completeness. The first stich of each stanza opens with the incipit from a verse of Song of Songs 7:12–8:13, which the poet works through sequentially; the second, with the phrase "dew of rest" (*tal menuchah*), underscoring the transition from the winter prayer for rain to the summer prayer for dew; and the final stich petitions the deity to bless the produce of the land. What is astonishing about these two units is precisely the catalogue of flora: thirty-five varieties of plants and thirty kinds of trees, all of which grew in the Land of Israel in late antiquity and all of which possessed some kind of utility, whether as foodstuffs, medicine, or both.[27]

At first glance, this catalogue may seem the height of mundanity: it sings the praises not of majestic cedars of Lebanon (not, after all, native to Israel) or resonantly allusive hyssop, but the most familiar and domestic items, plants easily at hand: wheat and lentils, mustard seeds and lettuce, pistachio trees and willows. In terms of appeal, this poem initially seems more akin to a child's posy than a dozen roses. The poem is jeweled with common spangles.[28] And yet, cumulatively, this poem possesses intrinsic force. Where in Yannai's poem, God (implicitly) sits in judgment over the adulteress, here God (explicitly) sits in judgment over the fate of the land and its inhabitants. In the first poem, the congregation constitutes the witnesses; in the second, the beneficiaries. But in both cases the poet needs to offer his listeners a compelling vision. In the first, Yanai paints a picture of the adulteress's brazen yet secret actions; here Qallir invokes garden imagery which is, on the one hand, mundane and familiar but, on the other hand, such a riot of abundance that it could never exist all in one place. Poem 5 begins:

Establish for me (Song 8:6) — Praise and make firm the Palace
Dew of rest — cause to course over the slice of pomegranate

26 Considered as a performed text, the question arises, to whom are these words said? To whom is "Take her out!" addressed?

27 The list of items in this poem resonates with the botanical catalogue of Symeon Seth, whose work enriched the symposium. The catalogue offers a kind of textual equivalent of the synagogal zodiac mosaics, where seasons are "compressed" into a single visual; or, to borrow a later example, the Unicorn Tapestries. These material artifacts enabled their audiences to imagine what they could never see. On the zodiac mosaics, see L. I. Levine, *Visual Judaism in Late Antiquity: Historical Contexts of Jewish Art* (New Haven, 2012), 319–36. With regard to the unicorn tapestries, Margaret B. Freeman notes, "The desire for accuracy on the part of the designers and weavers has not gone so far, however, as to restrict the showing of fruits and flowers to a particular season" (*The Unicorn Tapestries* [New York, 1983], 111).

28 I here refer, of course, to the idea of jeweled poetry, as laid out in Michael Roberts's classic work, *The Jeweled Style: Poetry and Poetics in Late Antiquity* (Ithaca, NY, 1989).

And may You bless	And multiply the laurel, and juniper, and storax, and bitter almonds, and plane tree

Waters (Song 8:7),	Holy waters will go forth from the recesses of the House
Dew of rest	make sparkle from briars and thistles
And may You bless	And blossom the grapevine, and fig, and pomegranate, and olive

The language here appeals particularly to sight: water courses over sliced pomegranates, dew sparkles on briars and thistles, the plants all evoke specific images in the mind. But they also suggest taste and scent, as many of the trees produce edible crops with distinctive flavors and aromas, and touch, as we imagine the texture of the pomegranate slice, the prick of the thistles, the transformation of grape into wine and olive into oil. Whereas the poem about the Sotah drew its force from the graphic vividness of its imagery, this poem derives its power from the sheer force of repetition. In every stanza we move from the heavenly realm to the fecund earth, with the dew of rest connecting the two. Reading these two poems side-by-side is like examining the closing arguments from two very different lawyers (trying two very different cases): Yannai is a prosecuting attorney who deploys dramatic, graphic, detailed reconstructions of a crime; Qallir makes his arguments in a civil court and counts on the sheer volume of his claim to persuade. Four species, twelve species, twenty-two species would suffice to structure a poem; a catalogue of sixty-five plant varieties overwhelms and dazzles. As vivid as Yannai's description of feminine sin was, Qallir almost overwhelms the sense with all the plants he lists: their clusters of scent, leaf patterns, produce, and flowers. Painting the image, plant by plant and tree by tree, the poet grows a multisensory, domestic garden out of words and invites his listeners to enter. If his rhetoric succeeds, for both humanity and God, by the time the sixty-fifth plant is planted, the garden is *real*.

Performance of Fantasy

The imagery and experiences in these two poems are beyond vivid, however, and go into the realm of the "performance of fantasy," a term I use to describe a rhetoric of sensory imagination, both positive (paradisiacal) and negative (even hellish), the language of which possesses the potency to distort the ways senses conventionally perceive reality. The rhetoric is aberrant. Empathy and, in particular, visual imagination are here pushed into a realm that requires the listeners to envision something beyond their own experience. In each case, the poet does not merely offer his listeners front-row seats to fantastical fates, both individual and communal; he draws them imaginatively into the experience of his vision. As a result, they see events through new eyes and find themselves reoriented toward the reality he conjures and the world into which they reemerge once the liturgy concludes.

The fantastical element of Yannai's piyyut becomes overt in the fourth unit, which focuses on "the woman"—Eve. Her sin is not disobedience but, as discussed above, seduction: she kindles masculine passion and causes "man" (Adam) to act against all reason. Her crime does not stop there: her wantonness sets the stage not only for adultery (with men her helpless victims) but for murder. Only a few lines after the recitation of the second blessing of the Amidah, celebrating God's power as Giver of Life, we have a portrait of Eve as demonic mortality: "In her eyes, death! / At her feet, death! / At her feet will dance the angel of death!" (poem 4, line 5).[29] In this imagery, simultaneously rich with appeals to the visual even as it defies easy envisioning, Death is Eve's self and her servant, and it clings to the presence of womankind. She whose name means "life" becomes an agent of destruction. The sound of the lines is sharp, impacting the ears even as it invokes and appeals to the eyes. As dramatic as Yannai's language is, we must remember that it occurs not on a theatrical stage but is

29 This line echoes and amplifies Sirach, "From a woman sin had its beginning, and because of her we all die" (25:24).

embedded in the middle of the central prayer of the liturgy, in a location which suggests that God and Woman wage a war between life and death, with men as the battlefield.

This ironic juxtaposition of life and death takes on added force in poem 5, where the woman, whose body should be a site of generation and fertility, graphically decomposes and rots as she is "uncreated" before the witnesses' eyes:

> The curves of her thighs will abruptly rot
> And the depths of her belly will empty out
> Her lovely face will yellow and her eyes bulge
> Her fingernails fall off and her sinews give way. (poem 5, lines 8–9)

The depiction of corruption appeals primarily to sight, but the sense of decay suggests stench and elicits a sense of almost tactile revulsion. The afflicted areas are those we might consider most visually and tactilely seductive: the face and eyes which attract a paramour, the nails and fingers that reach out to caress, and the thighs and belly, concealed until consummation.[30] The parts of her body through which she sinned are the parts of her body that are stricken. Before, Death danced before her; now Death consumes her from within.

The dominant rhetorical structure throughout the work, particularly in poems 5, 7A, and 7B, is measure-for-measure (*middah k'neged middah*, in Hebrew). This rhetoric of "poetic justice" has strong corollaries in apocalyptic texts and reflects a deep-seated sense of embodied appropriateness: the limb that sinned is the limb that suffers, and the behavior which seduced becomes an action that leads to shame.[31] Each element of the adulteress's transgression generates a parallel in terms of her punishment with one noteworthy inversion: the adulteress sinned actively but in her punishment, she is passive. She who acted autonomously is punished by being acted upon. Even poem 7B, which explores the possibility the woman might be innocent, focuses on the woman's potential for transgression, and this singular reticence from sin is rewarded twenty-two times in a singular fashion: fertility. In the end, just as the woman's seductive prowess reflects a masculine imagination of feminine power, her utter disempowerment here constitutes a kind of revenge fantasy that, in its graphically visual violation of norms of modesty, is itself fantastically deviant. The poet, in addition to acting as the attorney for the prosecution, becomes the tour guide for this vision of destruction.

If Yannai offers his community a waking nightmare, Qallir provides them with a delightfully vivid dream. Following the seductive catalogue of Edenic flora in poems 4 and 5, in poem 6 the poet transitions to a reality in which not only do the plants, nourished by dew, thrive, but human existence, nourished by the same dew, revives. Where Yannai creates a fantasy of destruction, Qallir paints a vision of renewal: the adulteress danced with death and died, but here Death itself is defeated. In this unit, the structure of poems 4 and 5 is adapted: as in those units, the first stich begins with a quotation from the Song of Songs—verse 8:14 parsed out, word-by-word—and the second opens with the phrase "dew of rest." Instead of beginning with "may You bless," however, the third stich of each stanza opens with a verb appealing to God to fulfill divine promises of triumph over death.

Mountains of	holiness will burst with joy
Dew of rest	will have drenched the most rotten of the rotten stones, to revive (them), and they will glisten
And announce:	Awaken, ye! "And from the summit of the mountains, let them rejoice!" (Isa. 42:11)

This stanza's imagery appeals to visual, tactile, and auditory registers: we can envision a

30 The catalogue of the woman's body here can be read as a negative counterpart to the similar catalogues of the woman's physique in the Song of Songs (Song 4:1–7, 6:4–10, and 7:1–9), a genre known by its Arabic name *wasf* or the English *blason*. Far less common is a description of the male body this way, as occurs in Song 5:10–16.

31 M. Himmelfarb, *Tours of Hell: An Apocalyptic Form in Jewish and Christian Literature* (Philadelphia, 1983). See especially chapters two, "Demonstrative Explanations and the Literary Content of the Tours of Hell" (pp. 41–67) and three, "Sins and Punishments I: Sins and Measure-for-Measure Punishments" (pp. 69–105).

mountain bursting, but also hear it and feel the force of air; we can feel the chill wetness implied by "drenched" and the crumbling of "rotten stones" even as the idea of "glisten" registers visually. The poet weaves dramatically personified yet ambiguous visuals—mountains burst, but do they feel joy?—with mundane ideas such as dew on worn rocks. The poet builds complicated images out of familiar objects routinely perceived. Like Yannai, Qallir crafts images at the border of the unimaginable out of raw material that doesn't even need to be imagined because it is right at hand.

In total, eight different assertions of God's power over life and death are recounted in Poem 6. Each stanza conjures its vision of this fantastical end-time with vigorous, physically compelling verbs that appeal to the embodied senses: the dead are those who have "been swallowed" (poem 6, line 2), who are "bowed in the dust" (line 5), and "suspended from the depths" (line 23). God will "create stunned wonder" (line 5) when He resurrects the dead but, tenderly, He will also "swaddle" (line 8) the newly alive like a midwife. The leitmotif throughout this unit, however, is—as throughout the poem—the life-giving moisture of dew. This new world glistens and sparkles in a vision of a marvelous dawning new day. This poem introduces the statutory second blessing of the Amidah, the prayer that God will revive the dead—the same blessing that preceded Yannai's invective against Eve. Where Yannai revealed to his listeners how human life constitutes a kind of battleground between life-giving God and the *femme fatale*, here the community, participating intellectually and viscerally in the imagined scenes of resurrection, affirms the utter truth of God's final triumph over Death.

One formal rhetorical element contributes to the otherworldly or even apocalyptic nature of the second half of the composition: its consistent, unwavering orientation toward the deity. While other parts of the poem consist of narration or reported speech, all three of these units, with their focus on the creation and restoration of a perfect world—an Edenic garden where death has once again been banished—speak exclusively in the second person. This persistent direct address, brimming with certitude in the truth of its own vision and spanning almost a hundred lines of poetry, echoes in its emphatic nature the power of deictic rhetoric in classical apocalyptic address. The final unit of the poem accelerates the aural dynamics of the poem by alternating narration in the stanzas with direct address in the benedictions. Whereas Yannai drew the attention of his listeners (human and divine) to the actions and comeuppance of "that woman" (poem 4, line 1), Qallir's rhetoric keeps his human audience oriented entirely toward the divine, even as it insists on the attention of the divine listener by appealing to him directly over and over and over again. Through the force of the poet's language, paradise becomes tantalizingly proximate—it can almost be seen, tasted, felt, and heard—but the realization of the imagined world will remain a fantasy, a reality deferred until the deity is moved to action.

Performance of Magic

If the performance of seduction and fantasy relies, ultimately, on powers of persuasion and an audience primed for empathy, the performance of magic indicates genuine empowerment of the human agents. This mode of analysis—as difficult as it is to tease out—suggests that the words of the poems, as embodied by a functionary whose "stage" is the potently charged setting of the liturgy and whose words are those of divine writ embedded in new settings, possessed some kind of intrinsic power in the world, a power shared between poet and congregation. The use of the term "magic" here connotes an efficacy of these poems as ritual texts: how they model the weaving and breaking of spells, particularly those associated with "erotic magic" or love-spells; and how the knowledge embedded in the poems empowers those who not only heard but actively participated in the experience of the piece. In the case of the suspected adulteress, Yannai enacts the nullification of her dangerous magic, unbinding that which—or he whom—she has bound and uprooting what she has planted; in Qallir's piyyut, by contrast, the poet weaves a spell upon his listeners, drawing them into the experience of joy that his poetry makes concrete and real.

Appeals with magical language are particularly overt in Yannai's poem on the unfaithful wife.[32] The poem functions, broadly speaking, as an antidote to the adulteress's erotic magic; it seeks to contain and purge the dangerous impulses the adulteress represents.[33] At the "macro" level of narrative and conceit, we see this in the way the poem deploys and imaginatively reenacts the entire (defunct) ritual of the bitter waters: the ritual itself cannot be performed, but as with so much else of the Temple cult in Jewish liturgy, the assertion of the act through words possesses the ability to transform the world in some concrete way. At the "micro" level, that of rhetoric and phrasing, we see the same desire to contain and purge adduced through the richly textured detail of the work, and even more so, through repeated use of imperative verbs demanding that God, the object of this speech, and one whose own ability to enact a new reality is particularly potent, respond to the memory of rituals in a tangible fashion.

The "magical" elements of the Sotah poem appear most forcefully in poems 3, 4, and 7A. Poem 3 opens initially on a forensic note (albeit in song rather than declamation), appealing to the omniscient deity to recall the flaws of human nature. In the final line, however, in language reminiscent of amulets, Yannai petitions God to "uproot [or bind] the Evil Inclination [*yetzer ha-ra*]" (line 4)—not an intellectual process but a demonic force—and thus eradicate the source of immorality.[34] And, indeed, in the very first line of poem 3, the Evil Inclination is personified and uniquely bound to humanity, described as "our afflictor / crouched always at our side" (line 1).[35] Immorality is thus both intrinsic to human existence and also something external; it is a demon that specifically plagues people and needs divine power to be purged.

Yannai develops the demonic subtext of the poem in poem 4, where "that woman" (line 1a)—Eve—becomes a death-bearing seductress whose hands must be "lashed and bound" (line 1b); she has become a Lilith figure from a contemporary magic bowl. Throughout the piyyut, the feminine is linked to fire: "She is fire and her name is fire and she is likened to fire // Woman-from-man: / She enflames the embers in the bosom of man" (line 2).[36] She cannot but lead a man to a fiery death. Read in this light, the dramatic imagery of line 5 becomes demonic: "In her eyes: death / At her feet: death // At her feet will dance the angel of death" (line 5). The only remedy for this feminine evil, which seems to be the master (or, rather, mistress) of death itself, is for God to "swallow up Death and uproot [or: bind] the Evil Inclination" (line 6a). Again, Yannai echoes the language of magical amulets as he implores God to purge not only the impulse to do evil but also its twin, mortality. God cannot unmake such powers but He can contain them and presumably expel them, and to do so God must act in highly bodily, transparently physical ways: ingesting and lashing, uprooting and binding. The language of Yannai's poetic exorcism evokes, and may well have elicited from the performer, physical gestures modeling the hoped-for actions, just as magic bowls bore images of demons bound

32 The latent potential of the Sotah ritual manifests even more concretely in magical texts that use the language and imagery of Num. 5, examples of which can be found in the Cairo Genizah. See N. Janowitz, "Water, Word, and Name: The Shifting Pragmatics of the Sotah/Suspected Adulteress Ritual," in *Literature or Liturgy?* ed. C. Leonhard and H. Löhr (Tübingen, 2014), 15–31.

33 It is worth noting both the prominence of demonic seductresses in texts such as the *Testament of Solomon* and the tradition that magicians summoned demons in part for sexual gratification; see S. I. Johnson, "The *Testament of Solomon* from Late Antiquity to the Renaissance," in *The Metamorphosis of Magic from Late Antiquity to the Early Modern Period*, ed. J. N. Bremmer and J. R. Veenstra (Leuven, 2002), 35–49. In the *Testament of Solomon*, Solomon is depicted as chaining, confining, and binding various demonic forces; he hangs Obyzouth (a Lilith-figure), for example, by her hair from the walls of the Temple, and he binds Enepsigos (who describes herself as a goddess and perhaps should be identified with Hecate) with a triple-link chain and the divine Name.

34 Aramaic amulets, incantations, and magic bowls use primarily the term "uproot" (עקר) rather than "bind" (עקד) to indicate the eradication or suppression of evil, but the iconography used to accompany many of these texts depicts demonic forces being tied up or bound. See J. Naveh and S. Shaked, *Amulets and Magic Bowls: Aramaic Incantations of Late Antiquity* (Jerusalem and Leiden, 1985); and, eidem, *Magic Spells and Formulae: Aramaic Incantations of Late Antiquity* (Jerusalem, 1993). On the demonic understanding of the Evil Inclination, see I. Rosen-Zvi, *Demonic Desires:* Yetzer Hara *and the Problem of Evil in Late Antiquity* (Philadelphia, 2011).

35 The language here echoes Gen. 4:7.

36 The phrase "woman-from-man: she enflames" echoes not only the creation of woman as depicted in Gen. 2, where she is fashioned from Adam's rib, but also aggadic tradition (b. Sotah 17a, PRE 12) which understands the terms "man" (איש) and "woman" (אשה) as related: the two common consonants (אש) mean "fire."

and contained. The performer embodied a ritual process which the congregation saw and heard.

Indeed, the poet does not merely seek a general exorcism; he details the process. In poem 7A, the poet offers a head-to-toe description of how the woman seduced her lover and a parallel head-to-toe infliction of comeuppance. Each of these has been discussed above, but taken together they effect of a kind of spell: the poet describes how the woman deployed her "feminine wiles" to work her erotic magic on the helpless man and then, in a kind of incantational reversal, he ensnares her in her own sin. The catalogue is comprehensive; no offending limb escapes mention. Yannai, depicting the efficacy of these imagination-generated rituals, underscores God's power to exorcise evil but he does not depict God directly as "doing" anything to the adulteress. Instead, he affirms the efficacy of human ritual using the Holy Name. Furthermore, the tightly parallel structure of the lines suggests that they were performed antiphonally, perhaps with a choir or even some form of audience participation, with the aural performance thus underscoring the potency of the rhetorical structure: one voice adjures, and the other makes it so.

Throughout the poem, evocative language conjures graphic images. Immaterial fire—suggesting vivid tactile and visual sensations—gives way to matched pairs of incantational vocabulary: binding and loosening, planting and uprooting, creation and annihilation. The demonic woman is loose, so she must be bound, and toxic, so she must be uprooted—imagery evoking depictions of Lilith and other feminine demons from magic bowls, where her hands are tied and her pudenda exposed and incantatory texts attempt to confine or expel her. She who ought to be a *genetrix*, a miraculous mother-of-life, instead decomposes in graphic detail—her thighs rot, her uterus falls out, her eyes bulge, her fingernails fall off, and her body gives way (poem 5, lines 8–9)—before actively involved and invested audiences (imagined, invoked, and congregational). In restoring the adulteress to the primordial ooze, the poet works his own kind of disturbing magical spell on his listeners. His rhetoric—deploying graphic and titillating visual imagery, still potent today and unsettling to imagine as part of prayer, presumably reinforced by body language—makes an imaginary scene visible and audible to his congregation (male and female), collapsing the boundaries between "then" and "now," as the community at prayer morphs into participants in the trial and punishment of "the woman" even as they pray that such impulses be expelled from their own midst.

If the ritual of the Sotah describes the consequences of erotic magic gone awry, Qallir's piyyut for dew works a very different kind of spell on its listeners. Where Yannai uprooted, Qallir plants. On the one hand, one could argue that as a poem for dew, this poem seeks to conjure through its sheer force of words the magical, life-giving benefit of dew for the land's crops, needed to sustain the life of the people. At the same time, in this poem, Qallir, like Yannai, seeks to create a "binding" of a deeper kind: not of evil so that it may be expelled but rather so that something good can take root. As the poet writes in the opening stanza of poem 1, "*Let Him kiss me me* / with a charm of delight and protection" (line 2); amplifying the words of the Song of Songs, the poem becomes an erotically transmitted amulet. Beyond the power of dew itself, in this work the poet seeks to realize through words his vision of restoration to the people even as he asserts the bond that yokes people and deity together. As with the Sotah poem, this poem about dew creates a realistic vision of fantastical and (as yet) unreal events, not merely to dazzle listeners with poetic virtuosity but to enact a tangible effect on and with his listeners. The poem's imagery appeals to its audience through vivid evocations of sound, sight, and touch. The "erotic magic" here lies in the ability of the poet—and, through the power of his words, the land itself—to entice the listeners away from powerlessness to hope through a vision that is both fantastic and plausible because it is both miraculous and mundane. Dew is both a manifestation of answered prayers and a symbol of the still-close bond uniting community and God.

The poet weaves his spell primarily through repetition. Repeated words and phrases imbue the work with an incantational element when performed. Almost every stanza of the piyyut contains the word *tal*, "dew," or the phrase *tal menuchah*, "dew of rest," as a structuring element. "*Tal*" is a short word, but with seventy-one repetitions its delicate presence becomes inexorable and inevitable: water wearing away stone, a trickle that becomes a torrent. Initially dew's powers are limited to those of "mere" terrestrial moisture, but by the end of the poem the dew resurrects dead individuals and a moribund nation. Each repetition constitutes a drop of the elixir of life. And most potently, it is likely that the community itself participated, actively, in the reiterations of this refrain, adding their voices to the poet's and transforming his words into something communally alive.[37]

Similarly, the botanical catalogues in poems 4 and 5, with their litanies of species and varieties of plants and trees, take on an incantational aural quality. There is a brute forcefulness in the power of the list: just as Yannai's head-to-toe description of the woman conjured a sense of comprehensiveness, Qallir's catalogue of flora connotes exhaustiveness through its ability to exhaust. Given the paucity of such vocabulary in the biblical text, the creative effort involved in compiling this list is particularly impressive, and even more so when one realizes that every plant on the list provides direct benefits to humankind, whether as food or medicine or both. If it is a garden of earthly delights, it is still a worker's paradise: nothing Qallir includes is exclusively ornamental. The poem thus seems to offer insight not only into how God, through dew, grants life (immediate and eternal) to His people but how, through the very nature of creation, the tools for living and healing have been placed in humankind's hands. Even as the poet weaves the spell, it is as if he shares clues for how one can conjure real remedies, and through his refrains and repetitions which directly invite congregational participation, aloud or sotto voce or simply in one's imagination, he shares with them the experience of conjuring. The borders between medicine, magic, and prayer are thin indeed.

In the end, Qallir's poem about dew becomes a poem about the magical, entrancing, and fragile promise of life itself. Where Yannai's suspected adulteress becomes a demonic, deadly, and otherworldly distillation of Eve, in Qallir's poem for dew the land—resonating in frisson with the Garden of Eden and the female beloved in the Song of Songs—becomes her opposite, her antidote. The feminine in this spell becomes a source of life, health, and happiness, something concrete and quotidian which thrives and engenders bounty rather than something toxic that consumes itself. The bitter waters of the Sotah's trial extinguish her transgressive flames, but the dew of rest actively heals.

As disparate as these two poems are, in themes, tones, and orientation, they can and should be seen as inversions of each other. It is worth noting that the concluding stanza of Qallir's paean to dew states:

"*He will lead me*" (Ps. 23:2)	and He will draw near With bridle and bit to muzzle the Evil Inclination
With dew	to bless the sown-seed of peace "*For He will speak peace*" (Ps. 85:9)

For Qallir, as in Yannai, death must be swallowed and the Evil Inclination restrained.[38] Demonic forces lurk in Qallir's world, as they do in Yannai's—it is just that Qallir writes of the triumph that will follow their destruction rather than of their destructiveness and destruction directly. Yannai's piyyut envisions overcoming demonic forces of evil; Qallir's poem, voiced by both performer and congregation, articulates a world from which those powers have been expelled. In the riotous fertility of Qallir's garden, evil will no longer be able to take root. Until such time as Qallir's vision comes to pass, however, this poem may serve all who heard it, and joined in its utterance, as an amulet against despair.

Concluding Analysis: A Body of Work

The fiery adulteress with the angel of death dancing before her; revivifying dew assuring life to land and people: these two poems could not seem less alike. And yet, for all the differences in the

37 Yannai's piyyut also contained a refrain in poem 6, but the manuscript is damaged and thus we do not know what it was, although it was almost certainly a phrase from the first or second verse of the Torah portion.

38 Note, too, the opening stanza of poem 8, which quotes Isa. 25:8, "He will swallow up death forever."

effects they conjure when performed (or read) the two works shared the same (liturgical) stage and came from the same world. Yannai's poem reveals an unpleasant underbelly of society: a demonic world of broken trust and lurid vindication; Qallir's piyyut paints an equally fantastic picture of paradise, a healing garden which remains recognizable even as it promises eternal bounty and life. Each poem inhabits an extreme, but each poet employs the same rhetorical tools. Each poet, responding to and exploiting the implicit, latent power of the biblical text and the propitiousness of his liturgical setting, deploys words in ways that make them potent and transformative, both when heard by the congregation and, even more so, when the community shares in their voicing. Through words—their own and those of Scripture, woven seamlessly together—the poets create experiences that, through their concrete appeals to an array of senses and experiences, have the potential to have real effects on their listeners.

The three rhetorical modes described here—the performances of seduction, of fantasy, and of magic—constitute a continuum of intensity, as all are ultimately forms of persuasion with increasing degrees of vividness and significance of consequence. *Seduction* exists at the realm of promise and plausibility, and in this register the poet engages his listeners as "objects"—he seduces them; *fantasy* offers an experience that is more tangible even as it becomes more desirable, and in this register the community comes to share the poet's perspective, to experience an alternative reality through his eyes; and *magic* makes something existentially or potentially "real," and draws its power not only from the poet's rhetoric but from the active participation of the community, not only through emotional and sensory sympathy but through performative integration by means of refrains. In all three registers, the poet persuades through appeals to an array of senses. To be sure, some senses—taste and scent—receive less emphasis in these works which, on the surface, appeal mostly to sight, touch, and sound. But particularly in these two compositions, all the senses receive some attention, and all the senses serve to seduce, reorient, and empower the community.

Touch, taste, and scent are embedded in these poems both through their evocative use of metaphorical language and their appeals to familiar items. Often the senses overlap in a kind of poetic and material synesthesia. Passion is a "flaming coal"—a visual image, yes, but also tactile: it causes pain and scarring. So, too, do the punishments of lashing, uprooting, and binding—they are felt as much as they are seen. Dew, by contrast, is often felt by feet before eyes perceive it. Its essence is moisture, something which affects skin more than eyes. Taste is also evoked: both the adulteress's sin and death are "bitter." Qallir's catalogue of plants lists only items that are edible or medicinal or both, and many of the items (particularly the spices, such as cumin, mustard, garlic, and coriander) affect both nose and palate. And in Qallir's poem, death is not bitter but dry, a sensation not of the tongue but of the skin. Indeed, Qallir's poem for dew is a prayer for the alleviation of thirst: the thirst of the land, the thirst of the body, and the thirst of the soul.

And yet, most obviously—at least for those of us who approach these texts as written works—they appeal to sight. The lines graphically depicting the adulteress's decomposition, for example, culminate with the effect this sight has on the witnesses who "will see her and say, 'Take her out!'" (poem 5, line 10)—take her away from our eyes. Visuals play a primary role in describing sexual transgression and its consequences, and the culmination of the ritual in public shaming—even taking place entirely in the imagination—relies on seeing what should be concealed. Qallir's poem for dew employs less vocabulary explicitly from the visual realm, and yet its catalogues of plants and trees create an implicitly graphic sense of abundance, one which relies on sight to imagine. And his descriptions of dew often invoke dew's subtle visual beauty: the ways it glistens and glimmers.

But we should not limit the consideration of sight to an appreciation of *ekphrasis*; we should remember that the performance of the poem itself had a powerful visual component. The performative elements of the poem are, without a doubt, the most difficult to reconstruct, but at the very least we must acknowledge that they existed and would have had interpretive significance. We can imagine, for instance, that the poet-performer would have drawn on the libraries of gestures familiar from theater and declamation, employing forensic postures and positions as he enacts (in song rather than speech) the accusation of the adulteress and vivifies her dramatic conviction.[39] By drawing on the body language of the court, for example, he would facilitate the visual experience of the listeners by appealing to cues that would create the sense that they were at a trial. The Qallir piyyut, by contrast, with its formal intricacy and highly patterned structures, opens up the possibility of complex styles of performance, with multiple speakers intoning various portions of a stanza, adopting different personae, gesturing to underscore the interplay between heaven and earth, or emphasizing biblical quotations. The performer's body (limbs, posture, voice) was, of necessity, some part of the performance; the question is only how he used it.

And, as a turn to performance reminds us, while we must not overlook the importance that sound plays in these works; as important as seeing a performance would have been, the auditory elements would have been even more determinative of the creation and conveying of meaning. The density of rushing-whispering-murmuring sounds when the adulteress's deceit is described (*ishah be-ishah / be-ma'al be-kakhashah // el kohen ye-khishah / u-ve-khakhash yakh-khishah* [poem 5, line 1]) underscores the conspiratorial nature of her sin, while the audible, emphatic parallels that articulate the consequences of her action underscore with physical force the parity between crime and punishment. In Qallir's poem, the manifold repetitions of key phrases and tightly repetitive structures, most acutely discernible only during oral performance, are precisely what lend the poem its almost incantational force, particularly when we remember that the community, attuned to these patterns and repetitions, almost certainly added their voices to the performer's throughout the poem.

Seduction, fantasy, and magic all work through the evocation of the senses to create an imagined alternative to the present reality. In both poems, the poets create a space apart from the mundane world, out of time: not exactly the biblical past and not quite the redeemed future. It is a separate realm, liturgical time, where past, present, and future overlap and intersect. Yannai's trial of the adulteress compels his audience's attention despite the unreality of the ritual it depicts; Qallir's description of abundance takes root even if the Edenic riot of produce exceeds the bounds of any garden in any season. The poets share and bring to life not merely a collective vision, but a shared experience that is both passively received and actively joined—and this sharing, this commonality, underscores the potency of such an experience, as it makes it ever more tangible and real.

The voices of Yannai and Qallir could not, on the surface, be more different: one revels luridly in trangessive and violent spectacle while the other exuberantly and joyfully envisions redemption on the smallest and largest scales. But upon closer examination, these two extremes reveal a broad middle ground of shared techniques and worldviews. The bitter waters of the Sotah ritual and the sweet dew of Sabbath rest are distinctive distillations of the same performative waters. The substance itself remains merely moisture, but its powers—amplified by context and shaped by imagination—are transformed by the poetic alchemy of words.

39 On the importance, symbolic and concrete, of gesture in antiquity, see A. Corbeill, *Nature Embodied: Gesture in Ancient Rome* (Princeton and Oxford, 2003), especially chapter one, "Participatory Gestures in Roman Religious Ritual and Medicine" (pp. 12–40).

I am grateful to Susan Ashbook Harvey and Margaret Mullett for the invitation to present this paper at the Dumbarton Oaks Spring Symposium, to Georgia Frank for her insightful comments on the draft, and for Joel Kalvesmaki's editorial diligence and sensitivity. I would also like to thank the anonymous reader, whose comments proved most helpful.

APPENDIX A

Yannai on Numbers 5, "The Suspected Adulteress"

This translation is based on the Hebrew text taken from the *Historical Dictionary of the Hebrew Language* database, compiled by the National Academy of the Hebrew Language (http://maagarim.hebrew-academy.org.il).

[poems 1 and 2, embellishing the first two blessings of the *Amidah* and the first two verses of the Torah portion, are absent]

POEM 3: *Meshallesh* (acrostic spells out "Yannai"—ינ״י)

י You know, O our Creator / our Evil Inclination
    That it is our afflictor / crouched always at our side
נ The adulterer is named as "lacking of heart" / the adulteress, "wily hearted"
    But You, Creator of the heart / probe deeply the heart's intentions
י O Yah, extinguish the coals / which burn within us
    Renew the heart of flesh / and remove the heart of stone
י Bind the Evil Inclination / and no longer shall You have to watch over
    The young women, should they play harlot / nor the brides, should they prove false

As it is written: "I will not punish your daughters when they commit harlotry, nor your daughters-in-law when they prove false; for they themselves consort with lewd women, and they sacrifice with harlots; and the people that is without understanding is distraught" (Hos. 4:14, first verse of haftarah).

POEM 4 (no acrostic)

From the time when that woman sinned through her hand
    You lashed and bound the hands of woman
She is fire and her name is fire and she is likened to fire
    Woman-from-man: / She enflames the embers in the bosom of man
She sinned and brought into being the bitterness of death
    Her sin was bitter as death / brazen is she, like death
No one masters the day of his death
    But all her pathways lead down to death
In her eyes: death / at her feet: death
    At her feet will dance the angel of death
Until You swallow up Death and uproot the Evil Inclination
    And remove the heart of stone from us
O Holy One . . .

POEM 5: *Asiriyyah* (acrostic from *alef* to *yod*)

A woman with her man / in deception, with deceit:
    Unto the priest shall he hasten her / and for (her) deception, let him accuse her
Into temptation and trespass— / oh, how sinfulness beguiled her!
    A curse he proclaims upon her / and an oath he makes her swear.
Indeed, just as she behaved like a beast
    So, too, is her offering that of a beast
Just as she walked "in the way of the Egyptian"

So, too, gird her hips with Egyptian rope
Just as in the presence of a stranger, concealed, did she stand
So, too, before the Pure One, exposed, the priest stands her
And just as she betrayed the nature of (her) Creator
He will make her drink curses from a created vessel
The mere mention of the Holy Name, written with holiness
Will be blotted out with holy water to put to proof the (un)holy woman
The curves of her thighs will abruptly rot
And the depths of her belly will there empty out
Her lovely face will yellow and her eyes bulge
Her fingernails fall off and her sinews give way
They will see her and say, "Take her out! That alien woman,
Before she renders the Temple Court impure!"
Please, God . . . Forever . . .

POEM 6 (full alphabetical acrostic, *alef* to *tav*)
. . . . [gap of eight lines, *alef* to *tet*] . . . .
She defiled her own purity without him
But the One Pure-of-Eyes (knows), for there is nothing without Him
He sees through. . . .
. . . [half line missing] . . .
All who would lie down besides the adulteress
Lie themselves down in sorrow
Before the Judge, the matter will not . . .
. . . [half line missing] . . .
From among a thousand, one can find a single man;
A single woman? Not among any of these
It was answered against her . . .
. . . [half line missing] . . .
She strayed from him, his lawfully wedded wife
She rejected him, his young maid
Concerning her, his jealousy consumed him
"Then he shall surely be jealous . . ."
His mason has torn down his fence
You will disfigure her beauty because of her breach
The Rock bound her to him when she entered his dwelling
Until he examines . . .
His bed is too short for stretching out
When a friend lies upon it with his wife
Her head shall be bared in disgrace
And from (her) body . . .
His recompense, if she did not steal seed
Nor any alien lie with her, plowing her with seed
She shall acquire and sow with seed
For a blessing . . .

POEM 7A: First *Rahit* (full alphabetical acrostic, *alef* to *tav*)
And thus, "She acted unfaithfully against him . . ." (Num. 5:12)
She bound jewels upon her head
Thus in shame she unbound the hair of her head

She grew proud and fastened fancily the braids of her hair
  Thus he judged she must hide her hair
She made herself pretty, for the sake of her sin
  Thus she became stupid and ugly, because of her sin
She was insolent and brazen of face
  Thus pale and green became her face
She soiled and defiled her flesh
  Thus thin and sickly became her flesh
She concealed her perversity within her
  Thus before the eyes of all it was revealed about her
She defied both curse and adjuration
  Thus she succumbed to both curse and adjuration
She rebelled against that which was written for her
  Thus her sins were revealed through a written text
She opened her thighs to the stranger
  Thus her diminishment came with the wasting of her thighs
She called to the stranger and he embraced her belly
  Thus decayed and bloated became her belly
She set her eye upon another
  Thus she shall belong to neither her husband nor any other

POEM 7B: Second *Rahit* (reverse alphabetical acrostic, *tav* to *alef*)
And thus, "If she has not defiled herself . . ." (Num. 5:28)
If she did not sin against her marital contract
  Let her be more blessed than the other women in her tent
If she did not revel like an alien woman
  Let her resemble a fruitful vine
If she did not show herself about outside the house
  Let her take root in the innermost house
If she did not play the harlot and ruin herself
  Let her bear sons instead of daughters
If she did not . . .
  Let her . . . and successfully sow seed
If she was not false against her marriage vows
  Let her . . .
If she did not rebel against him who rules over her
  Let her be comforted, [let] foreigners not rule over her
If she did not grow stubborn like a heifer
  Let her . . . if she shall be barren
If she did not spread her knees for the wicked
  Let her be justified through a blessed pregnancy
If she did not summon the alien to her belly
  Let her know the merciful reward of fruit in her belly
If she did not drink stolen waters in secret
  Let her be crowned with good favor in public and in secret

POEM 8 (transition to *Qedushah*)
For You, O God, dwell in secret / but everything before You is revealed and known / You give a man his tasks / and compensate him according to his deeds / the measure of affliction is diminished / and the measure of good amplified / in evildoing You take no pleasure / but rather doing justly do

You desire / and likewise . . . and giving thanks / bowing and bending knee and prostrating and praising / Your holy Name hallowing . . .

POEM 9 (the *Qedushah*: Isa. 6:3 and Ezek. 3:12)

From . . . and among those who surround the Throne, wings joined one to another
Holy, holy, holy is the Lord of Hosts! The whole earth is filled with His glory!

"Holy" from . . .
"Holy" from the sages of . . .
"Holy" from a place without any women or men

"Holy": From of old, . . .
"Holy": From of old, He decreed five afflictions for woman
"Holy": From of old, He had compassion and took pity on the honor of woman
The one toward the other . . .

"From His place": . . . a place of . . .
"From His place": From a place of modesty He took the rib to make Woman
"From His place": in . . .

Twice . . .

. . . persuading to stray; You taught us to suspect . . . They became drunk . . . In destruction, they were not wise . . . the head does . . . to see how the harlot dresses herself and hardens her face . . . They fell upon the harlot, "Much childishness causes it" . . . Impurity of the castrato . . . to our Lord singing . . . the Divine Presence . . . doing, the Moabite women . . . the straying ones will settle. . . a thousand they executed. . . for her beloved ones . . . who, most of them . . . her ways are the rejected way . . .

APPENDIX B

Eleazar berabbi Qallir, "The Power of Dew"[40]

This translation is based on the Hebrew text taken from the *Historical Dictionary of the Hebrew Language* database, compiled by the National Academy of the Hebrew Language (http://maagarim.hebrew-academy.org.il).

PRELUDE

"In grassy meadows	I will pasture My multitudes,"
	Said He-who-stands-in-My-camps
"With dew	to help My protected ones"
	"For today is a Sabbath unto the Lord" (Exod. 16:25)
	Blessed are You, O Lord, Shield of Abraham
He will pasture me	With pleasantness He delights you
	According to the decree of Him-who-dwells-in-your-shelter
With dew	To sprinkle, (at) your appointed hour of resurrection
	"For it is a sign between Me and you" (Exod. 31:13)

POEM 1: *Reshut* (Song 1:1–16)

The Song of Songs	I will chirp to Him who delights in what was leaped over
Let Him kiss me	with a charm of delight and protection
	I approached with additional offerings (*musafim*) in order to draw out (my) prayer
	The case of both parties I would speak with all my heart
As for the scent	You fattened the *'olah* and *minhah* offerings
Draw me after (You)	And my lowliness and my sorrow relieve
	Answer me, O Lord, with the dews of rest
I was darkened	(with) fear and with wearying hardship
Do not look at me	. . . weariness from the hand striking me
	I was filled with food for two days, dwelling in tranquility
	The Unique One to persuade with rejoicing and entreaty
Tell me,	As of old, of Your miracles, and in Your shade I will find tranquility
"If you don't know	For your own sake, O My sister, you rejoiced to find tranquility"
	Answer me, O Lord, with the dews of tranquility
"As a mare	I cast down the chariots of sorrow"
"Lovely are your cheeks	Glorious, as with lilies fenced"

40 For a fully annotated translation of this poem, with extensive commentary as well as the original Hebrew text, see L. S. Lieber, *A Vocabulary of Desire: The Song of Songs in the Ancient Synagogue* (Leiden, 2014), 264–316.

	He gives support to His creatures like a bed of spices
	Those borne by You have asked me to express my yearning to You
Bands of gold	The crown of Yah is the delightful one
Until	the Righteous One shall restore justice over you, to (your) delight
	Answer me, O Lord, with the dews of delight
A bundle of myrrh	You flung away enemies, shattering them
A cluster of henna	You held me tight like a cluster while I trembled
	Your whole ones were passed over with, "Go, select for yourselves a lamb"
	And may my roaring on behalf of those who are like the sheep of the flock be sweet [to You]
"Indeed, you are lovely"	You plucked (her) up from the oppressor
Indeed, You are lovely	You will delight her with the pleasures of happiness
	Answer me, with the dews of acceptance

As it is written in Your holy writings:
"May [the words of my mouth and the musings of my heart] be acceptable [to You, O Lord, my Rock and my Redeemer]" (Ps. 19:15)
"Blessed are You, O Lord, teach me Your laws" (Ps. 119:12)

Poem 2 (Song 1:17–4:4 and Ps. 92:1–93:1)

The beams	of a palanquin are a statute concerning (a time) which will be entirely Sabbath
I,	I will present the additional offerings of Passover and the burnt offering of the Sabbath
Dew of rest	strengthen those who delight in the Sabbath
	A psalm, a song, for the Sabbath day (Ps. 92:1)
Like a lily	among the thorns, I blossomed (with) expectation
Like an apple	among the trees of the forest, I luxuriated in dewy abundance
Dew of rest	is blessed, and it will flow over the poor and needy
	It is good to give thanks to the Lord, and to sing to Your exalted name (Ps. 92:2)
He brought me	My Redeemer, to the house of loving betrothal
Sustain me	(in) joy, this one becoming part of that one
Dew of rest	make strong, and we will triumphantly sing Hallel psalms
	To declare in the morning Your righteousness, and Your faithfulness at night (Ps. 92:3)
His left hand	lifted those who were passed over unto the Gate of Song, and the joyful to Nicanor's gate

I adjured — with a pitying whisper: the bereaved people will become [radiant]

Dew of rest — flourish those who make music with the summoning voice of the lyre

To the music of the lute and the harp, to the melody of the lyre (Ps. 92:4)

A voice — You revealed, to console Your supplicating people

It seemed — to be one, but the oath was heard twice

Dew of rest — He has made glisten, and (thus) you will blossom with joy and singing

For You have made me happy through Your deeds, O Lord, and the works of Your hands I sing forth (Ps. 92:5)

He answered — and gave precedence to doing over hearing, a nation craving Your responses

Indeed — Forever You promised him, "I will heal your affliction"

Dew of rest — summon him directly in front of Your dwelling

How great are Your works, O Lord, so very deep are Your thoughts! (Ps. 92:6)

The blossoms — You brightened with this rest

The fig tree — You purified as if it were to sprinkle upon a lintel

Dew of rest — bequeath to those who were entrusted with, "And even, also, this . . . "

The dull man does not know, the fool does not understand this (Ps. 92:7)

"My dove!" — You soothed her and You calmed her trembling

Cover — Her strong ones, concealed in the pasture of Bashan and Gilad

Dew of rest — distill for them, and the loins of their opponents make tremble

Though the wicked sprout like grass and the evildoers blossom, they are doomed to destruction forever and ever (Ps. 92:8)

My Beloved — You fitted me with the commandments of "this day, to celebrate it as a festival to the Lord"

While — we tasted "for today is a Sabbath to the Lord"

Dew of rest — drip upon those who delight in the Lord

And You are exalted forever, O Lord (Ps. 92:9)

Upon my couch — I became one with the One who refreshes me from the toil of brick-making

Let me arise — to trample those who laid snares for me, as heaps of straw are trampled

Dew of rest	will decree it, and a stone will crush an image *Surely, Your enemies, O Lord, surely, Your enemies perish; all evildoers are scattered* (Ps. 92:10)
The guards found me	Double a harlot's hire
Scarcely	Had He grown angry against me, and there was a flash of sharpened spear against them
Dew of rest	bedeck me in the beautiful tabernacle of tranquility *But You have amplified my strength like that of the wild ox; I am drenched in freshening oil* (Ps. 92:11)
"I adjured"	You taught me not to awaken the End (foreseen in) my vision
"Who	is mine in the heavens?" She blasphemed in order to falsify my scales
Dew of rest	Accompany me, and in my hand is vengeance, as when my villages ceased *My eye has beheld those who lie in wait for me; my ears hear of the evil deeds of those who would rise up against me* (Ps. 92:12)
Indeed	How good and how pleasant! The offspring in the dawn will thrive.
All of them	are blessed with fruitfulness to multiply greatly
Dew of rest	soften me, and during the watches of the night he will meditate upon You *The righteous will blossom like the date-palm, and thrive like the cedar of Lebanon* (Ps. 92:13)
A palanquin	is consolation, and the pillars of Ariel (the altar) will grant relief
Its pillars	forever make quiet, and no more shall they be wearied
Dew of rest	prosper them, and in Your delight they will find a balm *Those planted in the house of the Lord, in the courtyards of our God, will flourish* (Ps. 92:14)
Go forth and see	the wedding of the chosen one, at once serenity descends
"Indeed you are lovely	your blossom clusters to offer on the fitting night"
Dew of rest	sustain them, and in a well-watered garden they will be sated *In old age, they still bring forth fruit; they will stay sleek and verdant* (Ps. 92:15)
Your teeth	are garden beds to bind close, and no blemish shall be upon them

Like a scarlet thread	until your appointed times, He is a shield for all who trust in Him
Dew of rest	drip royal provisions, (as) upon the day when He rested *To declare that the Lord, my Rock, is upright, and there is no iniquity in Him* (Ps. 92:16)
Like a tower	He split the reeds, He is my refuge, I will not be shaken
Two	Blossoms He twinned, to lead from the traps of the (land of) shaking
Dew of rest	crown them, and their step will not stumble *The Lord is king, He is robed in grandeur; the Lord is robed, He is girded with strength. The world stands firm; it cannot be shaken* (Ps. 93:1)

[The final five stanzas of poem 2 and first seventeen stanzas of poem 3, covering Song 4:5–7:4, are missing]

Poem 3: Zodiac / Heavens (Song 7:5–11)

[*Your two breasts*]	. . .
[*Your throat*]	. . . to pierce . . .
Dew of rest	(For) those who delight in dew from the heavens . . . . . . to feed them, the heritage of Jacob

As it is written: "Then you shall take delight in the Lord[, and I will make you ride upon the heights of the earth; I will feed you with the heritage of your ancestor Jacob, for the mouth of the Lord has spoken]" (Isa. 58:14)

And it is said: "What shall I do with you[, O Ephraim? What shall I do with you, O Judah? Your love is like a morning cloud, like the dew that goes away early]" (Hos. 6:4)

"Your head is upon you like Carmel	to understand the delights of kingship;
"How lovely you are!	Anointed with the blood of the Passover and circumcision, in keeping with the teaching of the halakhah"
Dew of rest	anoint (with it) the Kid (*Capricorn*), one strong in kingship (Droplets) will drip, to settle in security those who rest from labor

As it is written: "Six days you shall do your work, but on the seventh day you shall rest; that your ox and your ass may have rest, and the son of your bondmaid, and the alien, may be refreshed" (Exod. 23:12)

And it is said: "Thus Israel dwells [in security, untroubled is Jacob's abode, in a land of grain and wine, under heavens dripping dew]" (Deut. 33:28)

"Such is your stature	Joyful for the day of delight"
"I said, 'I will lift up'	A nation delighted by the Passover offering and bitter herbs"

Dew of rest — spills out from the Bucket (*Aquarius*) (upon) the son of old age, delighted by a frock of many colors
May You [watch over] his progeny with the dew of clouds, then he will find delight in the Almighty

As it is written: "Then you will find delight in the Almighty[, and lift up your face to God]" (Job 22:26)
And it is said: "By his knowledge the deeps are split[, and the clouds drop down the dew]" (Prov. 3:20)

"And your palate — you will burst forth in song with 'A psalm, a song, for the Sabbath,' as the old sorrows are forgotten"
I am my Beloved's — with a melody to praise, joy expressed by ten expressions
Dew of rest — strengthen (Zion) through the Fish (*Pisces*) more than all other dwellings
"I will be like the dew to those who keep the Sabbath, settling them in quiet resting places"

As it is written: "I will be like dew [to Israel; he shall blossom like the lily, he shall strike root like the Lebanon]" (Hos. 14:6)
And it is said: "My people will settle in a peaceful habitation[, in secure dwellings, and in quiet resting places]" (Isa. 32:18)

POEM 4: Thirty-five species of grain/produce (Song 7:12–8:5)

Come, my Beloved! — Strengthen those who sanctify the Sabbaths
Dew of rest — give to those who call the sacred convocations
And may You bless — and heap up wheat, and barley, and lentils

Let us go early — to knock upon Your doors, (You who) seize the shutters
Dew of rest — pour forth from the Dwelling, rent asunder
And may You bless — and multiply millet, and sprouted spelt, and poppies, and split beans

The mandrakes — sing to You, (You who) are glorious over the lilies
Dew of rest — drip upon the undisturbed
And may You bless — and prosper white lupine, and yellow lupine, and white beans, and Egyptian beans, and horse beans

Oh, if only — He would cause a shoot to sprout from the southern corner
Dew of rest — bedeck those who keep far from deception
And may You bless — and coax forth the ears of fox-grain and purslane, and charlock, and sweet grass

I would lead you,	looking brightly from My Dwelling with dazzling heat
Dew of rest	make flourish those whose utterance is sweetest song
And may You bless	and enlarge sesame, and mustard, and cumin, and black cumin
I adjured	(and) I arrayed those who relinquish during the sabbatical year
Dew of rest	imbue them with splendor in their harv[est] . . .
And may You bless	And germinate fenugreek, and cress, and oats, and radishes, and wild peas
His left hand	sanctified the ones taken up like *ḥallah*
Dew of rest	distill upon the sacred seed
And may You bless	and fatten daucus, and lettuce, and sonchus-thistle, and eryngium, and endive
Who-is-this	May You sustain with abundant grain
Dew of rest	May You release for the redemption foreordained
And may You bless	and exalt vetch, and turnip, and garlic, and onion, and coriander
Our God and God of our Fathers:	

POEM 5: Thirty kinds of trees (Song 8:6–13)

Establish for me	Praise and make firm the Palace
Dew of rest	cause to course over the slice of pomegranate
And may You bless	And multiply the laurel, and juniper, and storax, and bitter almonds, and plane tree
Waters,	Holy waters will go forth from the recesses of the House
Dew of rest	make sparkle from briars and thistles
And may You bless	And blossom the grapevine, and fig, and pomegranate, and olive
A sister	borne, like dandled babes
Dew of rest	sate her, until the day breathes
And may You bless	and nurture the walnut, and sycamore, and date-palm, and . . . and apple
If she is a wall	she is prized by her parents
Dew of rest	to grant (her) joy; may her peace be like rivers
And may You bless	and ripen the pistachios, and sweet almonds, and the common oaks, and the boissier oaks of the hills

I am a wall Dew of rest And may You bless	I longed for the opening of the sack drip upon us when the fire grows hot and strengthen the white willows, the Syrian pear, and carob, and peach
There was a vineyard Dew of rest And may You bless	Its tendrils You tended, to strengthen (them) designate for it, after it has been rent asunder and beautify the citron, and pear, and the golden quince, and the crabapple
O My vineyard Dew of rest And may You bless	enter (and) spend the night, beyond the vault strengthen legs for the procession and nurture the tender sapling, and the quince, and the mulberry, and the sumac
She who dwells in the gardens Dew of rest And may You bless	gird her with dewdrops fortify her, O You who stand among the myrtles and root deeply the trees of the field and the groves of the orchards

POEM 6: Second Blessing of Amidah (Song 8:14)[41]

Flee Dew of rest	O majestic One, to Your resting place, O Glory! pour forth upon those who have been swallowed, for "to You belongs the glory" Then You will fulfill the saying, *"He will swallow up death forever"* (Isa. 25:8)
My Beloved Dew of rest	seek out "one whose dust cannot be counted" create stunned wonder by resurrecting those bowed into the dust And You will say, *"Awake and rejoice, O dwellers in the dust!"* (Isa. 26:19)
And show Yourself Dew of rest	Radiant One, who resurrects from dryness, with— Strong One, to swaddle them with wraps And You will make dew drip and moisten *"the dry bones"* (Ezek. 37:4)
As a gazelle Dew of rest	Will thrive through his own might give (it) moisture, to strengthen (it) And thus *"one bone will join to another"* (Ezek. 37:7)
Or a young stag Dew of rest	Hurry, for the sake of Your name . . . thundering . . . scatter, to stir up the crevices [that contain] my people

41 In the other passages, the quotations from the Song of Songs provided only the opening word or words of each verse; here each word of Song 8:14 is quoted.

And You will raise *"and I will bring you up from your graves, O My people"* (Ezek. 37:13)

Upon — Your city appear radiant, to awaken those sleeping within the earth

Dew of rest — Take care with it, to keep (it) clear from the carcasses of Dumah

And You will shine, *"And You will renew the face of the earth"* (Ps. 104:30)

Mountains — of holiness will burst with joy

Dew of rest — will have drenched the most rotten of the rotten stones, to revive (them), and they will glisten

And announce: Awaken, ye!, *"And from the summit of the mountains, let them rejoice!"* (Isa. 42:11)

Fragrant spices — You will gather, and the clouds will sprinkle from above

Dew of rest — You will give to those who are suspended from the depths, to raise (them) up

"Imposing death and giving life, casting down to Sheol and raising up" (1 Sam. 2:6)

For You are our God, who causes the wind to blow and the dew to fall
For a blessing and not for a curse,
For life and not for death,
(You who) puts to death and restores to life and causes redemption to sprout; none else resembles You.
Blessed are You, O Lord, who resurrects the dead

CONCLUSION (Ps. 23:2b and remaining blessings of Amidah)

Upon (Ps. 23:2b) — The valley of holiness He will delight us

Where once He looked down and judged our causes

With dew — The greatness of sanctifications . . . with our answers

"For today is holy to our Lord" (Neh. 8:10)

Blessed are You, O Lord, the Holy God

Waters — of the Curtain He will lift as He promised

From the treasure-house of goodness that is laid up with Him

With dew — of redemption, through which He gives strength

"For the Lord is pleased with His people" (Ps. 149:4)

Blessed are You, O Lord, whom we worship in awe

Tranquil waters — My multitudes are hasty for what is hidden
For respite from sorrow and grief
With dew — of song, a hymn of praise
"For David said: He has given rest" (1 Chr. 23:25)

Blessed are You, O Lord, to whom it is good to give thanks

He will lead me — and He will draw near
With bridle and bit to muzzle the evil inclination
With dew — to bless the sown seed of peace
"For He will speak peace" (Ps. 85:9)

Blessed are You, O Lord, who makes peace

CHAPTER SIXTEEN

The Spiritual Senses, Monastic and Theological

MARCUS PLESTED

If the doors of perception were cleansed everything would appear to man as it is, infinite. For man has closed himself up, till he sees all things thro' narrow chinks of his cavern.

—WILLIAM BLAKE,
The Marriage of Heaven and Hell

William Blake is just one representative of the long history of the doctrine of the spiritual senses—the idea that there are within the human being faculties corresponding in some manner with the five physical senses, yet capable of direct apprehension of spiritual and divine realities. In Blake's dazzling if decidedly *sui generis* mystical vision the cleansing of the doors of perception, the awakening of the spiritual senses, involves a shattering transformation of the physical senses which in and of themselves are profoundly limiting, affording "narow chinks" of reality at best. As the same poem puts it: "How do you know but ev'ry Bird that cuts the airy way, / Is an immense world of delight, clos'd by your senses five?" For Blake, this process of cleansing involved a good deal of spiritual struggle and mental fight, a dimension of his teaching circumvented in some of his epigones—witness Aldous Huxley's *Doors of Perception* or the eponymous Los Angeles rock group. But what is perhaps most significant in Blake for our purposes is his sense of the continuity between physical and spiritual perception—the spiritual senses are for Blake a kind of radical enhancement or unleashing of the physical senses, the kind of enhanced vision that enables one to see angels in the trees of Peckham Rye.

Blake's affirmation of the essential congruity of the physical and spiritual senses may be contrasted with much of the western mystical tradition in which spiritual sensation seems to involve the cessation or closing down of physical sensation. This strand of reflection has a long pedigree within the western mystical tradition, being implicit in the root μύω (close the eye), from which we have μυέω (initiate into the mysteries). Within the context of mystical experience this closing of the physical eye is necessary in order to open up that inner sight capable of apprehending the supreme reality underpinning and sustaining all things—ready, that is, to perceive the fullness of the transformative vision and experiences offered in the mystery cults and other religious contexts of antiquity. But even here we need not assume that spiritual sensation involves the complete cessation and negation of physical sensation. Physical sight was presumably a necessary precondition of spiritual seeing in, for example, the mysteries of Eleusis—one had to see the sacred ear of corn physically before apprehending its inner and more divine nature. Having said that, it is a given within much of the classical mystical tradition that spiritual perception is infinitely superior to physical perception and that the physical senses, where they do not actively militate against the mind's struggle to ascend out of the realm of materiality, serve at best as a kind of springboard or launching pad for the higher faculties of perception.

These non-Byzantine examples have been chosen not only to underline the fact that the notion of spiritual senses extends well beyond the realm of Byzantine theologoumena but also to flag some of the key questions that attend the notion, most notably the central question of the precise nature of the relationship between these two realms of perception. Questions attending the spiritual senses became a major area of interest and indeed contention within the Byzantine theological tradition. This essay serves as an attempt to discern the lineaments of the Byzantine understanding of the spiritual senses through a broadly diachronic discussion of some of the key expositors of the doctrine of the spiritual senses. But while focused perforce on explicit explorations of the subject at hand, this essay also aspires to give some hint of the all-pervading nature of theological considerations when it comes to understanding the Byzantine sensorium in all its fullness.

The doctrine of the spiritual senses is a constant within Byzantine theology and ascetic teaching. It is also deeply embedded within the liturgical and iconographic framework of the Empire. In the Byzantine world physical sense perception was only ever part of the story. Beyond the realm of the senses—separated only by the thin veil of materiality—lay a variegated world of heightened or transformed perception, a realm of divine encounter and struggle against the opposing powers. Robert Byron expresses this in inimitable fashion in his declamation, "in the eyes of the Byzantine, mortal life was a maze-like venture amid nonterrestrial forces, demoniac and divine, circling around him, imminent and overwhelming."[1] With every sight of an icon, every touch of a relic, every taste of the eucharist, every hearing of scripture or hagiography, every sniff of incense, the Byzantine man or woman was called out of the realm of everyday sense perception and into another world. Without assuming that every Byzantine man or woman was willing or able to respond to that invitation, the nature of that invitation is a question that preoccupied the minds of some of the greatest theologians of the age.

The doctrine of the spiritual senses is not univocal.[2] Various opinions exist within the Byzantine tradition as to the relation between the physical and the spiritual senses (depending here very much on the underlying anthropology and the extent which a given author has grappled with the implications of the incarnation). Similarly, various views exist as to the number of spiritual senses, whether spiritual senses are to be transcended at a certain point, whether the spiritual senses require the extinction or at least the transformation of the physical senses, or whether they are best construed as an intensification of the physical senses. I shall in what follows attempt to give some idea of the Byzantine doctrine of the spiritual senses as it unfolded over time, taking the story from Origen up to the Hesychast controversy of the fourteenth century, a period which saw the spiritual senses gravitate to the heart of the dogmatic enterprise of the Byzantine Church.[3]

Byzantine Writers on the Spiritual Senses

Origen of Alexandria

Origen is generally credited with having pioneered the doctrine of the spiritual senses.[4] It

1 *The Byzantine Achievement* (London, 1929), 155.

2 The seminal treatment of the doctrine of the spiritual senses in the modern era is A.-F. Poulain, *Des grâces d'oraison: Traité de théologie mystique,* 10th ed. (Paris, 1910), 93–125. His sources are, however, largely western (Dionysios the Areopagite being the chief exception).

3 This chapter builds in part on my earlier work on the spiritual sense(s), *The Macarian Legacy* (Oxford, 2004), especially 134–40 (Origen, Evagrios, Makarios, and Diadochos) and 236–37 (Maximos).

4 See K. Rahner, "Le début d'une doctrine des cinq sens spirituels chez Origène," *Revue d'Ascétique et de Mystique* 13 (1932): 113–45. Another prominent Roman Catholic theologian of the mid-twentieth century, Hans Urs von Balthasar, also picked up on the theme in the 1930s, building his understanding of the spiritual senses largely on his interpretation of Origen. See, for example, his anthology: *Origenes Geist und Feuer: Ein*

would, however, be quite misleading to regard him as the inventor of the notion. Origen was above all else an exegete and the doctrine emerges squarely from his close engagement with scripture.[5] In the first instance, the doctrine enables him to do justice to the multiple references in scripture to the sight, hearing, taste, smell, and touch of spiritual realties—whether by way of metaphor or by analogy. Second, the doctrine serves to explicate references to the vision or other sensory perception of God without lapsing into anthropomorphism or compromising God's transcendence. Third, there is undoubtedly an apologetic and polemical dimension: Origen is concerned to explain and defend the sensory and inescapably embodied language of Scripture in response both to the Gnostics and to pagan critics such as Celsus—neither of whom had much time for the body let alone for bodily language in respect of God.

Origen teaches that there is within the human being "a certain generic divine sense." His "divine sense" (αἴσθησιν θείαν) is grounded in the traditional Alexandrine (not the Septuagint) reading of Proverbs 2:5: "You shall find a divine sense."[6] This perceptive power operates in five principal modes analogous to the five physical senses: a sight to see invisible metaphysical realities such as the cherubim and seraphim, a hearing to hear that which has no objective existence in the air, a taste which is nourished by the living bread from heaven, a smell which smells spiritual things (cf. 2 Corinthians 2:15), and a sense of touch such as that of which the Apostle John spoke (1 John 1:1).[7] These modes are the divine or spiritual senses and convey something of the variegated nature of the soul's experience of the divine. As he puts it in his commentary on the Song of Songs:

> For those who have their senses exercised to the discerning of good and evil, Christ becomes each of these things in turn, to suit the several senses of the soul. He is called the true sight, therefore, that the soul's eyes may have something to lighten them. He is the Word, so that her ears may have something to hear. Again, he is the Bread of Life so that the soul's palate may have something to taste. And in the same way he is called spikenard or ointment, that the soul's sense of smell may apprehend the fragrance of the Word. For the same reason he is also said to be able to be felt and handled, and is called the Word made flesh so that the hand of the interior soul may touch concerning the Word of Life. But all these things are the One, Same Word of God, who adapts himself to the sundry tempers of prayer according to these several guises, and so leaves none of the soul's faculties empty of his grace.[8]

Elsewhere Origen asserts, again referring to Proverbs 2:5, that Solomon "knew that there exist in us two sorts of sense, one mortal, corruptible and human, the other immortal and intellectual, the sense he calls 'divine'." To see with the "eyes of the heart" (Ephesians 1:18), for example, is to grasp some intellectual or noetic reality by virtue of the intellect or νοῦς. It is the "divine sense" that sees God, the sight not of the eyes but of the "pure heart" (cf. Mt. 5:8), that is to say, of the intellect.[9]

Aufbau aus seinen Schriften (Salzburg, 1938). The spiritual senses became an important theme within his masterwork, *The Glory of the Lord: A Theological Aesthetics* (Edinburgh, 1982–). B. Fraigneau-Julien gives one of the best summaries of Origen's doctrine of the spiritual senses in his *Les sens spirituels et la vision de Dieu selon Syméon le Nouveau Théologien* (Paris, 1985), 29–43. More recently, M. McInroy has offered a thoughtful reassessment of modern scholarship on the matter, arguing that the theme runs throughout Origen's oeuvre, albeit with alternation between metaphorical and analogical usages. See his "Origen of Alexandria," in *The Spiritual Senses: Perceiving God in Western Christianity,* ed. P. Gavrilyuk and S. Coakley (Cambridge, 2012), 20–35.

5 This is not to say that Origen's doctrine of the spiritual senses is solely scriptural. John Dillon, in particular, has made a strong case for connecting Origen with analogous developments in Middle and Neo-Platonism. See his "Aisthêsis Noêtê: A Doctrine of the Spiritual Senses in Origen and in Plotinus," in *Hellenica et Judaica: Hommage à Valentin Nikiprowetzky*, ed. A. Caquot et al. (Leuven and Paris, 1986), 443–55. Cf., for example, Plotinus on intellectual perception in *Enneads* 6.7.6.

6 This is a reading known also to Clement of Alexandria. The LXX has "knowledge of God" (ἐπίγνωσιν θεοῦ). Origen is fully aware of the variant.

7 *Contra Celsum* 1.48 (GCS 2:98).

8 *Commentary on the Song* 2.9 (GCS 8:167–68), trans. Louth, in *The Origins of the Christian Mystical Tradition: From Plato to Denys* (Oxford, 1981), 68.

9 *De principiis* 1.1.9 (GCS 22:27).

Origen's commentaries on Scripture return to the theme with some frequency.[10]

Evagrios of Pontos

Evagrios takes up the doctrine virtually unchanged from Origen, speaking of the intellect's need for a spiritual sense in order to distinguish spiritual things.[11] He defines this spiritual sense as "the impassibility of the rational soul, produced by the grace of God."[12] Like Origen, he slides back and forth between one and five senses but without positing anything but an essentially adventitious connection with the physical senses. He speaks of the fivefold operation of the spiritual senses in some detail: "Sight shows [the intellect] intelligible objects nakedly; with the hearing it receives the *logoi* (underlying principles) concerning these objects; the sense of smell delights in the scent which is foreign to all dissimulation; the mouth receives the taste of these things, and by means of touch it is made steadfast, grasping the exact manifestation of things."[13] The spiritual senses are, in Evagrios, the faculties by which the contemplative intellect grasps the true nature of things and ascends toward theology—the summit of human life and experience—stripping away all images, perceptions, and sensations as it does so. In the realm of theology it seems that all the senses, spiritual and physical alike, are to be left behind: "Blessed is the intellect that has acquired complete freedom from senses (ἀναισθησία) during prayer."[14]

10 See also *Commentary on Luke* fr. 57 (GCS 49:308–9); *Commentary on John* 10.40 (GCS 10:218).

11 *Kephalaia gnostika* 1.33 (A. Guillaumont, ed., *Les six centuries des "Kephalaia gnostica": Édition critique de la version syriaque commune et édition d'une nouvelle version syriaque, intégrale, avec une double traduction française,* PO 28 [Paris, 1958], 33).

12 *Kephalaia gnostika* 1.37 (Guillaumont ed., p. 35). This and other uncredited translations are my own.

13 *Kephalaia gnostika* 2.35 (Guillaumont ed., p. 75), with Greek preserved in J. Muyldermans, *Evagriana: Extrait de la revue Le Muséon, vol. 44, augmenté de nouveax fragments grecs inédits* (Paris, 1931). The doctrine of the spiritual senses is also articulated in his *Advice to a Virgin* 55: "Virgin eyes will see the Lord. / The ears of virgins will hear the Lord. / The mouth of virgins will kiss the Bridegroom. / The nose of virgins is drawn by the scent of his ointments (cf. Cant. 1:3). / Virgin hands will touch the Lord."

14 *On Prayer* 120 PG 79:1193B.

Origen and Evagrios adopt an essentially spiritualizing approach, one which transfers or transposes the language of the bodily senses to the faculties of the soul. There is little or no perceptible continuity between the physical and the spiritual senses here, something that comes as no surprise given their own rather ambivalent approaches to physicality and materiality. The doctrine of the spiritual senses allows Origen and Evagrios to express the variety, immediacy, and reality of the soul's experience of God by analogy with the physical senses, but the principal function of the doctrine is as an exegetical and apologetic tool.

St. Gregory of Nyssa

We encounter a somewhat more embodied understanding of the spiritual senses in St. Gregory of Nyssa. Grappling more closely with the implications of incarnation than either Origen or Evagrios, Gregory cannot, for all his Platonic inclinations, regard the physical or material as being only analogically or adventitiously related to the spiritual or divine. In his commentary on the Song of Songs he takes the physical and sensory language of the Song as a kind of toehold for spiritual perception.[15] In Gregory's interpretation, the bridegroom (Christ) awakens the spiritual senses of the bride (the human soul) by means of the physical senses: "As light, he becomes beautiful to our eyes; and a sweet smell for our sense of smell; and life for those who eat of him."[16]

But for all the possible continuity between the physical and the spiritual senses in Gregory, physical sensory perception is certainly to be left behind. In the *Life of Moses* he writes:

15 I borrow the "toehold" from S. Coakley, *Powers and Submissions*, 138. Coakley also offers a limpid definition of the spiritual senses as "the transformed epistemic sensibilities of those being progressively reborn in the likeness of the Son." Ibid., 131. This bears comparison with Hans Urs von Balthasar, who argues that the spiritual senses are not "other" to the physical senses but rather are these senses "in so far as they have been formed according to the form of Christ." *Glory of the Lord,* 1:424.

16 *Comm. on the Song* GNO 6:117. For more on Gregory and the Song see H. Boersma, *Embodiment and Virtue in Gregory of Nyssa* (Oxford, 2013), 93–100.

> The contemplation of God is not effected by sight and hearing, nor is it comprehended by any of the customary perceptions of the mind. For "no eye has seen, and no ear has heard," nor does it belong to those things which usually enter "into the heart of man" (1 Cor. 2:9). He who would approach the knowledge of things sublime must first purify his manner of life from all sensual and irrational emotion. He must wash from his understanding every opinion derived from some preconception and withdraw himself from his customary intercourse with his own companion, that is, with his faculty of sense perception which is, as it were, wedded to our nature as its companion [σύζυγός πώς ἐστι τῇ ἡμετέρᾳ φύσει καὶ σύνοικος]. When he is so purified, then he assaults the mountain.[17]

The same applies *a fortiori* on the mountaintop:

> For leaving behind everything that is observed, not only what sense comprehends but also what the intelligence thinks it sees, the mind keeps on penetrating deeper until by its yearning for understanding it gains access to the invisible and incomprehensible, and there it sees God. This is the true knowledge of what is sought; this is the seeing that consists in not seeing, because that which is sought transcends all knowledge, being separated on all sides as by a kind of darkness.[18]

This theme of the divine darkness is certainly to be distinguished from the intellectual illumination taught by Origen and Evagrios. It may also be distinguished in terms of its assertion of an enduring role for the spiritual sense(s). Turning back to the commentary on the Song of Songs, we read that in the deepest and most intimate moment of divine encounter the soul "is encompassed by a divine night, during which her spouse approaches, but does not reveal himself. But how can that which is invisible reveal itself in the night? By the fact that he gives the soul some sense of his presence (αἴσθησιν μέν τινα δίδωσι τῇ ψυχῇ τῆς παρουσίας) even while he eludes her clear apprehension, concealed as he is by the invisibility of his nature."[19] Far from being transcended in the *unio mystica*, the spiritual sense, the sense of Christ's presence, is all we are left with.[20]

Dionysios the Areopagite

Dionysios the Areopagite, that most intriguing and perplexing of theologians, also offers a broadly anagogical approach, albeit one which envisages the cessation of all perception in the unio mystica. For Dionysios, the celestial and ecclesiastical hierarchies are alike geared to the reawakening of the spiritual senses, the cleansing of the doors of perception, by means of the foothold of the senses: "For it is quite impossible that we humans should, in any immaterial way, rise up to imitate and to contemplate the heavenly hierarchies without the aid of the those material means capable of guiding us as our nature requires. Hence, for anyone who reflects, the appearances of beauty become the signs of an invisible harmony. Perfumes, as they strike our senses, represent spiritual illumination. Material lights point to that immaterial light of which they are images" (*Celestial Hierarchy* 1.3 [121CD]). The spiritual senses operate, in Dionysios, in anagogical fashion. Using the physical senses as a foothold or, better, springboard, the angelic and ecclesiastical hierarchies invite us to ascend from the realm of materiality to the realm of the immaterial and invisible, putting aside sense perception as we do so, gathering us up ever higher until such time as we are embraced by the divine darkness of the one who is beyond being, beyond name, beyond affirmation and negation, and certainly beyond any kind of perception: "[The Cause of all] is neither perceived nor is it perceptible" (*Mystical Theology* 4 [1040D]). While Dionysios's intuition of the natural sympathy between material and divine things allows him to expound a doctrine of the spiritual senses, his teaching on the cessation of all perception in mystical union does point to an underlying weakness of his account—an inability to ascribe

17 *Life of Moses* 2.157 (SC 1 ter.) (trans. Malherbe and Ferguson, 93, lightly adapted).

18 *Life of Moses* 2.163 (SC 1 ter.) (trans. Malherbe and Ferguson, 93).

19 *Comm. on the Song* 11 p. 324.10 (trans. Louth, *Origins*, 67).

20 Presence is a key feature in Poulain, *Des grâces* (n. 2 above).

to the spiritual (let alone the physical) senses any kind of eternal significance or value.

Makarios (Makarios-Symeon, Pseudo-Makarios)

For a truly robust and unapologetically embodied understanding of the spiritual senses we must turn to Makarios (fl. 370s–390s), one of the key figures in the development of the Byzantine mystical tradition (and, it may be noted, an authority for St. Gregory of Nyssa).[21] Makarios has perhaps the most holistic anthropology of any writer of the patristic period, asserting an intimate and organic connection between the soul and the body, a connection rooted and grounded in the heart. There is in Makarios an intriguing reciprocity between soul and body, the soul being created in the image and likeness of God and the body in the image and likeness of the soul.[22] In this framework the spiritual senses may be interpreted not so much as an analogy drawn from the workings of the physical senses but rather it is the physical senses that reflect in some imperfect way the operation of the soul. Such considerations give Makarios's presentation of the spiritual senses an unusual centrality and firmness. Makarios can even define the very essence of Christianity in terms of the spiritual senses: "The reality of Christianity is this: the taste of truth, the eating and drinking of truth" (I 18.7.1–3).[23] We might note here that it is the faculty of taste that is privileged, taste being perhaps the most immediate of the senses. This experience is also frequently evoked in terms of the vision of God as light:

> The blessed Apostle Paul, the architect of the Church, forever anxious for the truth and not wishing that those who hear the word should be impeded by ignorance, indicated with great exactitude and clarity the goal of the truth and made known the perfect mystery of Christianity in every believing soul, this being to receive through a divine operation the experience of the effulgence of the heavenly light in holy souls in the revelation and power of the Spirit. (I 58.1.1)

Makarios routinely speaks of the drama of the Fall and Redemption in terms of the spiritual senses. The Fall has "blinded the eyes of the soul" (I 35.3) and caused us humans to lose the "intellectual and deathless senses" (I 58.3.3). It is significant that he uses αἰσθητήριον rather than αἴσθησις here. Makarios usually prefers the former term in preference to the latter for the physical senses. The choice of vocabulary seems to emphasize the correspondence between the physical and the spiritual senses. Through his incarnation, Christ reestablishes the "intellectual senses" of the soul (I 58.3.3). At Pentecost, the Holy Spirit uncovered the "eyes of the heart" of the apostles (I 63.1.5). The Lord came so as to allow the soul to see him "with its intellectual eyes" (I 28.1.4). Again and again this vision of Christ is construed in terms of the spiritual vision of the light of God shining in the soul (e.g., I 10.3.4). "As the sun on earth is to the eyes of the flesh, so is the glory of the Holy Spirit to the purified eyes of the inner man" (III 28.4.4). The soul's return to health is spoken of consistently in terms of the restoration of the spiritual senses, the reopening of the eyes of the soul, and the acquisition of the taste of grace. It is also, regrettably, necessary to taste the bitterness of the passions: "So that by the experience of the two natures, tasting frequently both the bitterness of sin and the sweetness of grace, the soul might become more perceptive and more vigilant, so as to flee evil entirely and to attach itself wholly to the Lord" (III 12.2.2).

It is vital to notice that in Makarios, by virtue of the centrality of the heart, spiritual sensation as it were overflows into physical sensation: "The heart governs and rules the whole bodily organ; and when grace takes hold of the

21 Citations to Makarios: I = H. Berthold, ed., *Makarios/Symeon, Reden und Briefe: Die Sammlung I des Vaticanus Graecus 694 (B)*, 2 vols., GCS 55–56 (Berlin, 1973); II = H. Dörries, E. Klostermann, and M. Kroeger, eds., *Die 50 geistlichen Homilien des Makarios*, PTS 4 (Berlin, 1964); III = E. Klostermann and H. Berthold, *Neue Homilien des Makarius/Symeon*, vol. 1, *Aus Typus III*, TU 72 (Berlin, 1961), given also in V. Desprez, *Pseudo-Macaire: Oeuvres spirituelles*, vol. 1, *Homélies propres à la Collection III*, SC 275 (Paris, 1980).

22 I 18.7.1–3. Cf. also II 4.9–10: "The soul, which is a subtle body, has enveloped the eye by which it sees, the ear by which it hears, the tongue by which it speaks, the hands. In short, the soul envelops the entire body and its members and is commingled with them, and through them accomplishes all the necessaries of life."

23 Cf. II 27.7.

pastures of the heart, it rules over all the members and the thoughts. For there is the intellect, and all the thoughts of the soul and its expectation, thus [through the heart] grace penetrates to all the members of the body" (II 15.20). And so while the vision of the divine light is in the first instance an experience of the spiritual senses, that vision is communicated also to the physical senses. Again the continuity between the physical and spiritual senses is made crystal clear.

Makarios also connects the doctrine of the spiritual senses to his curious theme of the "second soul," which is the work of the Spirit in us. In I 63.1.3 he writes, "There are other ears and other eyes and other cries and another mind and another soul, which is that very divine and heavenly Spirit which hears and cries and prays and knows and does the will of God in truth (cf. Rom. 8:26)." In this framework, the spiritual senses are to be construed as a divine operation.

Elsewhere, Makarios offers an alternative list of the five senses or faculties of the soul as understanding, knowledge, discernment, patience, and mercy (σύνεσις, γνῶσις, διάκρισις, ὑπομονή, ἔλεος) (I 49.2.3).[24] He proceeds to draw an analogy between the five senses of the soul operating as they should, that is, "receiving grace from above and the sanctification of the Spirit" and the five wise virgins of Matthew 25. Again, the spiritual senses are to be understood as awakened and actuated by divine grace.

In his trenchant insistence on the continuity between the physical and spiritual senses Makarios affords perhaps the closest thing to Blake—for all that he abhorred asceticism—that the Byzantine tradition has to offer. Makarios's robust and profoundly Christocentric teaching on the spiritual senses was to shape much subsequent Byzantine reflection on the topic.

St. Diadochos of Photike

St. Diadochos of Photike represents the chief witness in the fifth century to the doctrine of the spiritual senses. A mystical theologian of great stature with considerable impact on the later tradition, Diadochos abounds in the language of sense and sense perception. In this he is certainly drawing on Makarios.[25] Diadochos normally speaks of sense (αἴσθησις) in the singular.[26] The natural sense of the soul is single, but has been split into two by the Fall. The purpose of the ascetic life is to reunite the split disposition of the soul, now torn between heavenly and earthly aspirations. This reunion is effected by the Holy Spirit (*GC* 25, 29).[27] This inner sense is described as "intellectual sense" (αἴσθησις νοερά; *GC* 1, 7)[28]; the "sense of the intellect" (αἴσθησις νοὸς / τοῦ νοῦ; *GC* 24, 30, 61, 76, 77, 79, 83); the "sense of the soul" (αἴσθησις τῆς ψυχῆς; *GC* 14, 25, 29) and "sense of the heart" (αἴσθησις τῆς καρδίας; *GC* 14, 16, 23).[29] The variations in Diadochos's descriptions of the inner or spiritual sense do not imply a range of inner senses pertaining to the different constituent elements of the human being, nor do they correspond to the fivefold operation of the physical sense. The distinction is, rather, one of level. The sense of the intellect or the intellectual sense is the purest sense of our soul, and our surest guide in the spiritual life. When restored to its full vigor the intellect communicates the joy it

24 Note that Makarios's list here includes moral virtues as well as aspects of the operation of the intellect. The parallel text in II 4.7 omits the list of these senses but speaks of the "five *rational* senses" (emphasis mine). There is a connection between Makarios's exegesis of Matthew 25 and that of the second-century *Epistula apostolorum*, which speaks of the five wise virgins as representing knowledge, insight, obedience, patience and mercy. See R. Staats, *Gregor von Nyssa und die Messalianer: Die Frage der Priorität zweiter altkirchlicher Schriften*, PTS 8 (Berlin, 1968), 95 n. 9a (cited in C. Stewart, *Working the Earth of the Heart: The Messalian Controversy in History, Texts and Language to A.D. 431* [Oxford, 1991], 124) and M. Hornschuh, *Studien zur Epistula Apostolorum*, PTS 5 (Berlin, 1965), 21–29.

25 See my *Macarian Legacy*, 133–75. Much of the material in this section is drawn from this earlier work.

26 Hermann Dörries claims that Diadochos's understanding of just one spiritual sense represents one of the two significant departures he makes from Makarios's teaching, "Diadochos und Symeon: Das Verhältnis der *kephalaia gnostika* zum Messalianismus," in *Wort und Stunde*, vol. 1 (Göttingen 1966), 352–422, esp. 412. This is a position I have argued against elsewhere: *Macarian Legacy*, 134–40.

27 Note on references to Diadochos: *GC* = É. des Places, ed., *Diadoque de Photicé: Oeuvres spirituelles* (SC 5 ter.; Paris 1997).

28 The term αἴσθησις νοερά is first instanced in Makarios, who uses it to denote the faculty in man capable of spiritual discernment (I 2.10.5) and speaks of our advancing in this intellectual sense through gentleness (I 39.1.6).

29 He also speaks of the "sense of the spirit" or "spiritual sense" (*GC* 15 × 2), and "immaterial sense" (*GC* 24).

experiences from sensing the divine goodness to the body (*GC* 25)—even down to what Diadochos calls "very sense of the bones" (*GC* 14). The inner, intellectual, or spiritual sense is one whether related to the intellect, the soul, the heart, or even, by virtue of the overflowing of spiritual sensation, the body. In each case the term αἴσθησις designates the same reality, that inner faculty within the human being capable of perceiving, sensing, and experiencing the divine. It is through the cultivation of our spiritual sense that we enter into union with God: "love unites the soul with the excellences of God, seeking out the invisible by means of its intellectual sense" (*GC* 1).

While Diadochos prefers to speak of the spiritual sense, not senses, this does not rule out the use of language pertaining to the five physical senses when it comes to spiritual perception. In this connexion, Diadochos is most given to the language of sight and taste—just like Makarios. For example, Diadochos defines patience as the perseverance required "in order to see the invisible as visible with the eyes of the mind" (Defn. 3 [84.6–7]). Diadochos also describes the "eye of the soul" as being veiled by the body (*GC* 71).[30] Diadochos's language of taste is thoroughgoing and remarkable. The inner sense tastes the sweetness (*GC* 44, 63, 90), goodness (*GC* 24, 33, 89), and grace (*GC* 30, 36) of God. It is also possible for the theologian to taste the experience of spiritual knowledge (*GC* 72). This language of taste is, as we have seen, a stock in trade of the Macarian writings.[31] Taste is, as I have suggested, perhaps the most immediate of the spiritual senses, the most obviously suggestive of union with the object tasted.

Diadochos's language of sense is, of all its potential forerunners, most closely related to that of Makarios. Whereas for Origen and Evagrios the doctrine of the spiritual senses is essentially an analogy taken from the realm of the senses and transposed to the soul's apprehension of metaphysical realities, for both Makarios and Diadochos it is an expression of the unity of the human being—a unity founded upon and assured by the incarnation.

Maximos Confessor

Maximos Confessor achieved a definitive and creative synthesis of the Byzantine mystical and theological tradition. Naturally, the doctrine of the spiritual senses looms large in this synthesis. His approach can perhaps best be illustrated through an exploration of the Transfiguration of Christ on Mount Tabor—an event that was to assume an ever-increasing prominence in the Byzantine thought-world, as the debates over the character of that light (created or uncreated) came to dominate the Hesychast Controversy. *Ambiguum* 10, dealing with St. Gregory of Nazianzos's treatment of the ascent through materiality to God, presents the apostles' ascent of Tabor as very much an inward ascent: "And they passed over from flesh to spirit, before they had laid aside this fleshly life, by the *change in the operations of sense* that the Spirit worked in them, lifting the veils of the passions from the intellectual power that was in them" (*Ambigua* 10.17 [PG 91:1125D–28A]).[32] The apostles were taught that the all-blessed radiance that shone from Christ's face and which overpowered their physical sense-perception was "a symbol of his divinity which transcends intellect and sense and being and knowledge" (ibid.). As their spiritual senses were opened, Christ's garments, symbols of the words of Scripture, became clear to them, as did the underlying principles or *logoi* of creation (1128BC). The light of the Transfiguration becomes in Maximos a recurrent theme, as witnessed, for example, in his striking description of the state of pure prayer: "At the very onset of prayer, the intellect is ravished by the divine and infinite light and is aware neither of itself nor of any other created thing whatsoever, but only of him who through love has activated such radiance in it" (*CC* 2.6).[33] Needless to say,

30 The phrase "eye of the soul" is an ancient one. Origen criticizes Celsus for supposing that the Christians had not heard of it (*Contra Celsum* 7.39, GCS 3:189–90). Evagrios has "eye of the soul" in *Skemmata* 24 and "eyes of the soul" in *Schol. Prov.* 216. Makarios also speaks of the soul's eyes in I 63.2.4 and II 28.4.

31 For the taste of the sweetness of God in Makarios see, for example, I 5.4.4, 21.11, 33.4.4; II 14.2, 17.2. The most obvious Scriptural root for this is Ps. 33(34):8, "Taste and see that the Lord is good."

32 Emphasis mine. In his *Oration* 21, upon which this *aporia* is centered, Gregory Nazianzen had referred to matter and the fleshly as a cloud or veil.

33 *CC* = *Chapters on Love,* A. Ceresa-Gastaldo, ed., *Capitoli sulla carità,* Verba seniorum 3 (Rome, 1963). *QD* = *Questions*

such states do not come about without strenuous ascetic effort.

Maximos's use of the term αἴσθησις is worth dwelling in for a moment. In his works, the term usually refers to the physical sense or senses, often in a negative context.[34] Maximos does, however, also use αἴσθησις to denote understanding (*QD* 78 [59]) and in reference to the spiritual senses (*QD* 43; cf. Makarios I 58.3.3). The most interesting example for our purposes is perhaps Maximos's reference to the faculty of intellectual or spiritual perception, the αἴσθησις νοερά: "The Word enables us to participate in divine life by making himself food, as those who have received from him this intellectual perception (αἴσθησιν νοερὰν) know. It is by the taste of this food that they truly know in full knowledge that the Lord is good" (*LP* 34.128–132).

Maximos is here clearly drawing upon the language of spiritual sense perception—including the characteristic fascination with taste—articulated in Makarios and Diadochos. He stands, in short, as a supremely eloquent witness to the developed tradition of the spiritual senses in Byzantium—the spiritual senses as the principal motif by which the human person's ascent to divine encounter is articulated.

St. John of Damascus

We may also mention, at least briefly, another great synthesizer, albeit less creative a theologian than the Confessor. Here the prologue to the *Philosophical Chapters* is of particular interest—one of the few elements in that work original to the Damascene. Here, John enunciates a theory of embodied knowledge that makes full use of the notion of the spiritual senses:

> Now, since we do not live with our soul stripped bare, but, on the contrary, have it clothed over, as it were, with the veil of the flesh, our soul has the mind as a sort of eye which sees and has the faculty of knowing and which is capable of receiving knowledge and having understanding of things which are. Let us approach with attention and in all sincerity and proceed without letting the spiritual eye of our soul be dulled and let us not be satisfied with arriving speedily at the gate, but rather let us knock hard, so that the door of the bridal chamber may be opened to us and we may behold the beauties within. Now, the gate is the letter, but the bridal chamber within the gate is the beauty of the thoughts hidden behind the letter, which is to say, the Spirit of truth.[35]

Again one detects here the continuity between the physical and spiritual senses, a continuity founded on a profoundly holistic understanding of the human being.

St. Symeon the New Theologian

The doctrine of the spiritual senses erupts in a blaze of glory in the extraordinary figure of St. Symeon the New Theologian, the foremost apostle of the vision of divine light in the middle Byzantine period.

With regard to the physical senses, Symeon holds there is but a single sense of the soul, intellect, and reason (μίαν αἴσθησιν ἔχων ἐν μιᾷ ψυχῇ καὶ νοῒ καὶ λόγῳ) that operates in five ways or modes according to physical needs of the body. For example, it is not sight that sees but rather the soul that sees by means of sight. This is not a new point—Gregory of Nyssa, among others, says the same. Symeon does however appear to break new ground in what he has to say about the specifically spiritual senses:

> With regard to spiritual matters, however, the soul is no longer obliged to discern through the windows of the senses. It no longer seeks to open the eyes in order to see or contemplate some existing thing, nor the ears in order to admit discourse. Neither does it require lips or tongue in order to distinguish sweet from bitter, nor hands in order to know by means of them what is rough, or soft, or smooth.

and Doubts, J. Declerck, ed., *Quaestiones et dubia,* CCSG 10 (Louvain, 1982). *LP* = *On the Lord's Prayer,* P. Van Deun, ed., *Opuscula exegetica duo: Expositio in Psalmum LIX; Expositio orationis dominicae,* CCSG 23 (Louvain, 1991).

34 See for example the call to mortify sense (i.e., sensuality) (*LP* 35–36.161–62) or to restrain sense activity (*LP* 56.496–97).

35 *Philosophical Chapters,* ed. Kotter (PTS 7 53.14–54.41) (trans. Chase, 7–8).

> Rather perception goes outside of all of these and is gathered together wholly within the intellect, as being naturally consequent upon the latter and inseparably one with it. To put it more precisely, it possesses the five senses within itself as one rather than several.[36]

All this, I should note, comes as part of a developed understanding of the soul as the image of the Trinity. Symeon fleshes out what he has to say on the matter of the spiritual senses using the example of the "ineffable speech" (ἄρρητα ῥήματα) heard by St. Paul (cf. 2 Cor. 12:4):

> God is one, the creator of all. This one is therefore every thing which is good, as we said. The rational and immortal soul is one. This one soul is every perception, that is, it possesses the senses, as many as they are, within itself. Therefore, when the one God of all appears in revelation to the one and rational soul, every good thing is revealed to it and appears to it at one and the same time through all of its senses. He [God] is both seen and heard, is sweet to the taste and perfume to the sense of smell; He is felt and so made known. He both speaks and is spoken. He knows, and is recognized, and is perceived as knowing. For the one who is known by God knows that he is known, and he who sees God knows that God sees him.[37]

There is a palpable continuity here between the senses of the soul and the physical senses. This intimation of continuity between the physical and spiritual is given vivid illustration in his evocations of the new creation, the redeemed cosmos:

> All creation, too, once made new, will become spiritual, and together with paradise will be transformed into an immaterial, unchanging, eternal, and intelligible dwelling place. The sky on the one hand will be incomparably brighter, in a manner indeed quite new, other and brighter than our visible sky, while the earth on the other hand will take on a new and inexpressible beauty, an unfading verdure, ornamented by shining flowers, varied and spiritual. . . . The sun of righteousness will shine seven times more brightly, and the moon will gleam twice as bright as the sun which illumines it now. The stars will be like our sun—if, indeed, these are the same stars as are spoken of in the sublime thoughts of the wise. All things there are beyond speech, transcend thought, save only that they are spiritual and divine, joined to the intelligible world, and comprise another intellectual paradise and heavenly Jerusalem, made like and united to the angelic world, the inviolable inheritance of the sons of God.[38]

This understanding of the continuity between the material and spiritual cosmos in Symeon is also perfectly born out in his descriptions of the experience of the divine light. After only a brief period of prayer, Symeon recounts an overwhelming sense of joy and delight that gave way to a vision of God as light:

> A great light was immaterially shining on me and seized hold of my whole mind and soul, so that I was struck with amazement at the unexpected marvel and I was, as it were, in ecstasy. . . . I conversed with this light. The light itself knows it; it scattered whatever mist there was in my soul and cast out every earthly care. It expelled from me all material denseness and bodily heaviness that made my members to be sluggish and numb. What an awesome marvel! It so invigorated and strengthened my limbs and muscles, which had been faint through great weariness, that it seemed to me as though I was stripping myself of the garment of corruption. Besides, there was poured into my soul in unutterable fashion a great intellectual joy and perception and a sweetness surpassing every taste of visible things [ἀλλὰ καὶ χαρὰν εὐθέως πολλὴν νοεράν τε αἴσθησιν καὶ γλυκύτητα ὑπὲρ πᾶσαν γεῦσιν τῶν ὁρωμένων], together with a freedom and a forgetfulness of all thought pertaining to the things of this life. . . . Thus all the senses of my mind and my soul were

36 *Third Ethical Discourse* (SC 122:402) (trans. Golitzin).

37 *Ibid.* 122:402–4.

38 *First Ethical Discourse* (SC 122:218–20) (trans. Golitzin).

> wholly concentrated on the ineffable joy of that light.[39]

The Fourteenth-Century Hesychasts: The Two Gregories

The light mysticism so vividly expressed by Symeon (and indeed Makarios, Diadochos, and Maximos) was to bear spectacular fruit in the Hesychast controversy. The long and involved debates about the character of the light of Tabor—whether created or uncreated—and the minutiae of the attendant discussion of the distinction between the divine essence and the divine operations, activities, or energies fall outside the scope of this paper. For our purposes it is important to note that the Hesychasts routinely employ the notion of the spiritual senses to explicate the nature of the vision of divine light—whether on Tabor or in the experience of the monks of Athos and elsewhere. St. Gregory of Sinai makes this connection between the light of Tabor and monastic experience evident in his *Homily on the Transfiguration*. To grasp the mystery of the transfiguration one must, he exhorts, be "mentally transformed from flesh to spirit" and ascend the mountain together with the chosen disciples and "all the lovers of the divine vision who rejoice ecstatically in such a sight." The vision of God as light is "a vision of the brilliance of the godhead." And it is a vision that strains the conceptual categories of the spiritual senses:

> For when the mind is swallowed up by that ineffable light and comes to exist outside of the real world, it is removed from perceiving relationships, and [God] dulls the senses by the light of his power. Or else just the opposite happens: he separates the mind from the senses, and the senses from their relationships by his light, and makes it be preoccupied by divine love, thrusting away all the attraction that the mind has towards sensible things, through the very operation of the senses.[40]

Here we have two possibilities: the spiritual vision or experience of God comes about either through the suppression of the physical senses or through such an intensification and heightening of sense perception that the physical senses open up to the wider vistas of the spiritual senses. Gregory sees no need to resolve this antinomy.

The "other" Gregory, St. Gregory Palamas (ca. 1296–1359), tends to be rather more precise, writing as he does in an explicitly polemical context.[41] Palamas is careful to assert that the uncreated light of the transfiguration (and he is absolutely insistent on this uncreated character) is sensed and perceived by the spiritual senses. There is no physical light to be seen on Tabor—a bystander would have noticed nothing particularly out of ordinary (save perhaps the stricken postures of the chosen disciples). Palamas turns to Maximos for an assertion that the vision took place "by a change in the operation of sense" effected by the Holy Spirit.[42] It is by this transformation of the faculty of sense perception that the disciples are able to see the ineffable light. And it is this same transformation that allows the saints to see that same light in prayer—"with eyes transformed by the power of the Holy Spirit."[43] That said, Palamas does allow—on the basis of the unity of the human being, composed of body and soul, that spiritual perception is communicated in some mysterious way to the senses of the body—that, for example, a sensation of warmth or perception of visible light may accompany what is properly speaking an experience of the spiritual or intellectual senses. This is a teaching grounded squarely in Makarios. Indeed one finds in both Gregory and Makarios a clear sense of the sheer thinness of the veil between the material and the spiritual—in this context Palamas speaks of the veil between the two as a "crystal membrane."[44]

But, argues Palamas, even in this revelation of light there is always something that remains

39 *Discourse* 16 (SC 104:244–46) (trans. Cantazaro, lightly adapted).

40 *Homily on the Transfiguration* 13 (ed. Balfour 32), trans. B. Daley, *Light on the Mountain: Greek Patristic and Byzantine Homilies on the Transfiguration of the Lord* (Yonkers, 2013), 335.

41 *Homilies 34–35 On the Transfiguration* (ed. Chrestou 354–406), trans. Daley, *Light on the Mountain*, 355–78.

42 *Homily* 34.8, trans. Daley, *Light on the Mountain*, 360.

43 *Homily* 34.13, trans. Daley, *Light on the Mountain*, 363–64.

44 *Homily* 34.14, trans. Daley, *Light on the Mountain*, 364. Gregory also develops a rather intriguing notion of our having six senses (adding the faculty of language to the usual five) as a way of doing justice to the six days referenced in the Marcan and Matthean account.

invisible and unknowable in God, that is to say, the divine nature as opposed to the divine operation. Here a kind of analogy can be drawn with the sun. The sun provides the light by which we see but at the same time blinds us if we look at it directly. There is a very real sense in which the light of Tabor, the same light witnessed by the Hesychast monks in prayer, is also a kind of dazzling and overwhelming darkness—a darkness that points to the unsearchable, inscrutable, and unknowable nature of God, hidden from all sense perception—both physical and spiritual.

Conclusion

This survey will, I trust, have conveyed something of the richness of the Byzantine understandings of the spiritual senses. Let me now offer a few conclusions.

The contrast between five spiritual senses and one is more apparent than real. In practice evocations of the fivefold operation of the senses function as a way of expressing the variegated nature of human experience of the divine but do not rule out a unitary understanding of that experience.

Although there is within the Byzantine theological tradition a current of thought suggestive of the cessation of the spiritual senses in the *unio mystica*, the prevailing opinion is that the spiritual sense or senses represent the least inadequate way of conveying something of the overwhelming nature of human experience of encounter with the divine. Whether this be through a cessation or an intensification of the physical senses is perhaps less important than the fact of the endurance of the sense or senses in union with God.

While some understandings of the spiritual senses represent a mere transposition or transference from the realm of the physical senses, the dominant Byzantine tradition asserts a real continuity between the physical and spiritual senses. Far from being a poetic analogy or spiritualizing extrapolation from the sublunary sensorium, this tradition of interpretation asserts the essential connection between physical and spiritual perception and in so doing affirms in no uncertain terms the psycho-physical unity of the human person. In this respect, Makarios's intuition that it is the spiritual and not the physical senses that are primary is especially interesting. As inhabitants of the physical cosmos we are used to assuming that perception pertains in the first instance to the material, the sensible, and the phenomenal. Makarios prompts us to consider instead the primacy of spiritual and intellectual perception. What you see is, emphatically, not what you get.

The Byzantine theologians surveyed in this chapter offer a robust defense of the integrity of the material and the physical and a forceful assertion of the inescapably embodied character of human existence. At the same time they are in no doubt as to the potentially cloying effects of materiality and the need to penetrate beyond the realm of physical sense perception. While standing in a distinctly ascetic and theological tradition, the various voices treated here reflect a culture that was substantially more attuned to supra-physical sense perception than modern western society is. Few Byzantines, of course, could claim the kinds of experiences vouchsafed to a Makarios or a Symeon. But spiritual sensation, whether of grace or demonic activity, whether of saints, or angels, or God himself, was always a very real prospect within the Byzantine sensorium. The vision of light, the taste of grace, the hearing of ineffable words, the smelling of indescribable perfumes, the touch of an angel or saint—all these spiritual sense perceptions were far from being unusual features of Byzantine life. This was, after all, a world in which only a thin "crystal membrane" separated the physical from the spiritual, the material from the divine.

ABBREVIATIONS

AB	*Analecta Bollandiana*
AJA	*American Journal of Archaeology*
ArtB	*Art Bulletin*
BA	*Bollettino d'arte*
BASOR	*Bulletin of the American Schools of Oriental Research*
BCH	*Bulletin de correspondance hellénique*
BHG	*Bibliotheca hagiographica graeca*, 3rd ed., ed. F. Halkin, Subsidia hagiographica 47 (Brussels, 1957; repr. 1969)
BIFAO	*Bulletin de l'Institut français d'archéologie orientale*
BL	British Library
BMFD	*Byzantine Monastic Foundation Documents: A Complete Translation of the Surviving Founders' "Typika" and Testaments*, ed. J. Thomas and A. C. Hero (Washington, DC, 2000)
BMGS	*Byzantine and Modern Greek Studies*
BnF	Bibliothèque nationale de France
BSA	*The Annual of the British School at Athens*
BSl	*Byzantinoslavica*
BZ	*Byzantinische Zeitschrift*
CC	*Chapters on Love*, A. Ceresa-Gastaldo, ed., *Capitoli sulla carità*, Verba seniorum 3 (Rome, 1963)
CCCM	Corpus Christianorum: Continuatio Mediaevale
CCSG	Corpus christianorum, Series graeca
CCSL	Corpus christianorum, Series latina
CMJE	Center for Muslim-Jewish Engagement
CNRS	Centre national de la recherche scientifique
CSCO	Corpus scriptorum christianorum orientalium
CSCO Scr. Syr.	Corpus scriptorum christianorum orientalium, Scriptores Syri
DenkWien	Österreichische Akademie der Wissenschaften, Philosophisch-historische Klasse, Denkschriften
DOP	*Dumbarton Oaks Papers*
DOS	Dumbarton Oaks Studies
EI^{2}	*Encyclopaedia of Islam*, 2nd ed. (Leiden and London, 1960–)
EME	*Early Medieval Europe*
FGrH	F. Jacoby, *Die Fragmente der griechischen Historiker* (Berlin, 1923–58)
GC	É. des Places, ed., *Diadoque de Photicé: Oeuvres spirituelles*, SC 5 ter. (Paris 1997)
GCS	Die griechischen christlichen Schriftsteller der ersten [drei] Jahrhunderte
GRBS	*Greek, Roman, and Byzantine Studies*
HPar	*Hymns on Paradise*
HVirg	*Hymns on Virginity*
JEChrSt	*Journal of Early Christian Studies*

JÖB	*Jahrbuch der Österreichischen Byzantinistik*
JSAH	*Journal of the Society of Architectural Historians*
LP	*On the Lord's Prayer,* P. Van Deun, ed., *Opuscula exegetica duo: Expositio in Psalmum LIX; Expositio orationis dominicae,* CCSG 23 (Louvain, 1991)
LXX	Septuagint
MDAIK	*Mitteilungen des Deutschen Archäologischen Instituts,* Abteilung Kairo
NPNF2	P. Schaff and H. Wace, eds., *Nicene and Post-Nicene Fathers,* second series, 14 vols. (1890–1900; repr. Peabody, MA, 1994)
OCP	*Orientalia christiana periodica*
ODB	*The Oxford Dictionary of Byzantium,* ed. A. Kazhdan et al. (New York and Oxford, 1991)
PAM	*Polish Archaeology in the Mediterranean*
PG	Patrologiae cursus completus, Series graeca, ed. J.-P. Migne (Paris, 1857–66)
PL	Patrologiae cursus completus, Series latina, ed. J.-P. Migne (Paris, 1844–80)
PO	*Patrologia orientalis*
PTS	Patristische Texte und Studien
QD	*Questions and Doubts,* J. Declerck, ed., *Quaestiones et dubia,* CCSG 10 (Louvain, 1982)
REB	*Revue des études byzantines*
REG	*Revue des études grecques*
SBN	*Studi bizantini e neoellenici*
SC	Sources chrétiennes
SPBS	Society for the Promotion of Byzantine Studies
TM	*Travaux et mémoires*
TU	Texte und Untersuchungen zur Geschichte der altchristlichen Literatur (Leipzig and Berlin, 1882–)

ABOUT THE AUTHORS

SPYRIDON ANTONOPOULOS is an Honorary Research Fellow at City University of London, where he obtained his Ph.D. in Musicology in 2015, completing a thesis on the fifteenth-century Constantinopolitan composer and theorist Manuel Chrysaphes. A graduate of Brown University and the New England Conservatory, he is the Founder and Director of *Psaltikon* and a regular member of the internationally acclaimed *Cappella Romana*. His research interests include medieval Byzantine chant and liturgy, performance practice, and Greek musical styles of the nineteenth and twentieth centuries. He has spoken at dozens of international academic conferences and is currently a singer on Stanford's *Icons of Sound* project as well as a singer and researcher for UCLA/USC's *Soundscapes of Medieval Byzantium*—projects that are focused on the interplay of sound, space, and liturgy in late medieval churches.

THOMAS ARENTZEN is a postdoctoral research fellow at the University of Oslo and holds a doctoral degree in Church History from Lund University. He is the author of *The Virgin in Song: Mary and the Poetry of Romanos the Melodist* (Philadelphia, 2017), is coediting the book *The Reception of the Virgin in Byzantium: Marian Narratives in Texts and Images* (forthcoming) with Mary Cunningham, and has published articles on Byzantine hymns and homilies. Currently he works on a research project called "Bodies in Motion: Religion and Corporeality in Late Antiquity" and coedits the journal *Patristica Nordica Annuaria*.

A graduate of Cambridge University (BA and MA) and the Johns Hopkins University (PhD), MARTINA BAGNOLI is the Executive Director of the Gallerie Estensi, a cluster of museums located in Ferrara, Modena and Sassuolo, Italy. Before returning to Italy Bagnoli worked at the National Gallery of Art in Washington, DC and the Walters Art Museum, Baltimore, where she was Curator in Charge of Medieval Art and Manuscript. At the Walters, Bagnoli has curated a number of important exhibitions including *A Feast for the Senses, Art and Experience in Medieval Europe* (October 16, 2016–January 8, 2017) and *Treasures of Heaven: Relics, Saints and Devotion in Medieval Europe* (February 13–May 15, 2011).

DARLENE L. BROOKS HEDSTROM is Department Chair and Professor of History, and Director of Archaeology at Wittenberg University in Springfield, Ohio. She specializes in the archaeology of Byzantine Egypt with a focus on domestic archaeology, the built environment, landscape archaeology, and the archaeology of cooking. Her book *The Monastic Landscape in Late Antique Egypt: An Archaeological Reconstruction* is forthcoming from Cambridge University Press. A Fulbright scholar and a fellow at Dumbarton Oaks in Byzantine Studies, she has received fellowships and grants in Byzantine Studies and for archaeological fieldwork from Dumbarton Oaks Research Library and Collection; the National Endowment for the Humanities; and the Simpson Endowment for Egyptology. She is currently Senior Archaeological Consultant for the Yale Monastic Archaeology Project (YMAP)–North.

BÉATRICE CASEAU is professor of Byzantine history at the University of Paris-Sorbonne. She is the director of the research cluster LABEX RESMED (Religions and society in the Mediterranean world) and a member of the research center UMR 8167 Orient & Méditerranée. Her research interests concentrate on late antique and Byzantine Christianity, the cultural history of the senses, the history of childhood, and religious anthropology. She has published books or collected essays on Byzantine food culture (2015), on family networks (2012) and questions of inheritance (2014), on Eucharistic practices (2009), and on sacred spaces and pilgrimages (2006). She is currently preparing two collections of essays on antiquity and the middle ages, one on the senses in religious cultures and the other on food taboos.

KIM HAINES-EITZEN is the H. Stanley Krusen Professor of World Religions, Director of the Religious Studies Program, and Professor of Early Christianity in the Departments of Near Eastern Studies and Classics at Cornell University. A specialist in the religions of the ancient Mediterranean world, especially early Christianity and early Judaism, she has published *Guardians of Letters: Literacy, Power, and the Transmitters of Early Christian Literature* (Oxford, 2000); *The Gendered Palimpsest: Women, Writing, and Representation in Early Christianity* (Oxford, 2012); and essays on topics ranging from ancient book cultures, late ancient sacred fictions in Judaism and Christianity, and nineteenth-century scholarship about early Judaism. Her current book project, *A Sacred and Sonorous Desert*, explores how environmental sounds shaped late-ancient monastic ideology and practice.

SUSAN ASHBROOK HARVEY is the Willard Prescott and Annie McClelland Smith Professor of Religion and History at Brown University. She specializes in Christianity of the Byzantine and Syriac traditions and has published widely in academic venues on women in ancient Christianity, monasticism, the cult of saints, hagiography, hymnography, and religion and the senses. She is the author of, among other publications, *Scenting Salvation: Ancient Christianity and the Olfactory Imagination* (2006). Professor Harvey is working on a new book, *Women's Singing and Women's Stories in Ancient Syriac Christianity.*

LAURA SUZANNE LIEBER is Professor of Religious Studies at Duke University, where she directs the Duke-UNC Center for Late Ancient Studies and the Duke Center for Jewish Studies. Her primary field of research is Jewish liturgical poetry (*piyyut*) in late antiquity, read in light of Jewish, Christian, Roman, and Samaritan writings more broadly. Her books include *Yannai on Genesis: An Invitation to Piyyut* (Cincinnati, 2010) and *A Vocabulary of Desire: The Song of Songs in the Early Synagogue* (Leiden, 2014).

MARGARET MULLETT is Professor of Byzantine Studies emerita at Queen's University Belfast and Director of Byzantine Studies emerita at Dumbarton Oaks. She works on the borderlines of history and literature; on literacy, gender, social relations, funerary rhetoric; and now on tents, laments, and the *Christos Paschon*. She is General Editor of the new Routledge series Studies in Byzantine Cultural History. Currently Professor of Byzantine Social History at the University of Vienna, she is teaching "Thinking, perceiving, dreaming in Byzantium," there, and working with the Uppsala-Paris network on text and narrative.

INGELA NILSSON is Professor of Greek and Byzantine Studies at Uppsala University (Sweden). Her research interests concern all forms of narration and literary adaptation, and the tension that such procedures create between tradition and innovation. Such perspectives are at the center of a number of publications, including *Erotic Pathos, Rhetorical Pleasure: Narrative Technique and Mimesis in Eumathios Makrembolites' Hysmine & Hysminias* (Uppsala, 2001), the edited volume *Plotting with Eros: Essays on the Poetics of Love and the Erotics of Reading* (Copenhagen, 2009), and *Raconter Byzance: La littérature au 12ᵉ siècle* (Paris, 2014).

AMY PAPALEXANDROU's research has focused on how architecture and its context, especially spolia and monumental inscriptions, indicate ways in which space has been aurally experienced. Since 2010 she has turned to the soundways and sonic events of Byzantium, concentrating on the often overlooked sense of hearing, especially within churches, through chant and other sounds. This initial research provided the basis for a team project in 2014 to investigate the acoustic properties of Byzantine churches in Thessalonike as performative spaces. Her archaeological work has been focused in Greece and Cyprus, where she directs the Post-Classical research team of the Princeton University Expedition to Polis-tes-Chrysochou.

She teaches art history and archaeology at Stockton University, deep in the Pine Barrens of New Jersey.

GLENN PEERS is Professor in the Department of Art and Art History at the University of Texas at Austin. In 2013, he curated the exhibition *Byzantine Things in the World* at The Menil Collection, Houston. In 2014, he was a Senior Fellow at the Internationales Kolleg für Kulturtechnikforschung und Medienphilosophie, Bauhaus-Universität Weimar, and in 2015–16, Fellow at the Israel Institute for Advanced Studies, Hebrew University, Jerusalem.

MARCUS PLESTED is Associate Professor of Greek Patristic and Byzantine Theology at Marquette University. He was awarded his doctorate in 1999 by the University of Oxford (Merton College). He taught at the Institute for Orthodox Christian Studies (Cambridge Theological Federation) and the Faculty of Divinity of the University of Cambridge 2000–13. He has been a member of the Center of Theological Inquiry and the Institute for Advanced Study in Princeton, NJ, and has taught, lectured, and published widely in patristic, Byzantine, and modern Orthodox theology. He is the author of *The Macarian Legacy: The Place of Macarius-Symeon in the Eastern Christian Tradition* (Oxford, 2004) and *Orthodox Readings of Aquinas* (Oxford, 2012).

FELIPE ROJAS is an assistant professor of archaeology at the Joukowsky Institute for Archaeology and the Ancient World and the Department of Egyptology and Assyriology at Brown University. He has conducted archaeological fieldwork at various sites in Turkey and Jordan including Sardis, Aphrodisias, and Petra. He is currently assistant director of the Notion Archaeological Survey (https://sites.lsa.umich.edu/notionsurvey/) and is finishing a book titled *Inventing the Past in Roman Anatolia.*

D. FAIRCHILD RUGGLES is Professor in the Department of Landscape Architecture at the University of Illinois, Urbana-Champaign, with additional appointments in Art History, Architecture, and Medieval Studies. She is the author of two award-winning books on Islamic landscape history: *Gardens, Landscape, and Vision in the Palaces of Islamic Spain* (2000) and *Islamic Gardens and Landscapes* (2008), as well as nine authored, edited, and coedited volumes on Islamic art, cultural heritage, landscape history and theory, and the arts patronage of women in Islam and South Asia, and seven short films on Islamic art for the NEH Muslim Journeys Bookshelf project.

VALERIA SERGUEENKOVA is is an assistant professor in the Department of Classics at the University of Cincinnati. Her research interests concern ancient Greek and Roman historiography and science and focus especially on the interactions in antiquity between what we today think of as the "humanities" and the "sciences." She is finishing a book titled *A Science of the Past:* Herodotus' *Histories between Nature and Culture.*

GALINA TIRNANIĆ is Assistant Professor of Art History at Oakland University in Michigan. She received her PhD from the University of Chicago in 2010. In 2010-11 she was a Senior Fellow at the Research Center for Anatolian Cultures at Koç University in Istanbul. She specializes in the visual culture of punishment in Byzantium and has published essays on the relationship between instances of public punishment in the urban spaces of Constantinople and the visual and textual representations of imperial ideology, martyrdom, and Byzantine image theories.

RUTH WEBB is currently Professor of Greek at the University of Lille and a member of the UMR 8163 *Savoirs, Textes, Langage* (CNRS and University of Lille), having held previous positions in London, Princeton, and Paris. She is the author of *Demons and Dancers: Performance in Late Antiquity* (2008) and *Ekphrasis, Imagination and Persuasion in Ancient Rhetorical Theory and Practice* (2009) in addition to numerous articles on rhetoric and performance in postclassical Greek culture. She has a particular interest in ancient and Byzantine ideas about the uses of the word to evoke visual and other sensations.

INDEX

Page numbers in italics indicate illustrations. Specific manuscripts will be found under "manuscripts"; specific museum objects and paintings are under "objects and paintings." Written works will be under the author's name, unless they are anonymous, in which case readers should look up the title.